The Clinical Presentation of Parkinson's Disease and the Dyadic Relationship between Patients and Carers

The Clinical Presentation of Parkinson's Disease and the Dyadic Relationship between Patients and Carers: A Neuropsychological Approach

By

Barbara Politynska

CAMBRIDGE SCHOLARS PUBLISHING

The Clinical Presentation of Parkinson's Disease
and the Dyadic Relationship between Patients and Carers:
A Neuropsychological Approach,
by Barbara Politynska

This book first published 2013

Cambridge Scholars Publishing

12 Back Chapman Street, Newcastle upon Tyne, NE6 2XX, UK

British Library Cataloguing in Publication Data
A catalogue record for this book is available from the British Library

ISBN (10): 1-4438-4603-1, ISBN (13): 978-1-4438-4603-5

TABLE OF CONTENTS

FOREWORD

This book is an important and exceptional contribution to the neuropsychological literature on Parkinson's disease within the context of care-giving. It highlights the bond that emerges over the course of the disease between the person suffering from the condition and his/her carer, emphasising the significance of the dyadic relationship between couple in determining care-giving outcomes – a factor that has hitherto not been adequately appreciated. A novel approach taken by the author, building on these relationship factors, is in examining the carer's attitudes to the psychological changes occurring in the care recipient and demonstrating that these are of primary importance to determining care-giving outcomes.

In many countries there are increasing numbers of elderly people who are forming an ever greater proportion of the overall population. This poses many problems for society in general. One of these is that the prevalence of people suffering the health problems associated with ageing, is also increasing. In turn this leads to the problem of how to cope with a growing need to care for the elderly infirm. In the U.K. we are currently on the verge of introducing new legislation aimed at consolidating existing, somewhat piecemeal, laws to create a modern system for adult care and support, in which the disabled person and his/her family should be at the centre of service considerations.

Many relatives wish to care for their infirm or disabled family members themselves or with minimal contribution from the more formal methods of care provided by health and social agencies. Indeed these formal services would be unable to cope with the numbers of infirm elderly were it not for the often willing support provided by informal carers such as relatives, friends and neighbours.

There are two reasons why the problem of informal care needs to be addressed. The first, as indicated already, is that informal care is an essential feature of looking after the infirm elderly. It is important that relatives and others provide care in the best possible way. The second is that being a carer is not easy and creates problems for the carers themselves who may suffer a number of adverse consequences in carrying out their role. It is important that the problems experienced by carers are recognised and that, where necessary, addressed.

To date, the majority of work considering the problems experienced by informal carers of elderly people with infirmities has been based on dementia, not surprisingly because this is one of the most prevalent disorders. Here it has been found, for example, that carers experience various problems, particularly depression. Also depression in carers is more linked to the psychological changes in the person for whom they care rather than dealing with the physical disabilities or limitations of the sufferer.

Little attention has so far been given to the problems of caring for other disorders occurring in the elderly. This is especially true for Parkinson's disease which is the focus of the author's research. In the theoretical section of the book, the clinical presentation of Parkinson's disease, including both the motor and non-motor symptoms, is covered thoroughly and the detail in which the author has discussed questions of particular interest is impressive. Her comments on methodology demonstrate a competent grasp of the important issues.

In reporting the research study, the author has presented a clear justification for her research and has raised and made progress in resolving a number of issues relating to the psychological consequences of Parkinson's disease. These include the nature of depression in that disorder and the key factors causing distress in carers. She provides a clear summary of the findings with a competent discussion of their significance. In particular, she demonstrates an impressive ability to deal with a number of difficult methodological issues. To the best of my knowledge, it is the first sustained piece of research into this aspect of Parkinson's disease and as such constitutes a significant contribution to this field. As such it merits wide attention.

Edgar Miller
Emeritus Professor of Clinical Psychology,
University of Leicester.
Past President of the British Psychological Society.

CHAPTER ONE

INTRODUCTION

1.1 Parkinson's disease: a neuropsychological disorder

The study of Parkinson's disease (PD) and caring for someone with the disorder that is presented in the following pages is undertaken from a clinical neuropsychological perspective. Much has been written in recent years, particularly in the field of dementia, about the problems of caring for someone with a chronic and intractable disease and this is reflected in the exponential growth in the academic literature on the subject over the last thirty years. Far fewer studies have focused on other neuro-degenerative disorders, such as PD, and whilst this is an omission in its own right in need of repair, there is another reason, which from the neuropsychological perspective, highlights PD as a focus of interest. This is because PD has been aptly described as the "quintessential neuropsychiatric disorder" (Weintraub and Burn 2011). Although the condition is still primarily diagnosed from the perspective of a movement disorder, the high prevalence of accompanying non-motor symptoms in the form of neurocognitive and neuropsychiatric complications make it a unique model for the focus of research in neuropsychology.

Most attention to date has been devoted to the cognitive impairment characteristic of the condition and attempting to identify the neural substrate for dementia in PD. Cognitive impairments are recognised as a frequent accompaniment of the disorder affecting up to 25% of non-demented patients with PD (Aarsland et al. 2010). Dementia is considered to be a long-term complication, affecting up to 80% of patients as the disease evolves (Aarsland et al. 2003). Affective disorders on the other hand, in the form of depression or "melancholia", whilst having been recognised as a concomitant of the disorder since its earliest descriptions (Parkinson 1817), have generated a great deal of controversy and yet, as pointed out by Ponce and Lozano (2010), have received relatively little systematic attention. In recent years, agreement seems to have been reached that a more serious or "major" form of depression occurs with a frequency of 5-20%, but that milder forms (minor or subsyndromal depression) occur in an additional 35% of patients (Reijnders et al. 2008). However, there remains considerable debate surrounding the nature, profile and origin of the affective symptoms in PD. A main concern of the empirical study, which is described in later sections of this book, was to reach a better understanding of these features of the depressive disorder in PD and their relationship to the other symptoms of the condition.

Other clinically significant, neurobehavioural complications include anxiety symptoms, impulse control disorders, obsessionality, fatigue, disorders of sleep and wakefulness and apathy. The importance of these "non-motor" symptoms in PD is reflected in the growth of publications related to this topic over the last twenty-five years, primarily in the area of dementia and cognitive impairment (Weintraub and Burn 2011) and in the fact that it has increasingly been realised that improving the quality of life of people with PD and their carers demands extending clinical and treatment approaches from a primarily motor-oriented focus to include the non-motor features of the disorder (Cheng et al. 2010; Spica et al. 2013). It goes without saying that clinical neuropsychology has a clear contribution to make in the area of the cognitive and affective symptomatology of the condition in both the theoretical and clinically applied domains.

1.1.1 A brief note on terminology

A striking feature of neuropsychological approaches to distinct disorders is that they have traditionally tended to focus on cognitive impairments. Thus the neuropsychology of PD has largely been dominated by the study of attentional, perceptual, visuospatial, memory, language and more recently executive-type deficits (see chapter 4). Whilst behavioural disorders have also come within the realm of clinical psychology, disorders of emotion have traditionally been the sphere of psychiatry. As recognition has emerged that emotional disturbances, in particular disturbances of affect, are associated with neurological disorders such as PD, it has become increasingly common to refer to them as "neuropsychiatric" in origin. These divisions between neuropsychology and neuropsychiatry are somewhat artificial and this is reflected in the interchangeable use of the terms in the literature to account for cognitive, behavioural and affective symptoms. For example, Weintraub and Burn (2011) include cognitive deficits in their definition of the neuropsychiatric disorder in PD. Equally, neuropsychological approaches to the study of emotions are well-established (e.g. Damasio 1996; Grabowska 1999; Herzyk 1999, 2000a; Kądzielawa 1986; Konorski 1969; Luria 1976; Szepietowska and Misztal 1999; Watts 1993).

1.1.2 Clinical neuropsychological perspectives on Parkinson's disease

A widely accepted definition of neuropsychology is that it is the study of brain-behaviour relationships and traditionally, two main approaches have been discernable in this field as described by Miller (1984). The first has been concerned with delineating the kinds of functional disturbance that may occur as the result of lesions affecting specific parts of the brain in an attempt to specify the functions supported by defined anatomical substrates. Much of the early work in neuropsychology was of this kind, attempting to correlate focal lesions with observed deficits in higher cognitive functions. The second approach has had a more functional orientation, concerned with determining the kinds of change that may occur, for example in language or memory, following organic brain damage associated with specific disorders, such as Alzheimer's or Parkinson's disease. Here there has, until recently, been less emphasis on lesion location, largely because of technological limitations in identifying biochemical as opposed to anatomical lesions. Thus both anatomical and functional trends formed the background to the earlier understanding of brain-behaviour relationships in neuropsychology. However, over the last twenty years, dramatic advances in neuro-imaging techniques, especially those of a functional nature, have brought these trends together and are of considerable theoretical importance, both in furthering understanding of normal brain function, but also in providing explanatory models of how functions are integrated. PD has been at the forefront of research in these areas, as it has provided a unique model of a commonly encountered neurological disorder presenting with deficits in the motor, neuropsychological and neuropsychiatric fields of functioning, thereby enabling understanding of how functional processes are integrated and related to anatomical substrates in the human brain (e.g. Robbins 2010). However, despite the huge gains made in the theoretical understanding of conditions such as PD over recent years, this has not as yet, translated into significant improvements in pharmacological treatments or in advancing the possibility of a cure, which is understandably, the main desire of patients and is reflected in the key aims of patient organizations such as Parkinson's UK (2012a). This ultimate goal will doubtless be achieved in time, but in the interim, the majority of patients diagnosed with the condition must rely on their families for support and care in living with the consequences of this long-term neurodegenerative disease. A primary concern for clinical neuropsychology is to provide the empirical foundations for guiding practice in helping patients and their families to cope with the ensuing difficulties. This recognition provided the stimulus and motivation for the work reported in this volume, in the final part of the empirical study, which is reported in chapters 8-12.

It is self-evident that empirically guided, theoretical developments should lie at the heart of clinical practice. Without this core knowledge, proper diagnostic understanding and suitable treatment interventions are impossible. This has been demonstrated in the failure of a variety of allegedly useful interventions in PD, ranging from attempts to treat depression with pharmacological agents whose efficacy had not been adequately established in the condition to ill-fated surgical interventions ranging from thalamolysis to brain implants, which variously resulted in severe cognitive impairment and even premature death. Clinical neuropsychology, however, requires further elaboration and refinement of purely theoretical approaches. Here the questions raised demand answers that are of practical application, both in terms of helping to restore function in so far as this is possible, and to maintain the patient at optimal levels of functioning, preventing further deterioration within the limits imposed by the illness. This is usually seen as the task of neuropsychological rehabilitation and this field too, has developed significantly over the last thirty years (e.g. Pąchalska 2007; Sohlberg and Mateer 2001; Wilson et al. 2009). Clinical approaches in neuropsychology have been primarily patient focused and have gone a long way towards improving the quality of life of people with neuropsychological deficits in the wake of neurological disease and the disabilities consequent upon it.

1.2 Carers of people with Parkinson's disease

An underlying principle of the present work, in keeping with current concerns in health policy in the U.K. (Department of Health 2012a,b,c) and other member states of the European Union (e.g. Harkin 2011) is the notion that clinical neuropsychology not only has an obligation to the patient suffering from the condition that has brought him/her to the attention of the clinician, but also to his/her carer. The majority of neurological conditions involving neuropsychological assessment and intervention are long-term, intractable or progressive disorders, such as PD, in which the patient ultimately comes to depend on the care of a family member in order to be able to sustain functioning in his/her own home in the community. As a result, the carer becomes almost inextricably linked to the patient, embarking upon and sharing his/her journey with the disease, through all of its stages. It is inevitably a journey that has not been planned, heralds undesirable changes in the lives of both the patient and the carer and follows a singularly unpredictable course. Above all, the illness brings about an irreversible disruption, not only in the life of the patient, but also in that of his/her carer. For some way along their common course, they may be brought closer together by the illness experience, as they seek to adapt to its mercurial demands affecting both their lives, with the patient becoming increasingly dependent on the carer. In the main however, the changes wrought by the illness, especially those presenting in the form of neuropsychological and neuropsychiatric deficits, mean that from the carer's point of view, apart from increased problems with mobility, the patient may become more forgetful, disinterested and withdrawn and cease to be the source of support that s/he may have been in the past. As a result, the carer experiences a sense of loss and increasing isolation, and the couples' relationship comes under increasing pressure. This is further exacerbated by the patient's frequent unwillingness or inability to maintain social activities.

Not surprisingly, in view of the impact that caring for someone with a long term progressive illness has on the carer, a major theme running through the literature on care-giving is the emphasis on the highly stressful nature of the task. Models of care-giving based on stress (process) theories have predominated (e.g. Pearlin et al. 1990) with the consequent result that attention has focused on concepts such as the "burden" involved in the caring process (Zarit, Orr and Zarit 1985). For more than two decades, elaboration and refinement of this concept was the main preoccupation of the care-giving literature, with the consequent proliferation of instruments to measure burden. Many of these treated burden as a unidimensional construct in keeping with early conceptualizations (e.g. Zarit, Reever and Bach-Peterson 1980). Whilst the notion of burden was a useful concept from the point of view of providing a unifying approach to care-giving in diverse groups of older people, increasing experience and sophistication in this field of research has revealed its many limitations. First and foremost, researchers have achieved a better appreciation of the complexities of care-giving which are evident in the diversity of processes and outcomes in different groups of carers and care recipients. For example, it is becoming increasingly apparent that caring for someone with dementia differs in some important ways from caring for someone with other types of neurodegenerative disorder, such as PD (Hooker et al. 2000). However, the notion of burden has suffered not only from conceptual limitations in being too narrow, but was also found to lack empirical support. Only limited success was achieved in demonstrating that high levels of carer distress were linked to the "objective" demands of the care-giving situation, such as the physical tasks, time demands and financial responsibilities encompassed in the notion of burden. The idea of "subjective" burden (Hoenig and Hamilton 1966) was thus developed to account for the carer's appraisal of the situation and his/her perceived strain, which was conceptualised as the stress of care-giving and considered to be an outcome measure of the difficulties faced by carers. These approaches served to accentuate the perception of care-giving as a predominantly negative experience. In the late 1990s, the discovery that not only physical morbidity (Schulz et al. 1995; Vitaliano, Zhang and Scanlan 2003), but mortality rates were increased among carers (Schulz and Beach 1999) appeared to bring irrefutable validation to the growing concern that caring placed family members under intolerable levels of stress and required systematic and effective intervention procedures for the relief of carers. Alongside the relatively slow progression of research in this area towards finding successful remedial solutions, carers themselves formed support groups which were extremely effective in lobbying governments to recognise their role in caring for elderly and disabled relatives and to adopt policies that went some way towards meeting their needs. Nevertheless, the legislation relating to carers, which has emerged in somewhat piecemeal fashion over the last sixty years, is generally recognised as being ".... inadequate, often incomprehensible and outdated" (Law Commission 2012) and the funding of the care system as ".... not fit for purpose" and in need of "urgent and lasting reform" (Dilnot 2011). It is recognised that reforms, especially those involving substantial amounts of government funding will need to be carried out over a number of years, but at the time of writing a consultation process is being completed in relation to the draft Care and Support Bill (Department of Health 2012) which has proposals for making some significant and long-promised changes to help older and disabled people in need of care and support and their carers. A synopsis of this and other U.K. legislation in relation to carers is provided in Appendix A.

In spite of the stressful nature of caring, the majority of older people with a chronic and incapacitating condition are cared for at home, usually by their family. Families are willing carers, and their contribution is reflected in the not inconsiderable number of individuals who take on the role: over 6 million in the U.K. (NHS Carers Direct 2012a) and 65.7 million in the U.S.A. (National Alliance for Caregiving 2009). These numbers are likely to rise in the foreseeable future as developed countries experience a demographic shift, in which older people are living longer, but with the increased likelihood of suffering from poor health. One of the reasons for the success of carers' efforts probably lies in the individualized and high quality of care that they provide and their commitment to providing it. Yet this commitment finds itself in stark dissonance to the emphasis on the hardships of care-giving which have, to a large extent, been underlined by the stress models that have dominated the field of care-giving research. As Schulz and Williamson (1997, 123) pointed out over a decade ago: "Relatively little attention has been paid to the assessment of positive aspects of caregiving, the quality of care delivered by caregivers and the impact of caregiving transitions." Whilst a few attempts have been made to redress the bias in the presentation of caring as a wholly negative experience for carers (e.g. Nolan, Grant and Keady 1996) by drawing attention to positive aspects such as the satisfaction and recognition that some carers experience in their role, the negative focus has nonetheless predominated.

One explanation for this may be that it is natural to focus on difficulties in order to try to find solutions to the problems identified. Another, is that in attempting to drive policy decisions, a case has to made regarding the hardships involved. However, sometimes the impression given in the literature is that the strain on carers is such, that family care generally, is on the verge of breaking down. Apart from being misleading, this kind of stance is unhelpful in gaining a better understanding of care-giving. For example, an observation that has long been apparent to researchers in this field, is that given relatively similar care-giving situations, no two carers seem to manage and deal with the problems involved in the same way, and hence the outcomes they experience may vary considerably. Within the context of the stress process model, this observation elicited the search for intervening variables which might modify the care-giving situation and thus determine carer outcomes. These included differences in the coping mechanisms used by carers (Hooker et al. 2000) and varying degrees of social support available (Edwards and Scheetz 2002; Lai and Thomson 2011; Monahan and Hooker 1997), which were posited as being essential to modifying the outcome in terms of carers' well-being or contributing to the distress that they experienced. Nevertheless, factors that have traditionally been used to explain differences in stress processes have had only limited success in accounting for the difficulties of care-giving. For example, in one of the first studies to investigate the problems faced by carers of people with PD, Miller, Berrios and Politynska (1996) did not find any beneficial effect of social support on carer well-being.

Furthermore, the assumption at the heart of stress models of care-giving has been that the physical and mental disability of older care recipients, is the main determinant of deterioration in family carers' psychological well-being. As already mentioned, this has proved to have only partial justification and has led researchers in recent years to undertake a close re-evaluation of the problem and the way in which it has been conceptualised. An examination of the literature on care-giving carried out for the purposes of the present research highlighted an empirical observation that has not received a great deal of attention, despite being identified from some of the earliest studies in this area. This finding points to the fact that carer (and not predominantly care recipient) variables appear to be better in predicting psychological morbidity and deteriorating well-being in carers over time (Hooker et al. 1992; Hooker, Frazier and Monahan 1994; Hooker et al. 1998; Hooker et al. 2000; The Resource Implications Study Group of the Medical Research Council study of cognitive function and ageing [RIS MRC CFAS] 2000). This is an important finding which requires careful analysis and elaboration if it is not to be trivialised to the detriment of carers. Given its potential to characterise an essential aspect of care-giving, it formed an important background to the present study and determined an important line in the investigation of care-giving in PD that is described here.

It is important to understand carer characteristics as a complex set of interdependent variables that are only partially antecedent to taking on the care-giving task. Moreover, in the context of care-giving demands, it would seem unlikely that they should remain fixed or stable, as by its very nature, the care-giving situation requires adjustment and flexibility. However, the literature that has recognised the importance of carer variables to the outcomes of care-giving has tended to conceptualize them in terms of relatively constant characteristics such as personality variables (e.g. Hooker et al. 1998) and as reflecting the previous quality of the relationship with the care recipient (Murray and Livingstone 1998). Applied within the stress process model, these characteristics may be seen as determining different coping styles for dealing with the task of care-giving (Hooker et al. 2000). However, other potentially more important dimensions in relation to the way in which the carer is able to adapt and reconstruct his/her relationship with the care recipient in the light of the disability and its demands have largely been overlooked. In the early stages of PD, adjustment to the condition is likely to be a reciprocal task in which both the carer and the care recipient participate, albeit in different ways, through the process of coming to terms with any limitations imposed by the illness and undertaking adaptations that are perceived to be necessary. These processes are described in chapter 5 of the present study. However, at different stages over the course of the illness, the ability of both the carer and the care recipient to maintain these efforts may be challenged by evolving symptoms, especially in the area of affective and cognitive functioning, which diminish not only the patient's capacity to adapt his/her behaviour accordingly, but also alter his/her reactivity to situational needs. Hence the carer is likely to require a sensitivity to changes in the care recipient's possibilities for performing previously held roles and tasks, an ability to initiate changes in life-style in response to the needs of the situation and to come to terms with new responsibilities and limitations imposed by the care-giving situation. These adaptations, of course, are not one-way, as even passivity on the part of the care recipient may be an adaptive response within the resources that remain available. Thus a crucial dynamic involving both the carer and the care-recipient develops which is illustrative of the care-giving situation. This aspect of care-giving, namely that involving the interaction between the carer and the care recipient, has received relatively little attention, especially in the context of PD, but would appear crucial to achieving a proper understanding of care relationships in long-term, neurodegenerative illness. It requires a dyadic approach to care-giving (Lyons et al. 2002), which meets the long-expressed demand of both carers and care recipients for recognition, that is reflected both in the academic literature and more recently, has found recognition in U.K. government policies (Department of Health 2012b).

1.2.1 Dyadic approaches to care-giving

It is important to recognise, however, that dyadic approaches to care-giving require rather more than simply recognising the existence of carers. This, successive governments in the U.K. have done over the last decade or so, by introducing legislation expressly aimed at meeting the needs of carers, granting them the right to an annual assessment, introducing services for carers in their own right, together with direct payments in lieu of services that have been identified as lacking, and latterly involving them in decisions regarding the planning of local services and provision of individualised care packages, along with greater opportunities for respite care (see Appendix A). These measures form an indispensible and long-awaited foundation to establishing provisions for meeting the needs of carers, but they represent a mere starting point in terms of understanding the complexity of care-giving needs. This is reflected in the fact that attempts to support carers through a variety of intervention studies have frequently been disappointing in their results (Schulz, Martire and Klinger 2005; Torti et al. 2004). One reason for this is that they have been based, as indeed has the legislation, on a response to carers' appraisals of their own needs, but have been shown to lack support on empirical verification.

A classic example of this is the often cited need for respite care, prioritised once again in the recent legislative proposals. Although there can be no doubt that the restrictions and pressures of the care-giving task mean that carers frequently report detrimental effects on their health in the form of excessive tiredness, increased irritability and depression (Health and Social Care Information Centre 2012) and fulfil both objective and subjective criteria in requiring a break from care-giving, respite care is not taken up by carers in the numbers that might be expected to make use of this facility from an analysis of their expressed needs. The reasons for the failure to use these opportunities when they are made available are not adequately understood, but they seem to be related to the inflexibility and standards of the care on offer, which do not match carers' expectations of alternative care for their relatives (Lamura et al. 2006). However, clinical experience with patients and carers of people with PD also suggests that their desire for respite is a desire for respite from the disease itself, a yearning for the health status that preceded the onset of the disease, if only briefly. At the same time they realise that such expectations are unrealistic, and sometimes a break from their usual routine only serves as a reminder of this painful fact. It is not unusual for carers to report, that a period of respite care for their relative did not provide them with the restorative experience they had anticipated and that they missed the care recipient's presence, a fact that is reflected in their maintaining frequent visits to the patient in the respite care facility. The complexities of the situation can only be understood if a dyadic perspective is applied to care-giving.

Thus, in order to make a difference to the conditions and circumstances in which the patient and carer find themselves, it is essential not only to reach an understanding of their individual strengths and the difficulties that they face, but also to gain an appreciation of how they function in relation to each other. This relational approach advocating consideration of the mutuality of influences on care-giving from both the parties involved, allowing for greater flexibility and taking account of the multidimensional nature of the task, was first proposed by Kahana and Young (1990, 76) as a way of expanding on the "prevalent conceptual orientations to the study of caregiving". Research over the last twenty years has been slow to follow in the direction indicated. Indeed, most care-giving studies, especially those in areas that have received relatively little attention to date (such as PD), are unfortunately also failing to learn from the experience of research in related fields and remain fixed in the static, unidirectional outcome model, where focus remains on the carer, and, in the words of Lyons et al. (2002), the care recipient is reduced to little more than an independent variable and viewed as the source of stress to the carer. Apart from the limited empirical utility of this approach which has now been established (and which is discussed in greater detail in chapter 6), the conceptual framework for care-giving research, rooted as it has been in stress models, has emphasised the negative aspects of providing care for a dependent, elderly relative at home, and as mentioned above, virtually ignoring the fact that most families do and are happy to be engaged in caring for a loved one, finding satisfaction and fulfilment in a commitment they consider to be a natural part of family life (Nolan et al. 1996). This does not mean however, that they do not require support: the question that has still not been answered satisfactorily is what kind of support is likely to be most effective and how should it be delivered?

The task undertaken in the present study represents an attempt to use the applied methodology of clinical neuropsychology to understand the situation of both the patient and the carer in an effort to improve the care of people with long-term neurological illness. It is hoped that the dual focus adopted in accounting for both carer and care recipient outcomes will help to generate a meaningful conceptual framework within which to evaluate the various factors shaping care-giving in PD. This is a relatively new conceptualisation of the task in terms of a neuropsychological approach, where traditionally, assessment of the patient has been at the forefront of clinical concerns and work with the carer has essentially been of a supportive nature. Assessment of the patient's neuropsychological and neuropsychiatric performance continues to occupy a central place in any evaluation, but the purposes to which it is put, extend beyond that of diagnosis *per se*. It is also recognised that an evaluation of the carer's needs must be a prerequisite to any formulation of the care-giving situation. Depending on the circumstances, this may involve assessment of the symptoms of psychological distress, subjective feelings of self-efficacy and ability to cope, and attitudes (optimistic versus pessimistic) towards the future (Lyons et al. 2004). Whilst these components of the carer's perspective have received some attention in the literature, there is a further dimension, that appears as yet, not to have been considered, but which may be of importance as it may help to shape the characteristics mentioned. This relates to the way in which the carer perceives and subsequently interprets the care recipient's functioning in a variety of domains, including physical abilities, neuropsychological and neuropsychiatric performance. The latter two are of particular interest to the present study as there is evidence that the psychological symptoms of PD, in particular disturbances of affect, are of primary importance in influencing carer outcomes (Miller et al. 1996).

1.2.2 Carers' attitudes to the care-giving situation

Carers' attitudes to the care-giving situation are likely to be shaped by both emotional and cognitive factors, or indeed by an interaction between the two. There have been numerous explorations of care-giving based on theories focusing on emotional explanations, including attachment and familism (as described in chapter 7). Far less interest has been shown in cognitive factors, although it would be reasonable to expect that carers' perceptions of different aspects of the care-giving situation should influence their attitudes to caring and the way in which they cope. For example, if their perceptions of the physical and psychological changes in the care recipient are predominantly bleak, it is to be expected that frustration and depression might result. The same might be true concerning their relationship with the care recipient. Their attributions regarding these changes are equally important. Potential "cognitive biases" in the way in which the care recipient's physical ability, mood and cognitive performance are perceived, triggered by pre-existing cognitive schemata (Beck et al. 1979) would be expected to colour the carer's attitude to both the present and future, determining patterns of adjustment to the illness and feelings of self-efficacy.

The carer's view of the care recipient's functional performance may be important for two main reasons. Firstly, it may have a critical effect in shaping the process by which the care-giving situation evolves and determining the outcomes for both of the protagonists involved. For example, it has been observed that the amount of help that carers provide with the tasks of daily living, such as dressing, bathing, feeding etc. is relatively independent of the functional disability in PD and is more a feature of the carer's attitudes (Davies et al. 1999). This may result from differences in carers' perceptions of the extent of the disability in the care recipient, from a well-intentioned desire to be helpful and to provide assistance as an expression of affection for the patient or because they feel under pressure to complete the task at hand as quickly and efficiently as possible. In the latter case, this may be because of external pressures such as those of work or the need to keep to a specified timetable, or it may reflect impatience and intolerance of less than perfect performance. Whatever the cause, the consequences may be somewhat unpredictable (from the carer's point of view) and worse still, undesirable. An illustration of this comes from institutional settings, where it has long been recognised that certain patterns of behaviour on the part of care staff serve to reinforce dependency and result in learned helplessness in care recipients (M. Baltes and P. Baltes 1986). It is equally possible that family carers may activate a cycle in which care recipient dependency is potentiated, through behaviours which, while being well-meaning, result in the patient not attempting to do certain things which s/he is still capable of, because they are done for him/her. As a result, care recipient helplessness is reinforced and carer burden increased.

Secondly, needless to say, carer perceptions of care recipient functioning are also likely to influence the carer's ability to act as a proxy informant on his/her behalf, as may be required in certain circumstances for the purposes medical and needs assessments for care and support. It is important to understand that carers' judgements are likely to be influenced by a complex interplay between emotional and cognitive factors at different stages in the care-giving process.

The (mis)interpretation of care recipient psychological symptoms may take a variety of forms. Deficits in memory may be frustrating and annoying for the carer or may be "normalised" in terms of explanations of advancing age. More severe deficits are often poorly understood and may raise anxieties surrounding dementia. Some of the specific deficits associated with PD, such as apathy, withdrawal, depression, deterioration in communication or forms of impulse control disorders may be interpreted as "personality change" or as a rejection of the carer and his/her efforts to help. Carers are concerned at the lack of interest, refusal to see people, reluctance to engage in conversation, and even the failure to complain, that is characteristic of so many patients with PD. Occasionally they are startled by uncharacteristically hurtful comments or unusual behaviour. There is evidence to suggest that depression in the patient is particularly problematic for carers (Miller et al. 1996). One of the possible reasons for this, explored in the study, is that the misinterpretation of psychological symptoms, or their apparently brutal transparency in the minds of carers, wrecks havoc even with long established relationships, contributing further to the hardship of caring.

In view of the opportunities that exist for distortions in the perception of the care-giving situation, a priority of the present study was to examine carers' perceptions of the cognitive and affective state of their spouses, for whom they were caring. The primary purpose was to determine the extent to which carers' perceptions were in keeping with the formal neuropsychological and neuropsychiatric assessment of the care recipient. Establishing the extent to which there was concurrence between the two evaluations was deemed to be important for two reasons. The first was the possibility that carer perceptions of the care recipient's functioning (rather than the results of the neuropsychological assessment) might be more strongly associated with their own psychological well-being or lack of it. The second reason was related to the reliability of using proxy reports from carers in order to assess aspects of the care-giving situation. This is particularly important in view of the U.K. government's proposals to introduce new legislation in the form of the Care and Support Bill in 2013 (Department of Health 2012b), in which a commitment has been made to acknowledge carers as expert partners with formal services, ensuring that they have access to the integrated and personalised services they need to support them in their caring role. This recognition of carers answers a long-established charge from researchers in the field, calling for an acknowledgement of the dyadic nature of care-giving and the need to extend the focus of care services to include the carer, the wider family and formal care systems, whilst keeping the needs of the patient at the forefront of concerns (Kahana and Young 1990; Nolan et al. 2003; Zarit, Pearlin and Schaie 1993).

However, if acknowledging carers as "expert care partners" is to remain little more than a political slogan, there is a need for the care services offered to take an evidence based approach to the way in which goals are implemented for the fulfilment of this aim. There can be no doubt that carers have a unique perspective on the care-giving task, that cannot be matched in its richness of experience by other viewpoints. At the same time it has to be borne in mind, that theirs is the "insider" perspective of direct involvement, influenced by the emotional and perceptual factors referred to above. This involvement, whilst giving carers their unique expertise and invaluable insight into the complexities of caring for a disabled relative, also means that their perceptions are shaped by the actual experience of care-giving. Hence, they are very much part of the situation, involved in its evolution and the way in which it is constructed and relayed to others. Indeed, acknowledgement of this fact is the essence of the dyadic approach to caring that has been argued in favour of in the preceding section. However, it is in contrast to the way in which carers have typically been represented in the academic literature, that is, rather more as (albeit participant) observers, suffering the ill-effects and hardships of the toll exerted by the care-giving role, but essentially ignoring their ability to influence the process of caring and its outcomes at different stages, except through their practical efforts. It has rarely been acknowledged that their judgements and decisions are almost certainly influenced by their emotional, as well as cognitive state, sometimes leading to the observed disparities between their views and those of the person they help to care for. This is evidenced in the fact that carers frequently rate their care recipient's disabilities higher and their quality of life as much lower than does the patient him/herself (Fleming et al. 2005). Very little appears to be known about the way in which carers evaluate their care recipients' affective and cognitive functioning, still less about how these judgements may affect their own mental state. These considerations provide a salient reminder of the necessity for a comprehensive and evidenced based approach to understanding the caring process, in order to fully account for its multi-dimensional nature. Only then will it be possible to construct rational intervention procedures which have improved chances of success, as they are more likely to address the real issues at stake in care-giving. An attempt to understand how carers' perceptions of the mental state of their spouses with PD influenced care-giving outcomes formed an innovative part of the empirical work presented in this volume, providing an elaboration of the dyadic approach to care-giving.

1.3 Statistical approaches to the research

A specific feature of the research presented in this volume is in the use of multivariate statistical methods to identify relationships among the data. This has been identified by Weintraub and Burn (2011) as a priority for research in the area of PD, and was undertaken in the present work in an effort to capture the multidimensional nature of both the disorder and the complexities of the care-giving situation. The use of univariate statistical approaches to data still predominates in the field and it is sobering to be reminded that these problems of analysis were remarked upon by Alexander Luria in 1976 (85-86; author's own translation from Polish):

> It is necessary to mention the final direction in which neuropsychological research is developing, which in this case is more technical in nature. During our many years of research we have collected numerous observations and facts which form the basis of neuropsychological theory. These however need to be specified with greater precision, require further deliberation and in certain cases should be presented in the form of quantitative indicators, which would ensure their credibility.
>
> We are far from endorsing the view that measurement alone is the true criterion of science. The ordinary methods of medical statistics cannot be rated particularly highly, as they are able to do little more than to indicate the number of cases highlighting a particular symptom. In neuropsychology, as in other scientific disciplines in which the amount of material available for examination is relatively small, the centre of interest ought to be transferred to intercorrelations among symptoms and it is for these purposes that special mathematical methods need to be developed.
>
> There can be no doubt that this task can be realised by a single generation of scientists; indicating the necessary directions in which

developments ought to occur may help to undertake the necessary research activities.

In a field that is characterized by complex interdependencies among the many factors which combine to determine the well-being of both the person with PD and his/her carer, it is impossible to reach an understanding of the care-giving situation and crucial influences upon it, without adopting a more sophisticated approach to data analysis allowing for the covariance between key variables to be taken into account. These considerations were fundamental to the study conducted in three stages which is described in this volume.

1.4 Overview of the study

The model of PD as a neurodegenerative disorder was chosen for this study because the illness presents with symptoms in three distinct areas of functioning: physical, affective and cognitive, which provides the opportunity for examining how the three symptom domains relate to one another. It also allows a controlled way of determining how the effects wrought by the disabilities emerging from the impairment in these specific areas may affect not only the person suffering from the condition, but also his/her nearest relatives. In the case of the present study, the latter is the patient's spouse, and with the progression of the illness, s/he becomes increasingly involved in assisting with the day to day tasks of everyday living. The couple become entwined with the illness and both are affected by it, albeit in different ways. The resultant process, one of care-giving and care-receiving, is two-way and is based on a dyadic relationship between the patient and the spouse/carer.

The aim of the present work is to attempt a systematic approach to achieving an understanding of the various situational, clinical and relational interactions shaping different aspects of care-giving in PD, utilising a neuropsychological approach to the analysis. In order to do so, it is necessary to start by becoming acquainted with the current state of knowledge with regard to the three main symptom domains of PD. Hence chapter 2 provides a brief account of the nature of PD describing the key motor aspects of the disorder, its clinical presentation, and approaches to treatment of the condition. The two chapters that follow are concerned with the non-motor symptoms of PD: chapter 3 adopts a neuropsychiatric perspective, focusing mainly on the affective disorder which is the most common of these complications, but also providing a brief description of other psychiatric disturbances frequently present in PD. Chapter 4 provides an overview of the neuropsychological (cognitive) dysfunctions associated with PD. Both chapters 3 and 4 examine the mechanisms underlying the respective disorders and evaluate their aetiological status as arising from a common neurodegenerative processes or as comorbid conditions. In chapter 5 the effects of these three symptom areas on the disability in PD are considered along with the psychosocial adaptation that patients undergo in coming to terms with the condition. Consideration of functional adaptation to neurodegenerative disease processes forges a link between the patient and those closest to him/her, who through being involved in their relative's care, are also intimately involved in the experience of living with the condition from the perspective of carers. This is the subject matter of chapter 6, which provides the context to care-giving and critically examines different approaches to conceptualising care-giving outcomes before presenting the main theoretical models that have been applied to caring. A review of the research relating to care-giving in PD is presented in chapter 7 with a focus on identifying factors which lead to poorer outcomes in carers. Circumstances which may help to remediate some of the adverse effects of long-term care-giving commitments, with particular reference to the way in which adult attachment styles may affect the carer-care recipient relationship and help to promote relationship satisfaction, thus contributing to buffering the negative effects of care-giving are also considered in chapter 7. Other protective mechanisms reviewed include cultural expectations and family relationships. Chapters 2-7 form the theoretical basis for the research study, described in the later chapters. The empirical study is divided into three parts, parts I and II being concerned with testing specific hypotheses concerning the relationships among symptoms in PD. Affective symptoms, which as mentioned above, have hitherto received relatively little attention, were of special interest to the research, in view of the emerging evidence that they have particular significance for carer outcomes. Part III of the study focused on evaluating a model of the care-giving process, specifically taking into account carer perceptions of the patient's symptom presentation in the area of psychological functioning and the quality of the dyadic relationship between the carer and the care recipient. The justification for this approach is presented in chapter 8. Chapters 9 and 10 respectively, provide a description of the methods used and of the results obtained. Chapter 11 contains a discussion of the findings of stages I and II of the research which focused on the neuropsychological presentation of PD and chapter 12 presents a discussion of the empirical study of the dyadic relationship between the patient with PD and his/her carer, carried out in stage III of the research with reflections on the implications for clinical practice.

CHAPTER TWO

PARKINSON'S DISEASE: THE NATURE OF THE DISORDER

2.1 Introduction

The diagnosis of PD is made primarily on the basis of the clinical manifestation of the characteristic motor symptoms of the disorder. It is a progressive condition, with insidious onset, and the motor symptoms eventually give rise to the disabilities that seriously impair activities of daily living and lead to the need for care. This chapter provides an overview of the clinical presentation of PD in terms of the main symptoms and their clinical course, together with a classification of the disorder according to syndromes. There follows a discussion of the neural mechanisms underlying the disorder and a summary of the evidence regarding its possible aetiology. Finally the main forms of treatment, pharmacological and surgical, are presented.

2.2 Parkinson's disease – symptom presentation and clinical course of the disorder

PD was described for the first time by James Parkinson, a British physician, in 1817, and was originally known as paralysis agitans or the "shaking palsy". It is a sporadic (or idiopathic), degenerative disorder, once thought to affect only the central nervous system, but now known to be associated also with pathology of the peripheral and enteric nervous systems (Braak and Del Tredici 2008). It has thus increasingly been recognized as a multisystemic disorder, in which there is preferential obliteration of dopaminergic neurons in the nigrostriatal pathways of the basal ganglia. Clinically, the disorder is primarily associated with late age at onset and relatively slow progression of symptoms (Fahn 2003). There is general agreement that the condition presents with four cardinal symptoms, which include (i) a resting tremor and shaking of limbs, (ii) muscular rigidity, (iii) slowness and poverty of movement and (iv) postural instability (Caslake et al. 2008; Fahn 2003; Probst, Bloch and Tolnay 2008). The cause of the condition remains unknown, although some forms of the disorder show a slight familial tendency in patterns of occurrence (Lang and Lozano 1998) and a number of genetic mutations have been implicated, albeit in a minority of cases (Davie 2008; Weintraub, Comella and Horn 2008). The disorder stems from the degeneration of nuclei in the dopaminergic neurons of the brainstem, leading to depletion of the neurotransmitter dopamine in these regions. When dopamine production is reduced, the motor system nerves are unable to control movement and coordination. Patients suffering from PD are known to have lost 70%-80% of their dopamine-producing cells by the time that symptoms first appear (Kuran 2002; Martin 1998; Youdim and Riederer 1997). The discovery that PD was associated with dopamine depletion by Hornykiewicz in the 1960s led to the successful treatment of the disorder with the drug levodopa (L-dopa) (Górska and Majczyński 1997; Hornykiewicz 2006).

PD is the second most common neurodegenerative disorder, after Alzheimer's disease (DAT; Choonara et al. 2009; de Lau and Breteler 2006). The age at onset is typically in the sixth decade of life (mean age at onset is 60 years) with approximately 1-2% of the world's population in this age group affected by the disorder (Olanow, Stern and Sethi 2009; Post, Speelman and de Haan 2008). The condition is rare in people below 30 years of age, and risk for the disease increases with age. It is estimated that 5-10% of patients who have PD, experience symptoms before the age of 40 (Golbe 1991; Muthane et al. 1994). PD is common in the elderly and affects more than 3% of the population aged more than 75 years and 4% of those over the age of 80 (de Lau and Breteler 2006). The overall incidence rate, adjusted for age and gender, is estimated at 13.4 per 100,000, with a higher prevalence among males (19.0 per 100,000) than females (9.9 per 100,000) (Ben-Shlomo 1997; Van Den Eeden et al. 2003). Hence the relative risk for men of developing the condition appears to be approximately twice that for women, and other studies are broadly in keeping with these estimates e.g. Wooten et al. (2004) found a relative risk for men of 1.5 times greater than in women. There has been considerable controversy regarding variations in PD associated with race or ethnicity (Friedman 2006; Stern and Lees 1982), although in one American study, PD appeared to be higher among Hispanics than Caucasians, but less common among Asians and African-Americans (Van Den Eeden et al. 2003). There also appear to be geographical variations in the occurrence of PD: the frequency is greater in industrialized than in non-industrialized regions, and higher in Europe than in North America (Choonara et al.

2009), although rates in some countries (e.g. Poland) appear to be disproportionately low in comparison to other European countries (Friedman 2006). The disorder carries a risk of earlier mortality compared with the general population, especially for people with a young age at onset of the condition (Ishihara et al. 2007), although there is some evidence to suggest that the death rates among both men and women with PD have fallen in recent years in the U.K. (Mylne et al. 2009). There is also an increased risk of morbidity in persons with PD, which is associated with complications of inactivity, including poor nutrition, cardiovascular disease and pneumonia (Martin 1998).

2.2.1 The clinical presentation of Parkinson's disease

The main symptoms of PD usually develop over time; however patients do not have to present with the full symptom complex of bradykinesia, muscular rigidity, resting tremor and postural instability in order to be diagnosed with the disorder and indeed most patients do not develop the full range of symptoms that are associated with the condition (Zigmond and Burke 2002). Symptoms are usually lateralized at the start of the illness, but over time, gradually begin to affect both sides of the body. The rate of symptom progression is extremely variable; some patients become profoundly disabled whilst others continue to function relatively well, for up to ten years after the initial diagnosis. The symptoms of PD often show a great deal of fluctuation, often from day to day, but even from one moment to another. The reasons for this are often unclear, but are thought to be attributable to the disease process or to medication. Such fluctuations, when they occur, are difficult to manage clinically and are particularly problematic for patients.

2.2.2 Primary symptoms

The primary symptoms of PD, considered as being characteristic of the disorder, are tremor, rigidity, bradykinesia and postural instability (Caslake et al. 2008; Probst et al. 2008; Zigmond and Burke 2002). The description that follows is partly based on a classic and beautifully written text by Stern and Lees (1982), authorities in the field of PD, which is aimed at providing patients and their families with information about the condition.

The sign most frequently associated with PD, probably because it is so conspicuous, is that of tremor. It affects about 70% of patients with PD (Hoehn and Yahr 1967) and because it is perceived as being such an obvious departure from normal, it is usually the sign which first alerts patients to the fact that something is wrong and causes them to seek medical advice. Although tremor is a frequent source of embarrassment to patients, who may go to considerable lengths to try to disguise it, paradoxically it often proves to be the least disabling of symptoms, and forms of PD in which it predominates appear to follow a more benign course and have a longer therapeutic response to L-dopa (Martin 1998). Tremor is initially slight, and may occur intermittently, when the patient is tired or at times of emotional stress; some patients report that before it presents externally and is evident to others, it has occurred as a form of internal trembling for some considerable time. It usually begins unilaterally in the upper limbs and as the disease progresses, generally starts to affect the contralateral hand, but it may follow an ipsilateral course, affecting the lower limb, before it spreads to both sides of the body. In the long-term, tremor affects the hands, fingers, forearms and feet and is usually most severe in the limb in which it originally occurred. Although the tremor may be limited to one finger, more often it involves all the fingers and the thumb, giving rise to an oscillation of the thumb against the index finger, which is described as "pill rolling". Tremors of the mouth, chin and tongue are less frequently observed. The tremor of PD is described as a fine grain tremor, occurring with a characteristic frequency of 4-6 Hz, which distinguishes it from other causes such as anxiety or over-activity of the thyroid gland, which is associated with a much faster movement, and from benign essential tremor, which intensifies with movement. In contrast, in PD, the tremor tends to occur when the limbs are at rest, but not when the patient is performing a voluntary activity, so that the performance of skilled tasks may not be greatly affected, especially in the early stages of the condition. It disappears during sleep but even at later stages of the disease, may fluctuate considerably in intensity and duration, being exacerbated by stress and relieved during relaxation (Jankovic 2008; Kuran 2002).

Rigidity or muscle stiffness in PD is detected as a resistance to passive movements of the limbs, which is uniformly difficult to overcome in both the directions of flexion and extension (Zigmond and Burke 2002). The patient may be unaware of this difficulty, although sometimes the resistance is so great, that it is impossible to overcome and the patient is unable to completely release a limb. If rigidity is accompanied by tremor, the movement occurs in a regular, rhythmical jerking, which is known as "cog-wheel rigidity" (Youdim and Riederer 1997). Rigidity can be predominantly unilateral, affecting the arm and leg on one side of the body or it may symmetrically involve all four limbs. The degree of involvement and severity of rigidity varies considerably from one individual to another, but can usually be detected in a given limb when other limbs are moved vigorously. This strategy is often used by examiners in order to evoke evidence of the symptom clinically. As a result of rigidity, the muscles move more slowly and in the early stages of the illness this may give rise to pain, cramps and stiffness. Rigidity is also responsible for the characteristic profile of patients with PD, in which the torso leans forward slightly, the lower limbs are slightly bent at the knee, the upper limbs at the elbow, and the expressionless facial features remain immobile in a pattern known as "masking".

Bradykinesia is a term which refers to the slowness and poverty of voluntary movements and includes problems in initiating and completing movement once it is in progress (Jankovic 2008). In particular, difficulties in accomplishing rapid, repetitive movements are the consequence, accompanied by excessive fatiguability. Bradykinesia is considered to be the most incapacitating of all the symptoms encountered in PD and may be the cause of many of the frustrating problems encountered by patients in their everyday lives. An advantageous effect of the medication used in PD is that it is particularly effective in alleviating the symptoms of bradykinesia.

Postural instability occurs due to the impairment or loss of the reflexes that adjust posture in order to maintain balance, and precipitates falls which are very common in people with PD. There is also a distinctive, unsteady walk that is associated with the condition. The parkinsonian gait demonstrates a tendency to lean forward or backward unnaturally and to develop a stooped, head-down stance with drooping shoulders. Arm swing is diminished or absent and walking is characterized by small, shuffling steps (marche à petit pas) known as festination. There are problems with initiating walking and patients may appear to be falling forward as they walk; they may "freeze" in mid-stride and be unable to continue the movement or they may have difficulties with, and be unsteady when attempting to turn.

2.2.3 Secondary symptoms

Apart from these cardinal signs associated with PD, a number of secondary symptoms may also occur due to the progressive loss of voluntary and involuntary muscle control. Most patients do not experience all of these secondary symptoms and they vary in intensity from person to person. Indeed, even at diagnosis, the heterogeneity of symptoms is striking (Post et al. 2008). The secondary symptoms of PD include: small cramped handwriting (micrographia), a soft whispery voice (hypophonia) and a range of autonomic symptoms such as constipation, difficulty in swallowing (dysphagia) – saliva and food may collect in the mouth or back of the throat and cause choking, coughing or drooling, hypersalivation, excessive perspiration, scaling and dry skin on the face and scalp.

Non-motor symptoms have increasingly been recognised as forming an integral part of parkinsonian symptomatology (Chaudhuri et al. 2009). These involve loss of intellectual capacity, slowed thinking (bradyphrenia), sleep disturbances, impulse control disorders and affective difficulties such as anxiety and depression. The non-motor manifestations of PD are mentioned here for the sake of completion, but will be dealt with in separate chapters.

2.2.4 The clinical syndrome of parkinsonism

In order to understand PD, it is necessary to place the condition within the context of the broader syndrome of parkinsonism. Modern conceptualisations define parkinsonism according to any combination of the motor symptoms referred to above and some authorities further add loss of postural reflexes and the freezing phenomenon, in which the patient's feet seem to be transiently "glued to the ground" to create six cardinal features of the disease (Fahn and Przedborski 2005). All six of these features need not be present for the diagnosis of parkinsonism, but two are required, one of which should be either tremor at rest or bradykinesia (Fahn 2003). According to this conceptualisation, parkinsonism is divided into four categories (see table 2-1).

The present work is concerned with primary parkinsonism or PD. It is the most frequently encountered clinical category and one which has been the principal focus of research. The majority of cases (90%) of PD are sporadic, although in recent years a number of gene mutations have been identified as being causal. PD is distinguished from other forms of parkinsonism on the basis that it is not caused by acquired damage to the brain (as in secondary parkinsonism) and is not accompanied by other motor signs of neurological origin (as in the Parkinson-plus syndromes). These Parkinson-plus diseases usually progress more quickly than typical, idiopathic PD and there are subtle differences in presentation. Progressive supranuclear palsy is the neurodegenerative disorder most commonly confused with PD. It is associated with early postural instability, minimal tremor, paralysis of vertical gaze, prominent dysarthria and a subcortical type of dementia. In dementia with Lewy bodies, cognitive dysfunction precedes or presents very early in the course of the movement disorder and neuropsychiatric symptoms are prominent. Multiple system atrophy is a condition that presents considerable diagnostic difficulties and is most commonly confused with PD or progressive supranuclear palsy. It is characterised by early autonomic dysfunction and may include cerebellar signs. Cortical-basal degeneration is characterised by the presence of extreme asymmetric rigidity with patchy cortical cognitive defects such as dysphasia and apraxias and relatively frequent occurrence of the "alien limb" phenomena. The relationship between PD, PD with dementia and dementia with Lewy bodies might be most accurately conceptualized as a spectrum, with a discrete area of overlap between each of the three disorders (Cummings 2003; Fahn 2003).

Table 2-1. Classification of parkinsonism (after Fahn 2003).

Parkinson's disease (primary parkinsonism)
Sporadic (idiopathic)
Of known genetic aetiology
Secondary parkinsonism (environmental aetiology)
Drugs:
Dopamine receptor blockers (e.g. antipsychotic medication)
Dopamine storage depletors (reserpine, tetrabenzine)
Postencephalitic (viral)
Toxins, carbon monoxide, MPTP, cyanide
Vascular
Brain tumours
Head trauma
Normal-pressure hydrocephalus
Parkinsonism-plus syndromes
Progressive supranuclear palsy
Multiple system atrophy
Cortical-basal ganglionic degeneration
Parkinson-dementia-ALS complex of Guam
Progressive pallidal atrophy
Diffuse Lewy body disease
Heredodegenerative disorders
Alzheimer's disease
Wilson's disease
Huntington's disease
Frontotemporal dementia

Parkinson-plus syndromes do not respond well to L-dopa therapy (Fahn 2003) and patients may be extremely sensitive to neuroleptic medication, as demonstrated by exacerbation of motor symptoms. Differential diagnosis is important, because anti-cholinesterase inhibitors have been shown to have some effect in treating the neuropsychiatric symptoms of these disorders. Another condition commonly misdiagnosed as PD, as mentioned above, is benign essential tremor, but it lacks all other features of PD besides tremor, is not present at rest and is usually bilateral (Fahn 2003).

2.2.5 Establishing the diagnosis of Parkinson's disease

The diagnosis of PD is still established primarily according to clinical examination made by an expert clinician. The motor manifestations remain of paramount importance and the diagnosis of PD is based on the four cardinal clinical signs of tremor, rigidity, bradykinesia and postural instability described above (Hughes, Daniel and Lees 2001; Jankovic 2008; Kaasinen and Rinne 2002). Diagnostic criteria require that at least two of the four motor symptoms are present, one of which must be bradykinesia (Jankovic 2008; Litvan et al. 2003). Asymmetric onset of limb involvement and good response to L-dopa therapy are generally regarded as evidence in support of the diagnosis (Fahn 2003). There are no specific tests to establish the diagnosis of PD and neuroimaging techniques such as computerised tomography or magnetic resonance imaging (MRI), have until recently, been generally considered unhelpful (Cummings 2003). Structural changes in the substantia nigra in PD can now be recognised with more advanced MRI techniques (e.g. 7 tesla) and transcranial sonography can detect hyperechogenicity bilaterally from the lateral midbrain, which is increased in 96% of patients with PD (Brooks 2012). The latter is more a trait marker of susceptibility to the disease and does not correlate with the severity, as it has been shown to remain stable over five years, despite progression of symptoms (Berg et al. 2005). These imaging techniques are useful in discriminating atypical parkinsonian syndromes from typical PD on the basis of abnormal putamen signals (Brooks 2012). Functional imaging techniques such as positron emission tomography (PET) or single photon computed emission tomography (SPECT) using radioactively labelled tracers, which provide a marker of functional dopaminergic loss in the striatum, can support the diagnosis of PD by helping to discriminate it from atypical syndromes, including suspected early cases which do not progress on follow-up. Until recently, these structural and functional imaging techniques have been largely limited to a research setting, but are now recognised as being clinically useful for the differential diagnosis of degenerative parkinsonian syndromes (Brooks 2012).

Over the past decade there has been increasing recognition of the fact, that in the prodromal stages, PD is often characterised by non-motor symptoms, although there is substantial variability among patients (Wolters 2008). It has been known for a long time, that depression may precede the onset of motor symptoms (Rickards 2005), but autonomic dysfunction, sleep disorders, pain, fatigue and cognitive deficits are now acknowledged as equally likely precursors of the disorder (Wolters 2008). These symptoms however, do not form part of the diagnostic criteria for PD.

Diagnosis of PD can only be confirmed through documentation of salient clinical features and post-mortem verification of Lewy bodies, which are now considered to be the pathological hallmark of the disorder; some diagnostic uncertainty is thus unavoidable (Tessa et al. 2008). In one study, an alarming 47% of diagnoses made by a mixture of various specialists (geriatricians and neurologists) and non-specialists proved to be incorrect (Meara, Bhowmick and Hobson 1999). Post-mortem studies have shown an alternative diagnosis in up to 25% of patients with PD diagnosed by general neurologists (Hughes et al. 1992; Schrag, Ben-Shlomo and Quinn 2002) and fewer diagnostic errors (6-8%) appear to be made in expert movement disorders clinics (Hughes et al. 2002; Jankovic et al. 2000). An attempt to provide a systematic set of diagnostic criteria based on existing clinicopathologic studies is represented by the United Kingdom Parkinson's Disease Society (UKPDS) Brain Bank Diagnostic Criteria (Litvan et al. 2003) which have come to be accepted as the "gold standard" for diagnostic criteria in PD (see table 2-2).

2.2.6 Neural mechanisms in Parkinson's disease

PD is a disorder of involuntary movement associated with damage to the extrapyramidal nervous system. The core symptoms of the disorder, described above, appear to be mainly the result of decreased stimulation of the motor cortex by the basal ganglia, caused by depletion of the neurotransmitter dopamine. However, it is known that multiple cell types in many brain regions are afflicted and that deficiencies in other neurotransmitter systems also occur, namely GABA and 5-hydroxytryptamine, which predominantly exist in the striatum and substantia nigra (Androutsellis-Theotokis et al. 2009).

The basal ganglia are a large set of nuclear structures which connect to other areas of the brain and are functionally diverse, being involved, amongst others, in motor control. The nuclei involved in motor regulation include the caudate, putamen, and the globus pallidus, and they are functionally associated with the substantia nigra in the base of the midbrain and the subthalamic nucleus in the ventral thalamus.

Table 2-2. PD UKPDS Brain Bank diagnostic criteria (Litvan et al. 2003).

Step 1. Diagnosis of a parkinsonian syndrome Bradykinesia (slowness of initiation of voluntary movement with progressive reduction in speed and amplitude of repetitive actions) and at least one of the following (i) muscular rigidity, (ii) 4+6 Hz rest tremor and (iii) postural instability not caused by primary visual, vestibular, cerebellar or proprioreceptive dysfunction.
Step 2. Exclusion criteria for PD (i) History of repeated strokes with stepwise progression of parkinsonian features (ii) History of repeated head injury (iii) History of definite encephalitis (iv) Oculogyric crises (v) Neuroleptic treatment at the onset of symptoms (vi) More than one affected relative (vii) Sustained remission (viii) Strictly unilateral features after three years (ix) Supranuclear gaze palsy (x) Cerebellar signs (xi) Early severe autonomic involvement (xii) Early severe dementia with disturbances of memory, language and praxis (xiii) Babinski's sign (xiv) Presence of cerebral tumour or communicating hydrocephalus on CT scan (xv) Negative response to large doses of L-dopa (if malabsorption excluded)
Step 3. Supportive criteria for PD (three or more required for diagnosis of definite PD) (i) Unilateral onset (ii) Rest tremor present (iii) Progressive disorder (iv) Persistent asymmetry affecting side of onset most (v) Excellent response (70 + 100%) to L-dopa (vi) Severe L-dopa induced chorea (vii) L-dopa response for 5 years or more (viii) Clinical course of 10 years or more

Together they make a subcortical loop which links most areas of the cortex with groups of upper motor neurons in the primary motor cortex, the premotor cortex and in the brainstem. Normal initiation of voluntary movements is dependent upon the neurons in this loop, which respond in anticipation of and during movements, exerting their effects on upper motor neurons in the cortex (DeLong and Wichmann 2007). Damage to any of the structures within the basal ganglia or to any of the associated structures in this loop, leaves the patient unable to initiate and terminate movements smoothly. The resultant dysfunctional movements, characteristic of PD, are a consequence of abnormal upper motor neuron activity in the absence of the supervisory control normally provided by the basal ganglia (after Purves et al. 2001).

Two pathways are distinguished within the extrapyramidal system of which the basal ganglia are part: a direct pathway and an indirect pathway, both of which are involved in the regulation of movement. The direct pathway facilitates movement and is associated with the stimulatory activity of D1 receptors, which under normal circumstances, results in the activation of the motor cortex, whilst the indirect pathway inhibits movement, and is associated with the inhibitory role of the D2 receptors along the nigrostriatal pathway (DeLong and Wichmann 2007). Loss of dopamine in PD leads to inhibition of the direct pathway and excitation of the indirect pathway, giving rise to a hypokinetic movement disorder of the kind seen in PD. The lack of dopamine results in increased inhibition of the ventral anterior nucleus of the thalamus, which sends excitatory projections to the motor cortex, and results in the clinical picture of hypokinesia.

In all, there are four major dopamine pathways originating in the midbrain: the nigrostriatal pathway, referred to above, mediates movement and is the most conspicuously affected in early PD. The fibres of the nigrostriatal pathway form a thick network, projecting from the substantia nigra to the striatum. The mesocortical pathway connects the midbrain with the cerebral cortex, the mesolimbic pathway projects to the limbic system and the tuberoinfundibular pathway connects the hypothalamus with the pituitary gland. It is thought that disruption of dopamine along the non-striatal pathways is responsible for much of the neuropsychiatric pathology associated with PD (DeLong and Wichmann 2007).

The motor symptoms of PD are primarily associated with the loss of pigmented dopaminergic cells in the pars compacta region of the substantia nigra, a region with the greatest concentration of dopamine-producing cells. Post mortem studies demonstrate that in patients affected by PD, this part of the brain has lost between 60-80% of its neurones compared with the same region in unaffected individuals (Zigmond and Burke 2002).

Dopaminergic neurones project from the substantia nigra to the striatum and their loss leads to consequent depletion of dopamine in the striatum and the alterations in the activity of neural circuits within the basal ganglia that regulate movement, as described. Observations of these neuropathological changes led to the hypothesis that dopaminergic transmission along the nigrostriatal pathway may be the cause of the deficits in PD (Hornykiewicz 2006). This proved to be the first ever demonstration of the fact that brain disease may be associated with the loss of specific neurotransmitters, in this case, dopamine (Górska and Majczyński 1997).

The progression of pathological changes in PD has been shown to follow a pattern, with the earliest changes occurring in the medulla oblongata/pontine tegmentum and olfactory bulb. These have been defined as Braak stages 1 and 2 (Braak et al. 2006; Wolters 2008) and in these initial stages, patients remain pre-symptomatic from the point of view of motor symptoms. The early involvement of the olfactory bulb, which appears to be particularly prone to the deposition of Lewy bodies, is interesting as it correlates with the clinical picture of PD, in which disturbances of smell and taste often precede the onset of motor symptoms (Haehner, Hummel and Reichmann 2011). As the disease progresses, the substantia nigra, areas of the midbrain and basal forebrain become involved (Braak stages 3 and 4). Eventually the pathological changes begin to affect the neocortex. The pathological stages defined by Braak et al. (2006) are based on the distribution of Lewy bodies within the cell nuclei. Lewy bodies are cytoplasmic inclusions, consisting of a variety of proteins responsible for proteolysis, but their main constituent is alpha-synuclein, a protein of unknown function. Although Lewy bodies and Lewy neurites (protein formations comprising of abnormal alpha-synuclein filaments) are considered to be the classical neuropathological feature of PD (Davie 2008), they are not specifically indicative of the condition, as they also occur in Lewy body dementia (LBD; Cummings 2003), DAT (Hamilton 2000; Kotzbauer, Trojanowski and Lee 2001) and several of the Parkinsonism-plus syndromes, such as multiple system atrophy (see table 2-1; Jellinger 2007). It would appear that a spectrum of Lewy body disease exists, with the clinical presentation depending on the site of Lewy body formation and neuronal loss (Lowe, Mayer and Landon 1996). Idiopathic PD is characterised by the distribution of Lewy bodies throughout the substantia nigra and locus coeruleus, but they are also found in other brain regions such as the raphe nucleus, the nucleus basalis of Meynert, hypothalamic neurones and in areas of the neocortex, particularly the cingulate gyrus and entorhinal cortex (Cummings 2003).

Although the mechanisms underpinning the movement disorders associated with the basal ganglia are not well understood, it would appear that they might be attributed to a disruption in the balance between three different, but functionally linked neurotransmitter systems, which regulate basal gangliar activity. These include the dopaminergic system of the nigrostriatal pathway, the cholinergic system of the striatum and the GABA-ergic system which links the striatum with different parts of the globus pallidus and the substantia nigra. A very different clinical picture emerges of the movement disorder associated with dopaminergic depletion (PD) as opposed to that characteristic of cholinergic and GABA-ergic loss (Huntington's disease). The enzymes required for the synthesis of acetylcholine and GABA are greatly reduced in the latter condition and this may lead to an imbalance in the neurotransmitters, with a relative predominance of the dopaminergic system. This is in keeping with clinical observations, which demonstrate that the choreic movements of Huntington's disease increase after treatment with L-dopa. Equally, it is well known that the effects of treatment with anti-dopaminergic medication in such conditions as schizophrenia, can produce undesirable motor side effects, which are similar to the physical presentation of PD. At the same time, patients with PD have been observed to demonstrate involuntary movements, similar to the choreiform movements of Huntington's disease, when exposed to high doses of L-dopa. Taken together, these observations suggest that movement disorders may be the result of disruptions to an essential balance between the dopaminergic, cholinergic and GABA-ergic neurotransmitter systems (after Górska and Majczyński 1997).

2.2.7 The aetiology of Parkinson's disease

The aetiology of PD remains largely unknown. The majority of people with PD have the idiopathic form of the disorder, for which the pathological mechanism has not, as yet, been identified (Siderowf and Stern 2008). A number of different hypotheses have been proposed in attempting to account for the disorder in PD: these include genetic, environmental and acquired factors.

2.2.7.1 Genetic factors

Over the last decade, evidence to support the contribution of genetic factors to the aetiology of PD has accumulated (Bonifati 2005; Bonifati et al. 2003; Davie 2008; Elbaz et al.1999; International Parkinson Disease

Genomics Consortium 2011; Morris 2005). There are infrequent families throughout the world in whom PD is the result of a mutation in a single gene that leads to developing the disease. In these families, the risk of several individuals being affected by the condition is increased, but in all, such families account for only about 5% of people diagnosed with PD. Nevertheless, these families have proved an important source of information on how the disease develops.

The majority of people with PD, however do not have the familial genetic disorder, although it is considered likely that they may have an inherited predisposition for developing the condition. Whilst this susceptibility is also genetic in origin, it appears to be caused by changes in a variety of genes. A number of single gene mutations have now been identified which, whilst carrying a relatively low risk for PD, are thought to interact with environmental factors to increase the probability of developing the disease. The exception is the LRRK2 mutation, which is associated with 5-7% of cases of familial PD and 1.6% of cases with idiopathic PD. The clinical presentation is that of the typical features of PD associated with middle or late onset. The first gene mutation to be discovered, which it was believed played a central role in the aetiology of PD, was one that coded for the protein alpha-synuclein, the main constituent of Lewy bodies which are recognised as being characteristic of the neuropathology of PD. Early onset PD is associated with a point mutation of the alpha-synuclein gene in an autosomal dominant pattern. PD symptoms presenting in the fourth or fifth decade of life appear to be associated with duplications or triplications of the alpha-synuclein gene, leading to the speculation that over-expression of this gene may be a factor in the development of so-called "idiopathic" PD more generally (Davie 2008). More recently, a mutation located at the VPS35 gene has been found to be responsible for late onset PD (Vilariño-Güell et al. 2011). Still others are associated with an autosomal, recessive pattern of inheritance and different clinical manifestations of the condition. This is an intensive area of research which is rapidly yielding results in identifying the genetic changes thought to be implicated in PD.

Oxidative stress mechanisms have also been implicated in the neurodegenerative process in PD through the mechanism of gene mutation. It is considered likely that a mitochondrial defect might be responsible for the cell dysfunction and death that is characteristic of the disorder and a gene mutation has recently been identified which appears to account for the oxidative deficits in a familial form of PD (Chartier-Harlin et al. 2011). However, the role of genetic factors in the aetiology of PD may account for only a small proportion of cases of PD and for the majority (over 90%), causes for the disease process remain to be identified (Rappley et al. 2009). However, the possibility that gene mutations might be part of the pathological mechanism in PD has led to the search for environmental factors in the aetiology of the condition, that may have toxic effects for DNA and RNA.

2.2.7.2 Environmental factors

Attempts at identifying environmental factors that may predispose to the development of PD, however, have proved elusive. Although a number of studies have suggested that PD occurs more frequently in rural areas, the causal factor being attributed to toxins occurring in pesticides and metals such as manganese or iron, the evidence for this is controversial. One longitudinal study demonstrated that the incidence of PD was 70% higher in individuals who had been exposed to pesticides than those who had not (Ascherio et al. 2006). A number of studies have found increased rates of PD in people whose supply of water comes mainly from rural wells; it is thought that well water consumption is a proxy measure of exposure to pesticides (Koller et al. 1990; Wright and Keller-Byne 2005). Studies in agreement with this hypothesis have found a dose-dependent increase in PD in persons exposed to agricultural chemicals. A number of case studies have also linked solvent exposure, in particular trichloroethylene, to PD and a recent study has confirmed that the risk is significantly increased by an odds ratio of 6.1 (Goldman et al. 2011). Trichloroethylene is known to be the most common organic contaminant of groundwater, which may also explain the increased rates of PD associated with drinking water from rural wells. However, the fact that the appearance of the disorder predates the first synthesis of the chemical toxins attributed to causing PD indicates that these more recently synthesized compounds cannot be the sole cause of parkinsonism.

A famous example of exposure to toxins giving rise to a parkinsonian-like syndrome occurred in the USA (California) in the 1970s and was associated with the consumption of a substance called 1-methyl-4-phenyl-1,2,3,6-tetrahydropyidine (MPTP) by a group of young drug addicts. MPTP was produced as a contaminant in the illegal production of an opiate related to heroin and elicits a parkinsonian syndrome in primates and man which is caused by the destruction of dopaminergic neurones in the substantia nigra (Kapitza et al. 2008).

2.2.7.3 The role of head injury

It has been noted that patients with PD are more likely to report a past history of head injury in comparison to that occurring in the general population (Bower et al. 2003; Stern et al. 1991). The alleged association between PD and head injury is difficult to study, because of the strong possibility of a recall bias, as patients with PD may be selectively more likely to remember head traumas in a "search for meaning" when reflecting upon the antecedents to their illness, than control subjects not suffering from the disease. However, the research in this area does seem to provide support for the hypothesis that previous head trauma may be a more frequent finding in people suffering from PD. It appears that people who have experienced a head injury are four times more likely to develop the condition than those who have not (Bower et al. 2003). Moreover, the risk of developing PD appears to be associated with the severity of the trauma; in cases which required hospitalisation, the risk increased eight-fold and for those with a serious head injury, it was eleven times greater. The authors of the research caution that since head trauma is a rare event, the contribution to the incidence of PD is likely to be only slight. However, repeated head injuries, associated with certain sports such as boxing, are known to increase the probability of a form of the disorder which has earned its own name, and is referred to as pugilistic parkinsonism (Erlanger et al. 1999; Gibb 1988). In a study designed to overcome the methodological limitations which besiege research of this kind, Goldman et al. (2006) reported a similar risk (3.8) for PD to that of the study referred to above, increased susceptibility being associated with the severity of the injury and hospitalization. Nonetheless, the demonstrated relationship is a difficult one to disentangle, as it is not certain whether the head trauma actually contributed to the development of PD, or if the early symptoms of clumsiness associated with PD may have been a factor contributing to the increased likelihood of the head trauma.

2.2.7.4 Ageing as a causal factor

Age is generally considered to be a significant risk factor for PD, but this notion has limited explanatory value in itself. First of all, PD cannot be considered just a disease of old age as one in seven people develop the disorder in their thirties and forties (Stern and Lees 1982). Secondly, if the passage of time alone were to raise the risk of developing PD, then it would reflect little more than a process of normal ageing, in which most people would be expected to develop the condition if they were to live long enough. This is clearly not the case and there is now considerable evidence, as referred to above, to suggest that PD is associated with a specific brain pathology that is not characteristic of ageing *per se*.

Nonetheless, levels of dopamine are known to decrease with age even in people unaffected by PD (Youdim and Riederer 1997). Age related decline of dopamine receptors in the striatum has been demonstrated in a number of post-mortem studies and comparable reductions have been shown in cortical and thalamic dopamine (Kaasinen and Rinne 2002). However, the pattern and timing of dopamine loss is different from that which occurs in PD and hence it is unlikely that ageing has a direct role in the neurodegenerative process (Zigmond and Burke 2002). For example, lower levels of dopamine are associated with the caudate nucleus in ageing, whilst in PD there are greater reductions in the putamen (Hornykiewicz et al. 1989). Moreover levels of dopamine are not reduced in a homogeneous fashion in the various structures of the basal ganglia. For example, reductions of around 80% of dopamine in the striatum have been shown to be associated with a 50% drop in dopaminergic cells in the substantia nigra (Forno 1996). This suggests that the remaining cells are less efficient in the production of dopamine than normal. It implies that there must be an additional factor, independent of ageing, that gives rise to the progressive deterioration of these dopaminergic cells.

Neither can PD be considered a condition of abnormally rapid ageing of those parts of the brain associated with dopaminergic neurotransmission as has been suggested by some authors (Barbeau 1973). By the sixtieth decade of life, (when PD is most commonly diagnosed) about 40-50% of dopamine has been lost from the striatum, but this is not sufficient to elicit the clinical symptoms associated with the disorder (Friedman 1999). The symptoms of PD are only clinically evident when levels of dopamine have fallen by 70-80% or more in comparison to healthy individuals (Kuran 2002; Martin 1998; Youdim and Riederer 1997).

Friedman (1999) presents a number of arguments against the abnormal ageing theory of PD. For example, the clinical picture in early-onset PD differs considerably from that in late-onset (Friedman 1994). Late-onset PD presents more frequently with tremor, both as the first clinical symptom and in dominating the clinical picture. The response to treatment is also different for the two groups: younger-onset patients have a greater tendency to show dyskinaesias as a side-effect of L-dopa treatment, whereas the older-onset group have a tendency to suffer more from psychotic complications. This would appear to demonstrate a different sensitivity of dopamine receptors in the two forms of the disorder.

2.3 The treatment of Parkinson's disease

In view of the fact that the aetiology of PD remains largely uncertain, there is no cure and treatment of the disorder is based on symptom management. None of the existing pharmacological approaches to therapy has been shown to slow or reverse the progression of the disease and hopes for finding ways of bestowing neuroprotection have so far, proved futile (Singh, Pillay and Choonara 2007). Surgical ablative treatments, neural implants and more recently, deep brain stimulation techniques remain controversial.

2.3.1 The course of untreated Parkinson's disease

Although it is extremely unusual in the present day for PD to be untreated, the natural history of the disorder is a relentless and progressive deterioration in the patient's condition, such that the capacity for self-care is gradually eroded and the patient is reliant on the help of others in order to manage the activities of daily living, eventually becoming entirely bed-ridden. The course of the disorder is unpredictable, as are the symptom patterns that may dominate the clinical picture in any individual case. There is some evidence of clinical subtypes: patients with a tremor-dominant form of PD may show little deterioration over many years, and those with primarily unilateral symptoms may also have a relatively benign disease course. On the other hand, patients with an akinetic-rigid form of the disease have a worse clinical course in the long-term, characterised by faster rates of functional deterioration. A third, mixed form of PD typically presents with akinesia, tremor and rigidity and appears to take an intermediate course (Martin 1998).

2.3.2 Pharmacological treatment of Parkinson's disease

One of the first successful forms of pharmacological treatment for PD was instigated by Charcot in the late nineteenth century, well before the scientific basis for its action had been elucidated. Using plant extracts that were known to cause mouth dryness, Charcot initially attempted to exploit these substances in order to control the drooling of saliva in PD. He noticed that these, as it was later demonstrated, anticholinergic agents also alleviated stiffness and trembling. Elaborate herbal remedies were gradually replaced by synthetically prepared medications which are still in use. The most frequently prescribed include benzhexol (Artane) and orphenadrine (Disipal). It is now clear that anticholinergic medication has only limited efficacy in reducing rigidity and tremor and has potentially damaging side-effects in the form of significant memory impairments (Miller, Berrios and Politynska 1987). The action of anticholinergic drugs is effected through blocking the reaction of acetylcholine, which is in relative preponderance in PD because of the dopamine deficiency. Anticholinergic drugs thus serve to redress the balance between these two neurotransmitters. Although at one time they were usually prescribed as the first course of treatment, nowadays they are more frequently used as an adjunctive therapy in combination with L-dopa. This is due to their relative ineffectiveness compared to L-dopa as well as the undesirable side-effects they cause in the form of digestive, cardiac and neuropsychological problems such as memory impairment and confusion (Stern and Lees 1982).

2.3.3 Levodopa

For the last forty years levodopa has been the cornerstone in the treatment of PD (Weintraub et al. 2008). In combination with a peripheral decarboxylase inhibitor, which prevents the breakdown of L-dopa to dopamine before it crosses the blood-brain barrier and is decarboxylated to dopamine in the nigrostriatal pathways (Pallone 2007), L-dopa remains, in many respects the most efficacious drug treatment available. The proprietary preparations are called Sinemet, Madopar and Stalevo, and are available in different doses and with different types and combinations of inhibitor (Weintraub et al. 2008). L-dopa is most effective in treating bradykinesia and rigidity, but less so in reducing tremor and problems with balance. Its side effects, especially early in treatment, include hypotension and dyskinesias, but these can usually be managed through dose adjustment or taking medication with food. A good response to L-dopa, with a stable and predictable reaction in terms of motor improvement that can virtually be guaranteed, usually lasts for a period of up to 5 years and has been called "the honeymoon" period (Sławek 2008). A major drawback is that the response diminishes over time, with a characteristic end-of-dose "wearing off", when motor control is compromised and patients may experience abrupt and often unpredictable changes as they pass suddenly from a state of good motor control, sometimes to complete immobility, which is known as the "on-off" phenomenon. This has led to controversy regarding when it is best to instigate treatment with L-dopa in order to have optimal long-term benefit. No resolution to this problem has been achieved: some clinicians feel that it is better to delay treatment for so long as the symptoms of the disorder remain manageable with alternative medication, whilst others believe that there are few benefits to be gained from delaying treatment. Current clinical evidence does not support the fear that L-dopa itself may enhance the progression of PD; rather the opposite appears true i.e. that L-dopa may actually slow the progression of the disease (Halkias et al. 2007).

The range of responses to treatment with L-dopa is extremely broad and unpredictable. In general, patients report feeling more alert, appear more animated and notice definite improvements in ease of movement. In the early days of treatment in the late 1960s, spectacular results were reported in severely disabled individuals who had never taken levodopa previously, and who had gradually come to depend on other people for help in maintaining the activities of daily living (see Sacks 1999 for illuminating descriptions of the early days of treatment). Sometimes these therapeutic benefits of L-dopa are still seen today, though they are less dramatic, because treatment is usually started long before patients have deteriorated to the extent that was inevitable before the introduction of the drug. Early in the disease, all the signs and symptoms of the disorder may virtually disappear and even experienced physicians may have difficulty in diagnosing the condition, when the medication is taking effect. Most patients with PD gain useful benefit from L-dopa in the form of a smooth improvement in symptoms, by taking a divided dose of the medication three times daily after meals. With the passage of time, the therapeutic effect of the medication gradually decreases and after approximately five years (Weintraub et al. 2008) the benefit of an individual dose may wane after just half an hour, whereas previously a positive response might last for three to four hours. It is often possible to restore the original benefits of the medication by taking smaller doses at more frequent intervals. This feature is known as the "end-of-dose deterioration" and is thought to be due to the brain's inability to store dopamine. It occurs in about 40% of patients after five years of successful treatment with L-dopa. In general it is recognised that L-dopa has provided incomparable benefits in the treatment of PD and although it is far from being a cure for the condition, it remains the treatment of choice (Stern and Lees 1982).

2.3.3.1 The side effects of L-dopa

The side effects that used to occur with pure levodopa and included nausea and vomiting, gastric symptoms, hypotension and palpitations have now virtually been eliminated with the addition of the carboxylase inhibitor to L-dopa preparations. Most patients appear more animated with treatment, but there is little evidence that L-dopa has any direct effect as an anti-depressant (Choi, Sohn, Lee and Kim 2000). Occasionally patients may become mildly confused and increases in libido have also been reported, especially in men. Some patients develop more serious reactions which include intense restlessness, intolerable anxiety, or paranoid ideation. Confusion appears more likely in the elderly and delirium or disorientation may be provoked, along with vivid nightmares or visual hallucinations. The latter are more common in conditions of diminished ambient light and typically include "seeing" non-existent animals or human figures or experiencing the sensation that another person is in close proximity to the patient. These observations are systematic enough to conclude that L-dopa may have an effect on the non-motor as well as motor systems of the brain.

The most common complication of long-term L-dopa therapy is the appearance of abnormal, involuntary movements known as dyskinesias. The first signs of dyskinesias are usually observed by other people rather than the patient, in the form of fidgeting, twitching of the face and lips, raising eyebrows, grimacing, tongue protrusion or curling toes. They are particularly evident when the patient is mobile and is obtaining the maximum benefit from treatment. Although it is most common for dyskinesias to affect the face and mouth, in more severe instances the neck, upper and lower limbs may be affected by uncontrollable, writhing and jerky movements which are more distressing to the observer than to the patient. These dyskinesias are associated with peak levels of L-dopa in the blood and they usually occur about half an hour after each dose and may persist for up to three hours. At such times the patient has maximum relief from the symptoms of bradykinesia and rigidity and is at his/her most mobile both in motor and functional terms, as paradoxically, the dyskinesias do not appear to interfere excessively with normal day to day functioning. Indeed, patients often prefer to be in the dyskinetic rather than the rigid state. Dyskinesias are predominantly associated with the duration of L-dopa treatment (Schrag and Quinn 2000), and when they start to occur, they are evoked by doses that were previously uncomplicated by such adverse effects. It is now thought that they arise as a result of the intermittent stimulation of dopamine receptors (Davie 2008). L-dopa has a short half-life of just 60-90 minutes and treatment regimes which are based on divided doses throughout the day, result in the fact that the denervated striatum is supplied with L-dopa in fits and starts. This is thought to be an important aetiological factor in the development of dyskinesias. Furthermore, the greater the nigrostriatal neuronal loss, the sooner the effects appear after the instigation of treatment with L-dopa. Dyskinesias may be improved when the dose of L-dopa is reduced, but this is always at the cost of reinstating the symptoms of PD (Stern and Lees 1982).

With the progression of the disease, not only is the shortened duration of symptom relief from L-dopa medication and dyskinesias increasingly problematic, but individual responses may become erratic, and usually effective doses of medication may cease to bring benefit. Additionally patients develop unpredictable "on-off" fluctuations in which there is a sudden loss of drug effect and the patient goes from a state of good mobility and functioning to a state of immobility, with the recurrence of severe PD symptoms in just a few minutes (Weintraub et al. 2008). Up to 70% of patients suffer these motor complications after about nine years of treatment (Ahlskog and Muenter 2001). Postural instability may become resistant to therapy over time, resulting in falls and injury, despite otherwise good control of motor symptoms (Rezak 2007). Patients may also suffer from painful muscle spasms, especially after many years of taking L-dopa. These affect the toes and feet in particular, but may also occur in the jaw, making chewing and speech especially difficult. These difficulties with the use of L-dopa over time are difficult to manage (Pahwa et al. 2006) and a trade-off between treating the motor symptoms whilst keeping the motor fluctuations to a minimum, is considered to be the best solution in terms of preserving the functional independence of the patient and maintaining health related quality of life (Weintraub et al. 2008).

2.3.4 Dopamine agonists

Dopamine agonists exert their effects by stimulating the post-synaptic dopamine receptors, thereby increasing the availability of endogenous dopamine. They include bromocriptine, pergolide, cabergoline, lisuride, pramipexole, ropinirole, rotigotine and apomorphine (Davie 2008; Weintraub et al. 2008). There appear to be no significant differences in the clinical efficacy between the different dopamine agonists, although bromocriptine is now used less frequently because of its cost and adverse side-effects and others, such as pergolide and cabergoline are not recommended because of their adverse effects on cardiac function (Davie 2008; Weintraub et al. 2008). Pramipexole is reported to have an uncommon side-effect in the form of increased risk for pathological gambling (Voon et al. 2006; Imamura, Uitti and Wszolek 2006).

Dopamine agonists were originally introduced as an adjunctive therapy in combination with L-dopa for use in patients with advanced PD. Because of their efficacy in improving motor symptoms which allowed treatment with L-dopa to be delayed, and hence forestall the development of complications associated with L-dopa, they were later introduced as first-line agents in the treatment of PD.

In controlled trials, dopamine agonists alone have been found to produce a reduction in dyskinesias and in combination with L-dopa, to reduce the wearing off phenomenon. These improvements were maintained even when L-dopa was added to improve control of parkinsonian symptoms. However, dopamine agonists in isolation did not improve motor symptoms as efficiently as L-dopa, although the subjective evaluation of symptoms by patients did not differ between the two treatment groups. Nonetheless, dopamine agonists are less successful in controlling the motor symptoms of PD in the long-term and even if patients are initially helped by these preparations alone, almost all eventually require that L-dopa be added to the treatment regime (Weintraub et al. 2008). Dopamine agonists are also more likely than L-dopa to cause adverse cognitive effects in the form of confusion and hallucinations, (Lees 2005), although this risk is not greater for the elderly, as was once thought (Davie 2008).

Apomorphine is a dopamine agonist given subcutaneously in more advanced disease and because it is delivered systematically by pump, it has a greater potential to maintain steady levels of brain dopamine and thus to control resistant motor fluctuations. It is particularly useful in patients who have unpredictable off-times and failures to respond to normal doses of medication. A complication in the use of apomorphine (especially, it appears, with delivery by constant infusion), and indeed with L-dopa more generally, is in the addictive quality that it seems to have for some people with PD and indeed for some who do not (Borek and Friedman 2005). Excessive intake of L-dopa leads to agitation, confusion, hypersexuality, mania accompanied by dyskinesias and psychosis with delusions and visual hallucinations. Patients tend to increase L-dopa dosage even though they have good motor control at lower doses and in spite of the dyskinesias that accompany over-dosage. This suggests that they are gaining psychological rather than motor benefit and indeed, some patients report the subjective experience of feeling that they function better mentally under such conditions. The objective evidence for this is uncertain. This behavioural disorder is related to the misuse of L-dopa and most typically occurs in men with early onset PD, has been termed 'hedonistic homeostatic dysregulation' (Giovannoni et al. 2000). L-dopa addiction may be more frequent than has hitherto been appreciated: the author encountered three cases of dependency during the course of the present study.

2.3.5 Monoamine oxidase-B (MAO-B) inhibitors

MAO-B inhibitors have been considered to be useful in PD as a first line treatment, not only because of their proven efficacy in symptom improvement, but also because of their alleged neuroprotective effects (Parkinson's Study Group 1989). They exert their effects by preventing metabolism of dopamine in the brain, thus maintaining levels of endogenous dopamine (Weintraub et al. 2008). In this sense, their action is similar to that of the dopamine agonists. The most commonly used preparation is selegiline, which has been shown to have a modest effect on the incidence of motor fluctuations and to delay L-dopa therapy in PD, without causing significant side effects or increasing mortality (as was once suspected) (Davie 2008; Weintraub et al. 2008). However, the most beneficial effects are seen in the first year of treatment and there is little evidence in support of long-term benefits (Fernandez and Chen 2007). A more potent MAO-B inhibitor, rasagiline, that is available in the USA, has also been shown to be an effective monotherapy in early PD (Fernandez and Chen 2007; Siderowf and Stern 2006). Rasagiline has also been shown to have the additional benefit of controlling motor fluctuations in advanced disease by significantly reducing the amount of "off" time (Pahwa et al. 2006). There is however, little evidence to support the presumed neuroprotective effect of the MAO-B inhibitors (Davie 2008).

2.3.6 Catechol O-Methyltransferase (COMT) inhibitors

COMT inhibitors act in a similar way to the MAO-B inhibitors, preventing the action of COMT, a peripheral enzyme that metabolises L-dopa, thus serving to optimise L-dopa therapy (Davie 2008; Weintraub et al. 2008). They include entacapone and tolcapone which increase the half-life of L-dopa, resulting in greater and more sustained plasma and central nervous system levels of dopamine than with L-dopa and carbidopa alone, thus extending the duration of the antiparkinsonian effects of treatment with subsequent improvements in motor function (Rezak 2007). COMT inhibitors have a beneficial effect in smoothing out fluctuations in motor responses to treatment, reducing "off time", prolonging "on" time and allowing for reduced doses of L-dopa to be used. Their effect on dyskinesias has not been established (Davie 2008).

2.3.7 The role of surgery in the treatment of Parkinson's disease

The use of neurosurgical treatment in PD is not a new phenomenon. Before the availability of L-dopa, in the 1950s, ablative surgery of the thalamus was a procedure used to control severe tremor; this practice was gradually suspended with the introduction of pharmacological treatment and growing awareness that thallidotomy (or thalamolysis), especially bilaterally, resulted in severe impairment of cognitive function (e.g. Watkins and Oppenheimer 1962).

The complications of L-dopa treatment and the search for refinements in surgery which have been made possible by advances in technology, have caused clinicians to review the area of neurosurgical intervention. Lesion surgery was re-introduced in the form of pallidotomy which was shown to be useful for "off periods" and L-dopa induced dyskinesias (Davie 2008). A later development was the introduction of deep brain stimulation techniques, targeting areas within the basal ganglia, in order to produce functional, and reversible, inhibition. The procedure most commonly used is that of bilateral stimulation of the subthalamic nucleus, which is effective in reducing the core motor symptoms of bradykinesia, tremor and rigidity, but also helps to alleviate drug-induced motor complications such as wearing off, dyskinesias and dystonias (Kleiner-Fisman et al. 2006.) There is the additional benefit of a reduction in L-dopa dosage of up to 60%. Outcome of surgery is better in younger patients (Weintraub et al. 2008). There is considerable controversy however, surrounding the neuropsychiatric and neuropsychological consequences of deep brain stimulation, in particular in relation to its propensity to cause depression and decline in cognitive performance (for reviews see Massano and Garrett 2012; Takeshita et al. 2005).

2.4 Chapter summary

PD is a complex neurodegenerative condition associated with the depletion of dopamine levels within the basal ganglia, although it is now recognised that the balance of other neurotransmitters is also affected. It is considered to be a paradigmatic movement disorder (Seppi et al. 2011) and is diagnosed according to the clinical presentation of the motor symptoms, that characterize the condition. An understanding of the way in which motor functioning and the complications of treatment determine the overall disability of the person with PD, and the extent to which s/he gradually comes to depend on the help of another person, usually a close family member, is fundamental to the work described in the following pages and forms a background to the study undertaken.

It is, however, increasingly recognised that non-motor symptoms of PD form a very important part of the symptom complex being present in the majority of patients from early in the disease process (Erro et al. 2013) and virtually all are likely to experience them at some point over the course of their illness (Lim and Lang 2010). The non-motor symptoms include dysregulation of mood and affective disorders, cognitive dysfunction and dementia, psychosis, autonomic dysfunction and disorders of sleep and wakefulness. Some of these symptoms, in particular depression, may precede the motor manifestation of PD and several prospective studies have suggested that depression may be an independent risk factor for the development of PD (Aarsland, Marsh and Schrag 2009). Subtle cognitive impairments can also be present at diagnosis, indicating that non-motor symptoms may be part of the illness presentation (Barone et al. 2011). As the disease progresses and the non-motor symptoms become more prevalent, they are key factors in determining quality of life, progression of overall disability and nursing home placement (Hely et al. 2005; Schrag 2006). They are often also the greatest therapeutic challenge in the later stages of the illness (Seppi et al. 2011). Because of their singular influence in shaping the experience of PD for both patients and their carers, the mood and cognitive disorders associated with PD are discussed in chapters 3 and 4, that follow.

CHAPTER THREE

THE NEUROPSYCHIATRY OF PARKINSON'S DISEASE

3.1 Introduction

It is increasingly recognized that neuropsychiatric and neuropsychological disturbances are a frequent concomitant of the physical symptoms in PD. Indeed, the prevalence and impact of these non-motor symptoms has led to the description of PD as a prototypical neuropsychiatric disorder (Leentjens 2004; Weintraub and Burn 2011). They are often early predictors of disease onset (Ishihara and Brayne 2006; Lang 2011) and in themselves, constitute a significant source of disability in the disorder (Weintraub and Burn 2011). Mainly because of these characteristics, PD has been at the forefront of research concerning brain-behaviour relationships in recent decades and these approaches have led neuropsychology and neuropsychiatry to come together more closely with neurology within the neurosciences. The effect is seen in the major advances that these disciplines have contributed to understanding of neurological and psychiatric disorders, revealing the relationships between them.

The neuropsychiatric disturbances associated with PD include depression (for reviews see Cummings 1992; Reijnders et al. 2008; Slaughter et al. 2001; Veazey et al. 2005, Wichowicz 2009), anxiety (Pontone et al. 2009; Richard, Schiffer and Kurlan 1996; Skeie et al. 2013), psychotic disturbances (Forsaa et al. 2010), apathy (Kirsch-Darrow et al. 2006), fatigue (Karlsen et al. 1999; Alves, Wentzel-Larsen and Larsen 2004), sleep disturbances (Chaudhuri et al. 2010; Manni et al. 2007), obsessive compulsive disorders (Nicoletti et al. 2013) and impulse control disorders (Weintraub and Nirenberg 2013). Cognitive dysfunctions ranging from circumscribed cognitive impairments (Janvin et al. 2006; Weintraub, Moberg, Culbertson et al. 2004) to global dementia (Aarsland et al. 2001) are also recognised as a frequent complication, but these will be reviewed and discussed in a separate chapter. The neuropsychiatric disturbances are the focus of attention of this chapter, the aim being to present the current state of knowledge in this area.

3.2 Depression in Parkinson's disease

Over the past half century, many studies have addressed the relationship between PD and depression. More recent reports have developed a level of sophistication often lacking in earlier studies, i.e. with the use of standardised instruments, developing a greater awareness of the importance of reporting the population sampled with greater precision and demonstrating the need to account for symptom overlap between PD and depressive disorders along with a range of other methodological considerations that will be discussed. Despite significant improvements in methodology, controversies remain regarding the prevalence, classification of depressive symptoms and the pathogenesis of depression in PD.

The main focus of this chapter is the relationship between PD and depression, although other neuropsychiatric disturbances that frequently accompany PD are summarised at the end. The alleged association of PD with depression raises a number of questions, in the first instance whether, in spite of depressive symptoms being a relatively common occurrence in PD, there is actually a raised prevalence of depressive disorder in PD. The second question relates to the nature of the depressive symptomatology: does it constitute a depressive disorder of the same kind that is encountered in major depressive disorder (MDD)? A third and critical question, indeed one which has been a focus of interest since the earliest investigations into the relationship between PD and depression, relates to the aetiology of depression in PD; namely, is it 'reactive' or 'organic' in origin? In attempting to answer these questions, this chapter will review the literature on the subject in order to present a consensus view regarding rates of depression in PD and reasons for discrepancies in the estimates regarding prevalence figures will be discussed. A comparison of the symptoms which are considered to manifest as depression in PD will be made with MDD in order to identify any differences in presentation. Finally, the methodological issues central to a resolution of the argument about the aetiology of depression in physical disease will be addressed. Before turning to a discussion of these issues however, the reasons for the interest in affective disturbances in PD will be briefly considered.

3.2.1 The impact of depression in Parkinson's disease

It is clear from the earliest accounts of PD that researchers were aware of the possibility of an increased risk of depression being associated with the disorder. Indeed, James Parkinson (1817) himself appears to have recognised the association, describing 'melancholia' as a central symptom of the disorder. Over the last two centuries, treatments for PD have advanced, but understanding of co-morbid depression and other non-motor symptoms has not kept pace with these developments. Although it is now recognised that depression is by far the most common neuropsychiatric symptom presenting in PD (Rabinstein and Shulman 2001) it remains under-recognised in the clinical context and the likelihood that non-psychiatric specialists will recognize the mood disorder in PD is quite low (Shulman et al. 2002). This is of particular significance to the management of PD in general, as non-motor symptoms are thought to contribute significantly to the overall disability and morbidity in the condition. It has been shown for example, that depression in PD is associated with more rapid decline in the activities of daily living (Starkstein, Mayburg, Leiguarda et al. 1992), cognitive decline (Jellinger 2013; Klepac, Trkulja and Relja 2008; Kuzis et al. 1997; Marder et al. 1995; Norman et al. 2002; Starkstein and Robinson 1991; Stern, Marder et al. 1993; Tröster et al. 1995), reduced quality of life for both the patient (Kuopio et al. 2000; Schrag 2006; Yamamoto 2001) and the carer (Schrag, Hovris et al. 2006), excess motor disability (Weintraub, Moberg, Duda et al. 2004) and mortality (Hughes et al. 2004). Because of the wide-ranging co-morbidities associated with depression, it is clearly important that a better understanding of its aetiology, prevalence and significance in PD be attained for reasons of theoretical advances, as well as improvements in the clinical management of persons with PD. In particular, since depression in PD has been shown to respond to both pharmacological treatment (Ghazi-Noori et al. 2003; Menza et al. 2004; Veazey et al. 2005) and psychological treatment in the form of cognitive behavioural therapy (Dobkin et al. 2011), many of the problems associated with it can be reversed. Nevertheless, Bhidayasiri and Truong (2012) have drawn attention to the as yet, unmet need for determining the effectiveness of therapeutic interventions for the non-motor symptoms of PD.

3.3 Rates of depression in Parkinson's disease

Despite increasing awareness of the importance of affective symptoms in PD, there is no agreement with regard to incidence or prevalence rates for depressive disorders in the condition.

3.3.1 Incidence rates for depression in Parkinson's disease

Very little is known about the ***incidence*** rates for depression in patients with PD. An early study based in the USA and carried out in a tertiary referral centre and community hospital from 1983 to 1989, using a relatively small sample of patients with PD (N=129) arrived at an incidence rate for depression of 1.86 per year with a cumulative risk of 8.6% over a five year period (Dooneief et al. 1992). A smaller study (N=59) from Thailand in PD patients attending an outpatient neurology clinic reported a cumulative one year incidence of depression of 5.1% (Kulkantrakorn and Jirapramukpitak 2007). The highest incidence rate (13.8%) has been reported by Ravina et al. (2009) over a one year period in newly diagnosed, untreated patients participating in clinical trials. A more recent population based study using the General Practice Research Database in the UK has reported incidence rates of 2.6 per year for depression in PD, which is a two-fold increase compared to patients without PD from the same database (Becker et al. 2011). There are few published estimates of the incidence of depression in the general population for comparison, but a study by Copeland et al. (1992) reported an incidence rate of 2.4% for older people, and in the Lundby study from Sweden cited by Dooneief et al. (1992), the annual incidence of depression for people over the age of 40 years was 0.17% for both sexes (Essen-Möller and Hagnell 1961) and in another, known as the Stirling County study from the USA, for individuals over the age of 50 years it was 0.14% for men and 0.29% for women (Murphy et al. 1988). Thus the incidence of depression in PD would seem to be higher than in the general population with appropriate adjustments for age.

3.3.2 Prevalence rates for depression in Parkinson's disease

Much controversy still remains with regard to the ***prevalence*** figures for depression in PD. Estimates for the occurrence of depression vary greatly and range from 2.7% (Hantz et al. 1994) to 100% (Prado and Barbosa 2005). Such discrepancies justifiably give cause for concern as they are likely to reflect serious methodological differences and call into question the validity of the methods used to assess depression. The accurate determination of the true prevalence of depression in PD is complicated by the fact that there are no standardised assessment tools specifically designed for the assessment of depressive symptoms in PD. A number of studies have validated depression scales such as the Hamilton Depression Rating Scale (HAM-D; Hamilton 1960), the Beck Depression Inventory (BDI; Beck et al. 1961) and the Geriatric Depression Scale (GDS; Yesavage et al. 1983) for use in this patient population (e.g. Ertran et al. 2005; Leentjens, Verhey, Lousberg et al. 2000; Leentjens, Verhey, Luijckx et al. 2000; McDonald et al. 2006), but these instruments may over-diagnose depressive illness in PD, because they do not allow the physical and neurological symptoms of the condition to be sufficiently distinguished from depression. Although the validation procedures attempt to overcome this problem by raising the threshold scores for depressive disorder in PD, it may require more than a simple comparison with a "gold standard" to differentiate PD symptoms from those of an affective disorder in order to arrive at a diagnosis of depression in PD. In this case, it is recognised that the gold standard for the diagnosis of depressive disorders, which is usually taken to be the Diagnostic and Statistical Manual, Fourth Edition (DSM-IV-TR) of the American Psychiatric Association (APA 2000) is itself somewhat inadequate for the same reasons, and proposals for modifying the criteria in relation to PD have been suggested, with this in mind (Marsh et al. 2006). One proposal that has been put forward is to use clearly defined "inclusive" or "exclusive" scoring criteria (Marsh et al. 2006; Schrag et al. 2007), but this is not without its own difficulties, as discussed later in this chapter.

A figure of around 40-50% for the occurrence of depression in cross-sectional studies of patients with PD appears to have gained acceptance (Gomez-Esteban et al. 2009; Schrag et al. 2007), based on literature reviews which have suggested rates of between 30% (Slaughter et al. 2001) and 40% (Cummings 1992; Leentjens 2004; Lieberman 2006; McDonald, Richard and DeLong 2003) as being the most reliable estimates. Marsh et al. (2006) suggest up to 50% prevalence rates for mood disorders based on studies by Starkstein, Mayburg, Leiguarda et al. (1992) and Tandberg et al. (1996). Perhaps the best estimates have been provided by Reijnders et al. (2008); following a systematic review of the literature, using quality criteria for the selection of studies, they reported that the prevalence of MDD in PD is around 17%, that of minor depression is 22%, and of dysthymia,13%. Clinically significant levels of depressive symptoms, notwithstanding the presence of a DSM defined depressive disorder, occurred in 35% of patients. However, this apparent consensus is not based on well designed and properly controlled epidemiological research, but on a tertiary evaluation of existing studies in the literature, which are unlikely to have adopted standardised criteria either for the selection of patient samples or instruments to measure depression.

Thus, despite interest in the problem of PD depression and the publication of numerous studies addressing this issue over the last 20 years, no resolution of the differences in reported prevalence rates has in fact been reached, nor are the reasons for the large discrepancies in estimates properly understood. Clarification of these issues is important for reasons of clinical management as well as advancing theoretical understanding of brain-behaviour relationships and clarifying methodological issues in research. Thus, at a practical level a better understanding of the relationship between depression and PD would help to:

1. raise awareness of depression and its consequences in PD among non-psychiatric clinicians involved in the treatment of PD;
2. determine clinically and cost effective methods of screening for depression in PD in order to improve the recognition, clinical management and outcome of depression; and
3. help to arrive at optimal treatments for PD, including the treatment of any co-existing affective disorders;

and at a theoretical level, to:

1. improve understanding of the origins of depression in PD thus contributing to a better understanding of brain-behaviour relationships;
2. recognise symptom constellations for depression in PD and determine whether they differ in any significant way from patterns seen in major/minor depression; and
3. inform our understanding of the psychometric properties of instruments designed to measure depression and their usefulness in PD.

3.3.3 Reasons for discrepancies in prevalence estimates for depression in Parkinson's disease

The wide variation in estimates of the prevalence of depression in PD may be attributed to a range of methodological variations between studies including:

1. ***Sampling issues***: the study of unrepresentative samples (small samples, selection bias) and use of inappropriate control groups;
2. ***Appropriate definition of depression in PD***: diagnostic criterion differences arising from the confusion of depressive symptoms with syndromes; and
3. ***Validity of assessment methods used***: the failure to use standardised instruments for the assessment of depression. The introduction of standardised instruments for the measurement of depression, in general, has confirmed the association between PD and depression and it is probably fair to say, that nowadays, few would argue with the statement that PD leads to an increased risk of

affective disorder (e.g. Tan 2012). Nevertheless, the diagnostic criteria for depression in PD are a cause for concern, as is the appropriateness of using assessment scales, designed mainly for psychiatric or general populations, in patients with conditions such as PD which also present with physical symptoms. The latter concerns the largely unresolved problem of determining the validity of symptoms, particularly somatic ones, in the diagnosis of depressive disorders, when they are also a manifestation of the concurrent medical condition.

1. Sampling issues

Unrepresentative sampling has probably given rise to much of the variation in prevalence rates for depression in PD. For example, Mindham (1970) carried out a retrospective analysis of depressive symptomatology obtained from case notes, without patient interviews, in a sample of PD patients referred to a psychiatric service and reported prevalence rates of 90% for depression in PD. A clear bias in selection of patients and lack of standardised assessment instruments is likely to have been responsible for this high figure.

Gender bias is also likely to affect results. For example, Chen et al. (2007) studied only male veterans aged 55 or older with PD, and not surprisingly (rates of depression are known to be higher in women than in men), found lower rates of depression (18.5%) than reported in many studies. Furthermore, it appears from studies assessing the presence of depressive disorders in patients with PD, that the source from which patients are drawn is very important; the lowest prevalence rates are reported in population studies (10.8%), whereas studies in general practice, outpatient settings and nursing homes tend to report much higher prevalence rates (about 32-42%) and the highest rates are reported in inpatient clinical settings (54%; Reijnders et al. 2008).

When compared to various contrast groups of normal controls, PD patients have consistently shown elevated scores on a variety of measures of depression. The healthy control groups have included an age-matched volunteer panel (Gotham, Brown and Marsden 1986), a community sample (Horn 1974), patients attending an outpatient geriatric clinic, with exclusion criteria for neurological, rheumatological and oncological comorbidities (Veiga et al. 2009), the spouses of patients (Mayeux et al. 1981) and a diverse group consisting of hospital employees, physiotherapy patients without CNS disease and relatives of PD patients (Marsh and Markham 1973). The appropriateness of some of these control groups might be called into question: both the relatives (Arabia et al. 2007) and spouses of patients with PD (Miller et al. 1996) are known to have an increased risk of psychiatric morbidity. Furthermore, PD is a condition which manifests in later life, the peak age of onset occurring at 60-70 years, and the fact that depression rates are thought to be higher in the elderly (Rodda, Walker and Carter 2011) and in people with a comorbid medical condition (Nilsson et al. 2002) should be taken into account. Surprisingly few direct comparisons, controlling for the necessary variables have been made, but the rates of depression for patients with PD do appear to be higher than for older people in general. From a review of 34 studies which mainly included elderly people living independently in the community, Beekman, Copeland and Prince (1999) provide an estimate of all clinically relevant depressive syndromes as 13.3%. More recent studies using the 15 item Geriatric Depression Scale (Sheikh and Yesavage 1986), with a cut-off score of 5 or more, report levels of clinically significant depression among the elderly as 13.1% for a UK community based population over the age of 75 (Osborn et al. 2002), 16% for a German population (Wild et al. 2012) and 27% (with a cut-off score of 7 or more) in a Greek population living a rural town (Papadopoulos et al. 2005). Prevalence of depression increased with age, female gender and physical comorbidities. This may have accounted for the higher prevalence rates of depression in rural Greece, as it is likely that in the other countries studied, older people with physical disabilities and cognitive impairment were more likely to be institutionalised.

Given the raised prevalence rates for depression in older people with physical illness, it might be more appropriate to draw comparisons between depression in PD and other long-term medical conditions. Few studies have attempted comparisons of this sort, but those that have, generally report higher levels of depression in patients with PD than in those with other chronic diseases such as diabetes and arthritis, which do not affect the central nervous system, yet have an insidious onset, are of a progressive nature and engender similar levels of functional disability (Cantello et al. 1986; de Groot et al. 2001; Ehmann et al. 1990; Mayeux 1984; Söderlin, Hakala and Nieminen 2000). The rate of severe depression in PD appears to be twice that seen in other equivalently disabled patients (Rodin and Voshart 1986). A notable early exception to these findings was a study by Gotham et al. (1986), which found similar levels of depression for both patients with PD and those suffering from arthritis. However, it is important to note that results vary greatly depending on the criteria used to define depression (e.g. major depression versus other types deemed to be clinically significant, but not fulfilling the criteria for MDD) and on the instruments used for assessment.

2. Definition of depression in Parkinson's disease

One of the main difficulties in establishing a consensus with regard to prevalence rates for depression in PD have been diagnostic criterion differences i.e. the failure to use established criteria for distinguishing individual symptoms from symptom clusters which are recognized as forming distinct diagnostic categories. This is a problem which has occurred frequently in the neuropsychological literature, for example with regard to other neurodegenerative disorders such as multiple sclerosis (Berrios and Quemada 1990) and with conditions giving rise to less predictable patterns of organic brain damage such as head injury (Politynska, Mariak and Lewko 1999) and the sequelae to subarachnoid haemorrhage of aneurysmal origin (Politynska, Berrios and Lewko 1995). Although various symptoms of depression may frequently be observed in neurological patients, including those suffering from PD, their existence need not amount to a depressive illness, a consideration which has important implications from the point of view of management of the disability in PD. The fact that symptoms do not equal syndromes would appear to be so fundamental to the research in this area, that it is surprising that it still seems to be overlooked. As mentioned above, early studies not using standardised instruments, reported very high prevalence rates for depression in PD (e.g. Mindham 1970). Later research corrected this methodological failure; table 3-1 shows a summary of studies based on two of the most commonly used assessment scales to estimate the prevalence of depression in PD - the GDS and the BDI. None were specifically designed as epidemiological studies and sample sizes vary widely. More recent studies have also used DSM-IV-TR diagnostic criteria and the results are presented for the purposes of comparison.

Somewhat surprisingly, despite the adoption of standardised scales to measure depression, the results show a great deal of variability. One reason for this is that although studies addressing prevalence rates for depression in PD have utilised the same assessment instrument, comparisons are made difficult, because they have sometimes used different criteria to determine the definition of clinically relevant depressive disorders.

It can be seen from table 3-1 that there are considerable inconsistencies among studies in the cut-off scores for the definition of depression at mild, moderate and severe levels. These are not so great with the GDS as with the BDI. Nevertheless some authors do not provide information about thresholds for determining severe levels of depression on the GDS-30 (e.g. Gupta and Bhatia 2000a,b) and others do not differentiate levels of severity at all (Richard et al. 2001; Holroyd 2005). With the GDS-15 it is unusual for higher levels of severity to be differentiated, possibly because there are fewer patients in this category.

Table 3-1. Rates of depression in Parkinson's disease with respect to method of assessment and types of samples studied.

Study	Sample	N	Type/level of depression	
DSM-IV-R			**Minor %**	**Major %**
Weintraub, Moberg, Duda et al. 2004	o/p clinic	91	11.0	18.7
Weintraub et al. 2006	o/p clinic	148	9.4	12.2
Tumas et al. 2008	MDU	50	-	24.0
Gomez-Esteban et al. 2009	MDU	118	28.0	17.8
Veiga et al. 2009	o/p clinic	50	-	42.0
Inoue et al. 2010	o/p clinic	105	0.01	7.9
Thompson et al. 2011	cohort	214	7.5	14.0
Piccinni et al. 2012	MDU	122	-	53.3
Geriatric Depression Scale (30)			**moderate**	**severe**
Gupta et al. 2000a	o/p clinic	40	≥11 19.4	61.1
Gupta et al. 2000b	o/p clinic	40	≥11 37.5	52.5
Richard et al. 2001	PD clinic	16	≥10 44.0	
Rojo et al. 2003	o/p clinic	353	≥11 40.2	>20 16.7
Hely et al. 2005	Multi-centre	41	≥11 46.3	>20 7.3
Holroyd et al. 2005	o/p clinic	100	≥11 15.0	
Geriatric Depression Scale (15)				
Kang et al. 2005	community	193	≥7 13.0	
Meara, Mitchelmore et al. 1999	G.P.	132	≥5 64.0	
Caap-Ahlgen et al. 2001	o/p clinic	102	5-9 47.0	10-15 5.0
Weintraub, Moberg, Duda et al. 2004	o/p clinic	114	≥5 37.7	
Weintraub et al. 2006	o/p clinic	148	≥5 21.6	
Ravina et al. 2007	clinical trial	413	≥5 27.6	
Thompson et al. 2011	cohort	214	≥5 9.4	25.7

Sample source: MDU–Movement Disorders Unit, o/p clinic–outpatient clinic, G.P.–General Practice. Where possible, the percentage of patients falling within the mild, moderate and severe categories on the BDI is shown. The ranges (*italics*) used to define these categories are shown below the percentage figures.

Table 3-1. (cont'd) Rates of depression in Parkinson's disease with respect to method of assessment and types of samples studied.

Beck Depression Inventory			*%*	*%*	*%*	*%*
Study	***Sample***	***N***	***mild***	***mod***	***severe***	***overall***
Mayeux et al. 1981	No information	55	30.9 *10-17*	12.7 *18-24*	3.6 *25+*	47.2
Gotham et al. 1986	o/p clinic, post survey	187	40.0 *10-17*	17.0 *18-24*	12.0 *25+*	69.0
Santamaria et al. 1986	consecutive sample	34	18.0 *10-17*	20.0 *18-24*	6.0 *25+*	44.0
Taylor Saint-Cyr, Lang & Kenny 1986	No information	30	20.0 *?-7*	43.3 *> 7*	6.6	69.9
Brown et al. 1988	o/p clinic	132		27.3 *18+*		27.3
Ehmann et al. 1990	cohort study	45	40.0 *10-17*	16.0 *18-24*	2.0 *25+*	58.0
Tandberg et al. 1996	community sample	245		24.1 *17+*		24.1
Schrag et al. 2001	G.P.	92	36.1 *9-17*	10.3 *18-23*	9.3 *24+*	55.7
Shulman et al. 2001	o/p clinic	99		36.0 *≥ 10*		36.0
Richard et al. 2001	PD clinic	16		6.3 *≥ 16*		6.3
Shulman et al. 2002	o/p clinic	101	36.0 *10-18*	8.0 *19+*		44.0
Kirsch-Darrow et al. 2006	o/p clinic	80		26.3 *≥ 14*		26.3
Inoue et al. 2010	o/p clinic	105		38.0 *13+*		38.0
Van der Hoek et al. 2011	PD o/p clinic	256	36.3 *10-18*	12.9 *19+*		49.2
Rodriguez-Violante et al. 2012	o/p clinic	147		33.3 *16+*		33.3

Of the fifteen studies using the BDI, only four (Ehmann et al. 1990; Gotham et al. 1986; Mayeux et al. 1981; Santamaria, Tolosa and Valles 1986) used the same cut-off scores. Schrag, Jahanshahi and Quinn (2001) used similar, but not identical ranges of scores to define mild, moderate and severe depression and three studies used the BDI scores to produce a bimodal distribution of depressed versus non-depressed patients, but utilised different cut-off scores (Brown et al. 1988; Richard, Justus and Kurlan 2001; Schulman et al. 2002; Tandberg et al. 1996). Unfortunately, the varying criteria used for defining depression, inevitably affect estimates of prevalence, making comparisons difficult.

It is sometimes argued that thresholds for measuring depression should be raised to allow for the overlap between the motor and affective symptoms in PD; in some instances these decisions appear to be made on a purely intuitive level and researchers do not always justify their choice of threshold scores (Hughes et al. 2004). On occasion the decision is an empirical one, in which the performance of the scale is evaluated against a "gold standard" for the diagnosis of depression (i.e. DSM diagnostic criteria) and appropriate cut-off scores are established for use with patients with PD (e.g. Leentjens, Verhey, Luijckx et al. 2000; Silberman et al. 2006; Tumas et al. 2008; Visser et al. 2006). The latter approach is undoubtedly important in terms of helping to establish the validity of a particular depression scale for use in PD and providing adjusted cut-off points for greater accuracy in a population for whom the scale was not designed. However, a number of limitations should be borne in mind. Firstly, different studies are likely to recommend different cut-off scores for discriminating between depressed and non-depressed patients with PD, and this has indeed been found to be the case. For example, Leentjens, Verhey, Luijckx et al. (2000) recommended an optimal cut-off of 13/14, Silberman et al. (2006) of 17/18, Visser et al. (2006) of 14/15 and Tumas et al. (2008) of 17/18. Secondly, whilst these may appear to be similar, they span the entire range of scores normally used to differentiate mild from severe depression. Thirdly, the accuracy of these methods for establishing cut-offs is somewhat dubious, as they are often based on relatively small sample sizes, contravening the fundamental tenets of signal detection theory (Baird and Noma 1978), upon which they are based. And finally, using different scoring methods for defining depression in PD is likely to have a substantial impact on estimates of prevalence, especially with small samples.

Studies using self-rated measures of symptoms, such as the GDS and the BDI usually give the highest estimates of prevalence for depression in PD. Analysis of the data from the studies summarised in table 3-1 reveals that:

- for the GDS-30, rates of depression range from 15% to 90% with a mean rate of 57% (Holroyd, Currie and Wooten 2005; Gupta and Bhatia 2000b);

- for the GDS-15 the range is from 13% to 64% (Kang et al. 2005; Meara, Mitchelmore et al. 1999) with a mean of 36%.
- for the BDI, the proportion of patients estimated as having severe depression ranges from 2% to 12.0% (mean 6.6%), whereas those with mild to moderate levels range from 38% to 56% with a mean of 48% (Ehmann et al. 1990; Gotham et al. 1986; Santamaria et al. 1986).

Clinician rated scales which are based on structured interviews or assessments using recognised diagnostic criteria such as DSM-IV-TR generally give rise to the most conservative estimates for depressive disorders. From table 3-1 it can be seen that rates of minor depression are estimated between 7.5% to 28%, with a mean of 24% (Thompson et al. 2011; Gomez-Esteban et al. 2009). The estimates for major depression range from 7.9% to 24% with a mean of 16% (Inoue et al. 2010; Tumas et al. 2008). These rates are in keeping with the most recent review of studies in this area (Reijnders et al. 2008). It should be noted that this is not a systematic review, but that other studies in which relatively low rates of depression have been reported include Cubo et al. (2000) who found rates of 7.3% and Hantz et al. (1994) reported that 6.8% of their sample had a psychiatric diagnosis, but only 2.7% of them were considered to be depressed. These studies also used DSM criteria to define depression. Nevertheless, at least two studies have reported unusually high rates of major depression in PD; the reasons for this are unclear (Piccinni et al. 2012; Veiga et al. 2009).

Clinician assessments are equally open to unorthodox methods of classifying patients according to severity of depression and this may cause confusion in a way similar to that described for self-rated instruments. For example, Prado and Barbosa (2005), who reported a 100% prevalence of depression in their sample, studied 60 consecutive outpatients with PD from the Movement Disorders Unit (MDU) of a University Hospital and used the HAM-D for the assessment of depression. However, a closer look at their data shows that 82.6% of the patients scored within the "mild" range, which they defined as a score between 7 and 17 on the HAM-D and illustrates the point that symptoms should not be confused with syndromes. Giladi et al. (2000), who examined a sample of 172 patients from a similar source (MDU), reported a rate of MDD based on DSM-IV-TR criteria of only 18%, which is in keeping with a rate of 17.4% for moderate and severe depression (scores >17 on the HAM-D) in the Prado and Barbosa (2005) study and with the average rate for MDD reported in the Reijnders et al. (2008) review. The discrepancies between estimates for depression in PD are thus extremely wide-ranging and do little to clarify the discourse in this area. Moreover they are based on relatively few studies, often using different criterion reference values, some of which are confined to unacceptably small and unrepresentative samples. A straightforward way for overcoming some of these problems would be for researchers to apply the standardised criteria to depression rating scales, unless they have justified their reasons for doing otherwise.

Researchers need to be aware of these difficulties and to choose scoring methods on depression instruments to match the requirements of the task in hand. Clinicians too should be sensitive to these issues. The Global PD Survey of over 1,000 PD patients in six countries found that 50% of PD patients had clinically significant depression as measured on the BDI, but only 1% had revealed their depressive symptoms to a clinician (Global PD Survey Steering Committee 2002). Equally, in a movement disorders clinic, 34% of patients met the diagnostic criteria for a depressive disorder, but 65% of that proportion were not receiving any form of anti-depressant treatment (Marsh et al. 2006). Thus research is needed that establishes valid, reproducible criteria for depressive illness in PD and facilitates optimal treatment.

3. *The validity of assessment techniques used to measure depression in Parkinson's disease*

Another difficulty highlighted by this analysis concerns the validity of the assessment techniques used for the definition of depression in PD and other medical conditions; few studies have addressed this point directly and the question has not been given sufficient attention in the literature. As has already been mentioned, rates of depression appear to be higher in certain populations such as the elderly and those with concomitant medical conditions. This is due in part, to the non-specificity of certain symptoms, especially the somatic symptoms of depression, and their overlap with symptoms of physical disease and the restrictions of old age. Recognition of this problem has led to the development of scales for the measurement of depressive symptoms which have been specially adapted for use with the elderly, such as the GDS, and those with medical conditions, such as the Montgomery-Asberg Depression Rating Scale (MADRS) (Montgomery and Asberg 1979), and the Hospital Anxiety and Depression Scale (HADS) (Snaith and Zigmond 1986; Zigmond and Snaith 1983); there are also a few scales validated for specific conditions but there is none for PD in particular, that has received universal acceptance. Measurement of depression in PD is complicated by the fact that not only is it a condition in which many symptoms associated with the disorder itself, overlap with the symptoms of depression, but it is also a condition affecting people in later life. With depression scales standardised for use in the normal population, there may therefore be the risk of overestimating the prevalence of depressive disorders in PD. A number of studies have thus elected to use instruments, such as the GDS, which are designed to minimise this risk. However, in spite of this, from table 3-1 above, it can be seen that the GDS consistently delivers fairly high prevalence estimates for depression in PD in comparison to other scales. One reason for this may be that older people, in general, and patients with PD in particular, may endorse items on depression scales for reasons other than being depressed. Symptom overlap has already been mentioned as one potential cause, but others may include a tendency to withdraw from activities and reduce their investment in social interactions, which may not be connected with feeling depressed (Adams 2001). It is important to establish the underlying reasons for the systematic tendency of some scales to yield higher estimates of depression in order to improve the validity of methods for measuring and defining the depressive disorder in PD. In addition, variation in diagnostic approaches affects treatment decisions and research study design and it is therefore important to ascertain the properties of instruments to measure depression, when they are applied in contexts for which they were not designed, such as is the case with PD.

3.3.4 Problems associated with measuring depression in non-psychiatric patients

The assessment of depression in medical populations (non-psychiatric samples) raises a unique problem for researchers attempting to use instruments that have been standardised in psychiatric populations. Patients with chronic, progressive neurological illness such as PD demonstrate a wide range of symptoms which are not necessarily shared by either psychiatrically ill patients or those in the general population, albeit matched for age and gender. A different kind of approach to the assessment of depression is required under these circumstances, one that is essentially a method of screening for psychiatric symptoms in non-psychiatric patients. The need for modified procedures was recognised by Goldberg and Hillier (1979) in developing a special instrument, the General Health Questionnaire (GHQ), to help take account of such problems in evaluating psychiatric morbidity in people living in the community. Similarly, assessment procedures using the GDS (which is a screening instrument for non-institutionalised older people) have been modified for people living in nursing home and residential settings (Sutcliffe et al. 2000). These considerations are relevant to patients with PD, most of whom continue to live in their own homes and not in institutional settings. Nonetheless, the GHQ is not commonly used as a screening instrument for the detection of 'cases' of depression in PD samples. This may be because growing recognition of the fact that PD carries an increased risk of depression has led researchers and clinicians to feel there is justification for using instruments primarily designed for psychiatric populations. Indeed, because of its focus on the physical presentation of depressive symptomatology, the GHQ is probably not the most appropriate tool for screening for depressive illness in PD.

Unfortunately however, awareness of depression among clinicians in non-psychiatric settings remains limited, both in primary and secondary health care facilities (Cepoiu et al. 2008; Katon 1996). Depression is known to affect around 6% of individuals in the general population each year and in the course of a person's lifetime, the risk for the disorder is 15% (Pilling et al. 2009). It is the third most common reason for consultation in general practice/ primary care (Singleton 2001), although between 50-70% of cases go undetected (Timonen and Liukkonen 2008), because of the high rate of presentation with mainly somatic symptoms (Tylee and Walters 2007). The overlap between the symptoms of PD and the somatic symptoms of depression are only likely to exacerbate the problem of correct identification and attribution of symptoms in PD patients presenting to general medical practitioners and non-psychiatric hospital specialists. A practical way to implement routine screening for depression in PD is important, because there is evidence that it too remains substantially under-recognised and under-treated (Shulman et al. 2002; Weintraub et al. 2003).

These problems of "symptom overlap" as they have come to be known in the literature (e.g. Schrag et al. 2007), concern not only the commonality among the symptoms of PD and depression referred to above, but also those overlapping with manifestations of normal ageing. In screening for depression in PD it is important to take into account that patients with PD are likely to be elderly. PD is a disorder primarily affecting older people and many symptoms may coincide with those affecting physically healthy and normally ageing adults. For example, vegetative symptoms and medical comorbidity are common in the non-depressed geriatric population and may be associated with motor retardation or decreased levels of activity. In clinical practice it can be difficult to tease these symptoms apart and to know whether they should be attributed to physical disease or depressive illness. Moreover, even cognitive symptoms of depression, such as thoughts of death and hopelessness may have a different meaning for those in the later stages of life. Finally, comorbid cognitive impairment may affect concentration and cognitive processing. Thus scales especially adapted for use with the elderly (such as the GDS) are thought by some authors, to provide a better form of assessment for the depression of PD.

As mentioned above, a major problem for both researchers and clinicians attempting to measure depression in PD is that of trying to disentangle physical manifestations of the disease from various somatic symptoms of depression, which may have a similar presentation. This problem of symptom overlap is by no means unique to patients with PD. Research with other medical populations suffering from chronic progressive diseases such as multiple sclerosis, diabetes, cancer and arthritis is restricted by similar limitations in being able to discriminate illness related somatic symptoms from those of an affective disorder (Berrios and Quemada 1990; Leiber et al. 1976; Plumb and Holland 1977; Zemore and Eames 1979).

The problem is one of attempting to measure an affective construct which owes part of its operational definition to somatic symptoms, such as psychomotor retardation, anergia, flat affect and cognitive dysfunctions, in a population in which the core somatic features characteristic of PD, overlap with many of the features of depressive disorders. For example, the autonomic dysfunctions of PD which may give rise to vegetative symptoms such as fatigue, appetite and sleep disturbance, constipation and diminished sexual function, are also considered to be symptomatic of many depressive states. Equally, bradykinesia, the slowness of movement characteristic of PD or bradyphrenia, slowness of thought, may be classified as a symptom of depression. Furthermore, symptoms such as the mask-like facial expression observed in patients with PD, in which facial muscles do not respond owing to rigidity and fail to reflect emotional expression, may be interpreted as flat affect and so too, characteristic of depression. Some patients may withdraw from social activities because of embarrassment about their appearance and disabling dyskinaesias. Other symptoms that commonly occur in PD such as apathy, affective lability, anxiety, problems with sleep, concentration and attention also overlap with the symptoms of depression. The significance of these complications will be discussed later.

Given the lack of a validated scale especially designed for the measurement of depression in PD, authors have attempted to solve the problem of symptom overlap, which is essentially one of validity, by adopting, a priori, an explicitly inclusive or exclusive approach to the recording of symptoms. The inclusive approach advocates that all symptoms of depression should be recorded regardless of their probable origin, and should be considered as contributing to the diagnosis of depression. The inevitable result, especially when using rating scales for measurement, is that depression scores in PD may be inflated and there is the risk that patients will be evaluated as having an affective disorder in the absence of the core symptoms of depression (Levin, Llabre and Weiner 1988). The exclusive approach, explicitly excludes any symptoms that may be associated with the motor aspects of PD in the diagnosis of depression. Hoogendijk et al. (1998) used both of these methods to examine the effect of symptom overlap in PD on prevalence rates for depression. They evaluated 100 patients for major depression using a semi-structured clinical interview according to DSM-III-R criteria. In the inclusive approach, symptoms were scored irrespective of their possible origin, while in the exclusive approach, symptoms were not taken to be indicative of depression if they fluctuated along the same course as the signs and symptoms of PD or if they responded to dopaminergic medication. The inclusive approach resulted in a prevalence of 23% and the exclusive method in a prevalence of 13%, underlining the fact that the decision about how to rate these symptoms is not trivial and markedly affects study results. Moreover, scales that exclude overlapping symptoms, which may cluster with depression rather than with motor features may have poor criterion validity, particularly at the severe end of the spectrum (Starkstein, Preziosi, Forrester et al. 1990).

However, it is not only the physical/motor symptoms of PD that overlap with the somatic symptoms of depression thereby making the diagnosis of depression in PD more complicated. Other features of PD or the consequences that the condition brings about in the person's life may be indistinguishable from the presentation of depressive symptoms. Apart from the psychomotor changes, symptom overlap occurs in three other domains: as a result of cognitive impairments occurring in PD, due to the reportedly raised occurrence of other psychiatric symptoms such as anxiety and apathy and consequent upon the limitations imposed by the progressively disabling disease. The pattern of symptom overlap is presented in table 3-2 (adapted from Schrag et al. 2007). It is not an empirically derived list, but based on observation and common sense.

As we have seen, one approach to the problem of symptom overlap contaminating attempts to attain valid and reliable measures of depression in PD has been to suggest that the construct of depression should be measured without recourse to somatic symptomatology in order to avoid the confounding of physical and mental symptoms. Despite the consequent problems for rating severity of depression, for example, somatic symptoms are more common in severe depression (Schrag et al. 2007) this solution has generated considerable interest and led to the design of scales "tailor-made' for certain populations in whom the problem of symptom overlap is particularly acute. These include medically-ill populations for whom the HADS and the MADRS were especially devised, but also extend to other physically frail groups such as the elderly. The GDS was specifically developed with these conditions in mind, using essentially the same kind of reasoning with respect to elderly populations that the HADS relies upon in relation to medical patients, namely, focusing on the psychological aspects of depression and its social consequences, avoiding symptoms which overlap with medical disorders or the concomitants of ageing in general.

Table 3-2. Symptom overlap between depression and PD.

Features of Parkinson's disease	Features of depression
Parkinsonism: classic symptoms of motor impairment and autonomic failure	Diminished facial expression Psychomotor changes (slowness, motor restlessness) Fatigue or loss of energy Sleep disturbances Loss of appetite Weight loss
Cognitive Impairment	Slowness of thinking Diminished attention and concentration Memory difficulties Impaired executive functions
(Neuro-)Psychiatric symptoms	Anxiety Apathy (loss of interest, initiative and purposeful activity)
Consequences of having awareness of the progressive, disabling disease process	Social withdrawal Fearfulness Foreshortened future Hopelessness Helplessness

Although the elimination of somatic symptoms in the measurement of the construct of depression in medically-ill patients and the elderly may have a certain logic and thus appear defensible, there are a number of problems with this approach, as we have seen. A further difficulty lies in the fact that somatic symptoms are more prevalent among healthy elderly individuals compared to younger adults, as demonstrated by studies such as those of Zemore and Eames (1979). This observation questions the validity of entirely eliminating somatic symptoms from the assessment of depression in older people and indeed there are studies which warrant caution. Leentjens, Marinus et al. (2003) have shown that some somatic symptoms, such as loss of appetite and early morning wakening, may actually be crucial to the diagnosis of depression in PD. Thus, it is not surprising that measuring depression in elderly individuals with a chronic disease such as PD is particularly problematic.

One final point regarding symptom attribution needs to be made. Strictly speaking, use of DSM criteria for the diagnosis of depressive disorder in PD requires the attribution of specific symptoms to PD itself or to the depressive disorder (see table 3-3; section D). Thus, if strictly applied, Marsh et al. (2006) point out that DSM criteria for major depression and dysthymia would most likely result in around half of the patients with PD being under-diagnosed with respect to clinically significant depression. Such an approach allows for high specificity at the cost of sensitivity to the depressive disorder and it does not help to resolve the dilemma of how to recognize depression in PD.

Some authors have proposed a simple resolution to the problem of symptom origin, namely to ask the patient directly or to instruct him/her to rate their symptoms according to their own perceptions of whether they reflect low mood or physical disability. It would seem only parsimonious to assume that observers, or indeed PD patients themselves, may not be able to attribute all of the symptoms experienced in PD to their alleged origins with any reliable degree of accuracy. Given sufficient time and engagement with the patient an observer might well accurately conclude that the characteristic facial immobility often seen in PD patients is associated with the physical aspects of the disease, rather than being a sign of depressive disorder, but other symptoms may not be so readily classified. For example, it would seem logical to assume that many somatic symptoms such as tiredness, constipation or sleep disturbances are phenomenological experiences for the patient, detached of any obvious aetiological information. Hence merely asking the patient to determine whether his feelings are due to depression or physical illness is unlikely to yield reliable information.

Finally, it is also a possibility that symptoms of cognitive dysfunction may interfere with the diagnosis of depression in PD. Concentration and attention difficulties along with apathy and memory problems associated with dementia are at risk of being misdiagnosed as comorbid depression. This problem is frequently encountered in elderly populations and may require that depression assessment is accompanied by careful and sensitive neuropsychological assessment in such samples.

3.4 Instruments used to measure depression in PD

The instruments that have most commonly been used for the measurement of depression in PD samples have been the following (based on Schrag et al. 2007; Williams et al. 2012):

1. Hamilton Depression Rating Scale (HAM-D)
2. Montgomery-Asberg Depression Rating Scale (MADRS)
3. Beck Depression Inventory (BDI)
4. Hospital Anxiety and Depression Rating Scale (HADS)
5. Zung Self-Rating Depression Scale (SRS)
6. Geriatric Depression Scale (GDS)
7. The Unified Parkinson's Disease Rating Scale-Section 1 (UPDRS-Section 1)

Although not designed as an instrument for the measurement of depression, the Unified Parkinson's Disease Rating Scale-Section 1 (UPDRS; Fahn and Elton 1987) is also included in this review of instruments, as it is the most widely used rating scale to assess PD symptoms; it includes a single question on mood disorder (Schrag et al. 2007). In addition, the Leeds scales for the self-assessment of anxiety and depression (Snaith, Bridge and Hamilton 1976) are evaluated according to the same criteria as those used for the above-named scales, as they were used in the present study.

Although the instruments listed were selected by researchers because of their proven track record in the assessment of depression, they were designed to serve specific purposes, a fact which is reflected in the psychometric properties of each. An important consideration is that instruments to measure depression should be tailored to meet the requirements of the population sample being assessed. Of particular interest to the present study, was whether and for what purposes, these instruments might be considered useful in the assessment of depression in PD. For example, in the main, depression scales, have been designed to measure depression in psychiatric samples (e.g. HAM-D), and their sensitivity and specificity to psychiatric symptoms is adequate to the populations sampled for these purposes. It is not clear whether patients with PD, in whom a raised prevalence of depressive symptoms has been widely reported, should be assessed according to the same criteria as psychiatric samples or whether criteria used for the assessment of community samples, whose needs are more appropriately met by specially designed scales such as the GHQ would be better suited to the evaluation. Moreover, as PD is a disorder which typically manifests in later life, scales such as the GDS, which was specifically designed for the assessment of depression in elderly samples, may be more appropriate. Equally, the HADS, the MADRS and the SRS which were designed for use with physically ill samples may hold some advantages over other scales in PD populations. Although researchers have sometimes been aware of these considerations, relatively few studies have undertaken a formal investigation of these instruments to evaluate their suitability with respect to the needs of PD populations.

Another consideration is the purpose for which scales are designed. Some instruments such as the MADRS and the HADS were designed to be sensitive to change and thus provide good outcome measures in comparative studies; others such as the BDI and the HAM-D provide measures of symptom severity; still others, such as the GDS, were developed as screening instruments for depression. Furthermore, some instruments require that symptoms be graded by trained observers (HAM-D, MADRS) whilst others are self-rated by the patient (BDI, HADS, GDS, SRS) and there is some evidence that different results are obtained depending on how the data are gathered. It is important to remember that no single instrument can fulfil all of the criteria considered above. The purpose of this analysis is to evaluate the usefulness of the rating scales most commonly used to measure depression in PD and to determine their advantages and shortfalls with regard to the measurement of depression in this population.

3.4.1 Summary of main depression scales used in Parkinson's disease research

The "gold standard" or measure of **criterion validity** used in the literature examined on depression in PD were the DSM-IV-TR diagnostic criteria for MDD (APA 2000), which require the presence of depressed mood or loss of interest or pleasure (anhedonia) for at least two weeks, together with at least four other symptoms, in so far as they represent a significant change from previous functioning (see table 3-3).

A summary of the main instruments used in the scientific literature for the measurement of depression in PD, based on Schrag et al. (2007), is presented in table 3-4. Of the instruments described in table 3-4 the HAM-D and the BDI are the most widely used and accepted instruments for the measurement of depression both in PD and more generally (Schrag et al. 2007).

Table 3-3. DSM-IV-TR criteria for Major Depressive Disorder

Five (or more) of the following symptoms must have been present during the same 2-week period and represent a change from previous functioning; at least one of the symptoms is either (1) depressed mood or (2) loss of interest or pleasure *Note: Symptoms that are clearly due to a general medical condition, or mood-incongruent delusions or hallucinations should not be included* A:
Depressed mood most of the day, nearly every day, as indicated by either subjective report (e.g. feels sad or empty) or observation made by others (e.g. appears tearful). Note: In children and adolescents, can be irritable mood.
Markedly diminished interest or pleasure in all, or almost all, activities most of the day, nearly every day (as indicated by either subjective account or observation made by others).
Significant weight loss when not dieting or weight gain (e.g. a change of more than 5% of body weight in a month), or decrease or increase in appetite nearly every day. Note: in children, consider failure to make expected weight gains.
Insomnia or hypersomnia nearly every day.
Psychomotor agitation or retardation nearly every day (observable by others, not merely subjective feelings of restlessness or being slowed down).
Fatigue or loss of energy nearly every day
Feelings of worthlessness or excessive or inappropriate guilt (which may be delusional) nearly every day (not merely self-reproach or guilt about being sick).
Diminished ability to think or concentrate, or indecisiveness, nearly every day (either by subjective account or as observed by others).
Recurrent thoughts of death (not just fear of dying), recurrent suicidal ideation without a specific plan, or a suicide attempt or a specific plan for committing suicide.
B: The symptoms do not meet criteria for a Mixed Episode.
C: The symptoms cause clinically significant distress or impairment in social, occupational, or other important areas of functioning.
D: The symptoms are not due to the direct physiological effects of a substance (e.g. a drug of abuse, a medication) or a general medical condition (e.g. hypothyroidism).
E: The symptoms are not better accounted for by bereavement, i.e. after the loss of a loved one, the symptoms persist for longer than 2 months or are characterized by marked functional impairment, morbid preoccupation with worthlessness, suicidal ideation, psychotic symptoms, or psychomotor retardation.

Table 3-4 Scales used for the assessment of depression in Parkinson's disease

Properties of the scale	HAM-D	MADRS	BDI	HADS	SRS	GDS
Authors	Hamilton (1960)	Montgomery & Asberg (1979)	Beck et al. (1961)	Snaith & Zigmond (1986)	Zung (1965)	Yesavage et al. (1982/3)
Versions (no. of items):	HAM-D (21) HAM-D (17)		BDI-IA BDI-II[3]	Subscales for depression & anxiety	Original used most frequently, shorter versions exist	GDS(30) GDS(15) validated for age > 55
Rated by:	trained interviewer	trained interviewer	self rated	self rated	self rated	self rated
Purpose: severity measure	good	good	good	limited as excl. somatic items	good	Poor for individual items Overall-possibly
Screening instrument	questioned	rarely used for this purpose	yes	yes	Yes, limited in physical disease	yes
Sensitivity to change	good	good[5]	good[7]	good	questionable due to somatic items	questionable
Criterion validity: coverage of DSM-IV criteria	good but incomplete	good but incomplete[1]	very good for version BDI-II	limited: excl. somatic & suicide	good but incomplete	limited: excl. somatic & suicide
Face validity	high	high	high	moderate	high	high
Discriminant validity	acceptable		good	good	limited	acceptable
Sensitivity	high	high	good	good	good	good

Table 3-4 (cont'd). Scales used for the assessment of depression in Parkinson's disease

Specificity	high	high	good	good	good	good
Reliability: test-retest	good	good	high	good	good	good
Validity in cognitively impaired patients	yes	mild – yes severe – little	yes[9]	not known	not known	mild to mod good Severe conflicting
Correlation with biological markers of depression	yes	yes	yes[6]	not known	not known	not known
Symptoms represented: somatic	high	relatively few	several included	not included	high	not included
psychological	high	relatively few	weighted to Ψ	not included	included	weighted to Ψ
affective	yes	yes	yes	weighted		yes
Cognitive	few	few	yes	not included		yes
Cognitive complexity	determined by interviewer	determined by interviewer	high[8]	medium[8]	easily comprehensible[8]	easily comprehensible
Availability	Public domain	Public domain	Public domain	Public domain	Public domain	Public domain
Use for phenomenology	yes[2]	yes[4]	yes	Not suitable - low content validity	moderate	Not suitable - low content validity
Cognitive complexity				Poor for PD requires frequent concept shifting due to reverse coding	Poor for PD requires frequent concept shifting due to reverse coding	easily comprehensible; sensitive indicator of depression severity in cognitively impaired patients with PD

Table 3-4 (cont'd). Scales used for the assessment of depression in Parkinson's disease

Properties of the scale	HAM-D	MADRS	BDI-II	HADS	SRS	GDS	UPDRS Part 1
Proposed cut-off screening score for dPD[10]:	9/10 *(Naarding et al. 2002)* 11/12 *(Leentjens, Verhey, Lousberg et al. 2000)*	14/15 *(Leentjens, Verhey, Lousberg et al. 2000)*	8/9 *(Leentjens, Verhey, Luijckx et al. 2000)*	10/11 *(Leentjens et al. 2001)*	Not established		N/A: only one item to assess mood *Movement Disorders Society (2003)*
Proposed cut-off score for MDD[11] in dPD:	15/16 *(Naarding et al. 2002)* 13/14 *(Leentjens, Verhey, Lousberg et al. 2000)*	17/18 *(Leentjens, Verhey, Lousberg et al. 2000)*	16/17 *(Leentjens, Verhey, Luijckx et al. 2000)* 13/14 *(Visser et al. 2006)*	23/24 *(Leentjens et al. 2001)*	Not established	GDS-30: 9/10 *(McDonald et al. 2006)* GDS-15: 4/5 *(Weintraub et al. 2006)*	N/A: designed for PD pts: clinician & self rated versions
Purpose: severity measure	good	good	good	Limited as excl. somatic items reduced validity in severe depression	Limited: high in somatic items overlapping with PD	Not established; but excl most symptom overlap between MDD and PD	Not recommended/ cannot be assessed
Screening instrument	Adequate but overlap on somatic items	Rarely used for this purpose	yes	Moderately suitable	Limited: high level somatic items	yes	crude measure

Table 3-4 (cont'd). Scales used for the assessment of depression in Parkinson's disease

Sensitivity to change	Good	good	good	not known	Limited: high level of somatic items	Not established	yes
Correlation studies with PD scales	yes	yes	yes	not known	not known	Not established	Very limited
Use for phenomen-ology	yes	yes	yes	not suitable low content validity	No: validity in PD not established	not established; unlikely because of item exclusion	not suitable: low content validity
Correlation with biological markers of depression	yes	yes	yes	not known	not known	not established	not known
Discriminant validity for diagnosis of MDD in dPD	good	good	good	limited	not known	Adequate for cut-off: 9/10	Not recommend for this purpose
Sensitivity	good	good	good	good			
Specificity	good	good	good	Low for cut-off 10/11			

Adapted from: Schrag et al. (2007). [1] with the exception of psychomotor retardation/agitation, hypersomnia and increased appetite; [2]see Berrios & Samuel (1987) and Leentjens, Marinus et al. (2003); [3]includes agitation, concentration & loss of energy; [4]Leentjens, Marinus et al. (2003); [5]Leentjens, Vreeling et al. (2003); [6]Gold et al. (2004); [7]Richter et al. (1997); [8]Shumway et al. (2004); [9]Powell (2003) and Logsdon & Teri (1995). [10]dPD—depression in PD; [11]MDD—major depressive disorder

The HAM-D is completed on the basis of an interview carried out by a trained interviewer and obtaining reliable scores is dependent on this. It has good psychometric properties and its sensitivity and specificity have been shown to be superior to that of the BDI, the HADS and the SRS, but similar to the MADRS, most probably because the latter is also rated by a trained observer. Apart from the HAM-D and the MADRS, the remaining measures of depression are all self report instruments, of which the BDI has good reliability and validity compared to a DSM-IV-TR diagnosis of major depression in PD, superior to that of the other instruments.

As described above, scales in which somatic symptoms are heavily represented have been criticised by some authors as suitable screening measures of depression, especially in patients with physical illness (e.g. Bech 1993; Zimmerman, Posternak and Chelminski 2005). This is particularly so for the HAM-D, in which the overlap with symptoms of PD is considerable: almost 60% of the total items could be experienced by a typical patient with the condition (Schrag et al. 2007). Others, however, consider it to be a valid measure of PD depression (Leentjens, Verhey, Lousberg et al. 2000; Naarding et al. 2002). An important difficulty lies in the fact, that when somatic symptoms are excluded, as in the GDS and the HADS, these scales lose the propensity to meet validity criteria, as they do not cover the same range of symptoms as the gold standard in the form of DSM criteria. This may also mean that they are insensitive to the more severe ends of the spectrum of depressive symptoms, where suicidal ideation, psychotic features and vegetative symptoms are more prominent (Schrag et al. 2007). In spite of this, the sensitivity and specificity of the HADS for DSM criteria for MDD have been reported as good (Bjelland et al. 2002) and the GDS appears to have adequate discriminant validity for establishing a diagnosis of major and minor depressive disorder, performing comparably to the HAM-D (Weintraub et al. 2006). Nevertheless, diagnosis on the basis of these scales alone is not recommended.

An important characteristic of depression scales is that they should be sensitive to change, in order to establish possible treatment effects, amongst others. This attribute is also potentially extremely useful in PD, for example, to enable patterns in depression to be monitored in relation to changes in motor symptoms. All of the instruments represented in table 3-4, possibly with the exception of the SRS and the GDS, appear to have satisfactory qualities in respect of sensitivity to symptom change (Schrag et al. 2007).

Other properties of depression scales, making them particularly suited for use in PD, include their level of comprehensibility and validity for use with cognitively impaired older adults. Whilst the cognitive complexity of the HAM-D and MADRS can be adapted by a sensitive interviewer to the needs of the patient, certain of the remaining scales are likely to be particularly problematic for patients with PD, because of their construction. The HADS and the SRS, for example, employ items reversed for coding purposes and thus require frequent concept shifting, which may be especially difficult for PD patients with executive difficulties. Scales such as the MADRS have been shown to be valid in older patients with mild cognitive impairment (Gabrylewicz et al. 2004), though the data are sparse on patients with more severe impairments (Müller-Thomsen et al. 2005). Although the GDS appears to make a relatively low level of cognitive demand, there is conflicting evidence as to its suitability in severely cognitively impaired patients. On the other hand, the BDI, despite its multiple choice format, has been validated in patients with cognitive deficits. In view of the difficulties mentioned above regarding the cognitive complexity of the HADS and SRS, it is unlikely that these scales would perform satisfactorily in patients with cognitive impairments.

Finally, identification of scales that might allow a phenomenological analysis of depressive symptoms in PD is of particular interest to the present study, because of the attempt to clarify the existence of alleged differences in the symptom profile of depression in PD, which is discussed in the following section (3.5) of this chapter. The most appropriate in this respect would seem to be the two observer rated scales, the HAM-D and the MADRS, and the BDI. The remaining scales are unsuitable for these purposes because of their low content validity.

In summary, it would seem that the HAM-D is most suitable for assessing depression severity, for use in correlation studies with biological markers or other scales designed to capture the symptoms of PD and in the study of the phenomenology of depression (Leentjens, Marinus et al. 2003). Whilst the MADRS may be equally effective from a psychometric point of view, its performance in cases of severe cognitive impairment is more in doubt. As regards the self-report measures of depression, the GDS and HADS are generally considered to have the major advantage of avoiding the problems of symptom overlap in PD, because of the exclusion of the somatic symptoms of depression. Both instruments are short (though two versions of the GDS exist, the 30-item and the 15-item, with equally good psychometric properties), but the GDS is probably more easily understood, making it appropriate for use both in research and routine clinical practice as a screening instrument for depression in elderly patients with PD. There is however, insufficient evidence to recommend its use to assess depression severity (e.g. as an outcome measure, or in correlation studies with biological markers or other scales) or to determine the phenomenology of depression in PD. Although the psychometric properties of the BDI would make it suitable for most of these purposes, it would not be the ideal instrument for determining symptom profile in the depression of PD, as it is an instrument strongly weighted towards the psychological symptoms of depression.

One further instrument for measuring depression is considered here, although it was not included in the review by Schrag et al. (2007). In view of the almost unique position held by the HAM-D in the assessment of depression in general, and the fact that it is the only measure to satisfy virtually all of the criteria for an instrument for the assessment of depression in PD, a lesser known self-report measure, based on the HAM-D is also worthy of consideration. The Leeds Scales for the self-assessment of anxiety and depression (Snaith et al. 1976) were designed as self-rating scales to mirror the HAM-D and the Hamilton Anxiety Scale (HAM-A) and were validated against these scales. They are considered to have diagnostic potential in the sense of distinguishing between anxiety and depressive disorders. Two versions of the subscales for measuring depression and anxiety exist, one for use as a screening instrument, the other, to measure severity in patients with depression. Although the scales contain several somatic symptoms, they are weighted toward the psychological symptoms of depression and anxiety and have good concurrent and discriminant validity. Both scales have high test-retest reliability and internal consistency in a variety of patient groups. The depression subscale has been shown to correlate with biological markers of depression and to be sensitive to change (Snaith et al. 1976). The Leeds scales do not appear to have been used previously for the assessment of depression in PD. The scales would appear suitable for use in phenomenological studies of PD and so although no data exist for the Leeds scales in this respect, it may be justifiably assumed, that because of their even simpler multiple choice format than the BDI, the options should not cause patients undue difficulties.

The considerations outlined in the preceding section were drawn upon in choosing the instruments to measure depression in patients with PD assessed in the present study.

3.5 The nature of depressive symptoms in Parkinson's disease

Research on depression in PD has suggested that PD patients experience a qualitatively different form of depression from that of other adults, both young and old, and astute observers have reported distinctive characteristics in the depression related to PD. Few studies, however, have adopted a systematic approach and used all relevant control groups in order to evaluate whether the differences in depressive symptomatology are indeed specific to PD. These would ideally include age-matched control groups for depressed, physically disabled and healthy individuals. Moreover, few studies, have made direct comparisons between the symptom profiles for depression of depressed and non-depressed PD patients, with the notable exception of Pålhagen et al. (2008). Studies of this kind might help to elucidate which symptoms are crucial to determining a symptom profile characteristic of depression in PD. That such an approach is feasible is evidenced in studies which have reported that depressive symptoms experienced by younger adults are different from those experienced by older adults. Older adults are more likely to experience somatic symptoms (St. Pierre, Craven and Bruno 1986; Zemore and Eames 1979) and less likely to experience cognitive symptoms (Blazer 1989; St. Pierre et al. 1986) or depressed mood than are younger adults (Gallo, Anthony and Muthén 1994; National Institutes of Health Consensus Conference 1991/1992). Since PD patients tend to be older and appear to follow a similar symptom profile to older adults without PD, at least with respect to somatic and cognitive symptoms, it would be important to clarify, if their particular pattern of symptomatology differs in any substantial way from their older, healthy counterparts or if it is essentially reflecting the same kind of symptom clustering, which may be characteristic of ageing. A similar comparison with physically disabled patients would help to clarify differences in depressive symptomatology (if any) due to the effects of having a progressive physical illness which imposes significant limitations in everyday living. There are very few studies which have attempted this kind of comparison, but it has been reported that patients with arthritis (Gotham et al. 1986) endorsed significantly fewer cognitive symptoms and significantly more mood and somatic symptoms in comparison to other older adults. In this respect, the patients with arthritis closely resembled the PD patients examined in the study, both groups having a form of depression in which somatic and mood components predominated. Finally, patients with cognitive impairment demonstrate a symptom profile in which mood disturbances are particularly emphasized, with fewer somatic symptoms of depression than normal controls (Lazarus et al. 1987; Miller 1980); though not all studies have supported this finding (Greenwald et al. 1989). Levels of depression appear to be inversely associated with the severity of cognitive impairment, presumably because of an increasing lack of insight into personal mental health (Forsell et al. 1993).

However, the predominance of physiological symptoms in older adults, and in particular, in those who are medically ill, (e.g. Forsell et al. 1993; Zemore and Eames 1979) is problematic, for the reasons discussed in the previous section and it may not be a good indicator of depression in these groups. This has encouraged the development of assessment methods that minimise the contribution of these symptoms to the diagnosis of depression, as described above. Currently, however, evidence is accumulating to suggest that treating all somatic symptoms of depression in a collective manner may be an insensitive way of dealing with this difficult problem. A number of studies have demonstrated that some specific somatic features such as fatigue (Erdal 2001), loss of appetite and late insomnia (Leentjens, Marinus et al. 2003) are actually quite specific indicators of depression in PD. On the other hand, others have argued that sleep disturbances should not be considered indicative of depression as they are a common manifestation of PD and may be a side effect of PD treatment (Chaudhuri and Schapira 2009). These controversies indicate the need to elucidate these approaches further.

Another factor worthy of consideration as regards potential differences in the presentation of depression in PD is the consistency of responses shown by patients with depression. Clinical experience suggests that patients with primary affective disorders demonstrate poor reliability in reporting symptoms of depression, both during the course of clinical interviews and when asked to record symptoms using self-rated measures of depression. There is now a growing body of empirical literature to support this observation, suggesting that the recall of certain symptoms, such as anhedonia, sadness, confusion and suicidal intent are especially prone to negative distortions on retrospective recall by depressed people (Ben-Zeev and Young 2010). Non-depressed control subjects, on the other hand, show the opposite pattern of results in the sense that they appear to be relatively accurate in their recall of confusion, suicidal ideation and sadness, but demonstrate positive biases in their recall of anhedonia, helplessness, detachment and self-control. Patients and controls do not differ from each other in the negative bias they show in reporting symptoms of tension, difficulty concentrating, guilt and fear. The reasons for this remain poorly understood, but they may be a reflection of the indecisiveness that is characteristic of depression or of the cognitive deficits that occur in affective disorders (Bulbena and Berrios 1986;1993; also see Miller and Morley 1986, chapter 5 for what is still a very relevant, critical summary). These patterns of inconsistency do not appear to be so apparent in depressed patients with PD, which would be in keeping with the observation by Gotham et al. (1986) suggesting that diminished affect in the disorder is not associated, to the same extent as in MDD, with cognitive symptoms.

3.5.1 The phenomenology of depressive symptoms in Parkinson's disease

It is increasingly the case, that authors refer to the importance of identifying "true depressive illness in patients with PD" (Pålhagen et al. 2008), because of the similarity in many of the symptoms for both conditions. The intention of the authors is clear enough – it is the old problem of symptom overlap producing confounding effects in the classification of symptoms in PD. So long as the notion of "true" is applied to the concept of depressive *illness*, the position can be understood and the efforts to overcome the problem endorsed as we have seen in the foregoing discussion.

However, where authors refer to 'true' depressive *symptoms*, a complexity emerges which is not easily resolved using appropriately modified methodologies. The notion of "true" depressive symptoms becomes a phenomenological problem, namely is the anergia, weight loss, difficulty in concentrating etc. seen in PD, *experienced* in the same way by patients with PD as by patients with a diagnosis of MDD? It is unlikely that we can ever objectively know the answer to this question. DSM-IV-TR uses an operational decision to deal with the problem: at least one of the symptoms exhibited by the patient must be a feeling of sadness or anhedonia. This essentially establishes as a condition of the diagnosis, that the patient must admit to feeling depressed or attribute his/her symptoms to depression. Put another way, is it possible to have a depressive illness without feeling sad, experiencing low mood or no longer gaining pleasure from activities that were valued in the past? The question then arises, is it possible to be depressed without being aware of, or acknowledging the fact? A former diagnostic category, now largely abandoned, used to account for this phenomenon, was that of "masked depression". Although patients with PD would be excluded from this category because of having an organic disease, it is possible that something can be learned from examining a brief history of this concept.

3.5.2 Masked depression

Masked depression is a form of atypical depression. It was a diagnosis that was very common in the 1970s and 1980s for patients who presented with somatic complaints, but in whom no organic disorder to account for the symptoms could be identified. Such patients typically did not complain of the psychological and cognitive symptoms of depression, presenting a highly somatised view of their condition. It was considered that such disorders are due to the same, albeit unexplained, neurobiological causes as other unipolar depressive illness. However, the concept lost much of its clinical validity when it was dropped from the classification of depression with the introduction of DSM-III, which operationalised purely descriptive, as opposed to theory bound systems of classification, although the category of masked depression has been retained in the ICD10 classification of depressive illness (World Health Organisation 2010). A number of other problems were inherent in the concept of masked depression; firstly the diagnosis was expanded to include a wide range of different disorders, secondly the concept was lacking in clarity – namely the problem may have been one of under-recognition or under-reporting of depressive symptomatology and thirdly, it was never clear whether the lack of psychological symptoms was a pre-requisite for the diagnosis as opposed to forming the exclusion criteria for other diagnoses. Present day conceptualizations have reverted to emphasizing the somatic symptomatology of the disorder in these patients and are classified variously as somatisation disorder, somatoform disorder, psychosomatic disorder, conversion disorder, neuraesthenia or hypochondriasis. Nevertheless, some authors (e.g. Miodek et al. 2007) consider that the departure from the concept of masked depression in its variety of different forms is not fully justified on the grounds that it leads to inappropriate diagnosis and treatment in a significant number of patients and Bschor (2002) argues that it played a useful unitary diagnostic role in dealing with patients presenting with inexplicable and untreatable somatic symptoms and allowed justification for pharmacological treatment of these cases. Because of these difficulties the concept does not appear to have much to offer in terms of helping to resolve the problems inherent in understanding depression in PD. It is worth noting however, that a number of authors have argued that a characteristic of depression in PD is the relative lack of psychological symptoms of the disorder, making it similar to the specific presentation of masked depression (see section 3.5.4. below).

3.5.3 Phenocopies of depression

The speculation made above, that patients with PD may have many of the symptoms of depression, without sadness and anhedonia, leads to the possibility that they may demonstrate behavioural phenocopies of depression (Berrios, Campbell and Politynska 1995). There is some evidence for this: patients with PD tend to suffer from milder forms of depression (e.g. minor or subsyndromal depression) than that seen in MDD (Tandberg et al. 1996; Weintraub and Stern 2009). Indeed, not only are their symptoms frequently less severe, but the symptom profile appears to differ from major depression as described above.

There is some evidence that affective disorders seen in neurological conditions differ somewhat from those of MDD both in their symptomatology and in their response to treatment. Berrios and Samuel (1987) compared a group of neurological patients who were diagnosed as clinically depressed with a group of patients with MDD. There were no differences between the groups in terms of global scores on the HAM-D, but qualitative differences in symptomatology emerged. The group with MDD more frequently demonstrated a family and personal history of psychiatric illness, early morning wakening, guilt, suicidal ideation, shorter index episodes of depression and better response to treatment. At five year follow-up, the depressed neurological group continued to fare badly on the measures considered in comparison to the samples characterised by major depression and neurological conditions without depressive symptoms. The authors concluded that the presence of affective disorder in neurological patients has an adverse effect on prognosis.

Taylor, Saint-Cyr, Lang and Kenny (1986) noticed that the majority of PD patients exhibited signs of depressive affect during neuropsychological examination regardless of their BDI score. The most common symptoms were tearfulness, agitation and exacerbation of motor symptoms in response to direct probing of emotional status or frustrations that might accompany the motor problems. However they provide exceptional clinical insight in noting that unlike endogenously depressed patients who maintained a tense or apathetic state throughout the examination, the PD patients were responsive to encouragement and stimulation. Typically they expressed interest in the procedures, engaged spontaneously in conversation and maintained an appropriate level of rapport and interest throughout the somewhat lengthy psychometric test battery. Their mood state was reactive and responsive to the task in hand, fluctuating between expressions of distress when discussing disease related issues but resolving appropriately as topics changed. The impression was one of a certain lability in mood with depressive affect being sensitive to changes in context and resolving as novel events or interesting task demands were presented in an environment that was positively perceived. Situational stress, on the other hand, was able to quickly evoke low mood. Indeed, Taylor, Saint-Cyr, Lang and Kenny (1986) propose that a failure for PD patients to show this pattern of reactions (together with deficits in short-term memory) should be taken as indicative of the necessity for a psychiatric referral for the patient.

3.5.4 Symptom profile for depression in Parkinson's disease

No consensus exists as yet for the definition of a specific symptom profile for depression in PD. Nevertheless, astute observers of the condition have noted that the phenomenology of the depressive disorder differs from that encountered in MDD. An early observation was that of Friedrich Lewy (1923; cited in: Ehrt, Pedersen and Aarsland 2011), who noted that in their clinical presentation, depressed patients with PD tended to be moody, irritable and weepy. More recently, authors have suggested that the depression of PD does not follow a classical "endogenous" pattern (Osiejuk-Lojek 1998), being associated with fewer cognitive symptoms, such as feelings of guilt, self-blame, worthlessness, failure, punishment and negative self-referential statements, though thoughts of death and suicidal ruminations may be increased, with fewer actual suicidal attempts (Brown et al. 1988; Brown and MacCarthy 1990; Ehrt et al. 2006; Gotham et al. 1986; Huber et al. 1990; Prado and Barbosa 2005; Taylor, Saint-Cyr, Lang and Kenny 1986). On the other hand, as the foregoing discussion has demonstrated, somatic symptoms are prominent. However, not all of them appear to carry equal weight towards the diagnosis of depression in PD. Some, including loss of energy (Erdal 2001; Farabaugh et al. 2009, appetite loss and sleep disturbances (Koerts et al. 2008) are thought to be more pronounced. Weight loss (Brown and MacCarthy 1990) and diurnal variation (Merschdorf et al. 2003) on the other hand, appear less prominent.

Concentration difficulties (Koerts et al. 2008) and anxiety in the form of increased feelings of tension, restlessness and irritability are also common (Ehmann et al. 1990; Erdal 2001; Merschdorf et al. 2003; Schiffer et al. 1988; Starkstein, Preziosi, Forrester et al. 1990). The clinical picture of depression in PD is also reported to demonstrate greater levels of anxiety more generally (Menza, Robertson-Hoffman and Bonapace 1993) and higher levels of dysphoria (Brown et al. 1988) than typically occur in MDD. Most importantly, mood disturbances in the form of sadness, loss of interest, feelings of pessimism and hopelessness are also present (Cummings 1992; Gotham et al. 1986; Leentjens 2004; Slaughter et al. 2001), although some authors argue they are less severe than in MDD (Ehrt et al. 2006; Merschdorf et al. 2003). These findings are summarised in table 3-5.

Table 3-5. Symptom profile for depression in Parkinson's disease

Symptom profile	Symptom comparison: dPD vs MDD	Study
Sadness, dysphoria, depressed mood	More prominent in dPD	Brown et al 1988 Brown and MacCarthy 1990 Farabaugh et al 2009 Leentjens, Marinus et al 2003
	Less prominent in dPD	Merschdorf et al 2003 Ehrt et al 2006
	No difference	Erdal 2001
Anhedonia	More prominent in dPD	Leentjens, Marinus et al 2003
	Less prominent in dPD	Ehrt et al 2006
Loss of interest	More prominent in dPD	Brown and MacCarthy 1990 Leentjens, Marinus et al 2003
	Less prominent in dPD	Gotham et al 1986
Concentration difficulties	More prominent in dPD	Brown and MacCarthy 1990 Standaet and Stern 1993 Koerts et al 2008 Farabaugh et al 2009 Ehrt et al 2006
	Less prominent in dPD	Leentjens, Marinus et al 2003
Difficulty in making decisions	More prominent in dPD	Kanda et al 2008 Farabaugh et al 2009
Guilt, self blame	Less prominent in dPD	Gotham et al 1986 Brown et al 1988 Huber, Freidenberg et al 1989 Brown and MacCarthy 1990 Ehrt et al 2006 Taylor et al 1986[1] Prado and Barbosa 2005
Feelings of hopelessness	More prominent in dPD	Farabaugh et al 2009
Feelings of worthless-ness; negative self referential statements; sense of failure; self punishment	Fewer in dPD	Brown and MacCarthy 1990 Taylor et al 1986[1] Prado and Barbosa 2005

Table 3-5 (cont'd) Symptom profile for depression in PD

Suicidal ideation, attempted suicide	Decreased in dPD Increased in dPD	Taylor et al 1986[1] Brown et al 1988 Brown and MacCarthy 1990 Merschdorf et al 2003 Prado and Barbosa 2005 Kanda et al 2008 Koerts et al 2008 Kanda et al 2008
Irritability	More prominent in dPD	Brown et al. 1988 Brown and MacCarthy, 1990 Merschdorf et al. 2003
Anxiety	More prominent in dPD	Menza et al 1993 Schiffer et al 1988
Worrying, tension	More prominent in dPD	Brown and MacCarthy 1990 Koerts et al 2008
Constipation	Increased in dPD	Kanda et al 2008
Loss of energy, fatigue	Increased fatigue Low energy Fewer symptoms in dPD	Standaet and Stern,1993 Erdal 2001 Farabaugh et al 2009 Ehrt et al 2006
Concern with own health	More prominent in dPD	Gotham et al 1986
Reduced/poor sleep Early morning awakening	Increased problems in dPD Less prominent in dPD More prominent in dPD	Koerts et al 2008 Farabaugh et al 2009 Leentjens, Marinus et al 2003 Standaet and Stern 1993
Appetite loss	Less prominent in dPD	Brown and MacCarthy 1990 Leentjens, Marinus et al 2003
Weight loss	Less prominent in dPD	Brown and MacCarthy 1990
Diurnal variation	Less prominent in dPD	Merschdorf et al 2003
Delusions	Fewer symptoms in dPD	Merschdorf et al 2003 Prado and Barbosa 2005

Legend. dPD-depression in PD; MDD-major depressive disorder; Taylor et al 1986[1]: Taylor, Saint-Cyr, Lang and Kenny (1986).

Thus, leaving aside the controversial issue of somatic symptoms, PD depression follows a pattern of sadness without guilt or self-reproach, high rates of anxiety symptoms (Gotham et al. 1986; Schiffer et al. 1988), a relative lack of delusions and hallucinations (Brown and MacCarthy 1990) and a low suicide rate (Myslobodsky, Lalonde and Hicks 2001) despite a high frequency of suicidal ideation (Brown et al. 1988; see Lojek 1999 for review). These observations indicate that depression in PD may be subtly different from idiopathic or endogenous mood disorders. The pattern of symptoms is extremely interesting. In part it coincides with profiles of depression obtained for older people (Gurland et al. 1983) and may therefore be in keeping with the changes wrought by the ageing process.

If the symptom profile in PD is indeed qualitatively different from that in MDD, this may have implications for the conceptualisation and treatment of depression in PD. One possibility is that the characteristic profile for depression in PD is similar to that for depression in other (non-neurological) chronic illnesses, where raised prevalence levels with respect to age-matched healthy controls are well established (e.g. Detweiler-Bedell et al. 2008). An example is that of arthritis, where several authors have argued that patterns of depressive symptoms are similar to those in PD (e.g. Brown and MacCarthy 1990; Erdal 2001; Gotham et al. 1986). However, only two of these studies (the first and last) made a direct comparison between patient groups and only the former had large enough sample sizes to allow the necessary comparisons between individual items on scales to be made. Nevertheless, they provide initial support for the idea that patients with PD and arthritis do not differ on their symptom profiles for depression.

Another possibility is that it resembles the symptom profile in other chronic diseases, but this remains to be determined. It also raises the possibility that this pattern of symptoms is specific to PD, reflecting the underlying neurobiology of the disorder and endorsing the interesting possibility that these symptoms are a behavioural phenocopy of depression arising on the basis of a different substrate from that of MDD, but characteristic of the degenerative process occurring in PD. For example, the relatively high prevalence of somatic and anxiety related symptoms may be associated with the autonomic dysfunctions of PD (Berrios et al. 1995). Somatic symptoms form an essential and dominant part of the subjective experience of anxiety and it may be that in PD, dysregulation of the autonomic nervous system is the source of these unpleasant symptoms for the patient. Concentration difficulties, which are also prominent in PD, may be consequent upon anxiety.

It appears that the allegedly cohesive pattern of symptoms, differentiating a distinct profile for depression in PD has achieved some recognition (e.g. Weintraub and Stern 2009), though a conclusion of this kind is as yet unwarranted, as there is insufficient empirical evidence to support the notion. The best test of the hypothesis for differential symptom patterns in PD and MDD would be to make a direct comparison of depressive symptoms in patients with the two disorders. Only two studies appear to have attempted this: Merschdorf et al. (2003) and Ehrt et al. (2006), each of them reaching different conclusions. Merschdorf et al. (2003) found that there were no differences in depressive symptoms between the PD and MDD groups they examined, except that suicide attempts and delusional ideas were less frequent and the degree of affective flattening less severe in the PD patients compared to the MDD group. They argue against there being a distinct difference in the profile of depressive symptoms in PD.

On the other hand, Ehrt et al. (2006) found that depressed patients with PD reported fewer feelings of sadness and guilt and showed less anhedonia than elderly depressed patients without PD. As a result, they were less likely to endorse the DSM-IV-TR criteria for MDD. An unexpected finding in this study was that they also showed slightly less anergia – a symptom that is frequently reported as a feature of PD itself. Depressed patients with PD also had more difficulties with concentration. The authors argued that this represents a different profile of depressive symptoms in PD compared to MDD. However, a major difficulty with drawing conclusions from these studies is that they did not adequately control for symptom severity between the patient groups with PD and MDD. This is discussed in greater detail below.

In order to make comparisons of the individual symptoms of depression among different patient and control groups a number of criteria need to be met. The first of these has already been mentioned: that of sample size, which should be sufficiently large to ensure that the comparisons are reliable. Unfortunately, evidence of effect size is not always reported (e.g. Erdal 2001; Koerts et al. 2008; Merschdorf et al. 2003; Prado and Barbosa 2005). The second criterion is that PD samples should be matched for age and sex distribution with respect to control subjects, in view of the known variations in depression associated with these variables. Not all studies have attempted to satisfy this criterion, leaving uncertainties as to their interpretation. A third and critical criterion is that samples used for comparisons should be equated for severity of depression. This condition does not appear to have been adequately met in any of the studies reported to date and indeed, because of the lower prevalence rates of severe depression in PD, it is difficult to meet when making comparisons with patients suffering from MDD, as the overlap in severity between the two samples is relatively small. Making interpretations on the basis of comparisons between samples that have not been equated for severity of depression is predicated on the unwarranted assumption that the profile of depressive symptoms remains unchanged irrespective of the level of severity of the depressive disorder. Research evidence shows that this is not the case. For example, greater severity is associated with weight loss, insomnia, psychomotor agitation, indecisiveness, psychotic features, suicidal ideation and increased levels of vegetative symptomatology (e.g. Gaudiano et al. 2008; Schrag et al. 2007). Thus the allegedly qualitative differences in the depression of PD may derive from primarily quantitative phenomena. It is not surprising that when patients with PD are compared to normal, healthy controls or indeed patients with chronic conditions such as arthritis, in samples that are of mixed severity, but for which the overall group mean score for depressive symptoms does not exceed the threshold for mild depression, that no differences in patterns of symptomatology are found (e.g. Erdal 2001). Such comparisons are unlikely to have sufficient statistical power to demonstrate the effects being examined. Since it is generally accepted that most patients with PD who are depressed, fall into the DSM-IV-TR category of minor depression (Weintraub and Stern 2009), the appropriate comparison would be with a sample of non-PD patients with minor depression. However, this level of severity may still be insufficient to make comparisons across the full range of depressive symptoms, and in particular those such as suicidal ideation, that are of particular interest to the discussion. By definition this means that the sought-after comparison with the symptoms of MDD cannot easily be made. The definitive test of the proposed hypothesis that symptom patterns in PD are different from those of MDD requires a direct comparison of patients from both groups, matched for severity of symptoms, in order to maximise the possibility of the occurrence of the full range of depressive symptoms to enable a valid comparison. Anything other than this raises the possible criticism that any alleged differences in symptom profile are merely an artefact of differences in disease severity. It should be noted that it is insufficient to ensure that the mean scores on depression scales are equivalent for the samples being compared, as this might still include individuals who fall short of the cut-off for severe (clinically relevant) depression. An ideal way of matching would be to ensure that both PD patients and depressed controls meet the DSM-IV-TR criteria for MDD. However, this is extremely demanding in view of the relatively lower prevalence of PD patients with symptoms satisfying the criteria for MDD and would require large sample sizes to be screened in order to select patients meeting the required criteria. At a minimum, all patients should have depression scale scores which exceed the cut-off for clinical depression, and only then should their scores be matched with those of MDD patients. A comparison of this kind does not appear to have been made in the existing literature, but is presented in the empirical study reported later in this volume.

Probably because of the need for large samples, none of the studies examining the question of symptom profiles in PD and MDD have used evaluation scales such as the HAM-D, which is based on a clinical interview carried out by a trained clinician, for the comparisons. All have used self-rating scales and this too may have some influence on the results obtained. Indeed, some of the reports of differences in symptom profile are purely anecdotal and need empirical verification. Finally, it is questionable that the existing studies have used statistical analyses to the best advantage to test their hypotheses. The empirical study reported here represents an attempt to repair these deficiencies.

3.6 The aetiology of depression in Parkinson's disease

From a review of the literature on depression in PD, three main hypotheses concerning the aetiology of depression in the disorder can be distinguished:

1. Depression is considered to be an understandable reaction to having a progressive, chronic disease and the psychosocial stress of the consequent disability; thus it is seen as being *secondary* to the motor disorder.
2. Depression in PD is just one aspect of a multi-faceted disorder resulting from a deterioration in the functioning of specific brain systems; it is thus seen as being of *primary* origin in PD.
3. Depression is thought to be the result of the psycho-active medication used in the treatment of PD.

Needless to say, these three hypotheses are not mutually exclusively, as indeed is argued by various authors.

3.6.1 Depression in PD is reactive

The first hypothesis assumes that depression is *secondary* or "reactive" to the disability of PD. There can be no doubt that for many patients and their families receiving the diagnosis of PD may be a stressful life event of the kind described by Holmes and Rahe (1967). Adjusting to and managing a chronic and progressive illness is likely to add further strain as it may include dealing with the loss of a job, bring increasing withdrawal and isolation because of the physical disability and sometimes lead to heightened levels of marital discord. People suffering from PD are frequently concerned about the effects of their illness on their families, in particular their children, as they fear that the condition may be hereditary; they are only too well aware of the fact that there is no cure for the disease, that the treatment is only palliative and that it becomes less effective with time. Many of the older generation recall relatives and adults from their own childhood experiences who were suffering from PD and who left engrained in their memories, the sad picture of untreated Parkinsonism. So for many patients there may indeed be some aspect of a reactive depression, particularly around the time of diagnosis and it has been reported that this is one of the peak periods for depression in PD (Celesia and Wanamaker 1972; Schrag et al. 2001; Starkstein, Preziosi, Bolduc et al. 1990). Patients with early onset PD (i.e. below 65 years old) also show increased levels of depression (Cole et al. 1996; Kostíc et al. 1994) perhaps because they face more severe career and financial disruptions (Brown et al. 1988), as well as having to cope with the effects of their condition on children who may still be in their teenage years.

Nonetheless, there are now many lines of evidence that argue against depression in PD as simply a straightforward reaction to the severity of the physical impairment (Brown and Jahanshahi 1995). It is known that major depression can precede the onset of motor symptoms in PD by an average of about six years, and it is unlikely to be coincidental that positron emission tomography (PET) studies suggest that the onset of the disease process may predate the occurrence of motor symptoms by about the same length of time (Rickards 2005).

Another argument against the "reactive" view of the origins of depression in PD is that rates of depression are higher in patients with PD than in patients with other chronic diseases such as diabetes and arthritis, which do not affect the central nervous system, yet engender similar levels of disability, have an insidious onset and are of a progressive nature (Cantello et al. 1986; de Groot et al. 2001; Ehmann et al. 1990; Mayeux 1984; Murray 1996; Pluck and Brown 2002; Söderlin et al. 2000). The rate of severe depression in PD is twice that seen in other equivalently disabled patients (Rodin and Voshart 1986). Hence a straightforward reactive response in the form of depression does not seem to be a plausible explanation.

Furthermore, if the depression of PD were indeed secondary to the motor symptoms, a relationship would be expected between depression and levels of disability. However, most investigators have not found a relationship between depression and the duration of PD (e.g. Brown et al. 1988; Ehmann et al. 1990; Gotham et al. 1986; Hantz et al. 1994; Horn 1974; Tandberg et al. 1996; Warburton 1967a) and the natural history of depression in PD does not parallel the progression of the physical symptoms, suggesting that it is an independent process that might affect vulnerable patients (Brown and Jahanshahi 1995). When illness stage as measured with the Hoehn and Yahr scale (1967) has been used as an indicator of illness severity, some studies have reported no relationship with depression (e.g. Bieliauskas and Glanz 1989; Ehmann et al. 1990), whilst others have found greater levels of depression with more advanced disease stage (Huber, Paulson and Shuttleworth 1988; Starkstein, Preziosi, Bolduc et al. 1990). However, the presence of major depression (as opposed to minor or no depression) earlier in the disease process appears to be predictive of faster disease progression in terms of the motor symptoms (Starkstein, Mayburg, Leiguarda et al. 1992). Most studies have found only a weak relationship between absolute rates of functional disability and depression in PD (e.g. Brown et al. 1988; Cole et al. 1996; Ehmann et al. 1990; Menza and Mark 1994; Mindham, Marsden and Parkes 1976; Schrag et al. 2001; Tandberg et al. 1997). By contrast some studies have demonstrated a stronger correlation between the relative changes in disability and depression in individuals diagnosed over one year (Brown et al. 1988). A correlation between disability and depression late in the course of PD (Starkstein, Preziosi, Bolduc et al. 1990) has also been reported, as has an association between mood disorder and level of disability in a group of patients with "on-off phenomena" (Cantello et al. 1986). Motor symptoms in PD also appear to decline faster in patients with depression (Kuhn et al. 1996) and treating depression may improve motor function (Starkstein, Preziosi, Bolduc et al. 1990). Nevertheless no consensus has been reached regarding the association between depression and the physical disability in PD and as yet there is no evidence in support of a sub-type of PD that is characterised by depressive disorder.

3.6.2 Depression is part of the neurodegenerative process in PD

In recent years, the more favoured hypothesis concerning the aetiology of depression in PD is that it occurs as a *primary* consequence of the neurodegenerative process (Tandberg et al. 1997), although the pathophysiology of depression in PD remains obscure. Some authors have favoured multi-factorial models to explain depression (Brown and Jahanshahi 1995; Kamrowska 2009) whilst others postulate that the neurochemical abnormalities may be sufficient to explain depression in PD (Cummings and Masterman 1999).

The fact that depression often predates the motor symptoms of PD suggests a common aetiology for the two disorders (Looi, Matias and Ruzich 2005). A number of studies have also shown that patients with

MDD are more likely to go on to develop PD than other disorders such as osteoarthritis or diabetes (Nilsson, Kessing and Bowling 2001; Nilsson et al. 2002; Schuurman et al. 2002; Todes and Lees 1985) supporting the hypothesis that there is a close association between the two disorders. Additionally, PD is more likely to occur in patients with a main diagnosis of depression than in those with chronic medical disorders, such as osteoarthritis, and in comparison to the general population (Brandt-Christensen et al. 2007).

Some of the strongest evidence for the contention that depression in PD is related to the neurodegenerative disease process itself comes from post-mortem and imaging studies that have demonstrated an association between clinical symptoms of mood disturbance and disruption of the frontal cortex-basal ganglia-thalamic circuit in PD patients. Evidence from studies using PET show that patients with PD and depression have a greater decrease in metabolism in the striatum and orbital frontal cortex than PD patients without depression (Mayberg et al. 1990). Widespread dopamine deficiency is the main feature of PD, but other neurotransmitter systems are also depleted or altered by the degenerative process (Halliday et al. 1990). This results in an overall diminution of brainstem monoamine afferent neurones and a number of other subcortical nuclei are also involved in the process. Post-mortem studies of PD patients with a history of depression have revealed cell loss from the dorsal raphe nuclei (Paulus and Jellinger 1991); these are serotonin secreting neurones, thus implicating serotonin neurotransmitter mechanisms as the basis of depression in PD. However, a more recent study has raised doubts as to the existence of neuropathological differences in the raphe nuclei, amygdala and cortex between depressed and non-depressed patients with PD (Frisina, Haroutunian and Libow 2009). Studies have also demonstrated lower levels of serotonin metabolites in PD (Mayeux, Stern, Cote et al. 1984; Mayeux, Stern, Williams et al. 1986), but these are not specific to depressed patients either, as non-depressed patients with PD also show similar reductions (Guttman et al. 2007; Yamamoto 2001). Moreover, a number of PET/SPECT studies have failed to demonstrate a link between depleted serotonin levels and depression in PD, raising further doubts as to the role of serotonin in the depression of PD (e.g. Kim et al. 2003). It is perhaps therefore not surprising that the efficacy of selective serotonin reuptake inhibitors (SSRIs) in the treatment of PD depression remains inconclusive (Skapinakis et al. 2010).

The considerations outlined above have led researchers to review the possibility that the underlying pathology responsible for the depression of PD lies in other non-serotonergic neurotransmitter systems. The main ones implicated from neuroanatomical and neuropharmacological studies are catecholamine systems, involving noradrenaline and dopamine (Frisina et al. 2009). Here too, depletion of dopamine neurones in the ventral tegmental area and cell loss from the nucleus basalis, which leads to cholinergic deficits and loss of noradrenergic neurones from the locus coeruleus, have been found in post-mortem studies of PD patients with depression (Brown and Gershon 1993). Furthermore, reduced noradrenaline and dopamine outflow from brain stem regions such as the locus coeruleus to the limbic system and its projections, including the amygdala, ventral striatum and anterior cingulate cortex, have been confirmed with the aid of PET in depressed versus non-depressed patients with PD (Remy et al. 2005). Kostic et al. (2010) have demonstrated specific patterns of white matter tissue loss within these cortical-limbic pathways, which differentiate depressed from non-depressed patients with PD. Interestingly, these patterns of brain atrophy overlap with regions that have been implicated in MDD and indicate a specific role for the anterior cingulate cortex (Mayberg 2003). This is in keeping with earlier neuroimaging and metabolic studies of non-PD patients with MDD which revealed similar brain pathology to that of depressed PD patients (e.g. Berg et al. 1999; Ring et al. 1994). In addition, genetic association studies (e.g. Lesch and Mössner 1998) and biochemical studies of the basal limbic system (Chia et al. 1995) implicate similar changes in the underlying pathophysiology of PD depression and MDD.

The usefulness of tricyclic antidepressants, which block the reuptake of noradrenaline, is still controversial for PD-related depression (Ghazi-Noori et al. 2009; Weintraub et al. 2005) and while dopamine itself is not considered to have significant anti-depressive effects, some dopamine agonists (e.g. pramipexole and pergolide) have more recently been shown to be effective for the treatment of depression in PD (Rektorová et al. 2003; see Aarsland et al. 2012; Veazey et al. 2005 for a fuller discussion). Thus it appears that catecholamine deficiencies are more likely to account for the depression of PD, although changes in serotonin metabolism may also play a role. It is tempting to speculate that since the neuropathological findings for the PD patients in these studies who qualified as being depressed, resembled those of patients with MDD, they may share a similar vulnerability in the neural circuitry responsible for depression. On the other hand, in PD patients with subclinical levels of depression, a different underlying pathology, possibly associated with serotonergic neurotransmitter pathways, might be responsible for the milder symptoms. A corollary of this, is that different symptom patterns might be expected to characterise the two types of depression. Variability in the degeneration of subcortical structures in PD may account for the differences in clinical presentation, not only of the different types of depression, but of other non-motor symptoms, including dementia and psychosis. For example, Middleton and Strick (2000) have outlined a subcortical loop that involves the visual cortex and hypothesize that neurodegenerative changes to this loop may give rise to hallucinations. Loss of noradrenergic neurones from the locus coeruleus may affect regulation of mood and lead to problems with attention and concentration. Involvement of the putamen may be responsible for motor disability, whereas degeneration of the caudate nucleus is more closely associated with cognitive dysfunction. PET studies have demonstrated that there are two distinct processes in patients with PD which demonstrate disturbances of both affect and cognition. Patients with cognitive impairment and depression show decreased metabolism in the superior temporal lobe, whereas PD patients with depression alone have decreased metabolism in the prefrontal cortex (Paulus and Trenkwalder 1998).

It is difficult to evaluate the hypothesis that depressive symptoms accompanying PD are an expression of a common underlying neurodegenerative disease and thus an integral component of the PD process. Biological markers for depression such as shortened rapid eye movement (REM) latency, non-suppression of cortisol in the dexamethosone suppression test, decreased levels of serotonin markers in the cerebro-spinal fluid and decreased platelet imipramine binding are not sufficiently sensitive, specific or unambiguous diagnostic markers to resolve this question.

Finally, the relationship between the neurodegenerative process and comorbid depression is demonstrated in the correlations of depressive symptoms with specific clinical features of PD. Depression is higher in patients in whom the akinetic-rigid type of symptoms predominate as compared to the classic PD symptoms of tremor, rigidity and/or bradykinesia (Starkstein et al. 1998), in early onset PD versus age of onset after 55 years and in patients with right handed motor symptoms (Cummings 1992; Starkstein, Preziosi, Bolduc et al. 1990). So far, however, there is no evidence that depression occurs more commonly in a specific genotype of PD (Rickards 2005).

3.6.3 Depression and Dopamine agonists

The third hypothesis concerning the occurrence of affective disorders in PD, attributes mood disturbances to iatrogenic causes in the form of pharmacological management of the disease. The theory that depression may be medication induced has not been fully explored or documented, but it is unlikely to provide a sufficient explanation of the affective changes, since these were documented by researchers before the introduction of pharmacological agents in the treatment of PD.

Nevertheless, it may be the case that pharmacological agents accentuate neuropsychiatric symptoms. Although levodopa and various dopamine agonists (e.g. amantadine) have indeed been implicated in delirium, agitation, restlessness and other neuropsychiatric states, there is little evidence to suggest that they are involved in the development of mood disorders in PD. Furthermore, there is only limited evidence to support the view that they improve mood in PD (Marsh and Markham 1973; Veazey et al. 2005), although mood fluctuations related to "on" and "off" fluctuations in PD have been related to changes in affective state (Cummings 1992; Menza et al. 1990).

The main aim of this chapter has been to provide an analysis of depression in PD as a background to the study later to be described, in which affective symptoms are of primary interest. There are three main reasons for this: firstly because, as mentioned in chapter 1, affective disturbances have not, so far, been a major focus for the neuropsychology of PD, secondly because of the intrinsic interest they hold for allowing a better understanding of brain-behaviour relationships which may lead to better opportunities for treatment and thirdly, because of their impact on the well-being of the person suffering from PD and his/her carer. However, no review of the neuropsychiatry of PD would be complete without mention of the other neuropsychiatric symptoms that are characteristic of the disorder, and these are considered briefly, below.

3.7 Other neuropsychiatric symptoms in PD

3.7.1 Apathy

Apathy is defined as: "a decrease in goal-directed behaviour, thinking and mood" (Weintraub and Stern 2009). Studies variously refer to motivational deficits or decreases in emotional responsiveness as an essential feature of PD. Apathy is a state that is commonly confused with depression, but the descriptions of denial of low mood and absence of the typically cognitive symptoms of depression, such as guilt and hopelessness presented above, are considered to be more in keeping with apathy. The patient is usually unaware of this state of mind, but it may be a cause for concern for carers. Clearly, symptoms of apathy partly overlap with those of depression, but also with delirium and cognitive impairment and fatigue, though apathy may also occur independently (Starkstein, Mayburg, Preziosi et al. 1992). As with depression, there are wide ranging differences in the reported prevalence of apathy in PD, between 17% and 70%. Risk factors for apathy include dementia, an accelerated decline in speech, axial impairment and treatment for PD using unilateral deep brain stimulation of the STN or globus pallidus (Tan 2012). It is associated with increased levels of cognitive impairment and poorer performance in the activities of daily living. The neurobiological basis of apathy is poorly understood.

3.7.2 Anxiety

It is reported that up to 40% of patients with PD experience anxiety symptoms, which may be part of the clinical picture for depression, or form recognised disorders in their own right. These include generalised anxiety disorder, panic attacks, obsessive-compulsive disorder and social phobia (Weintraub and Stern 2009). Patients with PD may avoid public places and social gatherings due to embarrassment caused by their symptoms, in particular tremor and dyskinesias, voice changes and mobility problems; such behaviour however, does not meet the DSM-IV-TR criteria for social phobia (APA 2000). Anxiety has to date, been given relatively little attention in PD, but it has a propensity to be particularly disabling, because of the intensity of the symptoms, their frequently somatic presentation and tendency to exacerbate the symptoms of the disease itself, there being considerable symptom overlap, as with depression. Anxiety appears to be associated with the motor symptoms of PD, at least in so far as "off" periods are often characterised by increases in symptoms. Patients may describe a feeling of panic as they become increasingly "trapped" by immobilization, which resolves with the improvement of motor symptoms (Weintraub and Stern 2009).

3.7.3 Impulse control disorders

Impulse control disorders are recognised as a group of psychiatric disorders defined in the DSM-IV-TR (APA 2000) as a group of complex behavioural disorders, in which there is characteristic failure to resist an impulse, drive or temptation to indulge in an act that is harmful to the person or to others. Their clinical manifestation in PD occurs in a variety of forms, including: pathological gambling, hypersexual behaviour, compulsive behaviours such as shopping, eating and skin picking, problems with internet use, punding, which is a compulsive fascination with meaningless movements or activities such as collecting, arranging or dismantling objects, and walkabout, which is a form of excessive, aimless walking (Vilas, Pont-Sunyer and Tolosa 2012; Weintraub 2009). These disorders are thought to occur more frequently in patients with PD than in the general population (Avanzi et al. 2006) and they are the source of considerable distress to patients and their carers, because of the embarrassment and disastrous personal, financial and socio-familial consequences they may cause (Ceravolo et al. 2009). Inevitably, the potential for distressing or harmful consequences is great, when a behaviour is taken to excess. It is thought that behaviours related to impulse control disorders are underreported to clinicians for these reasons. Other behaviours that resemble those seen in impulse control disorders have also been reported in PD in the context of dopamine replacement therapy. For example, some patients have a tendency towards the use of dopaminergic drugs in doses that exceed the amounts required to control their motor symptoms and in spite of developing disabling dyskinesias (Giovannoni et al. 2000). These excessive doses of medication result in (hypo)manic episodes, characteristic of a mood disorder that the patient experiences as being highly pleasurable or may involve him/her in pleasurable activities. This condition is known as dopamine dysregulation syndrome and has a great deal in common conceptually with addictive behaviours (Ceravolo et al. 2009).

Sporadic reports of impulse control disorders associated with PD have been available since the introduction of dopaminergic therapy (e.g. Sacks 1999), although there remained doubt as to whether these were iatrogenic effects giving cause for concern, or no more than might be expected following the recovery of function from the frozen state imposed by the illness prior to the availability of pharmacological treatment (Stern and Lees 1982). Within the sample studied for the purposes of the present research, three patients, all of them male and with a younger age of onset of PD (below 60 years) were identified as having dopamine dysregulation syndrome. One of them was being treated with the aid of an apomorphine pump and this ability to control his own medication was particularly problematic. These patients demonstrated an appetitive urge or craving for dopaminergic medication, which had a hedonistic quality. They continued to administer excessive amounts of medication despite the negative consequences in terms of disabling dyskinesias and a constant preoccupation with their drug regime, which was particularly trying for their carers. They also demonstrated inappropriate sexual behaviours. As the effects of drug treatment wore off, they demonstrated end of dose withdrawal symptoms, such as dysphoria and anxiety and they were extremely reluctant to follow medical advice to cutback or stop their medication, even though it was clear that it was causing more problems than the illness for which it was prescribed. Attempts to manage the reduction of medication in an in-patient psychiatric setting proved unsuccessful, largely because of their refusal to cooperate with treatment. These patients suffered disproportionate impairments in virtually all areas of functioning in normal life, their personal lives were disrupted beyond repair and their carers were at breaking point.

In recent years, anecdotal reports of this kind have been complemented by a number of studies whose aim was to explore the epidemiology and neurobiology of impulse control disorders in PD. Although these studies are in their infancy, preliminary estimates of prevalence rates for an impulse control disorder range between 6-17% (Vilas et al. 2012), and specifically for pathological gambling, approximately 2.0-6.0%, for problematic sexual behaviour, 2.0-10.0%, for compulsive buying, 0.4-5.7%, and for compulsive eating, 4.3% (Ceravolo et al. 2009; Weintraub et al. 2010). A primary risk factor for the development of these disorders is treatment with dopamine agonists (Vilas et al. 2012) but levodopa is implicated too (Weintraub et al. 2010). Additional factors include being male, younger age, being unmarried, current cigarette smoking and a family history of alcohol addiction or gambling problems (Vilas et al. 2012). Thus there appears to be a clear role for the effects of dopaminergic stimulation in the occurrence of impulse control disorders, although the underlying pathology of PD is probably not important, as these disorders occur in other conditions treated with dopamine agonists, such as restless legs syndrome. However, only a minority of patients with PD develop these problem behaviours and so it is thought that they are the result of complex interactions between the pharmacological agents and the risk factors mentioned above.

On a neurobiological level, one hypothesis to account for impulse control disorders in PD, states that treatment attempts to restore dopamine in the dorso-striatal motor pathways, results in "overdosing" the ventral corticostriatal pathways involved in cognitive and limbic system circuitry. These central dopaminergic pathways form part of the brain's reward system and are involved in addiction. Dopamine receptors (D_1 and D_2) receptors in the dorsal striatum are thought to mediate the motor effects of dopamine replacement therapies, whereas D_3 receptors in the ventral striatum appear to mediate reward, emotional and cognitive processes. Certain of the dopamine agonists currently used in PD therapy have high affinity for the D_3 receptors and thus may cause these reward pathways to be over-stimulated, resulting in the behaviours associated with impulse control disorders (Vilas et al. 2012; Weintraub and Nirenberg 2013).

3.7.4 Psychosis

Psychotic symptoms in PD are, broadly speaking, classified according to two categories. The first of these is a "benign" hallucinatory syndrome, in which the patient typically experiences visual perceptual changes, including illusions, "passage" and "sense of presence" phenomena or hallucinations. These typically include animal or human figures, and patients retain insight into the hallucinations and are not disturbed by them. Auditory hallucinations and less frequently tactile or olfactory ones sometimes occur in this category. Because of their benign nature, they are tolerated well by both the patient and his carers, and may not require treatment.

The second category includes more complex psychotic symptoms, consisting of hallucinations and persecutory delusions, frequently in the presence of dementia. It is not usual for the patient to have any insight into these symptoms, which often occur towards the evening or when ambient light conditions are low. These symptoms are disturbing, especially to carers and require treatment.

Patients with PD also exhibit psychotic symptoms as part of sleep-related disorders involving vivid dreaming and rapid eye movement behaviour disorder. Equally, most patients with PD and psychosis also report sleep disturbances. Understandably, the overlap between these conditions makes it difficult to distinguish between the two (Weintraub and Stern 2009). It is unusual for patients with PD to demonstrate psychotic thinking in the context of depressive disorders (Cummings and Masterman 1999).

3.8 Neuropsychiatric symptoms in PD and the effect on the carer-care recipient relationship

A central aim of the foregoing discussion has been to show, that the neuropsychiatric symptoms associated with PD are an intrinsic part of the disorder, occurring in a large proportion of patients. Indeed, their significance is such, that PD is increasingly recognised as a neuropsychiatric disorder (Weintraub and Burn 2011) and has been at the forefront of research into brain-behaviour relationships (see chapter 4).

Evidence is emerging that the impact of neuropsychiatric symptoms for both patients and their carers (usually spouses) is considerable, exceeding that of the problems encountered as a result of the motor impairment (Leiknes et al. 2010; Miller et al. 1996). In some ways it is surprising that it has taken so long to recognise this fact, as there is considerable evidence to show that in couples without additional co-morbidities, where one person is depressed, the spouse or partner is more likely to be depressed in comparison to general population norms (e.g. Benazon and Coyne 2000). Furthermore, the association between depression and dysfunctional marital interaction is well documented (Gabriel, Beach and Bodenmann 2010), opening up possibilities for understanding the importance of the quality of the carer-care recipient relationship in spousal care-giving. These issues are discussed in greater depth in chapter 7 of this volume.

A further possibility is also worthy of consideration. One of the reasons that the recognition of depression has been so difficult in PD is not exclusively due to the problem of symptom overlap, but that the majority of patients who are depressed, do not suffer from major depressive disorder, but the minor form of affective disturbance. This, together with the suggestion that depression in PD presents with a different symptom profile, may have complicated the diagnosis for physicians and recognition that their spouses were suffering from a depressive disorder for carers. The patient's neuropsychiatric symptoms, such as apathy, withdrawal, disinterest, anhedonia and inflexibility may be misinterpreted by carers (see chapter 5) who react with sadness or anger or by distancing themselves from their spouse, who they perceive as having changed from a psychological perspective. During the course of the present study it was not uncommon to hear from carers that their spouse had changed to such an extent, that "he is no longer the person he used to be". It is this transformation, wrought by the neuropsychiatric symptoms of PD, with which carers find it most difficult to cope.

3.9 Chapter summary

Putting together the pieces of the complex puzzle represented by the status of depression in PD is a challenging task, yet to be resolved. Although it is acknowledged that depression is one of the most common non-motor symptoms of PD (Reijnders et al. 2008), controversies still surround the prevalence and nature of PD depression. A major difficulty arises from the problem of symptom overlap between the presentation of PD and that of neuropsychiatric and neuropsychological disorders. No adequate solution to this has been reached: excluding the somatic features of depression may lead to underdiagnosis, whereas the use of an inclusive approach may result in the overdiagnosis of the disorder in PD (Marsh et al. 2006). Considerable symptom overlap also exists between depression and apathy (Oguru et al. 2010) and cognitive performance, with the possibility that depression may present as pseudo-dementia (Bulbena and Berrios 1986).

The choice of instruments to measure depression in PD has important implications for clinical research, including epidemiological and treatment studies. None of the existing scales ideally meet the requirements for a depression scale in PD, but some have been shown to be preferable in meeting the psychometric properties required (McDonald et al. 2006; Reijnders et al. 2010). Nevertheless, the gold standard for their validation are DSM criteria for depressive disorders, which in themselves have raised concerns in the literature as an appropriate means for establishing the diagnosis of depressive illness in PD, because of the considerable overlap between the somatic symptoms of PD and depression.

Exclusion of somatic symptoms from the assessment of PD depression, which is one proposed solution to these problems, as exemplified in the HADS and GDS scales, is not necessarily a good one in PD. There is some evidence for example, that certain somatic symptoms, such as early morning wakening and appetite loss are a good means of discriminating between depressed and non-depressed patients with PD (Leentjens, Marinus et al. 2003). Furthermore, there continues to be a lack of consensus regarding the extent to which lowered mood states and anhedonia are as prominent in the clinical picture of depression in PD, as they are in MDD, where of course, they are central. A question of major importance relates to establishing whether the symptom pattern contributing to the profile of depressive disorder in PD is the same as that in MDD. A key issue here is that the severity of depressive symptoms should be controlled in making the appropriate comparisons between PD and the other groups of interest, as patterns of symptom presentation are thought to differ, according to age (St. Pierre et al. 1986; Zemore and Eames, 1979) and the severity of depressive illness (Gaudiano et al. 2008).

Finally, the relationship between depression and the other symptom domains of PD (motor and cognitive) was evaluated in the context of its meaning with regard to establishing the origins of depressive symptoms in PD.

This review of the neuropsychiatric aspects of PD, with its specific focus on depressive symptomatology, highlights the significance of non-motor symptoms in the presentation of the disorder. With a similar aim in mind, the chapter that follows will provide an account of neuropsychological functioning in PD, from mild cognitive dysfunction to the dementia associated with the disorder. Later chapters consider the effects of these non-motor manifestations of the illness for both the patient and close family members involved in his/her care.

The issues discussed in this chapter formed several of the questions of major interest to the present study and were formulated as follows:

1. What is the prevalence of depression in the sample of patients studied? How do prevalence rates differ according to the different methods of assessment used?
2. What is the symptom profile for depression in PD? Does it differ from that of MDD?
3. What is the relationship between the core motor symptoms and depression in PD?
4. What effect does depression in people suffering from PD have on their spouses, who are involved in their day to day care?
5. Are carers able to recognise the symptoms of depression in their spouses?

CHAPTER FOUR

THE NEUROPSYCHOLOGY OF PARKINSON'S DISEASE

4.1 Introduction

The presentation of PD from a neuropsychological perspective completes the description of the illness from the point of view of the triad of main symptom domains which characterise the illness. In parallel to the neuropsychiatric symptoms of the disorder, its neuropsychological aspects constitute the core non-motor symptoms and the study of these has brought PD to the forefront of neuro-scientific investigations of brain-behaviour relationships. As in the case of the affective disturbances discussed in the previous chapter, cognitive function in PD has been the subject of much controversy and debate. A form of dementia is recognised as being associated with PD (Aarsland, Beyer and Kurz 2008), but milder forms of cognitive impairment are thought to occur in the absence of dementia and to be present in about 25% of cases, from the earliest stages of the disease (Barone et al. 2011). Decline in cognitive functioning has a major impact on the everyday lives of patients and their carers (Aarsland, Bronnick et al. 2007; Schrag et al. 2006; Weintraub, Moberg, Duda et al. 2004) and thus forms an important background to the present study.

4.2 The historical background to cognitive deficits in PD

It is often stated that in his description of the disease that later came to bear his name, James Parkinson did not include changes in intellectual functioning. The much quoted phrase "the senses and intellects being uninjured" (Parkinson 1817) is taken as evidence of this. In an incisive historical account of Paralysis Agitans, as the disorder was originally called, Berrios (1995, 96) has pointed out that Parkinson's intentions were most probably to emphasize that cognitive dysfunctions were not involved to the same extent as in other neurological disorders, since at the time, they were considered to be intrinsic to other forms of paralysis, and his endeavour was to distinguish PD from these disorders (for a historical account of mental symptoms in PD see Berrios 1995; 1996). The patients reported by Parkinson were relatively young with a mean age of 60 years; today they would be classified as "early onset" (their disease duration is unknown). In view of present day knowledge about the cognitive impairment of PD, this may explain the absence of cognitive symptoms in the small sample reported; any that might have been present were probably quite subtle and would have evaded even an astute observer, as Parkinson himself undoubtedly was. Without treatment, these patients are unlikely to have survived long enough for any more evident cognitive deficits to become clinically apparent. This would be in keeping with the suggestion that dementia only began to be reported as a complication of PD after 1850, when anti-muscarinic agents were introduced as treatment (Berrios 1995). The early attempts to remedy the motor symptoms of PD may have prolonged the lives of patients long enough for the cognitive impairments to appear, or due to their anti-cholinergic effects, may themselves have been the cause of the deficits (Miller et al. 1987; see later discussion on drug treatments and cognitive impairment in PD).

Nevertheless, it took some considerable time for it to be accepted that mental changes do indeed occur in PD. In 1881, Ball (cited in Berrios 1996, 401) wrote: "... a large number of Parkinsonian patients present psychological disorders extending from simple irritability to psychosis; far from being an exception I would say that a slight degree of cognitive impairment (perturbation intellectuelle) is the rule." In the ensuing debate concerning the status of mental symptoms in PD, two opposing views emerged. That supported by Ball, Parant and others held that psychological disturbances, including intellectual loss were part of the disease, whilst others, including Charcot, appeared to believe that any association was coincidental (see Berrios 1996, 402). The latter, was essentially a "reactive" view of the mental changes accompanying PD. Berrios (1996, 402) cites Gowers: "The intellect may be unaffected throughout, except by the irritability which usually accompanies the physical restlessness, or by mental depression, which is chiefly the natural result of the physical ailment" and Wilson: "... on the intellectual side there may be noted some bradyphrenia or slowness of thought yet it is probably more apparent than real" as endorsing the reactive position. Charcot however, along with other French neurologists, appears to have held a more modified view, reflecting that: "at a given moment, intellect becomes blurred and memory is lost" (cited in Berrios 1996, 403). The trend towards recognising cognitive symptomatology continued throughout the first half of the twentieth century, with authors such as

Bebb (1925), Billenkamp (1959), Compin (1902; cited in Warburton 1967b), Critchley (1929), Diller and Riklan (1956), Lewy (1923; cited in Förstl and Levy 1991), Mjones (1949), Shrubshall (1927; cited in Reitan and Boll 1971), Schwab and England (1958) and Walshe (1955), all concurring that intellectual difficulties were to be seen in PD.

Thus, it can be seen that the relationship of neuropsychological impairments to PD has been a source of dissonance in the literature that can be traced back to the earliest publications. Not surprisingly therefore, much of the early work was concerned with establishing whether cognitive deficits are indeed an invariable part of the disorder, as both clinical impressions (Brain 1962; Patrick and Levy 1922) and empirical studies using controls (Talland 1962) did not always lend support to this view. Indeed, the presence of intellectual decline in patients with PD was used as a criterion for the diagnosis of so-called arteriosclerotic Parkinsonism and to distinguish it from the idiopathic form of the disease (Pollock and Hornabrook 1966). There was also much debate concerning the potentially confounding effects of such variables as the co-existence of depression, surgical and pharmacological treatment techniques, and the effects of normal ageing, in accounting for intellectual deficits (Lieberman et al.1979), but the evidence tended to support the contention that these were insufficient to explain the lowered cognitive performance of patients with the disease (Loranger et al. 1972). A great deal of controversy and confusion continued to surround the status of neuropsychological deficits in PD with regard to both their nature, prevalence and aetiology, nearly two hundred years after Parkinson had taken the first steps towards describing the disorder. This was to change quite dramatically towards the end of the twentieth century, as PD became the subject of intensive research investigations because of its potential for revealing the nature of important brain mechanisms relating to the basal ganglia and their role in mediating intentional and goal directed behaviours (i.e. willed behaviours).

4.2.1 Early views of the dementia of PD

Work in the second half of the twentieth century, based on neuropsychological test instruments with larger numbers of unselected patients, revealed the existence of a range of cognitive deficits in PD including memory and language disturbances, impairment in visuospatial processing and difficulties with attention and concept acquisition (e.g. Boller 1980; Boller et al. 1984; Flowers and Robertson 1985; Matison et al. 1982; Warburton 1967b). In some cases, these appeared to be quite generalised (Celesia and Wanamaker 1972; Loranger et al. 1972; Reitan and Boll 1971) and to take the form of dementia (Lieberman et al. 1979; Martilla and Rinne 1976; Pollock and Hornabrook 1966; Shaw, Lees and Stern 1980). Some authors contended that the underlying pathology responsible for the advanced dementia of PD was indistinguishable from that seen in DAT (Boller 1980; Boller et al. 1980; Braak et al. 1996; Ruberg et al. 1982), a position essentially arguing that intellectual difficulties were not associated with the pathology of PD itself and retaining the view that cortical pathology is crucial to dementia. Specifically, atrophy of the nucleus basalis of Meynert and the consequent loss of cholinergic innervations of the cortex was considered to be responsible. These positions held that PD and DAT were part of the same spectrum of disease (Rossor 1981) and were supported by evidence of clinical, histological and neurochemical similarities between the two diseases in their terminal phases (Lees and Smith 1983).

Others held that the clinical presentation of the symptoms of cognitive impairment in the two conditions was consistently and sufficiently different not to warrant support for the idea of a common underlying pathology for the dementia of PD and DAT (e.g. Huber, Shuttleworth and Freidenberg 1989). In support of this position, later studies were to reveal that the presence of degenerating neuronal processes in the form of Lewy bodies are the most sensitive and specific markers for PD dementia, whilst the histopathological hallmark for DAT, namely amyloid plaques and neurofibrillary tangles are less consistently present in PD (Cummings 2003; Dickson and Orr 2011). Furthermore, the pattern of grey matter loss in PD dementia most closely resembles that of a related clinical disorder, dementia with Lewy bodies (DLB), rather than DAT (Burton et al. 2004). This would appear to reflect the view that PD dementia is a separate clinical entity from DAT. From the point of view of present day understanding, these “either/or” positions have proved to be a gross over simplification. The neurodegenerative pattern associated with PD dementia is now known to generate dysfunction in multiple subcortical neurochemical projection systems to cortical and limbic regions, but is not necessarily sufficient to account for PD dementia, and combined DAT and PD dementia pathology is still implicated by some (Kalaitzakis and Pearce 2009). One of the reasons for the continuing controversy regarding the origins of dementia in PD is that there is considerable clinical heterogeneity in the presentation of cognitive deficits in the disorder and evidence is accruing that there may be distinct underlying pathologies associated with different patterns of impairment. PD dementia appears to be specifically associated with the genotype for the microtubule-associated protein tau (MAPT) H1/H2, which is also a common marker for DAT (Williams-Gray et al. 2009). Hence, there is a return to the notion that a common underlying mechanism is responsible for the neurodegeneration and protein aggregation that is recognised as being characteristic for both PD dementia and DAT. It remains unclear whether the origins of these lesions lie in different pathogenetic pathways or represent a final common pathway leading to the neuronal degeneration giving rise to the movement disorder and dementia alike (Jellinger 2010).

Early observations revealed not only qualitative differences (i.e. in terms of the type of deficits observed), but substantial quantitative differences between the presentation of PD dementia and DAT. Memory impairment is an important feature of cognitive dysfunction in most neurodegenerative disorders and PD is no exception, except that it is milder and does not dominate the clinical picture as in DAT, for example. Equally visuospatial disturbances occur in these disorders, but are more severe in patients with a cortical dementia, such as DAT. One hypothesis proposed to account for the differences between DAT and PD was in terms of a distinction between cortical and subcortical dementia (Cummings and Benson 1984; Huber and Paulson 1985). Cortical dementias occur in diseases in which degeneration predominantly affects the neocortical association areas with relative sparing of subcortical structures; DAT is the classic example of a cortical dementia. Cortical cognitive abilities have been traditionally conceptualised as serving intellectual functions such as perceptual and visuospatial abilities, language and memory and hence, cortical impairment leads to the classic neuropsychological deficits associated with agnosia, aphasia and amnesia. With the emerging understanding that subcortical structures also have an important role in cognitive function, the possibility of subcortical dementias gained credulity.

The term "subcortical dementia" entered the literature in the early 1970s (Albert, Feldman and Willis 1974), although the concept was originally described by Wilson in 1912. In contrast to the cortical abilities, subcortical abilities are those sustaining more fundamental functions such as arousal, mood and motivation. In subcortical dementia, the pathological changes affect deep brain structures, such as the basal ganglia, the diencephalon (thalamus and hypothalamus) and brain stem, with relative sparing of the cerebral cortex. Huntington's disease and PD are examples of conditions in which these subcortical structures are primarily affected. Patients with subcortical dementia are characteristically slower on tasks of information processing and present with relatively mild intellectual impairments affecting memory and problem solving abilities. Sometimes abnormalities of judgement also occur. Disturbances of mood, including depression and apathy are more likely to be in evidence as compared with cortical dementias. There are important qualitative differences in cognitive performance too. Severe language disturbances together with agnosia and apraxia are relatively rare in subcortical dementia and most patients retain insight and are aware of their diminishing mental faculties. Nevertheless, subcortical dementia has been characterised as leading to marked psychosocial incompetence (Dunne 1993; Turner, Moran and Kopelman 2002), which is likely to have profound effects for the carer - care recipient relationship in PD.

4.3 The neuropsychology of PD: current views

In recent years it has become established that alongside the cardinal, clinical features of PD in the form of resting tremor, bradykinesia, muscle rigidity and postural instability, non-motor complications are frequently encountered (Beatty et al. 1989; Chaudhuri, Healy and Schapira 2006). These include the neuropsychiatric symptoms such as depression, apathy, visual hallucinations and psychotic symptoms (Aarsland and Karlsen 1999) discussed in the previous chapter, as well as a heterogeneous range of cognitive impairments and dementia, which have damaging consequences for the prognosis of the condition (Aarsland et al. 2003; Riedel et al. 2008). The traditional view of PD as a paradigmatic movement disorder has thus given way to a view which acknowledges the neuropsychiatric and neuropsychological aspects of the disorder (Samuel et al. 2006). As a result of their frequent manifestation and impact on daily life, these non-motor symptoms add significantly to the personal and socio-economic burden of the disease (Riedel et al. 2008), are associated with more rapid disease progression, (Starkstein, Bolduc et al. 1990), affect the quality of life of both patients and their carers (Glozman 2004; Schrag, Jahanshahi and Quinn 2000) and are one of the main reasons for the breakdown of community care for the person with PD (Aarsland et al. 2000).

4.4 Dementia in Parkinson's disease

It is now generally agreed that the prevalence of dementia in PD is higher than in the general population of the same age (e.g. Aarsland and Kurz 2010; Aarsland, Zaccai and Brayne 2005; Bondi and Troster 1997; Cummings 1988). However estimates of the prevalence of dementia have been so disparate, as to be practically and theoretically of little use. For example, reported estimates have varied from 2% (Hietanen and Teravainen 1988) to 81% (Martin et al. 1973). These differences are most probably due to the criteria used for selecting patients, variations in the population samples studied (early versus late PD), the methods used for ascertaining cases, diverse methodologies for assessing cognitive decline and whether cross-sectional or longitudinal study designs are used. Results vary according to whether investigators have attempted to identify all patients in a defined region (e.g. Foltynie et al. 2004) or whether the study was based on convenience samples from hospital clinics and whether patients were studied early in the course of the disease, as in the Hietanen and Teravainen (1988) research or later, when symptoms were more advanced. Most studies have been cross-sectional, providing an estimate of the proportion of PD patients who are demented (point prevalence). In recent years, however, a number of longitudinal studies have been reported, which provide more accurate information regarding the frequency of dementia in PD.

4.4.1 The prevalence of dementia in PD

An early, but influential review by Cummings (1988), based on the results of 27 studies, estimated the mean prevalence for dementia in PD to be in the region of 40%. This figure came to be generally accepted, despite the wide variability in the studies upon which it was based. It may however, not have been representative of an unselected population of patients with PD as most of the studies were based on patients referred to specialist neurological clinics. Another complication is that in these early days, researchers would not have screened for the existence of cases of Lewy body dementia among the samples.

A more recent systematic review, covering 13 studies and using more sophisticated methodology, especially with regard to sampling methods, yielded a prevalence rate of 31.3% (Aarsland et al. 2005). Three studies which have been published in the wake of this review are broadly in keeping with its findings, reporting rates of dementia in PD of: 23% (Athey, Porter and Walker 2005), 22% (De Lau et al. 2005) and 48% (Hobson and Meara 2004).

In view of the fact that PD is a progressive, neurodegenerative disease, there is reason to believe that dementia may emerge with longer disease duration (Aarsland et al. 1996). Studies that have investigated the prevalence rates for dementia at different stages of the disease have indeed demonstrated, that the occurrence of dementia in newly diagnosed PD patients is lower (see Aarsland and Kurz 2010). However, the fact that dementia may exist early in the course of disease is considered by some authors to be problematic, as it may indicate the presence of multiple pathologies or be suggestive of an alternative diagnosis. For example, the U.K. Parkinson's Disease Society Brain Bank Clinical Diagnostic criteria state that "early severe dementia with disturbances of memory, language and praxis" should be an exclusion criterion for the diagnosis of PD (Litvan et al. 2003). Furthermore, it has also been recommended that the presence of dementia before or within one year of the onset of PD (the so-called "one year rule"), should be regarded as diagnostic of Lewy body dementia, though this is not based on empirical evidence (McKeith et al. 2005). In practice, as the following discussion will show, these decisions are very difficult to make. Mild cognitive deficits, which become evident on specialised neuropsychological investigation and evolve into a dementia syndrome as the disease progresses, together with the brain changes underlying these processes, suggest that dementia in PD is a continuously emerging process, rather than one which dichotomises patients into those that have, or do not have dementia (after Aarsland and Kurz 2010).

Patients with PD and dementia have a higher mortality rate than those without dementia (Boller et al. 1980; Levy, Tang et al. 2002; Marder et al. 1991; Nussbaum et al. 1998; Piccirilli et al. 1994), although there is at least one exception to these findings (see Papapetropoulos et al. 2005). Nonetheless, considering that the weight of the evidence points to dementia as being a risk factor for earlier death, point prevalence is an underestimate of the true frequency of dementia in PD. This is because estimates taken at one point in time are unable to account for a cohort of patients with PD, as they do not take into consideration attrition rates due to death and at the same time, include new cases which are continually being added; these latter cases may not yet have had time in which to develop dementia. They are thus unable to provide any information about what may happen to a cohort of PD patients over the course of the disease (Aarsland and Kurz 2010). This of course, is the really critical information sought, namely what proportion of patients is likely to develop dementia before they die. There appear to have been only two studies which have examined the cumulative prevalence of dementia in PD. One, a longitudinal study by Aarsland et al. (2003) reported a rate of 52% after four years, which had risen to nearly 80% after eight years. The other study, based in Sydney, Australia, followed a relatively small (N=136) cohort of patients for a period of 20 years. The results were equally discouraging. Altogether 75% of the patients had developed dementia prior to death and of the 30 survivors, 83% were demented (Hely et al. 2008).

4.4.2 The incidence of dementia in PD

For reasons concerning time and expense, there have been fewer incidence studies of dementia in PD. Based on longitudinal studies of community-based cohorts, it is estimated that approximately 10% of a PD population will develop dementia per year. The relative risk for developing dementia in PD is estimated to be 4-6 times that in the general population (Aarsland et al. 2001; Aarsland and Kurz 2010). One study has reported the incidence of PD dementia in the general population as 2-3% after six years (Yip et al. 2006) and the Rotterdam study found that 15% of those already diagnosed with PD at baseline developed dementia after a mean follow-up time of 6.9 years, whilst 4.9% of those with incident PD during the study, were diagnosed with dementia during a mean follow-up period of 4.3 years from disease onset. The hazard ratio for developing dementia for the PD prevalent group was 2.80 while for the incident group it was 4.74 (de Lau et al. 2005).

Following patients from the time of onset of PD is likely to provide a better estimate of the risk for developing dementia, because variations in disease duration may affect the observed incidence of dementia among cohorts (Aarsland and Kurz 2010). Most studies indicate that the mean duration from the onset of PD to the development of dementia is approximately ten years (e.g. Hely et al. 2008). In practice, wide variations are commonplace, and some patients develop dementia early in the course of the disease, whilst others may remain free of symptoms for twenty years or more, before they too show the apparently almost inevitable cognitive decline into dementia. There is evidence to show that the time to developing dementia is related to the type and extent of brain pathology present (Halliday et al. 2008). To date only the CamPaIGN study has taken on the arduous task of determining the rates at which dementia emerges in an incident cohort of patients with PD. Five years from the onset of PD, 17% had developed dementia and the incidence was 38.7 per 1000 person-years (Williams-Gray et al. 2009). This provides confirmation that the incidence of dementia appears to be lower early in the course of PD. However, after a mean duration to follow-up of 7.7 years, the proportion had doubled (34%) and the estimated mean time to dementia was 8.3 years. At ten years, 40% of the cohort had died, dementia being a risk factor for mortality, along with a past history of smoking and higher baseline severity of motor symptoms; only 21% of patients were without dementia or postural instability (Williams-Gray et al. 2012).

4.4.3 The impact of dementia in Parkinson's disease

These data, translated into the likelihood of developing dementia faced by individual patients and their families, suggests that unprecedentedly high levels of burden might be expected. The presence of dementia in PD is thought to contribute to a more malignant course of illness, increasing the risk of disturbing psychiatric symptoms such as apathy and visual hallucinations and faster progression of motor symptoms. These in combination lead to greater functional impairment which imposes a heavy burden in both personal and socioeconomic terms on the families of sufferers (Adler 2009; Huse et al. 2005), increases the need for nursing home placement (Aarsland et al. 2000) and has significant implications in terms of health economics (Findley et al. 2003).

4.4.4 The definition and measurement of dementia in PD

According to established criteria for determining dementia (e.g. DSM-IV-TR, APA 2000) memory impairment and deterioration in at least one of the following domains of cognitive functioning must be demonstrated at a level of severity to interfere with usual social or occupational performance: language, visuospatial skills, judgement or abstract thinking, and emotion or personality. There are many problems with this definition of dementia as a number of authors have pointed out (e.g. Cummings and Benson 1992). For example, memory impairment is not always a feature of dementing illness, especially in the early stages (e.g. Pick's disease and Lewy body dementia; Cummings 2003) and certainly it is not as pronounced in PD as DAT. On the other hand, as described in the following sections of this chapter, attention and executive dysfunction are relatively more impaired in PD than DAT (Bronnick et al. 2007). The question of severity is particularly problematic: it is theoretically possible for two patients with the same level of cognitive impairment to be classified differently, depending on the circumstances of their everyday lives – those in less demanding occupations, for example, might not be considered to have dementia. Moreover, as seen in previous chapters, the social or occupational difficulties of patients with PD may equally be affected by their motor and affective symptoms. Finally, a major disadvantage of the DSM-IV-TR is that it does not specify the grounds on which cognitive impairments are to be qualified as such.

These difficulties have been partially resolved with the acceptance of consensus criteria for the diagnosis of dementia in PD which require: a diagnosis of PD according to the U.K. Parkinson's Disease Society Brain

Bank Clinical Diagnostic criteria (Litvan et al. 2003); and a dementia syndrome with insidious onset and slow progression in which decline from premorbid levels has been established in at least two cognitive domains, and which leads to impairment in daily functioning (social, occupational or personal care) and is independent of the impairment ascribable to the motor or autonomic symptoms of PD (Emre et al. 2007). The cognitive deficits may arise in two of the following cognitive domains: attention (which may fluctuate), executive function, visuospatial function, memory (in particular free recall tasks which usually improve with cueing) and language abilities involving subtle changes such as word finding difficulties. The diagnosis is supported by the presence of neuropsychiatric symptoms such as apathy, changes in personality and mood, including depression and anxiety, hallucinations, delusions and excessive daytime sleepiness; however lack of these symptoms does not exclude the diagnosis of dementia. Validation of these diagnostic criteria remains to be demonstrated, requiring prospective, longitudinal studies.

An additional problem lies in the selection of appropriate instruments to measure the cognitive changes. In general, studies using standardised neuropsychological tests have reported the highest prevalence rates for dementia, those based on brief screening tests such as the Mini-Mental State Examination (M. Folstein, S. Folstein and McHugh 1975) have found somewhat lower rates and nonstandardised clinical examination has yielded the lowest estimates of dementia in PD (Cummings 1988).

It is likely that various neuropsychological test batteries focus on different types of cognitive dysfunction and may not be sufficiently sensitive to the types of deficits prominent in PD. In particular, the so-called "frontal" deficits which appear to dominate the neuropsychological picture may not be accessible to many of the traditional assessment procedures for dementia, which tend to be focused on memory and language deficits. For these reasons batteries especially designed for specific purposes, such as the Scales for Outcomes of Parkinson's Disease-Cognition (SCOPA-COG) (Kulisevsky and Pagonabarraga 2009), the Parkinson Neuropsychometric Dementia Assessment (PANDA) instrument (Kalbe et al. 2008), the Parkinson's Disease Cognitive Rating scale (PD-CRS) (Pagonabarraga et al. 2008) or those with well established psychometric properties, which have been shown to be sensitive to the cognitive impairments of PD, such as the Cambridge Neuropsychological Test Automated Battery (CANTAB) (Robbins et al. 1994; Sahakian and Owen 1992) and the Cambridge Cognitive Examination (CAMCOG) (Hobson and Meara 1999) may be preferable as diagnostic instruments.

Even more challenging is the criterion requiring that the origins of any difficulties with the instrumental activities of daily living should be determined, by attributing their source to either the physical or cognitive impairment in PD. This is essentially a problem of symptom overlap similar to that discussed for the occurrence of depressive symptoms in PD and shares many of the dilemmas raised in chapter 3.

4.5 Risk factors for dementia in PD

A range of demographic and clinical factors have been investigated as potential risk factors for dementia in PD. The factors that have emerged most consistently are the severity of the clinical symptoms, disease duration, patient age and the existence of mild cognitive impairment earlier in the disease process.

4.5.1 Motor symptoms and dementia in PD

An obvious line of enquiry has been to try to draw out any potential associations between the motor symptoms of PD and the occurrence of dementia. Higher risk for dementia has been reported in parallel with increased severity of clinical symptoms and more advanced PD (Aarsland et al. 1996; Levy et al. 2000). Studies have also suggested that neuropsychological test performance is significantly worse in patients in whom the rigid-akinetic form of the motor disability predominates (Ebmeier et al. 1990; Garron, Klawans and Narin 1972; Huber, Paulson and Shuttleworth 1988; Martilla and Rinne 1976); rigidity, postural instability and gait disturbance (PIGD) are reported to predict faster cognitive decline and more rapid onset of dementia. Tremor-dominant forms often evolve into the PIGD form. Recent studies have shown that in virtually all cases, dementia was preceded by the PIGD dominant form or by cases which had evolved from the tremor dominant to the PIGD type of PD, independently of age (Alves et al. 2006; Williams-Gray et al. 2007).

However, the association between rigidity and akinesia and dementia has not been universally sustained (Janvin 2006; Ogden, Growdon and Corkin 1990; Sahakian et al. 1988); for example, speech and axial impairments which are indicative of non-dopaminergic deficiencies have been found to predict incident dementia, whereas rigidity and akinesia did not (Levy et al. 2000). Atypical neurological features for idiopathic PD, such as early occurrence of autonomic failure, symmetrical disease presentation and only moderate response to L-dopa is also known to be associated with a higher rate and more severe symptoms of dementia (Aarsland et al. 1996).

One reason for the lack of consistency in demonstrating any relationships between motor and cognitive symptoms may be due to the possibility that cognitive deficits are quantitatively and qualitatively different at various stages of the disease process. Thus an association between the degree of bradykinesia and visuospatial deficits has been reported (Mortimer et al. 1982) and Taylor, Saint-Cyr and Lang (1986) found a correlation between the severity of the physical symptoms and neuropsychological performance. The alleged relationship, if it exists, is unlikely to be a simple one, since patients can fluctuate between extremes of motor disability, whilst aspects of cognitive function remain unaffected (Brown and Marsden 1984).

Although methodological differences make it difficult to draw comparisons between studies, deterioration of executive functions in PD appears to progress in parallel with motor degeneration (see Owen 2004 for discussion). Thus non-medicated patients in the early stages of the disease process, when clinical symptoms are relatively mild, have been shown to be unimpaired on a test of spatial working memory (e.g. Morris, Downes et al. 1988; Owen et al. 1992), whilst medicated patients, and in particular those with severe clinical symptoms, are frequently impaired (Owen et al. 1992). There is also evidence that some components of executive function may be affected before others i.e. spatial working memory appears to deteriorate before verbal and visual working memory. Although this may indicate that spatial processing is disproportionately affected in PD, it may also mean that spatial tasks differ with respect to others in terms of their underlying executive requirements (Owen 2004).

4.5.2 Patient's age

As is true for dementias in general, increasing age is one of the most consistently reported risk factors for dementia in PD (e.g. Stern, Marder et al. 1993; Aarsland et al. 1996). Older age at onset of the disease and duration of illness are also frequently implicated (Aarsland et al. 1996). However, age, duration of disease and age at onset are highly correlated in patient samples and it is difficult to separate their relative importance in contributing to dementia (Aarsland et al. 1996; Aarsland and Kurz 2010). One study has suggested that the key factor is age *per se* (see Aarsland, Kvaloy et al. 2007). Evidence of this kind has led some authors to argue that ageing plays an important role in the pathological processes in PD, interacting with the disease process and producing impairment in non-dopaminergic structures (Levy 2007).

4.5.3 Mild cognitive impairments

It is now well established that mild cognitive impairments (MCI) frequently accompany PD, even in the early stages of the disease and affect cognitive functioning in a variety of subtle ways (Foltynie et al. 2004; Janvin et al. 2003; Jellinger 2013; Levy, Tang, Louis et al. 2002; Levin and Katzen 2005; Muslimovic et al. 2005; Weintraub, Moberg, Culbertson et al. 2004). Selective deficits in the area of memory and executive functioning (Levy, Jacobs et al. 2002; Janvin, Aarsland and Larsen 2005) as well as MCI more generally (Janvin et al. 2006; Jellinger 2013) are associated with a higher risk of developing dementia than for patients without cognitive deficits. MCI, as with the risk for dementia, have been associated with severity of motor symptoms and higher levels of rigidity and akinesia (Janvin et al. 2003).

There is considerable heterogeneity in the range of cognitive deficits seen in PD and this is discussed below in greater detail. In particular, a characteristic executive-visuospatial impairment has been distinguished, which appears to be related to fronto-striatal dopamine depletion, along with a more memory specific impairment, which is thought to be related to posterior cortical dysfunction. There is some evidence that the different cognitive profiles are differentially associated with the risk of developing dementia (Janvin et al. 2006); those patients with primarily executive failures appear relatively protected (Williams-Gray et al. 2007), whilst those with deficits in posterior cortical functions, such as semantic fluency and visuoconstructional abilities, are at greater risk of dementia (Williams-Gray et al. 2012). This evidence from the CamPaIGN study is reinforced by a differential genetic pattern associated with the proposed clinical phenotypes. Specifically, the tau (MAPT H1/H1) genotype is linked to the posterior cortical deficit and an increased risk of dementia, while the COMT genotype is associated with executive impairment but not dementia.

4.5.4 Other risk factors for dementia

Other risk factors for dementia in PD include: low socio-economic status and education (Glatt et al. 1996), depression (Marder et al. 1995; Stern et al. 1993), the development of confusion or psychosis with L-dopa treatment (Stern et al. 1993) and visual hallucinations (Aarsland et al.

2003), the latter being associated with cholinergic deficits and Lewy body pathology in the temporal lobe. Although evidence is beginning to emerge that dementia in PD may be associated with a specific genotype as described in the previous section, the genetic contribution to impaired cognition is still not well understood and despite intensive interest in the genetics of PD over the past decade, this particular aspect has received relatively little attention. Both studies investigating the potential risk for developing dementia in families of people with PD and others exploring specific gene mutations have, as yet, yielded inconclusive results (Aarsland and Kurz 2010). The strongest evidence is in support of the MAPT genotype being predictive of dementia in PD (Williams-Gray et al. 2012).

It has become almost a popular myth, that smoking reduces the risk for PD through having a potentially neuroprotective effect. Since nicotinic receptors are known to have a role in learning and memory, it might be expected that smoking should protect against cognitive decline and dementia in PD. The evidence for this remains controversial (see Aarsland and Kurz 2010).

4.6 Mild cognitive impairment in PD

Although it is now recognised that a significant number of patients with PD follow a progressive cognitive decline into a dementia stage, which is distinguished from other forms of dementia and is termed PD dementia (Emre 2003; Aarsland et al. 2003; Williams-Gray et al. 2007), as in DAT, patients may also experience an interim stage between normal cognitive functioning and dementia, known as mild cognitive impairment (MCI), which may last for a number of years (Adler 2009; Jellinger 2013), and as described above, may herald the development of dementia. The MCI stage however, is clinically indistinguishable from PD without dementia, the latter also being associated with characteristic neuropsychological deficits.

These changes in cognitive functioning are accessible to neuropsychological testing, but may not be severe enough to interfere with activities of daily living or normal social functioning to any significant extent, especially in the early stages of the condition (Bosboom, Stoffers and Wolters 2004; Grujic 2007). For example, Lees and Smith (1983) recognised that during the first few years of the illness, patients may continue to hold down jobs and some may even retain high status positions without having to compromise in terms of the demands that continue to challenge them on a daily basis. They are able to enjoy intellectually challenging leisure activities such as listening to music, appreciate stimulating conversation and continue to write and compose poetry or music, as before the illness.

Any changes in cognitive function may only be apparent to those closest to the patient. They present initially as a slight lack of spontaneity, a tendency to repetition and a perceptible decrease in imaginative and creative thinking. This may be noticeable, as a previously skilled and fluent speaker has evident difficulties in maintaining conversation, for example. Some patients complain of a general tiredness and lethargy, mild forgetfulness and occasionally losing their way in unfamiliar surroundings. Another common symptom is inertia, which often presents as a lack of initiative and a reluctance to participate in previously valued activities and patients may acquire a characteristic placidity, that has been referred to as, "an air of mystical impassivity" (Lees and Smith 1983, 259). These changes are, at this stage, transient and can be overcome with determination on the part of the patient or encouragement from others (Lees and Smith 1983).

It may be, that despite their relative "silence" in functional terms, these neuropsychological symptoms are already beginning to affect the way in which the person with PD is able to manage and cope with the condition. They may also exert an effect on shaping the relationship with the carer, both directly, in the sense that the nature of the deficits makes it difficult for the sufferer to respond to and maintain his/her relationship with the carer with the same understanding and sensitivity as prior to the illness, and indirectly, as a result of his/her diminished ability to cope with, and regulate his/her behaviour. Thus the consequences of losing cognitive skills and flexibility may impinge on the relationship between the carer and the person with PD even relatively early in the disease process. However, because of the subtlety of these effects, it may be difficult for both carers and clinicians alike, to attribute them to the cognitive deficits characteristic of PD. Rather they may be interpreted as deliberate awkwardness and lack of co-operation on the part of the patient, which are frequently characterised by families as "a change in personality" and a "negativism" that was not typical of the patient's former self. Such perceived changes place considerable pressures on the relationship between the carer and the care recipient and may be an important factor in contributing to the strain of care-giving, a theme that is developed in section 4.11 below and formed an important element of the empirical study described later in this volume.

The recognition and assessment of cognitive impairment in PD is complicated by other aspects of the disorder, such as the frozen facial expression which masks any animation or evidence of alertness on the part of the sufferer. Performance on tests, especially those which impose time limitations, is often compromised by slowed cognition (bradyphrenia), fluctuations in attention and loss of motor skills. These difficulties may be compounded by depression and other neuropsychiatric symptoms, making it necessary to decide whether the cognitive deficits are a form of pseudodementia (Bulbena and Berrios 1986; Marder et al. 1995).

4.7 The nature of the neuropsychological deficits in PD

PD is associated with a fairly well-defined pattern of mild intellectual impairment even in the early stages of the disease. There has emerged a consensus that the deficits cluster around three main categories: (1) memory impairments (Warburton 1967b; Flowers et al. 1984; Helkala et al. 1988; Pillon et al. 1993; Sullivan and Sagar 1991; Williams-Gray et al. 2007); (2) visuospatial and constructional impairments (Boller et al. 1984; Bowen, Hoehn and Yahr 1972; Levin et al. 1991; Aarsland et al. 2003) and; (3) impairment of "executive" functions including working memory, planning, concept formation and attentional set-shifting ability (Harrison, Stow and Owen 2002; Owen et al. 1992; Owen, Roberts et al. 1993). Typical patterns of performance for non-demented patients with PD in each of the specific cognitive domains is presented in section 4.7.2. The extent to which these deficits can be understood as arising from disruption to a common underlying mechanism remains unclear and alternative sources of the cognitive heterogeneity in PD are considered next.

4.7.1 Sources of cognitive heterogeneity in PD

A great deal of heterogeneity has been recognised in the cognitive performance associated with PD (Foltynie et al. 2004; Levin and Katzen 2005; Osiejuk-Lojek 1998; Muslimovic et al. 2005) and the reasons for this are not well understood (Harrison et al. 2002). One factor may be that PD is a heterogeneous condition in itself, but since its causes remain largely unknown, grouping patients by aetiology is not possible. The population of patients with PD therefore consists of those with co-existing depression, dementia, other types of co-morbid illness (Parkinson's plus syndromes) and drug-induced cognitive deficits. When patients are sampled irrespective of these coexisting conditions and compared to a matched control group, poorer performance on cognitive tasks is frequently a feature of the PD group. In attempting to gain an insight into cognitive performance in "pure" PD, it might seem appropriate to screen patients carefully in order to remove the potentially confounding effects of the coexisting morbidities mentioned. However, as Harrison et al. (2002) point out, this raises further practical and theoretical problems. On the practical side, screening for such patients is likely to result in small sample sizes, making it difficult to demonstrate any "real" effects and may not be representative of the PD population as a whole. On the theoretical side, as has been argued in the previous chapter, some coexisting morbidity such as depression, or in this case, cognitive impairments may be an integral part of the disease process in PD and excluding such cases from analysis may therefore be unduly restrictive and inappropriate.

4.7.1.1 Comorbid disease

The absence of a diagnostic test for PD means that the condition is diagnosed on the basis of its clinical presentation as discussed in chapter 1, and this means that other disorders in which degeneration of the substantia nigra occurs may also mimic idiopathic PD. These include the Parkinson's plus syndromes such as progressive supranuclear palsy and multiple systems atrophy, as well as brain damage brought about by injury, infection and infarction of the substantia nigra. As a result, idiopathic PD has been shown to be misdiagnosed in up to 25% of cases on post-mortem (Hughes et al. 1992). Furthermore, studies show that Lewy bodies are present in up to 10% of control brains at post-mortem. Finally, it is increasingly considered likely that cognitive changes may occur early in the disease process, even before the so-called cardinal signs of PD are manifest. This brings into question the validity of using allegedly normal elderly controls for comparison, since a proportion of them may have "preclinical" PD along with the associated cognitive changes (Harrison et al. 2002).

4.7.1.2 Depression

As evidenced in chapter 3, the occurrence of depression in PD is relatively high compared to the general population and with respect to other patients with chronic or neurodegenerative disorders. Depression itself is associated with impaired cognitive functioning in both younger (Bulbena and Berrios 1993) and older people (Beats, Sahakian and Levy 1996); indeed, in the elderly, it may present as a specific form of cognitive impairment known as pseudodementia, which is reversible with appropriate pharmacological treatment. The cognitive deficits consequent upon depression affect executive functions such as attentional set-shifting, recognition memory and visuospatial functions (Bulbena and Berrios

1993; Beats et al. 1996) which overlap with the deficits primarily implicated in PD, thus confounding the situation further. Additionally, depression in PD is associated with executive dysfunction (Uekermann et al. 2003).

4.7.1.3 Dementia

As described above, the prevalence of dementia is raised in PD, although there has been considerable disagreement as to its origins. Three distinct positions have been discernible in the literature: the first, attributing the cognitive impairment to the same degenerative processes as in DAT (implying the co-existence of two pathologies); the second, arguing that it arises from the same neuropathological substrate as the motor symptoms, but the intricate connections of the basal ganglia with areas of the frontal cortex mean that neural degeneration in the former gives rise to characteristic patterns of cognitive deficits associated with the latter; and the third, that it is purely a manifestation of subcortical damage. Work carried out over the last two decades at the Unversity of Cambridge has helped to clarify these positions by differentiating the cognitive deficits in terms of their anatomical and neurochemical dependencies, their relationship to each other and to the disease process in PD. It represents a uniquely systematic approach to disentangling the complex pathways in the evolution of cognitive dysfunction in PD, accounting for individual differences, differential responses to pharmacological treatment and proposing a dual syndrome hypothesis, which distinguishes between a more benign course of cognitive dysfunction characterised primarily by executive deficits and more posterior cortical dysfunctions including semantic fluency, memory and visuospatial and constructional deficits which predict dementia in PD (e.g. Harrison, Stow and Owen 2002; Owen et al. 1992; Owen, Roberts et al. 1993; Williams-Gray et al. 2007; 2009; 2012; for discussion see Kehagia, Barker and Robbins 2013).

A long-held position is that DAT is co-morbid with PD, which is not implausible, given the age of the patients and the finding that plaques and tangles, which are pathognomonic for DAT, are often seen in the brains of patients with PD on post-mortem (Compta et al. 2011; Lewy 1923 cited in Förstl and Levy 1991; Förstl 1999). It is also well established that low cerebrospinal fluid levels of β-amyloid and abnormally high levels of tau protein are found in DAT and an argument has been made that these represent biomarkers of DAT-associated pathological brain changes (Tapiola et al. 2009). Similar changes have been detected in patients with PD, both newly diagnosed and in later stages of the disease when cognitive changes are evident, and so it is plausible that there is considerable overlap in the neurodegenerative process between PD dementia and DAT, with the possibility that the two pathological processes may even be synergistic. Moreover it has recently been shown that patterns of brain atrophy associated with DAT are also predictive of long-term cognitive decline in PD, with particular involvement of the hippocampus and parietal-temporal cortex (Weintraub et al. 2012).

Interestingly, these patterns fit with the clinical observations on neuropsychological testing that dementia in PD is associated with deficits in the more posterior cortical functions enumerated above (e.g. Williams-Gray 2012). These cognitive deficits appear to be acetylcholine-dependent, as it has been demonstrated that low doses of scopolamine impaired visual recognition memory in patients with PD, but not in control subjects (Dubois et al. 1987). In addition, the failure of levodopa to eliminate these deficits suggests that non-dopaminergic neurotransmitter systems are involved in PD dementia (Levy et al. 2000). Indeed in vivo imaging studies have confirmed cholinergic deficits in the cerebral cortex of patients with PD dementia and there is preliminary evidence to suggest that cholinesterase inhibitors may help to alleviate the symptoms of dementia in PD (Emre 2004).

However, a major obstacle for the theory that cognitive deficits in PD are caused by the same underlying neuropathology as in DAT has been the long established observation that the profile of cognitive deficits is different for the two disorders (Emre 2004), PD dementia being similar (some researchers claim virtually identical) to dementia with Lewy bodies (Galvin, Pollack and Morris 2006). A further complication is that while PD dementia is associated with diffuse limbic and neocortical Lewy body pathology (Aarsland, Perry et al. 2005), not all patients qualifying for a pathological diagnosis of Lewy body dementia are clinically demented (Emre 2004), but this is also true with regard to DAT pathology (Galvin et al. 2006).

In providing evidence for a dual syndrome hypothesis of the cognitive impairment in PD, the work from the Cambridge Department of Psychology (Kehagia et al. 2013) has extricated the field from some long-standing and major disagreements. In essence, it suggests that the dementia syndrome in PD presents with distinctive prodromal visuospatial deficits associated with more posterior cortical impairment, cholinergic neurotransmitter systems and tau protein pathology. On the other hand, there also exists a more benign form of cognitive dysfunction in PD characterised by deficits in executive functions and linked to dopamine-dependent fronto-striatal dysfunction. This distinct syndrome of cognitive impairment provides support for the second of the aetiological positions described above, but emphasising that a clearly defined pattern of "frontal" dysfunction is consistent with a disease process sharing the same underlying pathology as the motor and autonomic symptoms of PD. A position therefore seems to be emerging that dementia in PD may be caused either by DAT-type pathology or by Lewy body pathology which is indistinguishable from Lewy body dementia (Galvin et al. 2006), whereas typical PD-related pathology gives rise to milder cognitive impairments of an executive nature.

In the light of these findings, the third position positing the idea of a specifically subcortical dementia in PD (Cummings and Benson 1988) now seems oversimplified, but some authors continue to believe that there is sufficient evidence to support the view that subcortical pathology alone may be a sufficient cause of dementia in some patients with PD (Galvin et al. 2006; Hughes et al. 1993).

4.7.1.4 Drug induced cognitive changes in PD

Two main pharmacological agents are used in the treatment of PD: anticholinergic drugs and L-dopa combinations. Anticholinergic medication is reputedly efficacious in the management of tremor, but has been shown to have seriously undesirable side-effects in compromising cognitive functions, in particulary memory (Campbell et al. 2009; Koller 1984; Miller et al. 1987; Sadeh, Braham and Modan 1982; Syndulko et al. 1982) and other cognitive skills that are dependent on cholinergic neurotransmitter systems (De Smet et al. 1982; Dubois et al. 1990). As a result, anticholinergic medication, such as benzhexol (Artane) has largely been relegated in favour of preparations that supply dopamine precursors in the form of L-dopa or boost the availability of endogenous dopamine.

Nevertheless, potentially damaging effects on intellectual function were also claimed in respect of L-dopa, soon after its introduction in the treatment of PD (e.g. Barbeau 1971; Barbeau, Mars and Gillo-Joffroy 1971; Botez and Barbeau 1973; Sacks et al. 1972; Wolf and Davis 1973). These findings were in marked contrast to results published by other authors, who demonstrated improved cognitive functions following L-dopa therapy (e.g. Beardsley and Puletti 1971; Drachman and Stahl 1975; Loranger et al. 1972; Meier and Martin 1970). Yet others concluded that administration of L-dopa did not affect cognitive performance in PD (e.g. Markham, Treciokas and Diamond 1974).

Steps toward resolving these conflicting early findings with regard to dopamine supplementation have been taken in recent years and it has been demonstrated that the position is far from simple. Drug effects on cognitive function seem to depend on what have been termed "initial conditions" and studies with healthy volunteers have shown, that those with worse memory performance at the outset (before taking the drug) benefit most. However, the same dopamine enhancing drugs appear to worsen performance in healthy people who demonstrate optimal levels of performance at the outset (see Cools and Robbins 2004 for discussion). Thus administration of a dopaminergic receptor agonist (which produces similar effects to natural dopamine) enhances performance on complex tasks of cognitive functioning, only in those subjects who demonstrate poor baseline memory performance, having harmful effects when baseline performance is normal. Research evidence seems to indicate that the differences in baseline activity on cognitive functions may reflect quantitative variations in neurotransmitter function in individuals.

Dopamine is known to be critical for optimal performance on certain cognitive tasks, including working memory, future planning and cognitive flexibility. It appears that a complex "inverted U-shaped" relationship exists between cognitive performance and dopamine, such that not only insufficient, but also excessive levels impair working memory performance. In animal studies, the impairments following administration of dopamine enhancing drugs have been characterised as perseverative, suggesting that a "frontal-type" of deficit has been evoked. These interactions are highly complex as it appears that different types of cognitive processing, may require different optimal levels of dopamine. For example, optimal cognitive functioning requires information to be maintained continually within the cognitive system (i.e. the process of attention), but also requires a flexible updating process, responsive to novel task-relevant information. Complex cognitive tasks which require attentional flexibility appear to be particularly sensitive to the detrimental effects of excessive dopamine receptor stimulation in the prefrontal cortical area, although there is a suggestion that updating tasks may benefit. These cognitive processes are thus likely to require finely tuned maintenance, which is dependent on precisely balanced neurotransmission within the prefrontal cortex and basal ganglia, perhaps based on alternative modes of tonic versus phasic dopamine function (Cools and Robbins 2004). Such highly sophisticated mechanisms cannot, in the light of our present knowledge, be mimicked in the administration of dopaminergic replacement therapy for the relief of symptoms in PD. Although it is now recognised that L-dopa may relieve some of the cognitive impairments seen in PD (Lange et al. 1992; Moustafa, Herzallah and Gluck 2013), it is reasonable to expect, that like dopamine enhancing drugs in healthy volunteers, it may also bring about detrimental effects in other types of cognitive functions (Gotham, Brown and Marsden 1988).

The depletion of dopamine in PD does not affect all the nuclei of the basal ganglia in a uniform fashion, but follows a distinct progression starting, in the early stages of the disease, with the more dorsal parts of the striatum, later moving on to the more ventral parts. The dorsal and ventral striatum are strongly connected to the dorsal and ventral parts of the prefrontal cortex respectively in segregated fronto-striatal circuits (Alexander, DeLong and Strick 1986). Gotham et al. (1988) suggested that doses of medication necessary to relieve symptoms caused by severe depletions of dopamine in those brain areas already affected may bring about "overdose" effects in other brain areas where dopamine levels remain relatively normal. This hypothesis was later confirmed by a number of studies which demonstrated that medicated patients were indeed impaired on cognitive tasks supposedly subserved by the ventral striatum and ventral prefrontal cortex. Similarly contrasting effects on cognitive tasks associated with distinct fronto-striatal circuitry were found in studies employing controlled L-dopa withdrawal procedures (Cools et al. 2001, 2003). For example, L-dopa was shown to be associated with abnormally fast (impulsive) responses on a gambling task associated with the ventral prefrontal cortex, whilst at the same time alleviating the deficit in a task-switching paradigm, requiring patients to switch rapidly between two well-learnt tasks: letter naming and number naming. It appears therefore, that L-dopa may improve or impair mental flexibility, depending on the nature of the cognitive task and whether or not the brain area sustaining the task has been depleted of dopamine (Cools and Robbins 2004). It is thus reasonable to expect that, especially in the early stages of PD, it may have detrimental effects on cognitive functioning in some patients and that these effects may be difficult to predict as they appear to be dependent on patterns of dopamine loss in individual cases. This may also help to explain some of the heterogeneity seen in the cognitive dysfunctions associated with PD.

4.7.2 Profile of cognitive deficits in PD

As described above, the possibility that PD may consist of subtypes characterized by specific cognitive profiles is beginning to emerge. It has been proposed that within the MCI of PD, three distinct subtypes can be identified, based on explicit criteria associated with the domains of cognitive dysfunction described above (Janvin 2006). The first of these is an amnestic type, the second is one in which multiple domains of cognitive functioning are minimally affected and the third corresponds to an executive subtype. The latter is most commonly observed in PD and is likely to be associated with fronto-subcortical changes, whereas in the other two, cortical and hippocampal changes are more important. The division into these subtypes of cognitive impairment needs to be verified in PD and clinic-pathological studies are needed to explore how the neuropsychological profiles might be related to specific brain changes. Nonetheless this classification provides a potential path towards understanding the puzzling heterogeneity in cognitive functioning that has been observed for a long time and would have important implications for clinical practice. The following discussion starts with a brief consideration of language deficits and apraxia, which are widely considered to be mainly of cortical origin and relatively spared in PD. There then follows a description of the cognitive deficits that are highly characteristic of PD, namely memory, visuospatial and executive function impairments, which broadly speaking, are the constituents of the cognitive subtypes described by Janvin (2006).

4.7.2.1 Language deficits

Motor aspects of speech disturbances, such as dysarthria, are well recognised in PD (e.g. Cummings et al. 1988) and are particularly problematic from a psychosocial point of view as they interfere with normal communication and cause the patient a great deal of embarrassment and frustration (Miller et al. 2008). However, higher level language functions in the form of fully-developed aphasic syndromes do not appear to be part of the symptom profile in PD (Cummings et al. 1988; Levin and Katzen 1995). Indeed, the absence of aphasia has been considered to be a key criterion for defining the cognitive impairment seen in PD in terms of a subcortical dementia (Cummings and Benson 1992).

Nevertheless changes in both the syntactic and semantic aspects of language reception and production have been reported. For example, patients with PD without dementia have difficulties in comprehending more complex syntax and their spontaneous language output is syntactically simplified and the flow of speech interrupted, with longer pauses than normal. Aphasic symptoms are more pronounced in PD patients with dementia (Cummings et al. 1988; Galvin et al. 2006). However, some authors have argued that these changes are not reflective of a true language impairment, but are the result of attentional, executive and memory dysfunction (e.g. Bondi and Troster 1997).

Verbal fluency tasks have been the subject of much attention in PD; in the early literature they were interpreted in the context of language deficits (see Bondi and Troster 1997), but with increased theoretical refinement, a distinction has been made between phonemic and semantic verbal fluency, with PD patients being more impaired on the latter and implying that temporal lobe pathology might underlie the observed deficits (Henry and Crawford 2004). Performance on tasks of phonemic verbal fluency, on the other hand, is regarded as a reflection of "frontal-lobe" or executive function (e.g. Birn et al. 2010) and is discussed below in the section on the frontal-executive theory of cognitive deficits in PD.

Research related to visual confrontation naming in PD has generated widely discrepant findings. Some studies have reported mild naming difficulties even at the early stages of the disease (Globus, Mildworf and Melamed 1985), whilst others have found no deficits in this regard (Freedman et al. 1984; Levin, Llabre and Weiner 1989). One possibility is that as the severity of cognitive impairment in PD increases as the disease progresses, the likelihood of dysnomia rises accordingly (Cummings et al. 1988; Troster et al. 1996).

Performance on traditional vocabulary tests is less controversial and appears to be well preserved in PD (Huber et al. 1986; Matison et al. 1982; Loranger et al. 1972; Pirozzolo et al. 1982; Troster et al. 1996) as is general intelligence (I.Q.; Randolph, Mohr and Chase 1993; Troster et al. 1996). Patients with naming difficulties, however, are more likely to show poorer performance on vocabulary tests (Beatty and Monson 1989).

4.7.2.2 Apraxia

Few studies have examined apraxia in PD, which is generally considered to be of cortical rather than sub-cortical origin. Here too however, the evidence is inconsistent. Lees and Smith (1983) found no evidence of apraxia in PD patients, but others have raised the possibility of ideomotor (Goldenberg et al. 1986) and representational problems (Grossman et al. 1991) which are difficult to interpret in the light of current knowledge about the condition.

4.7.2.3 Memory impairment

Problems with memory are among the most consistently reported cognitive dysfunctions in PD. The specific profile of deficits in PD is thought to distinguish performance from that of DAT and to reflect a "frontal-lobe" type of memory impairment. It is characterised by poor free recall performance, with relatively better recognition. Semantic cueing or probing has been shown to remediate difficulties in immediate or delayed recall (Pillon et al. 1993), suggesting that the memory problems in PD may be due to a retrieval deficit (Aarsland et al. 2003; Jacobs et al. 1995; Stern, Richards et al. 1993). This is in contrast to DAT, where memory problems are considered to be due to deficiencies in encoding (Helkala et al. 1988; Kramer et al. 1989; Massman et al. 1990).

However, more recently it has been shown that a substantial subgroup of patients with PD demonstrate difficulties with both recall and recognition, a pattern that is typical for patients with DAT (Weintraub, Moberg, Culbertson et al. 2004). This has been interpreted as indicating that memory deficits in a significant proportion of patients with PD may be due to the same underlying pathology as in DAT, rekindling the approach taken by Boller et al. (1980). It is supported by the finding that hippocampal pathology is common in PD (Junqué et al. 2005; Tam et al. 2005). These patients may constitute the amnestic subtype proposed by Janvin (2006).

4.7.2.4 Remote memory

Memory for remote events is very difficult to test objectively, but a number of batteries have been developed in order to provide a reliable and valid procedure for examining memory for famous people or public events from the past. One of the best known of these was developed by Albert, Butters and Levin (1979) and required recall and recognition of information relating to famous individuals and events over the decades between the 1920s and the 1970s. A retrograde amnesia only became apparent in PD when decline in cognitive functioning overall had become severe and well established (Freedman et al. 1984; Huber, Shuttleworth and Paulson 1986). However, no temporal gradient was found for the information. This is in contrast to patients with DAT (Loranger et al. 1972), whose performance shows relative sparing of more distant events (Beatty 1994). Temporal gradients of this kind have been used to make inferences about the nature of the memory deficit in neurodegenerative disorders. For example, the sparing of remote memory in DAT has been interpreted in favour of an acquisition view of memory failure; this view contends that since old events can still be retrieved normally, the memory problem must be one with encoding or acquiring the information in the first place. For PD patients whose impairment appears to be the same across all decades, this would imply that the information had been normally encoded, but could not be retrieved as previously.

4.7.2.5 Explicit memory

Explicit or declarative memory is the type of memory assessed by traditional, clinical tests of recall and recognition. A distinction is made between episodic and semantic memory (Tulving 1983), based on the type of information stored. Episodic memory consists of information related to events in a person's life, set in a particular context defined in terms of time and place, whose retrieval depends on spatial and temporal cues. Semantic memory on the other hand, refers to information that is knowledge-based, context free and usually over-learned (Bondi and Troster 1997). These types of memory are discussed next in relation to PD.

4.7.2.6 Episodic memory

Until quite recently, the pattern of performance on tests of episodic memory in patients with PD appeared to have been established with remarkable consensus, even though the mechanisms underlying the deficits in memory and possible anatomical substrates for these impairments continued to be inadequately understood. It was generally agreed that patients with PD exhibited poorer performance on clinical tests of memory for word lists, prose passages, paired associates and pictorial designs, especially when the method used for testing retention was that of free recall (e.g. Lee et al. 2005; Loranger et al. 1972; Weingartner et al. 1984). However, the notion that recognition memory was preserved in PD was widely prevalent (e.g. Beatty, Monson and Goodkin 1989; Bondi and Kaszniak 1991; Breen 1993; Buytenhuijs et al. 1994; Cohen et al. 1994; Flowers et al. 1984; Helkala et al. 1988; Huber et al. 1986; Lees and Smith 1983; Levin et al. 1989; Mohr et al. 1990; Pillon et al. 1993; Taylor, Saint-Cyr and Lang 1986; Tsai et al. 1994). The inconsistency reflected in free recall and recognition paradigms led researchers to evaluate the possibility that other types of cognitive functioning, such as arousal, motivation or attention may have supported performance on these tests (Flowers et al. 1984; Wilson et al. 1980). Recognition memory may have appeared more robust simply because it required far less cognitive processing and so was less sensitive to deficits in other areas of cognitive functioning. Indeed, numerous studies have since demonstrated that recognition memory does not seem to be selectively spared in PD (e.g. Davidson et al. 2006; Sahakian et al. 1998) and this has been corroborated by a meta-analysis of studies on recognition in the disorder (Whittington, Podd and Kan 2000).

Equally, the recognition of events in remote memory was found to be relatively intact in PD, although PD patients had difficulty in dating the events, independently of the overall severity of their cognitive impairment

(Sagar et al. 1988). These authors suggested that the deficiencies in remote memory in PD might point to specific difficulties, such as temporal sequencing or recency discrimination, rather than to a retrieval deficit *per se*. Similar findings have been reported more recently, suggesting that failures in recognition memory are primarily due to an impairment of familiarity, i.e. a sense of *knowing* that something has been previously encountered (Tulving, 1983; for a review see Gardiner and Richardson-Klavehn 2000), rather than deficits in recollection (Davidson et al. 2006).

These early studies are significant in so far as they heralded developments in the cognitive neurosciences which led to a somewhat different concept of memory; one which recognised the complexity of the processes involved, in what had hitherto been viewed as a somewhat isolated and localised function. Research into PD has in no small part contributed to our current understanding of memory as being dependent on multiple interconnected processes which are supported by various neurocognitive circuits that can be disrupted by different types of brain pathology. According to these conceptualisations, different patterns of disruption to memory processes may arise as the result of disconnections between brain areas that have not traditionally been associated with supporting memory *per se*. In particular, many of the memory deficits in PD have come to be associated with disorder of executive functioning and thus with so-called "frontal lobe" dysfunctions (Robbins, Owen and Sahakian 1999).

4.7.2.7 Semantic memory

Semantic memory is usually assessed using the Vocabulary and Information subtests of the Wechsler Adult Intelligence Scale (WAIS; Wechsler 2008) which require oral responses in terms of word definitions and answers to general knowledge questions; verbal fluency tests using both letter and category cues; and visual confrontation naming tests.

Patients with PD, especially in the early stages of the disease, have been typically reported to fall within the normal range on the WAIS Vocabulary subtest (Huber et al. 1986; Matison et al. 1982; Pirozzolo et al. 1982; Troster et al. 1996). Performance with regard to general knowledge, however, has yielded more discrepant results: Pirozzolo et al. (1982) have reported impaired performance in PD on the WAIS Information subtest, whereas others have not observed deviations from the norm in PD patients (Randolph et al. 1993; Troster et al. 1996).

Findings in relation to verbal fluency are discussed in more detail below in the section on the frontal-executive theory of cognitive deficits in

PD. However, as already mentioned, there appears to be a dissociation between phonemic and semantic fluency, with PD patients being more impaired on the latter. Deficits in phonemic fluency are considered to be related to set-shifting abilities, reflecting impairments in executive functions (Robbins et al. 1999). Semantic or categorical deficits on the other hand may reflect difficulties in semantic memory and it is thought that temporal lobe pathology is more likely to underlie the observed deficits (Henry and Crawford 2004).

As mentioned above, visual confrontation naming has yielded inconsistent results in PD. A qualitative analysis of the error types and effects of cueing on semantic memory has shown that semantic errors predominate and that PD patients derived significant benefit from phonemic cues (Matison et al. 1982). This provides further support for the view that semantic memory deficits in PD are the result of retrieval rather than encoding failures and that the structure of semantic memory remains intact in these patients (Bondi and Troster 1997).

It also appears that there may be a subgroup of non-demented PD patients with naming difficulties, who also perform poorly on vocabulary (Beatty and Monson 1989); these findings have implications for supposing that PD patients may be classified into subtypes on the basis of their cognitive profile.

4.7.2.8 Implicit memory

Implicit memory refers to the ability to use information, of which the person is not consciously aware and explicitly denies knowledge of having (if asked), in guiding the performance of a task. Examples of implicit memory are classical conditioning, lexical and semantic priming and learning of motor and perceptual skills, the latter being an example of procedural memory, i.e. of "how" to do something (Schacter 1987; Squire 1987). In this kind of learning, performance is facilitated by exposure to the task and the individual does not have to retain a conscious or explicit memory for the stimulus materials or the occasion on which they were seen.

Implicit memory, as measured on tasks of priming, (e.g. Bondi and Kaszniak 1991) is preserved in both Huntington's disease and PD. Early views which considered these neurodegenerative disorders to be primarily the result of subcortical pathology, in contrast to the mainly cortical damage associated with DAT, emphasised the preservation of performance on implicit memory tasks in the former with respect to the latter (e.g. Bondi and Kaszniak 1991; Shimamura et al. 1987). Evidence of this kind was recruited in favour of the distinction between cortical and subcortical dementias, suggesting that they could be differentiated on the basis of neuropsychological test performance on such tasks (Bondi, Salmon and Butters 1994; Salmon and Butters 1995). However, another kind of implicit memory, namely skill learning or procedural memory has failed to give a consistent pattern in PD (see Salmon and Butters 1995 for a review). Patients with PD without dementia are unimpaired in some skill learning tasks such as reading in mirror reversal (Bondi and Kaszniak 1991; Harrington et al. 1990) and pursuit rotor learning (Bondi and Kaszniak 1991; Heindel et al. 1989), but may demonstrate impairments in tasks such as the Tower of London (Saint-Cyr, Taylor and Lang 1988; Owen et al. 1992), the skill learning component of the fragmented pictures task (Bondi and Kaszniak 1991) and on pursuit rotor tracking if learning is spread out across consecutive days, possibly as a result of greater susceptibility to the effects of interference from other motors tasks when learning practice is distributed (Harrington et al. 1990). An important determinant of PD patients' performance on these tasks has been shown to be due to difficulties with set-shifting; tasks such as pursuit rotor learning or mirror reversal reading involve a high level of predictability and thus do not result in impaired procedural learning. But when predictability is low, or shifts in the predictive value of information occur, PD patients demonstrate procedural performance deficits (Kaszniak et al. 1992). The difficulties in set-shifting which purportedly lie at the heart of these impairments and are considered to be secondary to an executive impairment, were found to correlate with performance on the Wisconsin Card Sorting Test (Hart et al. 1988), adding weight to the hypothesis (discussed below) that these deficits arise from a common dysfunction affecting the neuronal loops linking the basal ganglia with the prefrontal cortex (De Long, Georgeopoulos and Crutcher 1983).

4.7.2.9 Visuospatial memory

Visual memory is frequently impaired in PD (Loranger et al. 1972; Mortimer et al. 1982; Owen et al. 1993; Sahakian et al. 1988, although this is not an invariable finding (Flowers et al. 1984). An important early study by Sahakian et al. (1988) showed that medicated patients with PD in advanced stages of the disease were impaired on tasks of visual pattern and spatial recognition memory, whereas unmedicated patients, mildly affected by the condition were not. Both groups however, were impaired on a visuospatial paired associate learning task. This has proved to be a significant finding, because the latter task has more recently been found to be predictive of DAT in non-PD patients with mild cognitive deficits (Blackwell et al. 2004). Research also showed that brief, temporary withdrawal of L-dopa medication had no effect on PD patients' performance on tests of visual pattern and spatial recognition memory, visuospatial associative learning and simultaneous and visual delayed-matching-to-sample tasks, suggesting that the underlying functions were not sensitive to dopamine (Lange et al. 1992). In keeping with this, Owen et al. (1993) using the same tests, failed to find differences between patients with PD who were on low doses of dopaminergic replacement therapy and those who remained free of medication; only those with more advanced disease and taking medication showed deficits on these tasks. It thus appears that visuospatial memory deficits in PD are non-dopamine dependent (unlike spatial working memory; see section 4.7.3.5 below). It is thought that they are more likely to reflect cholinergic deficits in frontal and temporal cortex arising from pathology in the basal forebrain cholinergic nuclei and ascending pathways to these cortical areas, which are established early in the disease process in PD (Dubois et al. 1983).

Reviewing their input into this field of research over the last two decades, Kehagia et al. (2013) propose that the presence of visuospatial memory deficits represents a prodromal phase in the descent towards dementia in PD and is associated with depletion in cholinergic neurotransmitter systems. Visuospatial memory deficits are thus thought to be part of a distinct pattern of cognitive impairment in PD, specifically associated with dementia (Kehagia et al. 2013).

4.7.2.10 Visuospatial abilities

Although the universality of visuospatial impairment in PD was contested in the early literature (Brown and Marsen 1986) there followed a general consensus eventually agreeing that such deficits are consistently seen (e.g. Bentin, Silverberg and Gordon 1981; Montse et al. 2001; Passafiume, Boller and Keefe 1986; Pillon et al. 1991), even when motor involvement remains minimal (Hovestadt, De Jong and Meerwaldt 1987). To some extent, the deficits in question may not have been sufficiently distinguished from the visuospatial memory impairments described above and it remains to be determined whether the same patterns apply in relation to pharmacological manipulations and disease stage, and hence to the underlying neurotransmitter systems that support these functions.

4.7.2.11 Bradyphrenia

Bradyphrenia or a slowing of mental processes was considered by some investigators to be characteristic of cognitive performance in PD (Cooper et al. 1994; Mayeux et al. 1987), although this view was never universally endorsed. Some authors suggested that reductions in the speed of mental processing were not a feature of PD *per se*, but attributable to the depression and dementia suffered by some patients in unselected samples (Smith et al. 1998). More recent research, suggests that mental slowing, possibly secondary to attentional problems, may, in fact, be symptomatic in patients with Lewy body associated dementia (Janvin 2006).

4.7.3 The frontal-executive theory of cognitive deficits in PD

Early work investigating the nature of the cognitive impairment in PD focused on memory and visuospatial deficits. As described above, it consistently revealed that memory performance was characterised by impaired free recall, but relatively normal recognition and this has come to be recognised as the typical profile of memory impairment in PD (Beatty et al. 1989; Huber et al. 1986; Levin et al. 1989; Moss et al. 1986; Pillon et al. 1993; Talland 1962; Taylor, Saint-Cyr and Lang 1990; Weingartner et al. 1984). Patients with PD were also found to have difficulties with certain types of tests of short-term memory, exemplified by the Brown-Peterson test (Cooper et al. 1991; Sagar et al. 1988) and in tests of spatial working memory (Beato et al. 2008; Owen et al. 1997). This pattern of deficits in memory has been related to so-called "frontal-lobe" or executive dysfunctions (Robbins et al. 1999). The visuospatial impairment seen in PD is also thought to be attributable to frontal-executive dysfunction in addition to deficits in temporal and parietal cortices (Janvin 2006).

Our understanding of the contribution of the basal ganglia to cognitive function has been uniquely shaped by the work of Professor Trevor Robbins and his team at the University of Cambridge who have helped to define the contribution of these subcortical structures to the executive processes supported by the prefrontal cortex. This intellectually systematic approach, unprecedented in its ingenuity in terms of disentangling the component functions of neuropsychological tests, forms the basis for the following discussion.

4.7.3.1 Executive functions

Impairment of executive functions (defined as the ability to plan, organise and regulate goal-directed behaviour) is recognised in PD (Litvan et al. 1991; Pillon et al. 1993; Pillon et al. 1986) and is now thought to constitute the core feature of neuropsychological dysfunction in non-demented patients with PD (Kehagia et al. 2013). The term refers to impairment in concept formation and rule finding, problem solving, set elaboration and planning, set-shifting and set maintenance. These impairments are similar, but not identical (Owen et al. 1993) to those seen in patients with frontal lesions and are thought to represent a dysfunction of the fronto-striatal neuronal circuitry (Rogers et al. 1998; Rowe et al. 2002).

Executive function is a broad term used to describe a range of cognitive processes involved in the realisation of goal-directed, adaptive behaviour in response to new and challenging environmental situations. These processes represent cognitive mechanisms which are mobilised in order to optimise performance in situations that require a number of different mental operations to be carried out simultaneously (Baddeley 1986). Executive functioning is typically required for willed actions, when sequences of responses must be generated and novel plans of action formulated and then carried out, as in the pursuit of a long-term goal which requires that numerous sub-goals be met with appropriately targeted behaviours (Owen 2004). A variety of cognitive functions are under this kind of executive control, including directing attention to relevant stimuli and inhibiting irrelevant stimuli and responses, switching attention between different processes, coding and checking the contents of memory stores, initiation of activities, monitoring and feedback utilization, concept formation, abstract reasoning and planning (Bondi and Troster 1997; Grahn, Parkinson and Owen 2008; Smith and Jonides 1999). It has long been recognised that the frontal lobes play an important role in executive functioning.

A dysexecutive syndrome entailing circumscribed deficits in tasks which are thought to be sensitive to the integrity of the frontal lobes is held to be at the centre of the cognitive dysfunction observed in PD (Cools et al. 1984; Lees and Smith 1983; Owen 2004; Rogers et al. 1998; Rowe et al. 2002; Taylor, Saint-Cyr and Lang 1986), and often one of the earliest signs of cognitive failure heralding the disorder (Dubois and Pillon 1997). However, despite the apparent agreement in using the notion of a dysexecutive syndrome to encapsulate the cognitive dysfunction in PD, a note of caution needs to be added. There is some research evidence to show that a similar pattern of deficits may be observed in patients with damage to brain regions other than the frontal lobes (Morris, Downes and Robbins 1990) thus challenging the view that the prefrontal cortex is the "seat" of executive functioning. Even more damaging from the theoretical point of view is a challenge to the concept of a central executive (Stuss and Alexander 2008) and without a central executive, there can obviously be no dysexecutive syndrome.

4.7.3.2 Attentional deficits

Performance on simple attentional tasks, such as digit span, is not affected in PD (Huber, Freidenberg et al. 1989; Lees and Smith 1983; Pillon et al. 1986). The evidence with regard to more complex attentional tasks however, is more equivocal. Cognitive slowness or bradyphrenia has been demonstrated in information processing by some authors (e.g. Wilson et al. 1980) but not others (e.g. Rafal et al. 1984), which raised the possibility that bradyphrenia may not be associated with the dopaminergic deficit in PD (see Pirozzolo et al. 1993 for a discussion). However, later work was to show that demonstration of the existence of many of the cognitive deficits in PD appears to be related to a number of factors such as, disease stage, whether or not the patients are receiving medication (some cognitive deficits are responsive to treatment with L-dopa) and to the investigator's ingenuity in isolating quite subtle deficits in the complex tasks used for assessment (see Robbins et al. 1999). For example, on complex executive tasks requiring the internal allocation of attentional resources, patients with PD have been found to demonstrate impairments, but for different reasons than patients with frontal lobe deficits, for whom these tasks were originally designed. The fractionation of tests into their component parts has allowed these deficits to be revealed and has cast new light on the nature of the cognitive impairments in PD (see Robbins et al. 1999).

Thus, attentional deficits are now considered to be a prominent feature in PD; they usually occur in complex tasks requiring shifting or sustained attention (Downes et al. 1989; Lewis et al. 2005; Wright et al. 1990). The nature of the tasks in which attentional deficits appear, suggests that they too may be related to impairment in executive functions. Attentional problems are characteristic of PD dementia and Lewy body dementia and give rise to both diminished and fluctuating cognitive performance (Ballard et al. 2002). Although the underlying pathological cause for attentional deficits remains unknown, disturbances in metabolic activity (O'Brien et al. 2005) and cholinergic deficits in the thalamus (Ziabreva et al. 2006) have been proposed.

4.7.3.3 Set-shifting difficulties in PD: The Wisconsin Card Sorting Test

One line of investigation with regard to the "frontal-executive" hypothesis was to provide evidence demonstrating that patients with PD also had difficulties with tasks traditionally used to assess frontal function, such as the Wisconsin Card Sorting Test (WCST) (Bowen 1976; Downes et al. 1989; 1993; Lees and Smith 1983) and other tests with putative frontal components, including planning and short-term memory (Taylor, Saint-Cyr and Lang 1986). These deficits were present even in the early stages of the disease, prior to the initiation of treatment, and within the context of preserved intellectual functions and recognition memory. The initial interpretation of the difficulties in performance presented by patients with PD was in terms of an inability to elaborate efficient strategies spontaneously or to use internally guided behaviours in pursuit of a goal (Taylor, Saint-Cyr and Lang 1986). The observed pattern of deficits on tests of episodic and short-term memory was also explained in terms of more general difficulties in spontaneously generating efficient strategies in problem solving, secondary to frontal lobe dysfunctions. Executive deficits of this kind are particularly pronounced on tasks in which success is largely dependent on planning strategies that need to be initiated by the subject. Many memory tasks make demands of this kind on executive functions (Levin and Katzen 1995). It might therefore be expected that executive failures should affect memory performance.

It is now more usual for deficits on the WCST to be interpreted in terms of difficulty with set-formation, set-maintenance and in particular, set-shifting ability (Robbins et al. 1999); deficits of this kind are also evident on tasks not directly related to the WSCT. For example, Cools et al. (1984) identified a "diminished shifting aptitude" in PD patients who appeared to be impaired on motor and sorting tasks involving the ability to realign behaviour with changing task demands, especially if they had to rely on self-generated information for guidance. These set-shifting deficits came to be recognised as a feature of cognitive performance in PD and have probably been the most widely studied of all the executive dysfunctions in the disorder. They are known to affect both cognitive and motor domains (Cools et al. 1984; Downes et al. 1989; Owen et al. 1992; Van Spaendonck et al. 1996) and this kind of switching, which is considered characteristic of frontal function, was taken as further evidence in support of a "frontal" hypothesis in PD. Not all investigators however, accepted that this was a primary dysfunction of the frontal cortex, maintaining that the origins of the disorder in PD lay within the basal ganglia (Cools et al. 1984). This was to prove a well-founded reservation.

Set-shifting performance has been most extensively studied using tests of visual discrimination learning (e.g. Downes et al. 1989; Owen et al. 1992). Tasks of this kind require two types of switching behaviour. The first, a so-called "intra-dimensional shift" (IDS) requires the subject to stop responding on the basis of a particular criterion for a given stimulus dimension (e.g. "green" for the dimension of "colour") and to begin responding according to a new criterion (e.g. "red") for the same dimension. The second, is an "extra-dimensional shift" (EDS), which requires the subject to change a previous pattern of responding so that a novel exemplar of a previously irrelevant dimension becomes the new response criterion (i.e. a switch occurs from the colour "red' to "squares" representing the dimension of "shape"; see Robbins et al. 1999 for a full description). PD and patients with frontal lobe damage are more impaired when an attentional shift is required in the EDS condition (Downes et al. 1989; Owen et al. 1991; Roberts, Robbins and Everitt 1988) i.e. at the stage in which they are required to shift attention to a previously irrelevant stimulus dimension, rather than to a new exemplar of a previously relevant dimension (the IDS condition). Interestingly, other groups of patients with basal ganglia disorders (Huntington's disease, Steele-Richardson-Olszewski syndrome and multiple systems atrophy) follow a similar pattern, although Huntington's disease patients are also impaired in the IDS condition, because of a failure to inhibit perseverative responding, and in this, they were more impaired than patients with DAT (Lange et al. 1995; Robbins et al. 1992). Indeed, patients with mild DAT, who demonstrated significant memory deficits were no worse than controls on this task (Sahakian et al. 1990). These elegant and systematic studies produced a result that was of considerable significance in differentiating the specificity of deficits in attentional set formation and shifting for patients with basal ganglia disorders. Not only did they provide support for the hypothesis that these conditions have a profile of cognitive deficits that is similar to that seen in frontal lobe dysfunction, and distinctively separate from DAT, but they provided the impulse for the next stage in the research. This was to attempt to differentiate two cognitively distinct processes – that of "perseveration" and of "learned irrelevance" (Owen et al. 1993; Slabosz et al. 2006) in relation to the underlying brain pathology.

Perseveration has long been associated with frontal dysfunctions and has been interpreted as the inability to disengage responses from previously relevant, reinforced dimensions (Robbins et al. 1999). This is in contrast to the notion of learned irrelevance which refers to the inability to attend to, or to learn about, information that has previously been shown to be irrelevant (Grahn et al. 2008). For example, Robbins et al. (1999)

hypothesised that PD patients may be impaired on the WCST, not because they perseverate, but because they are reluctant to engage in strategies, or respond to stimulus dimensions, that have not previously been relevant. In a novel form of the set-shifting task patients with PD and those with circumscribed surgical lesions of the frontal lobes were compared on two EDS conditions: one which allowed perseveration but not learned irrelevance and vice versa (Owen et al. 1993). The patients with frontal lobe excisions showed greater perseverative errors, but no deficits in the learned irrelevance condition. The complete opposite of this pattern of results was found for the medicated PD patients, who showed no perseveration, but made more errors in the "learned irrelevance" condition. The pattern of performance in PD is reminiscent of a normal tendency not to respond to a dimension that has never previously been relevant, though to an abnormally inflated extent (Robbins et al. 1999). However, it should be contrasted with a group of PD patients at an early stage of the disease who had never received medication. These patients were impaired to an equal extent on both aspects of the task, i.e. in terms of failing to disengage from a previously relevant dimension (perseveration) and in their inability to switch their attention to a previously irrelevant dimension (Owen et al. 1993). Hence in the IDS condition, where it is required that attention be switched between stimuli, medicated patients with PD show no deficits, implying this task is sensitive to striatal dopamine. One explanation may be that L-dopa and related medication helps to reduce perseveration. In the EDS condition however, where switching is required between higher order perceptual dimensions, PD patients reliably demonstrate deficits in responding to category changes, whether or not they are receiving medication. Thus it seems that this type of higher order attentional control is not dopamine-dependent. These findings are in keeping with studies in animals which suggest that the EDS shifting component is under the control of noradrenaline systems. This is consistent with observations of early and significant degeneration of the locus coeruleus in PD (which also occurs in DAT). Additional support for this hypothesis comes from improvements in global cognition that have been observed in PD patients following administration of the noradrenaline re-uptake inhibitor atomoxetine in a placebo controlled trial and there is also preliminary evidence to suggest that executive function and attention may be specifically enhanced using flexible doses of the same drug (Kehagia et al. 2013).

4.7.3.4 Planning deficits: The Tower of London test

A second source of evidence in support of the frontal-executive theory of cognitive deficits in PD focused around the function of planning. Executive performance in PD appears to be compromised on "frontal-lobe" tasks which typically require the integration of multiple sub-goals in order to achieve a final end goal of behaviour (Grahn et al. 2008). Evidence shows however, that when these tasks are decomposed into their constituent elements, PD and frontal-lobe patients appear to fail for different reasons (Owen 2004). Studies using so-called "frontal-lobe" tests, which did not attempt to fractionate performance in this way, may have been insensitive to the subtle changes exhibited by patients with PD and hence yielded the diverse results frequently reported in the earlier literature on this subject.

One of the best examples of PD patients' failure in tasks of goal-directed action comes from studies with the "Tower of London" (TOL) test of planning (Shallice 1982). For details of this task see Owen et al. (1990), Robbins et al. (1999) and Grahn et al. (2008). Studies with "frontal-lobe" patients demonstrated that these patients had more difficulties on this task relative to a normal control group (Owen et al. 1990; Shallice 1982). They required more moves in order to solve the problem and took more time in thinking during the execution of the problem solution (Robbins et al. 1999). This pattern of performance appears to be specific to cortical frontal lesions since similar impairments are not seen in patients with temporal lobe damage (Owen et al. 1995). This test of planning appears to differentiate between patients in the early and late stages of PD (Owen et al. 1992). A "frontal like" impairment in arriving at a solution to the task was seen only in medicated patients in the advanced stages of PD (Hoehn and Yahr stages III-IV). On the other hand, both medicated patients with mild (Hoehn and Yahr stages II-III) and severe symptoms were slower than controls in initiating actions to solve the planning problems. In contrast to the frontal-lobe patients, neither group of PD patients took longer thinking time during the course of the task to reach the solution. Non-medicated PD patients with only mild clinical symptoms showed no impairments on this task (Robbins et al. 1999). The delay in initiating a planned action on the TOL represents the time spent in planning a solution and selecting between various sub-goals prior to its execution (Owen et al. 1992). This delay in initiating actions is what seems to be characteristic of the performance of patients, even with mild PD.

Additional support for this observation was also found in a study of eye gaze behaviour in PD. It was found that patients with PD do not use the initial planning period in the same way as control subjects to attend appropriately to the goals of the task (Hodgson et al. 2002). Functional neuroimaging has demonstrated impaired right caudate nucleus activity in patients with mild PD, compared to healthy controls, when engaged in difficult TOL problems, though frontal-lobe activity remains intact (Dagher et al. 2001). In contrast to patients with mild PD, patients with frontal-lobe damage do not demonstrate increased initial thinking times on the TOL task and they also require more moves to reach the appropriate solution (Owen et al. 1990). Furthermore, increased activity of the caudate nucleus is observed with functional neuroimaging when the difficulty of the task is increased in a conceptual sense, i.e. by increasing the number of sub-goals, but not when the number of moves *per se* is increased, the latter affecting activity in the putamen (Dagher et al. 1999; Owen et al. 1996).

These results confirm that whilst performance on an established test of frontal function in the form of the "Tower of London" test of planning is impaired in both frontal-lobe and PD patients, qualitatively different types of performance account for this. The slowed initial thinking time of PD patients was not prominent among frontal patients although it is consistent with the cognitive deficits described for subcortical dementia and the clinical symptom of bradyphrenia. Furthermore, this slower time to initiate an action is thought to be a dopamine dependent deficit in PD as it has been shown to be exacerbated by withdrawal of L-dopa (Lange et al. 1992). Severe deficits in the form of frontal-type inaccurate performance on the task are only seen in advanced PD. These qualitatively distinct features of PD performance on the TOL test are thought to reflect putative damage to the functioning of individual fronto-striatal circuits (Robbins et al. 1999).

The subtleties in performance on the TOL, differentiating between patients with neurosurgical lesions of the frontal cortex and patients with mild PD invites speculation about the role played by the caudate nucleus in cognition. Whilst it is thought that the frontal-lobes are involved in executive functions by setting up and monitoring strategies for action and evaluating outcomes, the fine differences observed in the behaviour patterns of patients with PD has led to the suggestion that the role of the caudate nucleus may be to identify optimal action schema and to select appropriate sub-goals, according to an evaluation of action-outcomes. Achieving optimal performance in goal-directed actions is likely to be dependent on the integral functioning of the processes supported by both the frontal cortex and the caudate nucleus (Grahn et al. 2008).

Following these analyses of the impaired performance on the TOL exhibited by PD patients, further exploration of the component processes which form the basis of planning abilities appeared warranted. Efficient problem solving appeared to be highly dependent on the formation of an appropriate attentional "set" and it was proposed that the ability to shift between competing possibilities played a crucial role in selecting the most appropriate solution. In keeping with this suggestion, the impaired performance of patients with PD on different cognitive tasks was attributed to problems with response shifting and, as might be expected, contrasted sharply with that of frontal-lobe patients (Robbins et al. 1999).

It was also suggested that these planning deficits might be a reflection of impaired memory function. Optimal planning on the TOL test is likely to place a heavy burden on spatial working memory as the range of possible solutions to the task is explored. This possibility was confirmed by analyses which showed that tests of spatial working memory are highly intercorrelated with tests of frontal function, including the TOL (Owen et al. 1992).

4.7.3.5 Spatial Working Memory

Medicated patients with mild PD show performance deficits of a similar kind to frontal-lobe patients on a test of spatial working memory, designed to be analogous to the radial arm maze used to investigate the role of working memory in rats (Olton, Becker and Handelman 1979). This test requires selection between, and sequencing of, a series of sub-goals in order to achieve successful completion of the task (Owen et al. 1990;1992). Whilst impaired on this task, the pattern of errors produced by patients with early PD is qualitatively different from that of frontal-lobe patients. Accuracy of performance was impaired in both frontal-lobe and PD patients irrespective of the severity of their impairments. However, unlike the frontal lobe patients, PD patients with both mild and severe clinical symptoms were unimpaired in terms of the strategy they adopted to tackle the problem and this has been interpreted as demonstrating that although PD patients are able to perform the complex searches required, using strategies similar to those of normal controls, they are unable to alternate effectively between important sub-goals (Grahn et al. 2008). The anatomical substrate for this and other types of working memory task has been shown to include both striatal and frontal lobe damage (e.g. Lewis et al. 2003). Controlled withdrawal of L-dopa in PD patients with marked clinical symptoms leads to further decline in spatial working memory performance (Lange et al. 1992), suggesting that a dopaminergic substrate is predominantly responsible for the deficits observed.

4.7.3.6 Verbal fluency

A general lack of fluency both on cognitive (Talland 1962; Wilson et al. 1980) and on motor tasks (Berardelli et al. 1986; Sheridan, Flowers and Hurrell 1987) has been noted in PD for many years, but formal tests of word fluency using standardised tasks have yielded widely differing results. Some studies have argued that only slight differences, if any, exist between patients with PD and normal control groups on letter fluency (Caltagirone et al. 1989; Lees and Smith 1983; Marsh, Markham and Ansel 1971; Matison et al. 1982; Miller 1985), semantic fluency (Gotham et al. 1988) or both (Hanley et al. 1990; Taylor, Saint-Cyr and Lang 1986; Weingartner et al. 1984). A number of reasons have been proposed to account for these reported differences. Since verbal fluency has been shown to be sensitive to the neurodegenerative effects of DAT (see Bayles et al. 1993) it was suggested that the deficits seen in PD occur only in the presence of concomitant dementia (Taylor, Saint-Cyr and Lang 1986; Troster et al. 1989) or reduced levels of verbal ability (Hanley et al. 1990), and resemble the pattern of deficits reported in patients with DAT (Bayles et al. 1993; Troster et al. 1998). This would suggest that poor verbal fluency may not be the result of either PD or of word finding difficulties.

Although it was once accepted that verbal fluency impairments are greater in DAT than in PD, this has not always been found to be the case (e.g. Stern et al. 1993). A large number of studies have indicated that non-demented PD patients are impaired on verbal fluency tasks, even when age, level of education, general cognitive abilities and articulation difficulties are taken into account (e.g. Flowers, Robertson and Sheridan 1995). The deficit in verbal fluency is most frequently reported when constraints are categorical (i.e. semantic categories), suggesting an impairment in semantic memory (for summaries see: Bondi and Troster 1997; Lezak, Howieson and Loring 2004; a large meta-analytic study: Henry and Crawford 2004; and empirical studies: Auriacombe et al. 1993; Beatty et al. 1989; Cooper et al. 1991; Cummings et al. 1988; Matison et al. 1982; Piovezan et al. 2007; Raskin, Sliwinski and Borod 1992). Some studies, albeit less frequently, have found deficits on verbal fluency in PD patients without dementia when lexical (letter or phonemic fluency) and semantic constraints are used (Bayles et al. 1993; Flowers et al. 1995; Gurd and Ward 1989). Few studies however, carried out qualitative analyses of performance on verbal fluency in PD as recommended by Raskin et al. 1992) until Flowers et al. (1995) demonstrated that although output is decreased in PD qualitatively, performance does not differ from that of normal controls in terms of the range and variety of words. This suggests that the reduction in fluency is not due to a restriction in the words available to the patients from semantic stores. Rather, Flowers et al. (1995) attributed the difficulty to slowness in accessing words, reflecting the bradyphrenia that is characteristic of PD and of the so-called 'subcortical' pattern of deficits.

However, the fact that PD patients are impaired on alternating fluency tasks (i.e. letter-letter and letter-category; e.g. Downes et al. 1993) suggests that impaired executive functions might lie at the heart of poor performance on tests of verbal fluency. Performance on tasks of verbal fluency is worse in PD patients who are depressed (Piovezan et al. 2007) and this, together with the suspicion that impaired executive function may be at the root of these difficulties, implicates fronto-striatal deficits as being the underlying cause (see later discussion). Since performance on these tasks is improved by cueing, some authors have interpreted failures in verbal fluency as being in keeping with a retrieval deficit (e.g. Downes et al. 1993).

4.8 The anatomical basis for the cognitive impairment in Parkinson's disease

The functions of the basal ganglia have long been considered to be related to motor control and this may have been part of the reason for the relatively late realisation that PD along with other basal ganglia disorders, such as Huntington's disease and Steele-Richardson-Olszewski syndrome are in fact, characterised by a specific pattern of cognitive impairment (Robbins et al. 1999). Increasing sophistication in neuropsychological assessment techniques, together with an improved understanding of functional neuroanatomy, has allowed a much clearer understanding of cognitive impairments in basal ganglia disorders, including PD. The nature and neural basis for these cognitive deficits was, to a large extent, elucidated by animal studies which prompted new hypotheses regarding the role of the basal ganglia. From these there emerged the notion of cortico-striatal circuits, which emphasised the intimate neural connections and the functional inter-relationships between the neocortex and the striatum (Alexander et al. 1986). Of particular significance to present-day understanding of the cognitive impairment associated with PD was the demonstration that the outflow from the basal ganglia was primarily targeted at the frontal lobes. This was to have major implications for the theoretical understanding of cognitive functioning in PD.

The main input nuclei to the basal ganglia are the caudate and the putamen, which receive axons from nearly all parts of the neocortex apart from the primary visual, auditory and olfactory cortices. Both the caudate and the putamen are connected with the substantia nigra in a reciprocal arrangement forming the nigrostriatal tract and output from the basal ganglia is sent via the substantia nigra and globus pallidus (see figure 4-1).

A model that has been greatly influential in shaping understanding of how the various nuclei which constitute the basal ganglia relate to one another and to the cortex, has been the concept of cortico-striatal loops (Alexander et al. 1986). This model emphasises the functional inter-relationships between the frontal cortical areas and the striatum which are sustained by complex neuronal circuits or "loops" linking the basal ganglia with the frontal cortex. These frontostriatal circuits are grouped into those subserving motor functions (i.e. the motor circuit and the occulomotor circuit) and complex (non-motor) circuits. The non-motor circuits originate in the dorsolateral prefrontal cortex, in the anterior cingulate cortex and in the orbitofrontal cortex.

Figure 4-1. The basal ganglia: connectivity diagram

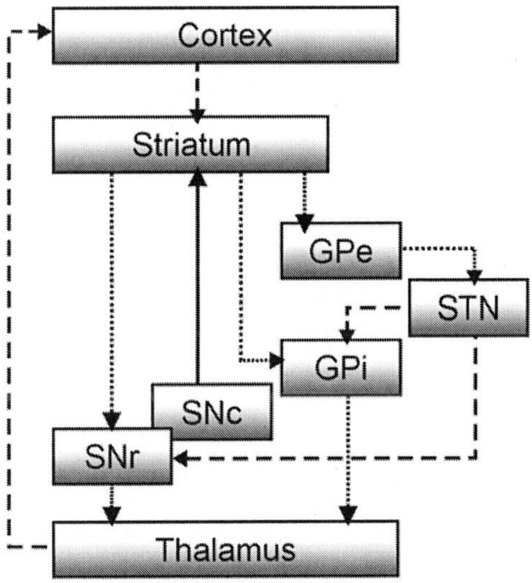

Legend: STN-subthalamic nucleus; GPe/GPi-globus pallidus; SNc/SNr-substantia nigra.
Glutamatergic pathways are shown with broken arrows, dopaminergic with a full arrow and GABA pathways with dotted arrows.

Andrew Gillies at http://en.wikipedia.org/wiki/Substantia_nigra

Each circuit projects to specific striatal regions preserving a strict topographical arrangement which remains segregated throughout the basal ganglia and the thalamus, allowing other areas of the brain to communicate with each circuit along the respective pathways (Zgaljardic et al. 2006). The frontostriatal pathways also receive inputs from dopaminergic, noradrenergic, serotonergic and cholinergic cell groups that modulate information processing (Tekin and Cummings 2002). Research efforts have now succeeded in verifying associations between each of the three respective prefrontal cortical areas and specific cognitive and behavioural functions. The anterior cingulate cortex is thus thought to regulate attentional processes such as response initiation, intention, inhibition and conflict monitoring, the dorsolateral prefrontal cortex is involved in cognitive executive functions such as set-shifting, complex problem-solving, retrieval abilities, organizational strategies, concept formation and working memory and the orbitofrontal cortex is implicated in aspects of decision-making based upon reinforcement/reward schedules, impulse control and, perseveration and mood (Zgaljardic et al. 2006; for review see Zgaljardic et al. 2003).

In relation to the neuropsychological basis for the executive deficits observed in PD without dementia, of particular interest is the fact that the principal target of basal ganglia outflow appears to be the frontal lobes (Owen 2004). Information is transmitted through the striatum via these complex loops to the frontal granular cortex, an area that has been implicated in supporting specific cognitive operations. According to this theoretical framework, the cognitive deficits in PD are the result of disturbed neuronal outflow from the striatum, in particular, the caudate nucleus (Taylor, Saint-Cyr and Lang 1986). Cognitive abilities dependent on the integrity of the frontal lobes would therefore be expected to be impaired in PD, due to the fact that the prefrontal cortex is not receiving appropriate input from the striatum.

From a detailed analysis of memory, visuospatial and executive functions Taylor, Saint-Cyr and Lang et al. (1986) concluded that there was no evidence of generalised disruption of cognitive processes in PD. Patients with PD differed from normal controls in so far as they were unable to spontaneously generate efficient strategies in tasks requiring self-directed, task-specific planning. The prefrontal cortex is considered to play an important role in self-directed behavioural planning. Thus, these investigators concluded that their results supported the notion of a neostriatal outflow model, in which dysfunction of the caudate nucleus has implications for the disruption of functioning in the prefrontal cortical areas. This interpretation is strengthened by findings of normal performance on tests which are believed to tap other areas of cortical functioning, such as recognition and most visuospatial skills (see Brown and Marsden 1986; Flowers et al. 1984).

A model positing disturbances to neostriatal outflow as the explanation for the deficits observed in PD would have to explain not only the lack of deficits associated with all but the frontal cortical area, but also intact performance on tasks associated with the frontal region (see for example, Lees and Smith 1983). The fronto-striatal impairment in PD does not present as a global impairment of all frontal functions and as described above, it is not exactly comparable to the impairment seen in so-called frontal lobe patients. This is not surprising as the frontal lobes are very large and represent around two-thirds of the overall cortical area, receiving input from other cortical areas and being strongly differentiated with regard to the functions that they sustain. The complexity of frontal tasks means that their resolution depends on a variety of underlying cognitive skills. When these skills crucially depend on internally guided strategies for planning a variety of motor, cognitive and emotional behaviours, a breakdown in function is observed in PD. These spontaneously generated strategies for guiding planning are thought to be disadvantaged by disturbed neostriatal outflow to the prefrontal cortex (Taylor, Saint-Cyr and Lang et al. 1986).

Numerous studies have led to the claim that the subcortical deafferentation of the frontal lobes caused by the disturbed neostriatal outflow in PD might also be responsible for the other cognitive deficits of PD patients in domains of cognitive functioning such as memory, visuospatial, perceptual and language skills (e.g. Bondi et al. 1993; Brown and Marsden 1984; 1986; Della Salla et al. 1986; Taylor, Saint-Cyr and Lang et al. 1986). Generally speaking, when the alleged "frontal" contribution on tasks was statistically controlled, by taking covariances into account, non-demented patients with PD did not perform any differently to normal age-matched controls on tasks of memory and visuospatial function (e.g. Bondi et al. 1993). Thus frontal system dysfunction appeared to account for many of the apparent failures on other cognitive tasks.

4.9 Functional neuroimaging and cognitive performance in PD

In recent years, functional neuroimaging studies using PET, SPECT and functional MRI have made it possible to correlate patterns of cortical and sub-cortical activation with different aspects of cognitive processing in both patients with PD and appropriate control groups. These techniques measure increases in oxygenated blood flow to the local vasculature that accompanies neural (synaptic) activity in different brain areas. A description of neuroimaging techniques is beyond the scope of the present work, but see Grahn et al. (2008) for a full discussion.

Suffice it to say that those neuroimaging studies that have focused on the striatum have demonstrated that caudate function is implicated in various executive processes, but in particular, in tasks that require processes critical for goal-directed action. A vital component of goal-directed action is the expectation (before a course of action is embarked on, or during it) that a specific outcome will occur. The expectation of specific consequences following an action is crucial to the shaping of intentional or willed behaviour and evidence is accumulating that the caudate plays a role in this process (Grahn, et al. 2008). Many studies have also implicated the caudate in the type of set-shifting abilities that are essential to successful performance on tasks such as the WSCT. Shifting strategies are involved in processes by which actions are chosen based on expectations and their consequences. These studies would appear to lend support to the view that the caudate is involved in goal-directed learning as it is sensitive to action contingencies and evaluation of subsequent outcomes.

A study by Owen et al. (1998) observed abnormal blood flow in the basal ganglia in patients with PD during performance both on the TOL planning task and the spatial working memory test described above. Both tasks have been shown to activate the caudate nucleus and dorsolateral cortex in healthy controls. The abnormal striatal activation pattern in the PD patients was accompanied by a performance deficit similar to that seen in patients with frontal lobe damage, although no abnormalities in regional blood flow were seen in the prefrontal cortex. This observation suggests that the striatum (specifically the caudate nucleus) is the likely neural substrate for the deficit observed in patients on these tasks. This study was replicated by Dagher et al. (2001). Moreover PET studies have also confirmed a correlation between caudate dopamine loss and neuropsychological performance in PD (Marie et al. 1999) suggesting the important role of the dopamine system in the cognitive impairments seen in PD (Ito et al. 2002). Another study compared two groups of PD patients selected according to whether they demonstrated executive deficits or not (Lewis et al. 2003). Results revealed selective impairments in working memory associated with reduced activity in the caudate nucleus in the executively impaired sub-group but not in the unimpaired one. This again suggests that the caudate contributes to executive performance by guiding the selection of responses necessary to achieve the goals of the task in hand, by initiating the required action contingencies and evaluating subsequent outcomes (Grahn et al. 2008).

Neuroimaging studies have also identified cortical changes associated with cognitive dysfunction in PD. PD patients with MCI have been shown to have limited atrophy in the temporal, parietal and frontal cortex, which was accompanied by neuronal loss in the bilateral caudal hippocampi, amygdala and right putamen. PD dementia patients demonstrated similar patterns of cortical loss, although it was more extensive, affecting larger areas of the temporal lobe, posterior cingulate gyrus, frontal regions and bilateral caudate (Beyer et al. 2007; Melzer et al. 2012). Numerous studies suggest that atrophy of the medial temporal lobe and limbic structures, with some frontal lobe involvement, precedes the onset of observed cognitive impairment in PD. More extensive atrophy of cortical and subcortical structures probably proceeds in relation to subsequent decline in cognitive functions. Regional volumetric brain changes are thought to be reliably related to cognitive performance in non-demented PD patients, but whether they are sensitive predictors for risk of dementia has yet to be established (Silbert and Kaye 2010).

A variety of measures reflecting changes in brain volume, perfusion and metabolic activity have been confirmed by neuroimaging studies in PD. These are particularly pronounced in PD dementia and involve multiple neurotransmitter systems, including dopamine and acetylcholine dependent ones. This indicates widespread neurotransmitter deficiencies in the dementia of PD. The abnormalities seen in PD dementia are of a similar pattern and magnitude to those of Lewy body dementia, but show some differences in relation to DAT (see Silbert and Kaye 2010 for a more complete discussion of these findings).

4.10 Cognitive deficits in PD and the effect on the carer-care recipient relationship

A conclusion that emerges from the foregoing discussion is that frontal lobe dysfunction in the form of executive impairments becomes evident in PD at a very early stage of the disorder. The dysfunction does not signify a frontal lobe lesion, but is rather the remote effect of more distant and diffuse damage to the frontostriatal circuits originating in the basal ganglia. It is an example of what Hughlings Jackson (1884) meant when he referred to his law of "evolution and dissolution", namely that the phylogenetically youngest parts of the brain are the first to succumb to the disruption of brain disease, even though they may be far removed from the origins of the problem.

As might then be expected, those parts of the brain that have been the most recent to evolve, support functions that are more complex in their construction – a characteristic that has been embodied in the notion of the central executive function of the frontal lobes. Failures in the central executive, especially when they are relatively circumscribed as would seem to be the case with PD (in contrast say, to patients with surgical ablation of the frontal cortex) result in deficits that are subtle and elusive in their manifestations. The changes in attention, initiative, planning and foresight, interest in the surrounding world and an inability to make decisions, which are the day to day neuropsychological manifestations of cognitive impairment in PD, are unlikely to be recognised as such by carers and perhaps even by professionals. These changes in the patient's mental processing capacity are often attributed to "personality" or "depression" and the loss of mental flexibility which is characteristic of neuropsychological performance in PD is perceived as a kind of "obsessionality" or stubbornness on the part of the patient. The disease deprives the mental processes of their former agility and dynamism and although their individual, component parts remain relatively intact (language, memory, visuospatial abilities) the ability to manipulate these skills is affected and the patient presents as lacking in mental flexibility, apathetic and disengaged. In addition, patients with PD often seem to be relatively unaware of their mental limitations, presenting with a kind of anosognosia which is associated with damage to the right frontal lobe, in particular. This too may be reflective of impaired executive functions: in the patient's inability to compare the outcome of his/her actions with his/her original plans and to notice any disparity between them.

Few reports in the literature have examined the possibility of an association between the neuropsychology of PD and the effects on the carer-care recipient relationship. There is evidence that carers' distress is associated with neuropsychiatric symptoms, including cognitive impairment in the care recipient with PD (Aarsland, Larsen, Karlsen et al. 1999; Shin, Youn Kim et al. 2012), but there do not appear to have been any systematic attempts to delineate which aspects of the cognitive impairment, if any, cause greatest difficulties. Neither does there seem to have been any investigation of the so-called "personality" changes of PD from the cognitive perspective. The heterogeneity of the cognitive deficits in PD, with the possibility that these may cluster to form specific subtypes of the disorder (Foltynie, Brayne and Barker 2002; Janvin 2006) also raises the question of whether certain of these subtypes may be associated with greater distress for carers. A study of patients with PD dementia, by Aarsland, Bronnick et al. (2007) identified five subtypes: patients showing symptoms of psychosis and agitation had the lowest scores on the MMSE and their carers demonstrated the highest levels of distress. It is difficult to draw clear-cut conclusions from these findings, however, as it is likely that the neuropsychiatric symptoms may have been primarily responsible, not only for the increased levels of carer distress, but also for the poor cognitive performance of the patients.

The cognitive deficits of PD and PD dementia patients demonstrate characteristic differences that differentiate them from other types of MCI and dementia. Although carers may not recognise the MCI stage of PD as detracting from the patient's normal intellectual performance or they may be prepared to accommodate minor lapses (e.g. of memory) as part of the normal process of ageing, they may misinterpret other failures in terms of "personality" changes or depression, as described above. Such interpretations may place strain upon the carer's relation with the care recipient, especially if s/he takes the view that the patient has become deliberately "awkward", "stubborn" or "intransigent". Equally, the very subtle nature of the cognitive impairment, may in itself mean that it is frequently unrecognised as such and therefore be more difficult to come to terms with, than the overt changes associated, for example, with DAT. An important question, that does not appear to have been explored to date, is the extent to which carers are indeed capable of recognising cognitive failures in the patients with PD that they help to look after. This is an area that is still much in need of systematic investigation.

4.11 Chapter summary

Over the last decade or so, the research evidence on the neuropsychological status of patients with PD has converged in support of the view that cognitive deficits largely resemble those executive dysfunctions that follow fronto-striatal impairments. Detailed studies of the performance of PD patients on a variety of tests which allow the fractionation of the component cognitive abilities of executive function have revealed the existence of subtly important qualitative differences in comparison to patients with frontal-lobe disorders, DAT and other neurodegenerative disorders associated with subcortical damage. This suggests that the cognitive functions supported by neurochemical activity in the individual cortico-striatal loops is differentiated and highly specific. The evidence supports the notion that executive dysfunctions are differentially affected at the various stages of PD, increasing in severity and broadening in range as patients show increasing clinical disability. Only those with the most severe clinical symptoms come to resemble frontal-lobe patients on tests of executive function. The pattern of cognitive impairment in PD emerges and subsequently progresses according to a defined sequence that evolves in parallel with the motor deficits that characterise the disorder (Owen et al. 1992; 1993). Along with the motor degeneration there is thus a progression on tests that are known to emphasise different aspects of executive functions. Some of these deficits appear to be responsive to L-dopa therapy, adding support to the notion that they are caused by dopamine depletion in the various functional subsystems supported by the complex pattern of cortico-striatal connectivity.

It thus appears that some of the heterogeneity in the presentation of PD (motor, cognitive and affective symptomatology) may be explained by differential depletion of dopamine in the various functional subsystems supported by the complex pattern of cortico-striatal connectivity. Nevertheless, there is also evidence that dysfunctions in other neurotransmitter systems (cholinergic, serotonergic and noradrenergic) may be responsible for some of the non-motor symptoms recognised in PD. In particular, PD dementia appears to be characterised by attentional and visuospatial memory deficits arising from more posterior cortical lesions and dependent on cholinergic neurotransmitter systems.

There is a rich literature on the problems of caring for someone with DAT, which allows certain parallels to be drawn with PD, at least in so far as building the expectation that the process is likely to be demanding and stressful for the carer. Far less is known about how the MCI and dementia stages of PD are likely to impact upon the carer. It would be unduly optimistic and reflect a naivety with regard to the mechanism involved in contributing to carer distress, to assume that because the profile of cognitive impairment in PD is different and the severity of the deficits lesser, at least to some degree, that the strain experienced by carers of people with PD would be less than that reported for carers of people suffering from DAT.

A number of considerations raised in the foregoing discussion of cognitive dysfunction in PD formed the basis of the research questions posed in the present study. These included:

1. What is the prevalence of cognitive dysfunction in a sample of patients with PD, selected to avoid the presence of dementia?
2. How do the cognitive symptoms of PD relate to the other symptoms of the disorder?

3. What is the impact of the cognitive dysfunction on the carers of people with PD?
4. In view of the subtlety of presentation of some of the cognitive deficits in PD, are carers able to identify these disturbances in their spouses?

CHAPTER FIVE

THE PSYCHOSOCIAL FUNCTIONING OF PEOPLE WITH PARKINSON'S DISEASE

5.1 Introduction

Fundamental to the purpose of this research, which is concerned with gaining a clearer picture of the relationship between the carer and the care-recipient in the context of a chronic neurodegenerative disorder such as PD, is an understanding of how the experience of living with a condition of this kind affects the psychosocial functioning of both sufferer and carer. The experience of chronic illness modifies their respective roles as partners in a long-term (marital) relationship, and begins a process of adaptation in which they gradually adopt the roles of carer and care-recipient. It is thus incumbent upon a research study of this kind to examine the experience of chronic ill-health from the point of view of both the sufferers of PD and their carers. The focus of this chapter is the subjective experience of PD and how it affects the psychosocial functioning of the person with the condition. The chapters that follow examine the effects for carers of living with a close family member suffering from a neurodegenerative condition such as PD.

Much work over recent decades has gone into describing the experience of illness (e.g. Anderson and Bury 1988) and although initially the main focus was on acute conditions, more recently the literature has expanded to include living with a chronic condition (Lubkin and Larsen 2006) and dementia, in particular (e.g. Kitwood 1997; Livneh and Antonak 1997). So far, little attention has been given to other neurodegenerative illnesses, which like Alzheimer's disease also tend to be long-term and incurable, so the following discussion represents an attempt to draw upon the existing literature with a view to gaining a better understanding of the implications for living with PD.

One reason for the failure to develop models of illness experience for chronic conditions until relatively recently is that chronic illness is essentially a twentieth century phenomenon, certainly in terms of the overwhelming problem that it represents (Smith 1996). Improved sanitation and advances in medical knowledge and management of illness have contributed to the fact that chronic illnesses have replaced infectious diseases as the major challenge to healthcare; people are living longer and thus opportunities for chronic illnesses to emerge have increased (Gerhardt 1989). Around 60% of the population in the U.K. are estimated to be living with a chronic health problem and in those aged 75 and over, the proportion rises to 75% (Department of Health 2004). Chronic conditions are thus a part of everyday life and although not directly life-threatening, are frequently disabling and present a serious challenge to individuals and their families.

As we enter the 21st century, the problems of chronic ill-health are certain to increase among the ageing populations of the western world, where they also present a serious challenge to healthcare providers and policy makers. A major difficulty is that healthcare systems throughout the developed world remain firmly entrenched in a model designed mainly for episodic and acute care, where the task can be defined in three main stages and in ideal circumstances, is self-limiting (Lubkin and Larsen 2006). Within this model, firstly the underlying disease process is identified through the process of diagnosis, secondly the cause(s) is treated and thirdly, there is the expectation of a cure. When this model is applied to chronic illness a serious mismatch occurs, as stages two and three, are, quite simply, incompatible with the definition of chronic disease, in which frequently only symptomatic treatment may at best be available, and a cure is impossible in the absence of a known cause. Chronic conditions are thus more than disease processes, which arise out of disruptions to normal physiological functions and neatly fit a biomedical model. They occur against a background of considerable uncertainty regarding causality and optimal treatment, usually predict progressive underlying pathology and functional deterioration and therefore herald considerable psychosocial consequences for the patient and those most closely involved with his/her welfare.

One of the key characteristics of PD that appear to be particularly relevant to a discussion of this kind is that it is a chronic and progressively degenerative condition, which does not reduce life expectancy to any significant degree (Mylne et al. 2009). It is a condition with a relatively late onset in life (the peak being in the sixth decade; Olanow et al. 2009), and one that the person may expect to live with for an average of 10-15 years, although the range of illness duration is very broad (R.G. Martilla, Rinne and R.J. Martilla1991; Schelosky and Poewe 1994; Zhao et al. 2010). The majority of people suffering from PD continue to live in their own homes in the community, usually with the support of a spouse or close relative. It is these characteristic features that primarily form the background to the experience of PD which is explored in the first part of the discussion that follows. The second part deals with the processes of adaptation to a chronic illness such as PD.

5.2 Definitions of chronic illness

Researchers have been influenced by different theoretical and practice perspectives in attempting to define chronic illness and consequently support for a single, uniform formulation has not been established. Bury (2000) has proposed a definition that appears to be consensual with regard to the main characteristics involved (O'Halloran, Miller and Britt 2004; Thrall 2005) and could almost have been written with PD in mind, at least in relation to the three essential features that he describes:

1. The illness has an insidious or subtle onset and the early symptoms may not even be recognized by the individual
2. The course of the illness has a fluctuating trajectory and will include "highs" and "lows" and even plateaus of little or no adverse effects
3. Illnesses that are chronic have uncertain outcomes.

PD is indeed a condition with an insidious onset, in which the early symptoms may not be recognized as such by the person concerned; moreover, diagnosis is sometimes very difficult and frequently requires specialist knowledge. Secondly, the illness often takes a fluctuating and unpredictable course, there being periods when the symptoms are well controlled and others when their management poses seemingly insurmountable problems; there are also periods of more rapid deterioration interleaved with plateaus in which the condition is relatively stable (Zhao et al. 2010). Thirdly, uncertainty frequently characterises the course of PD, it being difficult to predict the progression of symptoms, rates of deterioration in motor functioning and the likelihood of occurrence of non-motor manifestations of the disorder in specific cases.

Other conceptualisations of chronic illness, when applied to PD, endorse the characteristics referred to in Bury's (2000) definition, though giving a different emphasis. For example, Stewart and Sullivan (1982, 1397) further elaborate the first characteristic mentioned, when they refer to the "non-disabling and vague" quality of the initial symptoms which are "not easily recognisable by lay people or most physicians". At the same time, in drawing attention to the "permanent and continuing nature" of these disorders and the fact that "effective diagnostic and treatment strategies do not exist for many chronic diseases" they reflect the consensus established in the literature in relation to duration and prognosis, as discussed above. Nursing perspectives are more likely to emphasize the consequences of living with a chronic condition, for example, Curtin and Lubkin (1995, 5) provide the following definition of chronic illness, describing it as:

> the irreversible presence, accumulation or latency of disease states or impairments that involve the total human environment for supportive care and self-care, maintenance of function and prevention of further disability.

This definition recognizes the differentiation between disease, illness and disability (World Health Organization 1980) and the totality of the effects of chronic illness on everyday living, not least because of the permanence of such conditions and the ever-present possibility of further deterioration. Emphasis here is placed on sequelae, in terms of functional aspects, and on dependency as critical features of chronic conditions. This reflects an important shift in emphasis in the understanding of chronic conditions, in which both the sick person and his/her family become the unit of care (Raudonis 2006). This is especially pertinent to the present discussion, as family carers provide supportive care during the entire course of chronic illness in all care settings and for all types of needs (McMillan 2005). It is reasonable to expect that carers will experience ever increasing burdens as more and more complex healthcare is moved into the home setting in future decades. Most people with PD continue to live at home and research evidence indicates that this is by far the preferred option both for them and their families (Oxtoby 1982). Levels of dependency on the carer increase with disease progression (Tison et al. 1997) and these are not confined to the sphere of physical incapacity such as requiring help with the activities of daily living. For example, higher levels of care dependency are also associated with concomitant depression in PD (Riedel et al. 2011). Many people with PD also withdraw from a range of other activities such as managing their financial affairs, retreating from social contacts and dropping many of their former interests, and in this their behaviour is characteristic of that observed in other types of chronic illness (Bury 1982). Various explanations have been proposed to account for such behaviour, including obvious functional limitations (Bury 1982), apathy and depression (as discussed in chapter 3) and stigmatisation (to be discussed later in this chapter). These sequelae – if indeed they are such – elicit secondary problems that both the sufferer and carer are required to cope with, which in turn conspire to form part of the illness experience of PD. For people with PD themselves, there is another dimension which forms part of the illness experience. Research based on qualitative methodology (though not specific to PD) has revealed that neither the nursing focus on functional status nor the medical focus on treatment of symptoms were considered by sufferers to provide an adequate account of their experience of chronic illness (Ironside et al. 2003). Rather, the focus on these aspects of the condition was seen as detracting from equally important discussions of meaning in the context of chronic illness. The notion of meaning refers to the person's readiness to accept the illness and to integrate it into their life context, reframing its implications positively so that they can continue to lead a personally meaningful life (Baker and Stern 1993; Whittemore and Dixon 2008).

5.3 The subjective experience of Parkinson's disease

Although not specific to the condition of PD, the definitions derived from different perspectives referred to in the preceding section serve to highlight a number of the effects of chronic illness for the person with PD and his/her family. Firstly, they point to the possibility that initial symptoms may not be recognised for some time and hence raise the possibility for potential conflict between the sufferer and the physician with regard to their recognition in the early stages of the disease process. Difficulties with diagnosis are likely to be a considerable source of stress to the patient and his/her family (The Global Parkinson's Disease Survey Steering Committee 2002) and might therefore be expected to elicit a variety of coping behaviours, including ones that are dysfunctional in the long-term, such as denial. Secondly, in reflecting a picture of chronic conditions that often leaves more questions unanswered than clarified, the definitions serve to highlight the uncertainty of a chronic illness such as PD and the lack of control over their lives that people with the disorder experience (Nijhof 1996; Pinder 1988;1990). In order to resolve these uncertainties, patients might be expected to develop their own expertise in relation to the health problem, by seeking information wherever possible, from health professionals, by reading and joining associations of people with similar problems or via the internet (Kennedy 2003). Thirdly, the illness and the way in which it is received by the patient and his/her family is likely to have implications for the patient's self concept (Charmaz 1983) and relationships within his/her family and wider social network (O'Shaughnessy, Lee and Lintern 2010). Fourthly, a consequence of these early problems might be, that the diagnosis, when eventually established, is greeted with initial relief by the patient and his/her family, followed by a period in which there is a coming to terms with, and adjustment to, its implications and the meaning that it has for the patient (Pinder 1992). These considerations have important implications for how people construct their illness experience and cope with more existential questions such as "why me?", "why this?" or "why now?" Finally, considerations arising out of the uncertain illness pattern and prognosis (Bury 1982; 2000; Stewart and Sullivan 1982) in PD and the emergent functional and dependency issues (Curtin and Lubkin 1995) are likely to generate a range of problems with adjustment to the condition, including learning to accept the day-to-day symptom fluctuations, managing treatments, coming to terms with having to rely on others for help (Freidson 1970) and psychological issues such as learning how to manage changes in personal image associated with chronic illness and dealing with any perceived labelling and stigmatisation that may occur (Young 2004).

In the discussion that follows, an attempt will be made to contrast the predictions based on these definitions with the evidence that is available from patients themselves regarding the experience of PD. The issues raised are organised around the points highlighted above and recurrent themes emerging from the discussion. It should be emphasised that the underlying aim was not to undertake a qualitative study of PD in order to arrive at a better understanding of the components of the experience that constitutes living with PD. This would have required a completely different research paradigm and methodology from that used in the present study. Hence this chapter is in no way an attempt to construct a phenomenology of the experience of living with PD. Its aims are modest, namely to present a brief account of how patients (mainly those participating in the study) described their experiences of living with PD against a background of the literature on chronic illness. Quotations from people involved in the study are used merely to illustrate certain theoretical points. They are not intended to represent constructs derived from a qualitative analysis of the interviews carried out with people suffering from PD and their carers.

5.3.1 Biographical disruption in Parkinson's disease

Bury (1982) contends that illness in general, but chronic illness in particular, has a major, disruptive effect on everyday life, in which even the most fundamental, taken-for-granted aspects of daily living are severely threatened. Chronic illness "involves a recognition of pain and suffering, possibly even death, which are normally only seen as distant possibilities or the plight of others" (Bury 1982, 69). The disturbance is so intense, that it is seen as a "biographical disruption" affecting three main spheres of functioning. In the first place, as the person's usual taken-for-granted assumptions and behaviours are interfered with by the advent of illness, he or she becomes aware that something is wrong and cannot be explained in simple, common-sense terms. The point of realisation that something may be amiss provokes intense monitoring of bodily states and raises the potential need for professional help. Secondly, according to Bury (1982), the explanatory frameworks that a person normally uses undergo a fundamental challenge, causing him/her to totally reconsider his/her biography and brings about alterations in self-concept. Questions that typically arise at this time include "why me?", "why now?" or "what have I done to deserve this?", reflecting the need to make sense of the illness experience in the context of one's own life or what might be described as a search for meaning. Finally, the response to this disruption in practical terms demands that resources are mobilised to meet the needs of the altered situation (Williams 2000). The notion of resources includes the physical, social, financial, medical and cultural support that is available to people in adverse circumstances.

5.3.2 The decision to seek help and learning the diagnosis

The point at which the individual can no longer ignore the worrying signs and symptoms of the encroaching illness and comes to a decision about seeking help is the first stage in the biographical disruption described by Bury (1982). Clearly there are different individual thresholds determining both the action taken and its timing, but certain symptoms such as pain and advice from family and friends (so-called lay referral networks) are known to influence decisions regarding medical consultation (Helman 1994).

Once the decision to seek help has been taken, there follows a period of further uncertainty of variable length, depending on the pattern of symptom presentation. Where motor symptoms dominate the clinical picture of PD, establishing a diagnosis is usually relatively straightforward; where non-motor symptoms predominate, the task is more difficult and the uncertainty prolonged. These initial difficulties with establishing a diagnosis can be distressing, as patients feel that their concerns may not be adequately acknowledged, yet are fearful that something is seriously amiss. Initial reactions to hearing the diagnosis may include shock, disbelief, anger and a sense of betrayal. Since patients are frequently able to trace the onset of symptoms back several years before the diagnosis, they sometimes describe feelings of initial relief, which they see as confirming their long-held suspicions that "something was wrong". Several of the patients in the present study described this in terms of putting an end to the uncertainty of their knowing that their health was deteriorating, but not being able to account for their problems. Others have used the metaphor of "dropping the bomb" to describe the life-altering experience that learning the diagnosis and coming to terms with its physical and emotional impact had for them (Phillips 2006). One female patient described the experience as follows:

> I was in deep shock. I tell you ..... my world had turned upside down within half an hour..... . After a couple of hours of weeping and wailing "why me?" I was still in shock the rest of the day.
> (Female patient cited in Fleming, Tolson and Schartau 2004).

For people with PD, the biographical disruption brought about by the illness is evident in a number of ways. Those still working may do everything they can to continue in employment, in an effort to retain control over their lives: "I was absolutely determined to carry on working. For me, it was a way of fighting the illness. I wanted to show that I was still capable" (male patient, aged 54, cited in Gisquet 2008). This may occur in spite of functional limitations, which patients strive to hide from others, in what may become unrealistic efforts to maintain normality. Thus denial that "there is anything wrong" may be used as way of trying to maintain continuity with the past, against the biographical disruption caused by the illness, as in the example cited. Alternatively it may be an attempt to convince even oneself that the illness did not have the power to overturn one's life, as in the following example: "I didn't have to give up work at this point, although I could have gone on health grounds. I took early retirement so that I could continue to write, but on my own terms" (male patient, aged 57, participating in the present study). Others seem to feel that the biographical disruption caused by the disorder has overshadowed their entire lives: "Parkinson's disease ruined my life. I don't have friends anymore" (female patient, aged 69, cited in Gisquet 2008).

5.3.3 Uncertainty in Parkinson's disease

Uncertainty is likely to accompany the experience of PD from the very beginning. It has been described as the universal experience of chronic illness (Mast 1995). In a certain sense, of course, it is a feature of normal human life, but in chronic illness much of what people take for granted in their ordinary lives can no longer be relied upon. The orderly and predictable nature of the world is turned upside-down and fundamental issues such as the meaning of the illness experience and questions related to the person's identity in sickness come to the fore (Charmaz 1983; Pinder 1990). As an extension of this, the person, his/her family and wider social networks are forced to re-examine the changing nature of their relationships, as the increasing dependency of the affected individual disrupts the normal rules of reciprocity and mutual support.

For some people, these questions, and the impossibility of finding answers to them, constitute a crisis that further adds to the burden of chronic illness. For others, the ongoing uncertainty of chronic illness becomes part of the long-term struggle and anxiety is a common outcome, which has to be managed along with the other tasks of living with chronic ill-health. Even when the diagnostic label has been acquired, people are confronted with new uncertainties. Their concerns appear to centre around the following issues:

- How PD may affect their present lives and priorities
- How their lives might be expected to change in the immediate future (i.e. with the instigation of a medical regime)
- How the condition may affect their capacity to work and maintain family relationships
- What is to be expected in the future.
  (Based on Pinder 1990; Hayes 1994).

However, there is a deeper question underpinning many of the doubts expressed above, which although not voiced explicitly, is at the heart of the reappraisal frequently described by people in terms such as "what to make of life now that this has happened" (Pinder 1990).

With conditions such as PD, which until recently, have not occupied a prominent place in public discussions, many patients may have only heard of the illness in passing and their knowledge of it may be vague and imprecise. They may never have known anyone with the condition and this leaves them feeling lonely and isolated, not knowing what to expect of the future. In recent years the availability of numerous internet websites dedicated to specific conditions such as PD has gone a long way to providing people with support and information, as has the publicly voiced encouragement of well-known media figures such as Michael J. Fox, who themselves suffer from the condition and have written about their experiences (Fox 2002). This in itself is acknowledgement of the fact that people with a long-term condition such as PD seek knowledge of the shared experiences of others in an effort to make sense of their own situation. This is, in essence, the search for meaning described by Bury (1982) and others.

5.3.4 The search for meaning in chronic illness

The search for meaning appears to be a natural outcome of the biographical disruption. Bury (1991, 453) identifies two kinds of meaning associated with chronic illness, the first being related to its practical consequences for individuals and their families and the second, to its symbolic significance. As regards the first, the onset of symptoms may have a disruptive effect on everyday life affecting both home, work and leisure activities. The individual may need time to recognise the pattern of symptom presentation and how best to manage symptoms with medication and alterations in lifestyle. Problems may arise in relation to the accessibility and costs of treatment; for example, this is especially relevant to younger people with PD living in England, who despite the progressive nature of the condition, are not exempt from prescription charges.

Pierret (2003) points out that at a different level of understanding, the symbolic significance of the condition to the individual may be the key to understanding its meaning. Ordinary explanations are often insufficient in the face of chronic illness and patients often reach for a range of interpretative devices such as metaphors, cognitive representations and images to explain their experiences. These appear to provide a better account for the perceived alterations in the person's sense of self and identity that the illness has wrought through a variety of themes that gradually become established as part of the illness experience.

It appears that an important task in the process of adaptation to ill-health is finding an explanation as to why the illness chose the individual concerned as its victim. This search for meaning appears to be a common response to trauma of various types (Lifton 1988), which might include being diagnosed with long-term, progressive neurodegenerative condition. A starting point seems to be trying to find the reasons for becoming ill. One commonly encountered assumption is that stress is the causal factor in a variety of conditions and another that trauma may be responsible. Even patients who "know" that the origin of their illness is unknown, may nonetheless attribute their condition to: " ... a bang on the head, when I fell off a ladder, just a few months before it started. I've never felt quite right since" (male patient with PD, present study). Culturally held beliefs appear to be particularly strong in influencing the way in which people think about causality (Salmon 2002).

Meanings are sometimes extended not just to causal explanations, but to the overall experience of the disease. Some common interpretations are that the illness is intended as a test or challenge of some kind, or even as a punishment for previous misdemeanours. Negative reasoning of this kind is sometimes characteristic of depression (Beck et al. 1979) and may reflect clinically significant mood changes in patients, which in turn need to be addressed.

5.3.4.1 Meaning imposed externally: labelling and stigmatisation

Originating from a sociological perspective, labelling theory (Lemert 1967) and its later refinements (Link et al. 1987) held that the meaning attributed to the manifestations of chronic illness depended upon the way in which they were perceived in society. Under certain circumstances, the illness label may be stigmatising or stereotyping, as has been extensively discussed in the literature on mental illness (e.g. Goffman 1963). The extent to which any condition becomes stigmatised depends on various factors, including notions such as whether or not the individual is held responsible for the condition, the impact of the illness on others, outward manifestations of the illness and the extent to which it brings about changes in the person's functional competence. The person with the stigmatising condition is often labelled with the negative social meaning applied to the illness and this becomes part of the illness experience.

Although PD may not immediately come to mind as a stigmatised condition, many of its manifestations, particularly changes in outward appearance and loss of functional competence, meet the criteria for stigmatisation outlined above. Few studies appear to have addressed these issues, but there is evidence that the perceived stigma inherent in PD has not been recognised sufficiently (Burgener and Berger 2008). Motor fluctuations and dyskinesias appear to cause sufferers greatest embarrassment and humiliation (Karlsen et al. 2000; Pahwa et al. 1997; Rosser 1988; Scheife et al. 2000). PD may also be stigmatised because a number of the symptoms may be associated with other, more negatively regarded conditions. For example, patients will often go to extreme lengths in attempting to hide the signs of the movement disorder for fear that it might be misinterpreted (e.g. as drunkenness) and lead to their rejection (Karlsen et al. 2000; Nijhof 1995):

> The "off" comes on with increasingly little warning. One can adopt strategies to save oneself from various kinds of embarrassment; I have a radio taxi account or if one goes "off" badly in the street, one holds onto a lamp-post until a taxi comes past. ... I find that an aluminium walking stick

> is useful. It's a sign that something is wrong and holding onto a lamp-post is not necessarily because one is drunk.
> (Male patient with PD, aged 57, participating in the present study).

Since PD is also associated with the risk of developing cognitive symptoms, stigma related to mental impairment may become apparent with disease progression (Link et al. 1987). Moreover, the association with ageing can in itself be a cause for stigmatisation (Kahana et al. 2005).

Thus PD, because of its physical and mental limitations may cause patients to be aware of the negative labels associated with it. Moreover, identification with and internalization of these labels inevitably results in negative consequences for the patient, including lowered self-esteem, and altered perceptions of self. Labelling interactions also result in social rejection of the person with PD, as others respond with fear, uncertainty or embarrassment regarding his/her continued performance in the workplace and other spheres of social functioning. Fearful anticipation of these reactions means that patients often seek to hide the signs of their illness for as long possible, but this only serves to accentuate their feelings of insecurity, internalized shame and social isolation, which along with social rejection are conceptualised as the four dimensions or consequences of the labelling or stigmatising process (Burgener and Berger 2008). Apart from their loss of health, they thus also risk losing social support and earning capacity and must adapt to alterations in family relationships, which only increases their vulnerability to the illness (Hutchinson and Wilson 1998).

A survey of public attitudes to PD showed that those interviewed were more or less equally divided on the question of whether stigma was associated with the condition and these views were unrelated to respondent's age, gender, education or income level. Negative attitudes towards the illness were associated with the potential consequences, such as being a burden, the likelihood of mental deterioration and becoming dependent on others, while social issues such as the attitudes of other people, sexuality and loneliness were considered less important. Negative attitudes to PD were predicted by (younger) age, the expressed belief that PD is more unpleasant than other diseases and that it is stigmatised; they were also associated with a decreased likelihood of knowing someone with the condition and with poorer knowledge of the illness (Moore and Knowles 2006). This last point appears to be important: there is some indication that the "insider" and "outsider" views of PD are somewhat divergent. When asked to predict which aspects of the disorder would be most worrying for them, people unaffected by the condition focused on issues of dependency and becoming a burden to carers. For those suffering from the condition the priorities were somewhat different. Hence it appears that outsider attitudes to PD, which may be taken to represent the views of society at large, and thus influence stigmatisation, may focus on aspects of the condition that are quite different from those that make up the illness experience. Nevertheless, through contributing to the process of stigmatisation, they have a "rebound" effect on the illness experience and so need to be taken into account. Understanding these processes and the contribution they make to the illness experience is important, because they can help to inform public education campaigns about the nature of PD, which aim to modify attitudes and beliefs and thus to reduce the stigma associated with the condition, which in part, at least, is based on lack of experience and ignorance of the condition.

5.3.4.2 Meaning internalised: shame

Nijhof (1995) drew attention to the fact that stigmatisation has undesirable effects for the social construction of PD for sufferers. In a qualitative study focusing on patients' interpretations of the meaning of PD, shame was found to be a significant feature, accounting for their tendency to withdraw from many aspects of life. Words such as "shame", "embarrassed", "awkward" and "disgrace" featured prominently in the accounts patients gave of their illness:

> I feel ashamed about the way I'm sitting here talking, totally different. ... Well, I don't talk anymore when I'm in a large group, because of the fact that the words come out so awkwardly, don't you think?
> (patient with PD cited in Nijhof 1995).

Stigma and shame also have repercussions for carers and other family members, in particular children. Younger patients, whose children are still living at home are faced with having to explain their limitations and account for what may be perceived as their "strange" or "clumsy" behaviour (e.g. drooling, slurred speech). Sometimes patients felt that their children were repulsed by the symptoms of the disease and did not want to discuss it: "It's embarrassing for both of us" (female patient with PD cited in Fleming et al. 2004). Another patient felt that her daughter had stopped bringing friends home, because she was embarrassed by her mother's condition:

> My daughter wouldn't really bring her friends round to the house so much, she went out to other people's houses more. Although she probably wouldn't say so herself, I feel it was to do with the Parkinson's. Quite embarrassed about things.
> (Female patient with PD cited in Fleming et al. 2004).

Stanley-Hermanns and Engebretson (2010, 358) provide the following example:

> The number one complaint my family has is they said that I always look like I am mad. My left side of my face tends to freeze, like a zombie type and I can't talk sometimes and they always think I am mad or something.

One area of human behaviour that is particularly prone to inducing embarrassment and shame is sexual activity, especially when this is perceived as having exceeded "normal" limits. Increases in sexual interest and libido are known to be side effects of anti-parkinsonian medication (Ahlskog 2011; Ivanco and Bohnen 2005; Klos et al. 2005; Uitti et al. 1989), but less frequently reported are paraphilias, including zoophilia (Fernandez and Durso 1998; Jiménez-Jiménez et al. 2002), cross-dressing behaviour (Riley 2002; Shapiro et al. 2006) and internet pornography (Dodd et al. 2005; Shapiro et al. 2006). Marital infidelity has also been reported (Dodd et al. 2005; Shapiro et al. 2006). Abnormal sexual behaviour may be improved by altering antiparkinsonian medication (Riley 2002). However, embarrassment and shame prevent patients and their families from openly discussing aberrant behaviours of this kind with their clinicians. This means that there is likely to be considerable under-reporting of these problem behaviours and this may be further complicated by the fact that patients and their families do not appear to associate them with treatment. Inevitably, other interpretations are sought, with consequent strains for relationships. Although difficulties of this kind appear to affect a relatively small proportion of people with PD (see chapter 3), when they do occur, they often overshadow other concerns, because of their possible social repercussions in the form of the associated stigma. In the sample of patients interviewed for the purposes of this study, difficulties associated with hypersexuality came to light in two patients and with paraphilia in one, requiring extremely careful management in order to defray the consequences of stigmatisation.

However, changes in sexual activity appear to be the norm for couples, even in the absence of sexual dysfunction (Wermuth and Stenager 1995). One woman in the sample of people with PD reported in the present study commented that in view of her increasing dependence on her husband with regard to self-care activities, including help with managing menstrual hygiene, she did not find it surprising that: "... he seems to have gone off sex completely" (female patient with PD, aged 52, participating in the present study). She felt that this and the symptoms of rigidity, which severely restricted her mobility, had made her unattractive to him.

The consequences of stigmatisation in the form of embarrassment, repulsion, shame and rejection are a sequential step in the cascade of events that comprise the illness experience. They in turn, lead to changes that are even more fundamental to the sick person's image of themselves and to their own identity.

5.3.5 Altered perceptions of self

A person's self-concept is not something that is seen as being stable across the life-span, nor is it conceived of in terms of growth or maturation; rather the view is that there are many self-concepts: past, present and future, which retain their individual identities. For someone with PD, past selves may represent the person before the illness and at its different stages of progression. Future selves may be many and reflect the person's notions of what s/he might become, what s/he would like to become and what s/he fears s/he might become. These future selves reflect the person's expectations in terms of hopes and fears, challenges and threats, viewed both from the pre-illness perspective and following it. The expectation of future selves may provide an incentive for behaviour, but equally the realisation that certain expectations are never likely to be met as the result of illness, may cause the person to abandon their aspirations and resign themselves to a less-challenging view of themselves in the future. Current views of self are likely to be modified in view of the evaluative and interpretative context set by the future view of self (Markus and Nurius 1986; Frazier, Cotrell and Hooker 2003).

The consequences of the biographical disruption wrought by a chronic, neurodegenerative illness such as PD, may lead, as has been illustrated, to alterations in life-style (e.g. social withdrawal) and decreased role fulfilment (e.g. being forced to give up work or unable to carry out certain tasks such as driving or domestic maintenance). This in turn, may lead to diminished feelings of self-worth, depression and shame. If these persist and are reinforced, with time they may become so much a part of the person's self-image that an altered perception of the self comes into being: "I'm no longer the person I once was. I can never go back to the old me. It's taken me some time to come to terms with this, but I think I've finally accepted it now" (male patient, aged 60, participating in the present study).

This does not necessarily imply that patients' representations of themselves are diminished with respect to the number of possible domains, but that all domains become imbued by the illness (Frazier et al. 2003). Nevertheless, specific domains of self appear to gain particular significance, depending on the nature of the illness. Perhaps not surprisingly, patients with Alzheimer's disease appear more focused on their "cognitive-related selves" and those with PD on their "physical-related selves" (Frazier et al. 2003).Women in particular, often express having become more self-conscious of the changes to their bodies as the result of illness. Brearley and Birchley (1994, 78) comment that:

> Women who have become disabled may feel unattractive or even repulsive. Limitation of movement or pain or deformity (.......) can all attack a woman's self-image to a destructive degree. When a woman's sexual identity depends on feeling physically desirable disability may negate her feelings of femininity.

Several authors have suggested that patients with PD share a number of common characteristics such as being less talkative and flexible, but more cautious and suspicious than age matched healthy individuals or those with other chronic illnesses (e.g. McNamara, Durso and Brown 2003). Observations of this type have even led to the notion of a "Parkinsonian personality" characterised by such features (e.g. Eatough et al. 1990). More recently, these changes have been conceptualised as alterations in the sense of self in PD, characterised by harm avoidance and lower novelty seeking type behaviours, the former allegedly being associated with the co-existence of affective disturbances, while the latter is thought to be related to the dopaminergic types of "frontal" cognitive dysfunction described in chapter 4 (McNamara, Durso and Harris 2008; Poletti and Bonuccelli 2012).

Patients' future view of themselves is also likely to be affected. Frazier et al. (2003) found that patients with PD were especially concerned with future loss of independence and feared becoming dependent on others. They also perceived less distance between their current self and the feared self envisioned in the future. Nevertheless they reported a healthy balance between their hoped-for and feared illness-related selves, reflecting good levels of adaptation, which the authors suggest may have been achieved through mechanisms of social comparison to others who may be better or worse off than the patients themselves.

According to Charmaz (1983, 168) the dissipation of self-image in chronic illness arises out of the illness experience itself and constitutes "a fundamental form of suffering in the chronically ill". Charmaz delineates four consequences of chronic illness which impinge on the person's sense of self, and in the absence of opportunities to rebuild equally valued alternative self-images, contribute to the sense of loss and suffering experienced in long-term, progressive illness: (1) living a restricted life, (2) experiencing social isolation, (3) being discredited and (4) burdening others. These sources of suffering do not represent mutually exclusive categories; they both follow on from one another in a cascading effect and produce reciprocal effects on each other. For example, having to give up various activities as the result of mobility problems in PD inevitably leads to a more restricted lifestyle, which in turn causes greater social isolation, restricting opportunities for social validation of oneself. Social isolation imposes further limits on the person's lifestyle, by means of a negative feedback loop and the gradual erosion of mechanisms that sustain a normal life, eventually narrows down the opportunities for maintaining intact perceptions of self.

A sense of control over one's life and the ability to take specific actions, which are referred to in cognitive theory as a sense of mastery (Beck et al. 1979), are considered to lie at the heart of the self-concept (Charmaz 1983). The way in which this sense of mastery is affected by the sources of suffering referred to above and leads to a loss of self will be discussed next in relation to PD.

5.3.6 Living a restricted life

Many people with PD feel that their lives have become narrow and restricted by the illness, contrasting sharply both with their previous lifestyle and aspirations, and those of their peer group without the disease. The condition assumes a pivotal role in their lives, which are increasingly structured around the demands of the illness, as loss of mobility, fatigue and decline in physical capacity exert their effects on accomplishing everyday tasks, which may be considerably slower and more laboured, occupying both the sufferer and the carer. Activities that the couple valued and enjoyed in the past often become severely restricted. Having to adhere to treatment regimes, G.P. visits, clinic attendance and the need to "fall in" with the dictates of the illness eventually replace former routines, both occupational and recreational. The immobilising effects of PD mean that holidays, travelling independently and (often) in the company of others, driving, sports and hobbies, shopping and leisure activities outside the home are gradually curtailed. One patient described this as follows:

> Parkinson's disease has gradually taken over my whole life. Everything I want to do has to be done around the illness. Trying to plan things and then keep to the plan is just a waste of time. I may want to do something, but then my legs won't let me. Sometimes, it seems that the more I want to do it, the worse it is. I feel a bit like a prisoner, at the mercy of the illness. I feel quite useless.
> (Female patient, aged 66, participating in the present study).

70% of those with PD in the U.K. are aged 70 and over (Mutch et al. 1986), and these restrictions are often considered to be a normal consequence of ageing, exacerbated by the disease. Older people may not suffer the effects of these restrictions so keenly as younger ones. It also seems that if people feel they have retained some choice in pursuing valued activities and are still able to exercise freedom of action in following those choices, their lives are not perceived as restricted, their suffering is less acute and their image of themselves is preserved (Charmaz 1983). A familiar figure in Cambridge in the 1980s was a male lecturer with PD, who although retired from teaching, prided himself on a rigorous jogging regime, which he believed helped to maintain his mobility. He also wrote a book about his experience of living with PD, which according to the constructivist perspective, allowed him to reconstruct his illness as a worthwhile and challenging experience, thus helping to build a new and valued self-image (see Vaughan 1986). Conversely, having to surrender a driving licence on account of the limitations imposed by PD was a significant step for a number of patients, as it symbolised loss of independence and with it, the loss of many taken for granted activities. It was often a source of friction in families, who feared for the safety of the sufferer, but had difficulty in persuading him/her to accept these limitations. Resistance from the sufferer's point of view, can be understood as his/her struggle to remain in control of important aspects of his/her life.

The restrictions imposed by the necessity for various physical aids, such as a wheelchair or lifting equipment in the later stages of the disease are even more significant, as they are a visible sign of the disability to the outside world. Hence they often meet with resistance and may be rarely used in order to preserve the vestiges of independence. Several patients encountered in the present study would only agree to using a wheelchair when away from home, where the risk of meeting acquaintances was diminished and they felt that their anonymity made their disability less obtrusive, thereby preserving the integrity of their self-image.

Medication is another difficult issue. The relative value of treatment is often weighed up against the losses it allegedly induces. For some this involves striking a balance between good mobility and feeling mentally alert and competent. One man in the sample studied felt that although L-dopa improved his motor control, it compromised his intellectual capabilities to an unacceptable degree. In an effort to achieve what he considered to be optimal cognitive performance, he was known to titrate his medication in a particularly idiosyncratic way, not always with the knowledge of his neurologist. His efforts at maintaining control of the situation in this way led him to be seen as a "difficult" patient, which from the point of view of his doctors, he undoubtedly was. His behaviour however, should also be understood in terms of his struggle to retain control and not to be "at the mercy of his medication" (male patient, aged 45). Negative or unpredictable experiences with medication remind the patient of how distanced they have become from their past life, especially when dependency characterises the present. Experiences of this kind may also amount to another chip in the gradual etching away of the person's image of themselves.

Charmaz (1983) suggests that another kind of restriction on peoples' lives may come about as a result of not receiving sufficient information and treatment. Although a great deal of effort has gone into improving communication in this area over recent years, in large part due to lobbying from patients' organisations such as Parkinson's U.K., a major concern on the part of patients' and their families is that they may not be fully informed about innovations in treatment; inequalities in access to certain services, such as rehabilitation and speech therapy are also recognised as an on-going problem (All Party Parliamentary Group for Parkinson's Disease 2009; Hatano et al. 2009).

Some people restrict their lives voluntarily, because of the anxiety and uncertainty they feel as a result of their condition. They may stop travelling "for fear that something might happen", give up driving "to avoid stress", or change their place of residence for ease of access or "to be nearer their children" (female patient, age 62, present sample). Such changes in lifestyle may appear pragmatic and sensible, but when they are not in keeping with any realistic threats, rather an expression of anxiety, they do not serve to eliminate problems. One sufferer's daughter remarked:

> She moved here a few years ago because she wanted to be closer to us, but it hasn't really made any difference. We still don't see much of her unless we go to visit her. She's so reluctant to go out on her own, even though the illness doesn't really stop her doing so. Physically she's quite well on the medication. But she's full of nerves, worries about almost everything. She won't be reassured. People tried at first, but they have stopped going round to see her. Even the children don't want to, because she just complains all the time, nothing seems to cheer her up.
> (Re: female patient, aged 62, present study).

These observations would appear to confirm Charmaz's (1983, 175) view that: "the greater the loss of control, ... the more likely that the individual's self-concept suffers and he or she will restrict his or her life voluntarily".

Finally, the financial burden imposed by chronic illness may be a major factor in restricting peoples' lives. For example, changing accommodation may be forced on people by financial circumstances, resulting in loss of friends and neighbours and giving rise to social isolation. Although this appeared less of a concern for older people in the sample studied, their financial positions being relatively stable, it was more likely to affect younger sufferers and their families, where the impact of losing social support might be potentially more serious as it extends to a larger number of family members, including children. Younger sufferers were also more affected by the financial burden of being forced to resign their jobs because of the illness. These fundamental restrictions to peoples' lives, whether voluntary or enforced, are likely to detrimentally influence their image of themselves.

5.3.7 Social isolation

A major consequence of leading a restricted life is social isolation. Since people normally live in social networks and derive their sense of self from social relationships, social isolation is a major contributor to losing one's self-concept. For most people social relationships are built around their work and leisure activities, and the two frequently overlap considerably. Losing the ability to participate in just one of these areas of life is thus severely restricting and generally leads to feelings of isolation (Charmaz 1983).

In chronic illness such as PD, peoples' social networks are often reduced to contact with their families, as sufferers withdraw from former social circles, often taking their spouse-carers with them (Miller et al. 1996). Lack of reciprocity in established relationships on the part of the person with PD may be one reason for increasing social isolation, as former friends and even relatives sense that they are no longer welcome. A reason for this may be that the sufferer does not have the energy or concentration to sustain these relationships. Difficulties in communication and the Parkinsonian mask-like appearance of facial features only serve to strengthen these impressions and cause others to withdraw. Some people, a minority in the present study, complained that they felt "abandoned", left to cope by themselves, whilst others reported a singular form of isolation, feeling as if they were alone in being affected by the disease. Stanley-Hermanns et al. (2010) have reported similar impressions among their patients. The majority, however, despite sometimes quite evident social isolation, did not complain. They saw their situation as being: "par for the course, under the circumstances" (male patient, aged 65).

A number of people remarked that when they first revealed their condition to their family and friends they were met with concern, interest and demonstrations of assistance if required. With the passage of time, however, this interest dwindled to just a few members of their immediate family.

On occasion, sufferers feel isolated even though in the presence of others. This occurs when the attitudes expressed towards the patient, albeit unwittingly, are infantilising and embarrass, ignore or otherwise devalue the patient. This has been described as the "does he take sugar?" syndrome, (BBC Radio 4: programme title for those with visual impairments) in which questions concerning the patient are not addressed directly to him/her, but through his carer, as if the person was not able to understand and respond to them normally. Not surprisingly, patients feel alienated by this approach, but may not have the resources to protest, and so choose to withdraw and isolate themselves voluntarily. Again, Charmaz (1983) reflects that feelings of lack of control and consequent changes in the person's self-image are almost inevitable under these circumstances.

Social isolation affects not only the patient, but the carer too. As the number of people in contact with the couple decreases, so too do opportunities for social support and all that it offers. One carer described this as follows:

> Support. Here is where your research will, I hope, produce the greatly needed improvement. You refer to the need of support from 'informal sources'. How right you are. By far the greatest trauma for me has been the discovery of how friends, even of long standing, will back off, 'might get involved' withdrawal, even if one has done a lot for them. We have lived in this little road for 26 years, and are 'friends' with all; my wife, an SRN ... has always helped the sick here, and even laid out the dead, yet now, about half the road keep their distance. Inexplicably .... But destructive as this has been to me, how many cases I come across of family and *EVEN* spouses who just do not want to know. That must be devastating indeed.
> (Male carer of spouse with PD, aged 72, participating in the study; original emphasis).

With time, the carer may feel worn down by the task of caring and in the absence of support from others, may communicate this to the sufferer. This is reflected in the following words of one carer:

> ... the "carer" (horrible expression, or word, isn't it? I would prefer a more neutral word like "minder" or something more truthfully reflecting the sufferer's housekeeper/nurse/victim);

She goes on to speak of:

> ... the reality of being boxed up with an advanced PD case...;

and refers to her husband as "Sir":

> ... (I) can't imagine anything worse than being boxed up with Sir at some "special" nursing home-type accommodation, entirely surrounded by PD "couples"!! ... . I would willingly take my husband on holiday, if he wanted to go anywhere, but NOT a "special" holiday.
> (Female carer of spouse with PD, aged 74, participating in the study; original emphasis).

This carer's euphemistic use of language and the scorn that she pours upon the idea of spending time in a specialised facility set up for people with PD to take a break, accompanied by their carers, reflects her desire to distance herself from the situation. From her point of view this can be seen as a form of denial and therefore as a means of coping. From the sufferer's perspective, it serves to deepen the sense of isolation, strengthening feelings of being a burden and consequent guilt and depression. Equally, however, the person with PD may become so absorbed in their own condition that they fail to recognise the effect that it is having on others:

> He just sits there, all day. Nothing seems to interest him anymore – not even the grandchildren, so they've stopped coming round. No-one really visits anymore. It's impossible to talk to him, to have a conversation like before. It's like he's there in body, but he's not himself anymore;
> (Female carer of spouse with PD, aged 68, participating in the study).

In consequence, carers frequently experience social isolation themselves, as the sufferer withdraws into the illness (McRae et al. 2009).
Charmaz (1983, 179) writes:

> Visibility of obvious suffering typically causes friends and acquaintances discomfort since obvious suffering rips away the previously known public, sociable presentation of self, thereby making sociability problematic.

The stooped, shuffling figure of someone with PD, tremorous and drooling, having difficulty speaking, a mere shadow of his/her former self is almost a stereotype of old age and disability. Even the language used in the description suggests that loss of self lies at the heart of the person's suffering. People often use language of this kind to make their point: "He's just not the same person he once was" (female carer, age 60, participating in the present study).

The loneliness of social isolation is most acute for people with PD who live alone. Even the most trivial of social contacts, such as deliveries from the postman or the milkman, often take on exceptional significance, making the person feel valued and supported:

> Oh, the milkman always stops for a little chat on the doorstep when I pay him. It's something I look forward to, you know, seeing his cheery face. It helps when you live alone and don't get out as much anymore.
> (Female patient, age 69, present study).

Contacts of this kind, though brief and intermittent are re-valued and provide a welcome interlude in the person's daily routine, giving them something to look forward to. Routine clinical appointments may take on a special significance, around which the person's life is planned, as they take priority over everything else. The sense of this is rarely, if ever, questioned, unless a collision arises with an exceptional family event such as a wedding:

> I really don't know what to do – my grandson's getting married in April, and it just happens to be the date of my next appointment at the clinic. I'll have to ring up and ask to have it changed – I hope they won't mind. (Female patient, age 66, present study).

Patients who are socially isolated may also vest doctors with special authority, which assumes an extraordinary significance for their self-image (Charmaz 1983). The images of self reflected by the clinician begin to occupy the patient, sometimes for lengthy periods of time; they are chewed over, elaborated and, if the opportunity arises, discussed with others. They form the substance of self-appraisals which modify the person's image of themselves and can often have immense importance for their future wellbeing:

> When ill persons receive positive reflections of self in interaction and take them as credible and real, they are more apt to regard themselves positively. But when demeaned and discredited by those to whom they attach significance – even during the briefest of interactions – then maintaining a positive self-image becomes problematic (Charmaz 1983, 181).

Patients frequently emphasize their need to be treated "as a person"; a female patient, aged 40, with early PD writes of her family doctor:

> She encourages and supports my endeavours and always has time to listen. Depression can be a big part of Parkinson's, and I know that somehow she

> understands. She is there rooting for me to pick myself up and get going again. Just knowing that she is there, available when needed, is reassuring. I depend on my family doctor more than she realises. It would have been nice if she could have been there at the beginning, but I'm thankful she's here now. ... If my doctor can't give me what I really want, which is a cure, she can do the next best thing. She can be there when I need to talk or work something out; she can make the time to listen carefully. She can make me feel like a real, feeling person, not just an unusual statistic. And I am very lucky, because she does (Hayes 1994).

It is of course, not always the case that clinicians are regarded as having such unquestionable authority and psychological rather than social factors may be responsible for this. Nevertheless, the cases cited provide an illustration of how social isolation may influence a person's self-concept in PD.

5.3.8 Discrediting definitions of self

Views of the self which are critical and demoralising arise not only from interactions with others, but also from the person's own unmet expectations (Charmaz 1983). Stigmatisation, which has already been discussed, is an example of the former. Failure to achieve one's aspirations, along with the realisation that illness has barred the way to their future realisation, constitutes the latter.

People with PD may suffer discrediting forms of stigmatisation in a number of different forms. Patients may feel that their actions are being watched and evaluated by others, without a proper understanding of their cause. A common theme in PD is an unsteady gait being judged as a sign of inebriation. Others include inappropriate interpretation of the tremor characteristic of the disease as well as rigidity, freezing, facial immobility and incomprehensible speech all of which may be disconcerting to others and cause confusion socially, thereby eliciting negative responses. The significance of such discrediting encounters depends on their perceived magnitude, the situation in which this occurs, the relative importance of the person involved in the discrediting behaviour and how often such behaviour takes place (Charmaz 1983). If the person with PD is already particularly vulnerable or feels compelled to accept the disparaging definitions of him/herself, the intensity of the experience is magnified.

One of the most acute influences likely to shape the sufferer's self-concept is in relation to significant people in his/her life with whom s/he shares an intimate relationship (Schneider and Conrad 1981). For most people with PD this is usually the person's spouse or partner, but it may also be their children and occasionally it may be other relatives or friends. Precisely because of their close intimacy with the sufferer, spouses (or children) are involved in the mainstream of caring and it has increasingly been recognised that their experiences of the situation of chronic illness are often stressful, taking a toll on their physical and mental wellbeing (see chapter 6). Carers often lack support at times when the demands on them intensify significantly. The mental and physical exhaustion that they experience may prevent them from being able to maintain the sufferer's morale by sustaining positive images of the (sufferer's) self. At times they may even discredit or abuse them (Smith et al. 2011). The reasons for this are complex, but they often lie in the sufferer no longer being able to meet the carer's expectations, whether or not these are realistic (Charmaz 1983). For example, the wife of a sufferer in the present study who was considerably older by some twenty years, admitted: " I would never have married him if I had known that he would go on to develop Parkinson's disease *and* if I had known then, what Parkinson's disease is really like" (female carer of spouse with PD, aged 47, participating in the study; original emphasis). Such extreme reactions are very rare and from observation of this couple's situation, it seemed unlikely that she would have confronted her husband with this information directly. But it is likely that, at times, she put this message across to him in other ways. Had she done so directly, the ensuing crisis would have led us to draw the conclusion that she was indeed, under extreme stress. This carer was unable to come to terms with the range and intensity of the limitations that had been imposed on their lives by the illness and the disappointment she experienced may have been intensified by her relatively younger age and the expectations she had of married life, companionship, sexual relations, meeting the demands of domestic life and her own personal and career aspirations.

Carers' inability to recognise or accept certain aspects of PD may account for the fact that the sufferer is sometimes unable to fulfil the carer's expectations in the areas mentioned. The attitude respected in British society, of "soldiering on, no matter what" may put pressure on people with PD to try to "carry on as before." Their inability to function normally is then interpreted in terms of poor motivation rather than their physical condition and develops negative connotations, which are perceived as an attack upon their sense of self (Charmaz 1983).

By contrast, carers can help to maintain sufferers' continuity with their pre-illness self. It was not unusual in the course of the present study to interview carers who were sensitive to the needs of their spouse, respecting their autonomy, but offering support when needed. This is exemplified in the way a number of carers showed no irritation or impatience with their spouses, whose speech was slow and laboured, but allowed them to speak for themselves during the interviews. They did not interrupt, and when speaking themselves, engaged their husband or wife in the conversation. They exercised tact, rather than overriding their partner, when disagreements arose. These attitudes conveyed the respect and dignity in which carers held the person they were caring for, and at the same time, reflected their coming to terms with their own position, showing an understanding of the sufferer's behaviour in the context of the illness and the adaptations they had had to make to their lives in order to cope with it. By making efforts to maintain their ongoing relationship with the sufferer, and emphasising the positive aspects of their lives in the present, these carers effectively ensured that their partners were not discredited.

People without supportive carers appear more vulnerable to this kind of demoralisation and become particularly susceptible to attempts to discredit them, whether it be at the point of diagnosis, where they may get the impression that their concerns are not validated by clinicians, or during the course of the illness, because they feel that their complaints regarding ill-health are not taken seriously by those looking after them.

Charmaz (1983, 184) summarises the conditions that make it more likely that discrediting definitions will be adopted by the patient as follows:

> when (1) the ill-person feels vulnerable, (2) the ill-person identifies with the individual(s) who discredit him or her, and (3) the discrediting validates a hidden fear or recasts the ill person's self-images in new unattractive light.

Discrediting may occur in a variety of different forms, some of which are quite subtle. This happens when people are devalued or discounted as a result of their condition, as if they were no longer human or adult and able to take responsibility for themselves. Examples are when the patient's views are overridden or trivialised, mocked or quite simply not taken into account. It occurs when people feel they are being treated as "cases of Parkinson's disease" and not as individuals who happen to have PD: "The neurology clinic I attend is renowned for its expertise, but I'm just a number. Basically I don't like going there" (patient with PD cited in Hayes 1994, 507). Being discounted in this way, not only diminishes the person's status, but also leads to emotional isolation.

When people become unable to assert their personal significance in the usual ways valued by society, i.e. through different forms of action, but appear frail and incapacitated, affirmation of a positive self-image that is acceptable to and valued by others becomes difficult. Charmaz (1987) has described how chronically sick people are involved in a constant struggle to lead valued lives and maintain definitions of self which are positive and worthwhile. Social and cultural conventions are extremely powerful and patients feel humiliated by attempts to make light of the fact that they have been granted special exemptions from meeting them, by virtue of their illness. Thus hearing from others that they are fortunate to be exempt from certain duties, such as doing housework, may be good-naturedly acknowledged, but only serves to remind the person with PD that his/her limitations are readily recognised and taken as evidence of the fact that they can no longer participate in the real business of everyday life.

People may also feel discounted when care arrangements are introduced that draw attention to those areas in which they have become most incapable. Such arrangements may then be viewed as invasions of privacy or unnecessary indulgences. For example, home care arrangements may be resented by a wife who has managed a home for many years and she may protest that she is "... perfectly capable of looking after this small flat, especially when you compare it to the house we used to live in" and the person whose driving skills are in question, may complain that a taxi is an "unjustifiable expense" (female patient, aged 62, present study; male patient, aged 59, present study).

Several strategies can be identified, which appear to represent attempts on the sufferer's part to maintain positive evaluations of themselves whilst continuing relationships with others. Sometimes these involve negotiating positions with carers in order that the sufferer still feels s/he is making a valued contribution to the relationship. For one couple interviewed for the present study this was evidenced in the fact that although the carer husband had taken over many of the domestic duties, he was happy to let his wife continue in what he light-heartedly referred to as the "managerial role" in which she decided upon what shopping was required each day, the menu for meals and other such household matters. Although at times this must have been trying for him, he patiently encouraged her involvement without forcing her to live up to unrealistic expectations of her past self, thus validating the positive aspects of her current existence. As a result they continued to share important aspects of their daily lives together and not just those centred around care-giving activities which helped to maintain the continuity of their pre-illness relationship.

Another example is the couples' readiness to take part in research of the kind described in the present study. The refusal rate was very low (see chapter 9) and people were keen to share their experiences openly and gave generously of their time, despite the tribulations of the disease. They frequently expressed the view, that they were willing to help in this way, in the hope that their contributions might ultimately be of some value to others in similar circumstances. The extent to which the illness had touched their lives and caused a fundamental re-evaluation of their sense of purpose was reflected in the fact that carers of people with PD frequently volunteered their assistance, even after the death of their spouse.

Not all forms of discrediting are external. Sometimes, when the person with PD is no longer able to take for granted some valued aspect of his/her functioning which is viewed as an essential part of positive self-image, for example sexual functioning, self-discrediting occurs. Sufferers feel extreme disappointment, that despite their best efforts to come to terms with chronic illness, and their willingness to accept certain restrictions, the illness has nonetheless deprived them of something that they did not feel able to sacrifice to it. With the accumulation of discrediting events which have eroded away their self-image, people begin to lose faith in their own abilities and to lack confidence in the likelihood of future achievements. Their perception of themselves is redrawn in terms of being a burden to others. Eventually overwhelmed by the hopelessness of the situation as they perceive it, they cease any attempts to reconstruct the self that has emerged and accept a discredited self-image (Charmaz 1983, 188).

5.3.9 Becoming a burden

The concern that one is, or may become, a burden is frequently voiced by people with all types of chronic illness. According to Charmaz (1983) it is associated with losing hope and becoming resigned to the fact that positive self-images are irretrievably a thing of the past. People with PD worry that they are becoming a burden as they grow increasingly dependent and lose mobility. This is in keeping with Charmaz's (1983) observation that concerns about burden are, in the main, related to the need for physical care. Sufferers are less likely to acknowledge the burden of psychological and financial care for their carers: they may be surprised when, and if, recognition of the former eventually dawns. Indeed, this did not appear to be a major concern for the sample of the population with PD interviewed for the present study.

The sense of becoming a burden from the sufferer's point of view in PD is a degrading experience, dominated by uncertainty and feeling that control has been lost over the more fundamental aspects of their existence. Sufferers may acknowledge the burden for their carers, at the same time, expressing the fear that they never have the certainty that something will in fact, get done:

> I know that my wife does her best for me, but I still worry about the medication. You see, if I don't get my tablets on time, I'm likely to go off, and there's no knowing when I'll get right again. I have to have the medication on time just to be able to do things. It's very important. But my wife doesn't really see that. She says that 5 minutes here or there won't make any difference.
> (Male patient, aged 68, participating in the present study).

Concerns of this kind are often reinforced by the inflexibility of thinking and obsessionality that is frequently seen in PD. Equally, for the carer, knowing that the daily routine had to be completed, no matter what, with the awareness that the sufferer was particularly anxious about this happening, was often an additional source of stress.

In resigning themselves to being a burden, or at least recognising that they may be becoming one, people with chronic illness become aware of the fact that their conditions are now the most important determinant of their social identity. People with PD become "Parkinsonians" or "Parkinson's patients"; terms such as "sufferer" and "patient" have also been criticised as they are seen as serving to identify the person in terms of their illness. The negative consequences of these labelling effects are well-known and have been discussed in detail by Goffman (1963).

The illness experience for people who feel that they have acquired the negative status of being a burden also means distancing themselves from former images of themselves. Their former identities, which were once based upon their occupation and social position, community and leisure activities, are of the past. For them, the sense of being a burden is also associated with not being able to fulfil the obligations that were implicit in these different roles and they may be riddled with guilt and shame as a result. Others attempt to carry on beyond what could be reasonably expected of them, in an effort to avoid burdening others more than is absolutely necessary and in an effort to conserve their self-image.

Feelings of uselessness are frequently expressed by people with PD, particularly in relation to giving up significant roles in their lives. Most commonly, this is in relation to work, especially for men, but women too may feel that they are no longer able to fulfil the demands of being a grandmother, for example, as they no longer feel competent to have responsibility for children in their care. Concerns about being useless may be particularly acute for younger people with PD disease, as the strain of the disease is increasingly a burden on the carer. Few of those interviewed for the present study had any outside help, either formal or informal, and so responsibility for caring for the sufferer usually lay with one person, in the case of the present study, with the spouse. The impact of this is discussed in the chapters that follow.

This account of the experience of PD emphasizes the disadvantage and deprivation that results from chronic illness. It paints a bleak and depressing picture because PD is associated with a diminution in quality of life for both sufferers and carers (Chaudhuri 2011; Rahman et al. 2008). However, the universality of the deprivation experience as characteristic of chronic illness, has been challenged by a number of authors in recent years, including Charmaz (2006) herself, and it was by no means the most pervasive impression gained of living with PD from the present study. The way in which people adapt to and cope with their illnesses to a large extent determines the quality of their experiences. Processes of adaptation are discussed next in the final section of this chapter.

5.4 Theories of adaptation to chronic illness

Theories concerned with adaptation to chronic illness recognise ill-health as a natural and inevitable part of life which requires that the sick person adapt to the illness, a demand which is particularly apt in the case of chronic conditions. Psychosocial views of adaptation see it as a transactional process, shaped through psychological, cultural, social, institutional and biomedical mechanisms of interaction; illness events, when evaluated from this perspective, are seen as an on-going, dynamic process or "sickness career" (Twaddle 1973). This terminology has two major advantages: firstly it serves to emphasize that the adaptive process is drawn out and not confined within a limited time scale. It is thus suited to descriptions of chronic illness. Secondly, the notion of a sickness career is not intended to be pejorative in the sense of emphasizing that patients with chronic illness relish their situation because of the benefits it brings in releasing them from the duties and obligations of "normal" life. Rather, the notion of career is intended to describe "a conventionally patterned sequence of social events through which people pass" (Freidson 1970). Its main advantage is in recognising that the experience of having a chronic condition is a process in which the patient's behaviour is continually being redefined according to his/her perceptual view of the illness; this in turn determines a variety of responses such as the choice of carer, the success of the doctor-patient interaction, patterns of adherence to treatment regimes and the degree of functional adaptation (see Young 2004 for a full review).

The notion of "adaptation to disability" refers to an individual's ability to acknowledge and accept his or her current health status, including the physical, emotional and cognitive aspects of his condition which determine his/her strengths as well as limitations with regard to independent-living, interpersonal relationships and employment prospects. It also reflects the individual's ability to set appropriate goals and plans within the constraints imposed by his/her illness and its consequences (Livneh and Antonak 1997). Research suggests that for people with congenital disabilities the process of body image and identity development is likely to be similar to that of children without disabilities (Livneh and Antonak 1997) so that the adaptation process appears to be a natural part of development. However, people who experience later-onset, chronic illness or acquired disability are likely to find that their internal equilibrium and sense of self is considerably shaken, as described above. Learning to live with chronic illness or disability is one of the developmental tasks of later life for many people, who often describe the onset of ill-health as a major "turning point" in their lives (Frazier et al. 2003), or in terms of the "biographical disruption" described by Bury (1982). They may be required to contend with significant changes in their social and familial relationships and adapt their roles in life, whilst at the same time having to deal with the psychological distress, physical pain, prolonged medical treatment and functional limitations imposed by the illness (Charmaz 1983). One of the tasks of rehabilitation research has been to try to understand this process of adaptation and to devise effective clinical interventions that may help to facilitate its evolution. Attention has been particularly focused on understanding why some people appear to get "stuck" along the way (Wright and Kirby 1999).

Recent research however, has challenged the view that a biographical disruption is the inevitable consequence in chronic illness. Studies are emerging which appear to suggest that the context in which chronic illness occurs, i.e. in terms of the person's age and lifetime experience, is important to how it is perceived. It seems that older people are more likely to accept illness (for example, arthritis) as a normal part of old age (Sanders, Donovan and Dieppe 2002). Equally those whose lives have been characterised by adversity in the form of health and social problems are less likely to view the onset of a serious interruption to health in the form of cancer (Sinding and Wiernikowski 2008) or stroke (Faircloth et al. 2004) as a singularly disruptive event in their lives. The stoicism exemplified in their attitudes reflects a frequently cited commitment to avoid "dwelling" on the illness. The interpretation of this position is radically different depending on the theoretical perspective taken. The sociological position using health narratives would most likely interpret the biographical continuity as evidence of the fact that the illness experience is, to a large extent, shaped by the context, or the society, in which we live: "broad cultural and moral discourses, patterns of social interaction and structures of power combine to foreclose older women's accounts of disruption" (Sinding and Wiernikowski 2008, 389). An explanation derived from psychological theory would be more likely to emphasize "how individual efforts to manage distressing problems and emotions affect the physical and psychological outcomes of stress" (Somerfield and McCrae 2000, 620). From this perspective, the impact of an event depends on how the subject perceives and interprets it (Lazarus and Folkman 1984) and on the defence and coping mechanisms used to adapt to the disruption that it causes (Salmon 2002).

There do not appear to be any published studies on biographical disruption in PD and so direct evidence is not available. Nevertheless, the maintenance of continuity experienced by older people in spite of the onset of chronic or life-threatening illness suggests that older people with PD might also be protected from the effects of the disruption. The corollary of this is that the disruption might be greater for people in whom PD starts at an earlier age and there is preliminary evidence that this is the case (e.g. Schrag and Schott 2006). Adaptation to chronic illness in general, and to PD in particular, may be facilitated by circumstances such as those mentioned, in spite of the adversities described in the foregoing discussion.

5.4.1 Theories of psychosocial adaptation

In the wake of decades of research dedicated to understanding the dynamics of psychosocial adaptation, it is disappointing to find a lack of conceptual clarity and limited agreement concerning fundamental questions, such as the nature of the process of adaptation (Frank and Elliott 2000). Bishop (2005) points out that the early approaches to understanding the process of psychosocial adaptation were drawn on medical or psychopathological models which held that: "specific types of disabilities brought about specific types of personality characteristics or psychological problems" (Shontz 2003, 178). It was believed that there existed "a direct relationship between the condition and the psychosocial impairment" (Elliott 1994, 231). An example of this was the so-called "homilopathic" personality disorder described by Kraepelin (1915), which was supposed to pertain to "invalids" and reflected their alleged "separateness" in psychological terms, producing difficulties in psychosocial adaptation and in particular, in their inability to function normally in a variety of social roles e.g. family, sexual, professional, social (Garett and Levine 1962). This diagnostic category is no longer recognised as many of the characteristics associated with it have been subsumed under the notion of personality disorder. Moreover the simplistic attribution of certain personality traits to people with disabilities is clearly unwarranted and indeed, has gone a long way to be damaging, by fuelling the negative stereotypes of chronic illness and disability which persist in society and which Goffman (1963) termed “stigmatisation”.

These early attempts at a theoretical conceptualisation of adaptation to chronic illness were doomed to failure as they did not reflect either the individuality of the disabled person, or the complexity of the process of adaptation. Neither did they take into account the interaction between the individual and his or her social and physical environment. Indeed, later studies were to show that neither diagnosis nor degree of impairment were good predictors of outcome as far as psychosocial adaptation was concerned (Williamson et al. 1994). These early theories were thus shown to be lacking in empirical support and clinical utility (Bishop 2005).

5.4.2 Stage theories of adaptation

The theories that followed were sequential or stage theories which implied that adaptation to chronic illness followed a predictable, developmental path through different levels of adjustment, ending in a so-called stage of adaptation. Full adaptation was to be achieved by passing through a hierarchical sequence of stages, in which coming to terms with the tasks required in each preceding stage of the adaptation procedure was the prerequisite for moving on to the next stage. This developmental aspect of the models was one of their greatest assets, as it emphasised the dynamics of the adaptation process. Numerous stage models have been proposed, all of them essentially viewing adaptation to chronic illness as a process of coming to terms with the loss of health and hence similar to the grief experienced after the loss of a loved one (e.g. Kubler-Ross 1969). There were considerable differences among the various models proposed with regard to the total number of stages involved in the process of adaptation, but they generally had three stages in common as typified by the model described by Shontz (1975). The first of these was that of initial “shock”, when the person is bewildered, especially if the diagnosis was unexpected, and reacts almost automatically, without the possibility of more considered analysis, or perhaps with denial, as if unable to take in the full meaning of the disclosure. This initial phase is gradually transformed into an "encounter" reaction, where the individual is overcome by emotional distress, characterised by feelings of loss and despair. The third and final stage is that of acceptance and represents the point of adjustment to the illness. Other variants included additional reactions (e.g. guilt, hostility), but the models were less consistent in this regard (Kendall and Buys 1998). Stage models mostly retained Parson's sick role model as a central tenet, but built upon it, by acknowledging the fact that living with chronic illness involved a long-term extension of the doctor-patient relationship and perceiving adaptation in terms of the patient's return to socially normal functioning (e.g. Suchman 1965). Shontz's model, and other linear models of this kind, implying a defined trajectory towards adaptation that must be traversed, had many shortcomings. Not all patients follow the path defined, nor is it a path that once trodden, delivers the person to his/her final destination in the secure knowledge that the journey is complete. Progressive illnesses bring further losses and the path to adaptation inevitably becomes well-trodden as new challenges present themselves (Charmaz 1995). For a fuller discussion of stage theories see Pąchalska (2007) and Livneh and Antonak (1997).

As a result of these deficiencies, the underlying assumptions behind theories of this kind have been questioned in recent years. A major criticism is that it is unrealistic to conceive of a final stage of adjustment and to define exactly what is required of the patient in order to achieve this (Parker, Schaller and Hansmann 2003). In addition, Kendall and Buys (1998) have drawn attention to the fact that since these theories are sequential and recognise depression and denial as normal in the adaptation process, using them to guide practice carries a potential risk, in that clinicians might be inclined not only to refrain from referring patients to specialist services in the belief that this was an inevitable step in the adaptation process, but that they might actually anticipate and encourage such responses. Such theories imply that adaptation cannot be achieved unless the stage of depression and/or denial is "worked through" and where these reactions are not apparent, the patient may be deemed not to have successfully completed the transition. A more realistic view is that depression is likely to recur at different stages in long-term illness and denial may be a coping mechanism that is invoked at various points in the process. Adjustment is therefore a goal that has to be achieved repeatedly throughout the person's lifetime. Stage theories have thus been criticised as lacking empirical validity (Parker et al. 2003) and having insufficient complexity to accurately represent the adaptation process, particularly where progressive conditions are concerned (Kendall and Buys 1998).

5.4.3 Interactionist models of adaptation to chronic illness

The next phase in the development of psychosocial adaptation models came with a more comprehensive approach in which emphasis was placed on the interaction between the individual and the environment in which s/he lives. According to Livneh and Antonak (1997) adaptation outcomes are influenced by four groups of variables: social-demographic, disability-related, personal attributes and physical/social environment. This represents an attempt at forming a comprehensive and interactive model which takes into account the fact that psychosocial adaptation is not only a highly complex, but also individual process.

One particular form of interactionist theory takes a specifically psychological or cognitive approach to adaptation, acknowledging it as a recurrent process. This view suggests that the path taken by an individual in adapting to chronic illness is likely to be guided by his/her system of beliefs and understanding of the world more generally. These cognitive dimensions are conceptualised as schemas and they serve to filter and interpret a person's experiences, particularly at times of stress (Beck et al. 1979). Pre-existing schemas are likely to be challenged in the context of chronic illness, but patients' tendencies to persist in using them, despite their inadequacies, is used to explain the phenomenon of denial or distortion of reality. Alternatively, awareness of their insufficiencies may lead to depression. With time, however, as new information is assimilated, schemas can be modified, allowing a more realistic stance in which a more balanced view of the person him/herself and of the future can be formed. The process of adaptation to chronic illness is seen as following a recurrent cycle in which new schemas are developed, modified and restructured in line with the individual's changing needs over the course of the illness (Kendall and Buys 1998). Three specific areas of need have been identified and these include (1) the search for meaning in chronic illness; (2) the need for a sense of mastery and control over the illness and the future; and (3) the need to protect the person's sense of self and post-illness identity (Barnard 1990). Researchers have described the process of adaptation in these areas as a pendulum motion, swinging between two extremes, which eventually settles at an optimal centre point over time (Yoshida 1993). At one extreme, the person's perceptions are associated with a pre-illness identity, in which they attempt to function as their former selves, or even in an above normal capacity, as if trying to prove to themselves that illness need not be a barrier to fulfilment. This apparent lack of accommodation to the reality of disability is referred to as "denial", but within a recurrent model of adaptation it may also represent an attempt to retain the meaning, control and identity that was associated with pre-illness cognitive schema. Charmaz (1983) views this as an essential phase in schema reconstruction which facilitates the emergence of a valued post-illness identity and helps to contradict negative images of illness and disability. Initially, before these new schema are formed, confrontation with the former self and the demands placed upon it are likely to result in disappointment, forcing the pendulum to swing towards the "disability" extreme, in which individuals see themselves only in a negative light, leading to diminished self-worth, self-recrimination and severe depression. This is a point of extreme vulnerability in the adaptation process, leading to the formation of negative self-schema, which if not curtailed, may precipitate a downward spiral into helplessness, persistent depression and other chronic psychosocial problems. However, with time and the accumulation of new experiences, the need to prove oneself diminishes, reducing opportunities for failure and allowing more positive schema to emerge to the fore. Although the illness continues to be evaluated negatively, it no longer dominates the person's schema as in former swings. Instead, it gradually becomes dissociated from other characteristics of the self, at the same time being integrated into the person's schema, allowing them to recognise the permanent limitations imposed by the illness (Kendall and Buys 1998). This is evidenced in situations where the illness takes on a persona and patients may refer to various aspects of living with "Mr Parkinson" (Phillips 2006).

This more ecological approach embodied in interactionist models, however, does not overcome the difficulty of stage models, namely that they remain more descriptive than predictive. They also fail in explaining why some individuals manage the transition towards adaptation and defining the characteristic settings in which this occurs, despite having to overcome a range of problems, whilst others do not. Adaptation is a uniquely subjective process (Bishop 2005). Individuals show significant variation, both within their own performance and in comparison to others, in the adaptation process (Kendall and Buys 1998). Thus neither the condition itself, nor specific characteristics of the individual and his/her environment are predictors of outcome as far as adaptation is concerned. It appears that a complex interaction of the individual's subjective appraisal of his/her situation, and availability of resources in the form of individual coping styles and possible benefits derived from the environment, such as social support, seem to guide the process of adaptation (Lazarus and Folkman 1984). In particular, appropriate access to resources appears to facilitate the emergence of more positive cognitive schema in the face of life-altering circumstances, such as those accompanying chronic illness. These in turn generate effective coping strategies which result in improved psychosocial well-being (Lazarus 1993). Kendall and Buys (1998) speculate that "individuals with higher levels of resources will progress through the adjustment cycle at a faster rate with better outcomes and fewer recurrent problems than those with low levels of resources." They consider personal resources such as self-esteem or social skills and environmental resources, such as social and family support and financial security to be key elements in the process of adaptation, which they view as a cyclical, recurrent process rather than in terms of the traditional sequential paradigm. Models of adaptation to chronic illness and disability thus need to take account of adaptation as an individual and personal response to disability or illness-related disruptions across a wide range of life domains. These disruptions may be experienced for example, in interpersonal relationships, in interaction with the physical environment and as changes in psychological health and function (after Bishop 2005).

5.4.4 Psychometric approaches to adaptation

A number of psychometric approaches have been used to define and measure adaptation outcome. Those in common use have been criticised for their unidimensional and atheoretical nature combined with conceptual vagueness (Livneh and Antonak 1997). Adaptation is reduced to a unidimensional construct, in which, for example, the presence of psychopathology (usually depression or anxiety), physical or behavioural complaints, changes in productivity or reduction in performance and the degree of acceptance of the disability are often treated, in isolation, as the sole indicators of the success or failure to adapt to chronic illness. Needless to say, these limitations mean that approaches of this kind are unable to capture the complex and multidimensional nature of the individual's experience, including those associated with gender and culture (Bishop 2005).

Moreover, the predominantly negative perspective that permeates this field, marginalises any positive aspects of the experience of living with a disability, and hence they do not have a place in the theoretical models or the instruments used to measure various aspects of adaptation. This is an important factor to bear in mind, as the majority of people do in fact adapt to chronic illness, taking the demands of the process of adaptation in their stride (which is not say that they do not experience difficulties) and despite chronic illness and disability, manage to derive as much satisfaction from life as healthy people (Salmon 2002). This is evidenced in the fact that people disabled by PD consistently evaluate their own quality of life more positively than do their carers (Fleming et al. 2005).

Thus as Bishop (2005) concludes, two main lessons emerge from the literature: first that adaptation is a multidimensional construct, and second, that it is a highly individualised process. As regards the first of these, it is clear that chronic illness and disability affect a range of psychological, physical, environmental and social areas of functioning and so adaptation must be measured using a multidimensional approach. Thus adaptation to chronic illness has been conceptualised in terms of management of psychological and behavioural symptoms (Sohlberg and Mateer 1989), the acquisition of new skills in vocational and social situations (Pąchalska 2007), and attitudes regarding the condition (Livneh and Martz 2007). In similar vein, Livneh and Antonak (1997, 8) have characterised adaptation as a process of: "active participation in social, vocational and avocational pursuits; successful negotiation of the physical environment; and awareness of remaining strengths and assets as well as existing functional limitations".

Most authors (e.g. Livneh and Antonak 1997) would probably accept that the following abilities need to be examined in order to evaluate a person's level of adaptation to chronic illness:

1. The individual's capacity to make a realistic appraisal of current abilities and deficits
2. Willingness to utilise compensation strategies
3. Progression through the grief and mourning process (denial, anger, depression) related to recognition of current abilities and deficits and acceptance of the situation
4. The patient's level of emotional stress, defensiveness or denial when confronted with current deficits or estimated possibilities of future functioning.
5. The severity of symptoms of depression, including preoccupation with loss and negativity about the present and the future.

If individuals appear not to have managed to negotiate a resolution in certain of these areas, treatment efforts might be effectively addressed to one or more of the particular points.

5.5 Adjustment

In the context of chronic illness, especially in the form of neurodegenerative conditions, the notion of adjustment cannot be conceived of as the achievement of a final, optimal stage in the process of adaptation. As noted in the foregoing discussion, the aim of treatment and management in a chronic condition is not the same as in acute disease. A recovery to full health and reintegration into a person's societal roles is not possible in a way similar to that which existed before the onset of illness and the person's view of the future is entirely changed. The aims of managing a chronic condition are consequently quite different. The individual concerned must be helped to understand the condition and to live successfully with it, as far as this is possible. A particularly valuable source of support in this regard has been from individuals themselves suffering from chronic illness (e.g. Fox 2002; Rosenbaum 2006; Vaughan 1986 and numerous websites, (e.g. http://www.healthinsite.gov.au/ topics/Personal_Stories_about_Parkinson_s_Disease) in which people with PD have given detailed accounts of their experiences and made their own recommendations about the management of the condition. There has been a proliferation of publications of this kind both in the form of advice and handbooks and via the internet on websites specifically devoted to the discussion of the illness experience in PD. The interest in them suggests that case studies of this kind are helpful in improving understanding of what it means to live with a chronic disabling disorder and that they are useful to individuals with similar problems. There has also been a very rapid expansion of lay associations in the form of self-help groups, patients' organizations etc. for specific conditions and these groups have become indispensable as an adjunct to the health-care system in many countries, providing high quality practical and information, engaging in advocacy work on behalf of people with specific conditions and sponsoring various forms of activity such as scientific and welfare research, and organising educational and support meetings etc. in an effort to meet the needs of their members. Many of these organizations (e.g. Parkinson's UK) are non-governmental organizations which play a significant role in lobbying government on behalf of their members and exerting an influence on policies affecting their welfare.

5.6 Chapter summary

The aim of this chapter has been to provide a focus on the experience of living with PD, following on from the description of the symptoms of the illness, which have been presented in the preceding chapters. It is impossible to do justice to the reality of living with the condition, in these few pages. The magnitude of the task, from accepting the initial diagnosis, through the many vicissitudes of the illness, its gradual progression and the toll that it takes in terms of physical and mental functioning is belied even in patients' own descriptions of the illness, which allow us rare glimpses into the subjective experience of PD. The evolving nature of the condition demands that adaptation to the illness follows a recurrent cycle in which the person's emotions and cognitions are continually modified and restructured in line with changing needs over the course of the illness.

In most instances, adaptation and adjustment is required not only on the part of the person with PD, but also from those who are in close contact with him/her, including family, friends, employers and others. The extent to which these associated people are able, or indeed willing, to make this adjustment, may to a large extent, affect the success with which the person is able to adapt to his/her situation. A vital role is played by carers of people with PD, whose presence is in evidence in the run-up to diagnosis and whose support is a guarantor of the patient's adaptation to the challenge of chronic illness. It is to the effects of having to support a close family member with PD that the discussion now turns in the chapters that follow.

CHAPTER SIX

THE CONTEXT OF CARE-GIVING IN NEURODEGENERATIVE CONDITIONS

6.1 Introduction

Over the last fifty years considerable gains in life expectancy for older people have emerged in developed countries, although they are often accompanied by longer periods of ill-health and disability (Olshansky et al. 1991). Governments have responded to the healthcare demands of their increasingly ageing populations by placing a much greater emphasis on community based programmes for the care of elderly and infirm sufferers. A series of policy reforms have directed this approach in the U.K. from the Department of Health (DOH) White Paper "Caring for people" (Secretaries of State 1989) to the "Vision for Adult Social Care" (DOH 2010b) which has given rise to the draft "Care and Support Bill" (DOH 2012b) and at the time of writing, is undergoing pre-legislative consultative procedures (for a full description of relevant legislation see Appendix A). All have relied to a large extent on the mobilization and maintenance of informal support systems for their implementation. It is estimated that in Britain (Pickard et al. 2000) and other countries of the OECD (Fujisawa and Colombo 2009) between 70-90% of the help and care services for people with long-term health problems are provided by informal carers, mainly spouses and adult children. It is increasingly recognized that, in order to be effective, community oriented services need to work in close liaison with families providing informal care. There has long been evidence that maintenance of an elderly demented person in the community is related to the degree of family support (Bergmann et al. 1978; Poulshock and Deimling 1984), and the decision to place a relative in long-term care is often determined primarily by the attitudes and well-being of the carer, rather than the level of disability of the care recipient (Bond and Clark 2002; Colerick and George 1986; Cousins et al. 2002; Deimling and Poulshock 1985; Gaugler, Kane, Kane and Newcomer 2005; Gilhooly 1986; Gilleard 1987; Gort et al. 2007; Greene and Timbury 1979;

Haupt and Kurz 1993; Okamoto, Hasebe and Harasawa 2007; Pot, Deeg and Knipscheer 2001; Yaffe et al. 2002; Zarit, Todd and Zarit 1986).

6.2 The context of care-giving

There has been some debate in the literature concerning the definition of who may be regarded as a carer. Broadly speaking, carers are acknowledged as being the primary unpaid helpers of people residing in the community, who need assistance with one or more of the basic tasks of everyday living. These are daily routine tasks involving either the activities of daily living (ADL; Mahoney and Barthel 1965), such as mobility, eating, bathing and using the toilet or the instrumental activities of daily living (IADL; Lawton and Brody 1969) such as doing housework, managing finances or medication and providing help with transport. The Carers (Recognition and Services) Act 1995 describes a carer as "someone who provides, or intends to provide, a substantial amount of care on a regular basis for a disabled, ill or elderly person." The basic elements of this definition are echoed in that used by Parkinson's UK (2012b), the U.K. charitable organisation for people with PD and their carers, which describes a carer as: "..... anyone who provides unpaid care and support to someone with Parkinson's".

The majority of people aged 65 or older who need help in performing these daily tasks rely exclusively on the help of their closest family, and to a lesser extent, their friends for their long-term care needs. Hence the terms "family" or "spousal" carers have been adopted to distinguish between different care situations and the term "child" carer is used to describe non-adult children who are the primary carers for their disabled parents. All of these terms have been subsumed under the more general description of "informal carers" which is increasingly used in the academic literature and in policy documents, but is perceived by carers themselves as failing to acknowledge the actual impact that caring may have on an individual's life and diminishing the importance of their contribution. It may also be an inadequate term, as in emphasizing the lack of formality attached to the caring role, it fails to recognize a number of the realities of becoming a carer, such as the lack of realistic alternatives and the extent to which many relatives feel that they are duty-bound to provide care to the sick and frail members of their families. In being viewed as "informal" rather than "professional", it might also be taken to infer that the care provided is of low intensity or even of low quality. None of these assumptions are likely to be true, as Twigg (1992) has pointed out:

> Informal care normally occurs in the context of the family or marital relationships, and is provided on an unpaid basis that draws on feelings of love, obligation and duty. Informal care does not imply that the care is provided on a casual or easy basis;

and carers are often unwilling to use formal services, because they are perceived as not being able to meet the needs of those that they look after to an acceptable standard (Lamura et al. 2006).

The number of carers in the U.K. is estimated at 6.8 million (based on the most recent General Household Survey (GHS) carried out in 2000 which addressed issues of informal care (Maher and Green 2002). This represents just over 11% of the population and is a figure that is set to increase into the twenty-first century (Brink 2004 cited in Duxbury, Higgins and Schroeder 2009). Informal carers do not constitute a homogeneous group, not least with regard to the intensity of care provided. Lighter involvement has been described in the social policy literature as "informal helping" as opposed to more demanding forms of assistance, described as "heavily involved caring" (Parker 1992). Carers defined as the latter are usually involved in providing long hours of care (in excess of 20 hours a week), they share the same household with the care-recipient and take responsibility for a range of personal and domestic tasks. It is estimated that approximately 1.8 million (27%) carers are providing more than 20 hours of care per week (Maher and Green 2002).

Carers' relationship to their care-recipients are also varied and as a result, their characteristics and needs differ considerably (Parker 1993). The majority of carers (approximately 75%) are looking after older people, who may be parents, parents-in-law or spouses. Those caring for parents and parents-in-law are usually in paid employment and this raises complex issues concerning the management of work and care responsibilities. Spouse carers are often elderly and may have health problems themselves. The most recent estimates of the numbers of people caring for an older person in Great Britain, using the 2000 GHS data, suggest that there are over a third of a million spouse carers and nearly half a million children caring for an older parent/parent-in-law for 20 hours a week or more (Pickard 2002).

Studies of the families of frail, elderly people have found that provision of informal care can have profound consequences for the carer and the experience has been described as one of "enduring stress and frustration" (Butcher, Holkup and Buckwalter 2001). It has increasingly been acknowledged that carers are placed under great strain as a consequence of their intensive involvement in care provision, which often constrains their social participation and necessitates their withdrawal from employment (Evandrou 1995; Joshi 1995; Parker and Lawton 1994). Other adverse effects of caring, for a significant number of carers, include the erosion of their physical and mental health (e.g. Aneshensel et al. 1995; Bauld et al. 2000; Butcher et al. 2001; Gilleard 1984a; Gilleard et al. 1984; Grad and Sainsbury 1966; Greene et al. 1982; Hoenig and Hamilton 1969; Rabins, Mace and Lucas 1982; Schulz et al. 2006) and some studies have alleged that mortality rates are higher among carers (Schulz and Beach 1999). It has been claimed that the extent of the problem is extreme: carers have been described as "hidden patients" (Fengler and Goodrich 1979) and a general consensus has emerged pressing for the need to provide carers with assistance both in the physical and psychological aspects of their task.

6.2.1 Policy initiatives with regard to carers

In many developed countries, governments have responded to the growing awareness of the needs of carers by introducing legislation which aims to recognize the role of family care as providing the mainstay of care provision for older and disabled people, enabling them to continue living in the community. In the U.K. the earliest of these initiatives took place two decades ago and was concerned mainly with community care reforms embodied in the NHS and Community Care Act (House of Commons 1990) which was preceded by the White Paper "Caring for People" (Secretaries of State 1989). A key objective set by the White Paper for service delivery was that "service providers make practical support for carers a high priority" (Secretaries of State 1989, 1.11). For the first time carers were recognized for the essential role that they play in supporting older frail and disabled people in the community. This was a crucial step in the formal appreciation of the fact that they needed and deserved support in carrying out their difficult, but immensely significant task and above all, families were acknowledged as partners with the State in the provision of care to older people (Baldwin and Parker 1989). As Twigg and Atkin (1994, 1) commented: "Carers have moved out of the shadows into the policy arena." Indeed, the acknowledgement of carers was central to the community care reforms in which there was a change in emphasis away from institutional to community services (Wistow et al. 1996, 161). In the words of one policy researcher: "Carers have become recognised as one of the building blocks of community care" (Twigg 1998, 133).

The way in which legislation and policies related to the provision of health and care services has evolved in the U.K. is summarized in Appendix A to this volume, and it reflects a number of important facts pertinent to carers. To a large extent, it is indicative of the way in which carers' groups (e.g. Carers Trust and Carers U.K. along with other charitable trusts representing specific disorders, such as Parkinson's U.K.) have been able to recruit carers' experiences of caring and research evidence in this field in order to serve their cause, in lobbying for changes to the law, so that the role of carers has finally been recognized. As a result, it has been acknowledged that informal family support systems provide an alternative to institutional care of older and disabled people. Indeed, demographic changes and financial constraints have evolved in such a way over the last fifty years, as to make it plain that current health service policies could not function without informal carers, whose contribution in economic terms is estimated at being in the region of £119 billion per year in the U.K. (Buckner and Yeandle 2011). It is hardly surprising therefore, that an important instrumental concern of policies relating to carers has been primarily to ensure the continuation of informal care provision (Pickard 2001). It is now evident that the work of carers is far more than a desirable option, in so far as the majority of people prefer to be cared for at home, but is in fact indispensible to the system of care provision. This is reflected in the consultation procedure taking place at the time of writing with a view to introducing the major care reforms outlined in the "Vision for Adult Social Care" (DOH 2010b) which are to be enacted in the form of legislation in 2013. One of the main aims of the proposed policy changes is to promote individual wellbeing and for carers this is to be guaranteed by equating their right to an assessment with that of the person they care for. Previous legislation had slowly evolved to recognise carers and whilst acknowledging their contribution, was widely criticised as doing little more than paying "lip-service" to their existence, despite their being the mainstay of community care. It is to be hoped that the imposition of a duty to assess carers independently, will translate into a right for them to receive support appropriate to their needs. This is to be ensured through providing essential services, financial assistance and linking the care recipient to formal resources in the community as a systematic response to the needs of both. Carers are to be offered greater choice and control over the resources available to them and the person they care for through the provision of personal budgets (see Appendix A). It would seem therefore, that current policies with regard to people with long-term disabilities are also concerned with the interests of their carer *per se* and with endeavouring to enhance his/her sense of well-being (Pickard 2001). Of course, the extent to which this is actually achieved is a matter of future experience and empirical investigation.

6.3 Identifying the needs of carers

The latest legislative proposals in the U.K. if implemented would go some way beyond the mere recognition of carers in helping to identify and meet their needs, especially if the measures recommended by the Dilnot Commission on the Funding of Care and Support (2011) were to be instigated. This however is unlikely to happen before 2015.

There is nothing new or surprising in the fact that families have always provided care for their older and disabled members and to quote one carer: "they do so, because they want to." They have always been willing, and have made themselves available, sometimes at considerable cost, (by giving up employment, sacrificing current earnings and a future pension) to deliver services to their relatives in need of care (Doty, Jackson and Crown 1998; Duxbury et al. 2009; Krach and Brooks 1995). If anything, in light of the likely demands for care into the twenty-first century, the concern of governments is to strengthen the commitment of families to providing care and to re-establish local neighbourhood and community ties where they may have become weakened, in order to support people in the community:

> The vision sets out a new direction for adult social care, putting people, personalised services and outcomes centre stage and returning social care to its foundations of reciprocity and constructive action by individuals on behalf of the whole community (DOH 2010b).

The provision of financial assistance to carers might be seen as satisfying only the most fundamental of carer needs, but all the more necessary for that reason. Physical burdens too are frequently managed with the aid of formal services such as assistance from community care nurses and nursing assistants, day care provision and help from charitable agencies. One need that has consistently been identified is the opportunity for carers to take regular breaks from the daily activities of care-giving, having time for themselves and being secure in the knowledge that the care-recipient is receiving high quality respite care, in an attempt to alleviate the negative psychological consequences of care-giving.

The need for solutions to the problems of carers of disabled people living at home is evident not only in the number of organizations for carers that have proliferated and that are engaged in a range of activities from lobbying for the rights of carers to supporting them in their day to day work with disabled people, but also in the amount of legislation in recent years that has addressed caring issues (see Appendix A). Furthermore, over the past twenty-five years, a wealth of empirical studies on the psychological effects of care-giving has been published, most of them focusing on the difficulties experienced by carers and frequently referred to as “carer burden” or “carer stress” (Pinquart and Sorensen 2003a). Evidence in support of the fact that carers are indeed under immense pressures as a result of caring is well established, but in the light of the efforts that have been expended in this area of research, it is difficult to understand why so little progress has been made beyond that of the bland conclusion that carers are in need of support. A variety of carer intervention studies have failed to produce convincing evidence to demonstrate that we know how to make things better for carers and those in their care (see Callahan 1989; Sorensen, Pinquart and Duberstein 2002 for reviews). Nevertheless new publications each year continue to add to the now well-established data base bearing witness to the fact that carers experience considerable levels of hardship. But relatively little is still known about the characteristics of carers who need support and how they might optimally be identified, or about the kind of help they need, when they need it most and what precisely, it is hoped to achieve. Without a proper understanding of these issues even the best intervention packages may fail, because they set out to address perceived needs as declared by carers and endorsed by formal services, without first verifying the extent to which perceived needs are indeed actual needs. And actual needs they may be, but there may be serious impediments to their realization, which also need to be explored. For example, it is probably for this reason that opportunities for respite care often fail to be taken up by carers, though many studies show that it is high on their “wish-list” of priorities. Lack of clear knowledge of the factors that may contribute to stress and well-being in particular care-giving situations makes the implementation of intervention strategies purely intuitive and it is not surprising that many such attempts have failed to give the expected results. The academic literature has been slow to provide theoretically-based approaches that might help to advance understanding beyond the merely descriptive accounts of carer stress and burden. This continues to be a major drawback for understanding in this area.

6.4 Ways of conceptualizing care-giving outcomes

A wide variety of concepts have been used in an attempt to define the outcome of the caring process for carers across studies. These include notions such as burden, stress, well-being and quality of life among the most frequently used, but a number of other terms intended to convey an equivalent meaning are also in operation in the literature and these reflect the ambiguity of the definitions: stress effects, care-giving consequences, care-giving impact (Montgomery 1989) as well as notions of strain and satisfaction (Dorfman, Holmes and Berlin 1996). The use of specific terms and the way in which they are used, both as independent or dependent variables, reflects the varying theoretical positions of different researchers, although these are rarely explicitly stated. Moreover, the use of terms in this area lacks consistency and is only loosely based on theoretical models.

An examination of the main examples of the concepts used (which have been influential in guiding the literature) is a worthwhile exercise, as it throws light on the theoretical approaches taken and highlights the differences between them, making it possible to fully understand the implications of using specific concepts as descriptors of what is happening to carers.

6.4.1 The concept of care-giving burden

The term carer or care-giving "burden" is probably the most widely used in the literature on care-giving to describe outcomes for carers and the concept has been intensively researched for more than 30 years (Stull, Kosloski and Kercher 1994; Zarit, Reever et al. 1980). George and Gwyther (1986, 253) defined care-giving burden as "the physical, psychological or emotional, social, and financial problems that can be experienced by family members caring for impaired older adults". To the extent that definitions of this kind emphasize the adversity of the care-giving experience and the costs borne by carers, they concur with the notion that caring has a significant impact on the carer, and continue to be used to the present day (e.g. Bullock 2004; Savundranayagam, Montgomery and Kosloski 2011) having been adopted in the legislation referred to above, and in relation to specific disorders such as DAT (Werner et al. 2012) and PD (e.g. Martinez-Martin et al. 2008; Stella et al. 2009).

As with much of the work in the field of caring for older and disabled people, the conceptualisation of care-giving burden has not been theoretically driven, but developed in the context of intervention programmes which were aimed at helping family carers contending with everyday care situations (Zarit et al. 1986). A review of the literature demonstrates that there is no generally accepted definition of care-giving burden in operation (e.g. Beeri et al. 2002; Gonyea et al. 2005; Montgomery 1989; Montgomery, Stull and Borgatta 1985; Price and Levy 1990; Stuckey, Neundorfer and Smyth 1996) although for some, the notion of burden has become so well-established, that they do not even attempt to define it (e.g. Campbell et al. 2008). Care-giving burden thus remains subject to wide variations in conceptualisation and operational measurement throughout the literature (Chou 2000; Montgomery 1989; Tindall and Huebner 2009), although it is still widely used to convey the notion that in taking on the role of caring, the individual is adversely affected in a variety of life-domains and suffers enduring personal consequences as a result of the impact of caring on his/her life (Horowitz, 1985a). It is essentially a psychological concept, involving a subjective interpretation by carers of the extent to which the care-giving experience impacts on their health, social life or financial status (Roland, Johnson and Jenkins 2011).

Care-giving burden originally emerged as a concept in the psychiatric literature in relation to mental health patients being discharged into the community, as an attempt to describe the consequences for their families and thus to gain a better understanding of the care-giving experience (Grad and Sainsbury 1963). In these early studies there was no attempt to measure burden in terms of the additional tasks and responsibilities incurred by families as a result of having a mentally ill member living with them, nor in terms of any subjective consequences for them relating to the difficulties that this imposed. It was simply assumed that under such circumstances carers were inevitably exposed to certain costs in relation to societal attitudes and stigma which they had no alternative but to bear (Montagu 1989). The first investigators to measure the costs of caring were Grad and Sainsbury (1963) in their seminal work on the burden of community care for elderly psychiatric patients discharged into the community. They conceptualized burden as “any costs to the family”, by which they meant, any negative consequences arising out of care-giving, a definition which assumed the oppressive nature of burden, thus setting the stage for many subsequent studies in this area and shaping the way in which caring was, and frequently still is, perceived.

The definition of burden in relation to the care of people with neurodegenerative diseases (e.g. DAT, PD) is further complicated by the fact that work in this field developed largely without reference to what had been achieved earlier in the literature, concerning care of psychiatrically ill patients living in the care of their families (Herz, Endicott and Spritzer 1976; Hoenig and Hamilton 1967; Platt and Hirsch 1981). Thus the conceptualization and measurement of carer burden particularly in the area of dementia care, occurred in parallel and did not avoid, but rather added to, the proliferation of confusion surrounding the terminology used to refer to the consequences of care-giving. Apart from the notion of burden, other terms have also been used to describe the outcome for the carer, including caregiver strain (Cantor 1983; Greene et al. 1982; Robinson 1983), costs of care (Cicirelli 1981), care-giving impact (Poulshock and Deimling 1984), role strain and carer overload (Campbell et al. 2008), care-giving consequences (Bass, Noelker and Rechlin 1996), personal strain and role strain (Whitlatch, Zarit and von Eye 1991), stress effects (Pearlin et al. 1990), carer well-being (George and Gwyther 1986) and morale (Fengler and Goodrich 1979). Despite the lack of consistency in terminology there is a degree of overall uniformity in the way in which the consequences of care-giving have been conceptualized. There appears to be general agreement between studies in assuming that the responsibilities of care-giving are causally related to negative effects on the health or well-being of the carer. Indeed, these negative effects have played a central role in the evaluation of the effects for carers of people with DAT and later, PD.

The notion of burden implies a load that has to be borne, a heavy and difficult weight that must be carried, or something oppressive and overwhelming, that is difficult to accept (Collins Dictionary 1992). This use of language has largely determined the perception of caring that has been promoted in the literature. It is not necessarily an accurate picture, as will be shown in the following discussion. Furthermore, the two meanings conveyed in the dictionary definition of burden (the former objective, the latter requiring an evaluation on the part of the subject) have frequently been interpreted as being complementary, but they do not have to be so. A carer may be laden with extra duties and responsibilities, but does not have to see them as onerous or oppressive. As Montgomery (1989, 202) points out: "a subjective judgement is involved in the determination of whether a load or responsibility is oppressive". Hence care-giving should not be viewed as intrinsically and exclusively detrimental to the health of the carer. It may objectively place greater demands on the carer, but the carer's appraisal of the situation, his/her subjective response to it, determines, at least in part, the final outcome.

6.4.1.1 Objective and subjective aspects of burden

The notion of "objective" and "subjective" aspects of burden was first introduced by Hoenig and Hamilton (1966) in applying an important distinction to evaluating the burden of care for families with a relative suffering from a psychiatric illness. The notion of "objective" burden refers to the physical and behavioural changes in the care recipient and the ensuing practical problems for the carer, such as providing physical care and having to adapt to changes in daily routine (e.g. financial costs, giving up work to look after the disabled person, costs in time). Lazarus and De

Longis' (1982) description of "daily hassles" is related to this, encompassing the multitude of trivial but irritating and frustrating events which conspire together to make up the daily grind of caring (Gilhooly 1986). "Objective burden" also includes "caregiving impact" (Poulshock and Deimling 1984) which describes the social effect on the carer's daily life, such as changes in family relations, employment and health (Rabins, Mace and Lucas 1982). This conceptualization of burden in "objective" terms has much in common with the notion of the "load to be carried" described above, and is seen as the source (whether directly or indirectly) of the emotional reactions of the carer.

"Subjective burden" on the other hand, refers to the emotional reactions of the carer, which have been described in the form of increased psychiatric morbidity (Bergman and Jacoby 1983), reduced morale (Gilhooly 1984), anxiety (George and Gwyther 1986), depression (Morris, Morris and Britton 1988b) and the way in which the carer perceives the strain of care-giving (Machin 1980, cited in Gilleard 1984a; Rabins et al. 1982). The distinction classifying burden in terms of objectively and subjectively quantifiable aspects was also found to be useful in the dementia care-giving literature (e.g. Cicirelli 1981; Hooyman, Gonyea and Montgomery 1985; Montgomery, Gonyea and Hooyman 1985) as it was considered to add clarity to the debate, since the causes and consequences of the two types of burden could be quite different (Montgomery 1989).

Although research in this area has frequently treated burden as a unitary construct, it is evident not only from these definitions, but from its earliest conceptualizations, that the multidimensional nature of burden was indeed recognised (e.g. Grad and Sainsbury 1963). This has not always been reflected in the measures used to quantify burden, however (e.g. Cameron et al. 2002; Lamura et al. 2008; Robinson 1983; Zarit et al. 1980) so that the various dimensions of care-giving hardships have not always been differentiated and subjective and objective aspects have been combined in the same scale (e.g. Montgomery et al. 1985), leading to a lack of clarity in what is being measured. Many of the scales devised for measuring burden simply summate the responses to a diverse catalogue of items in the form of a single score, which is referred to as a measure of carer strain (Robinson 1983), burden (Zarit et al. 1980), stress (Pearlin et al. 1990) or care-giving consequences (Horowitz 1985b), costs (Kosberg and Cairl 1986), appraisal (Lawton et al. 1989) impact (Cameron et al. 2002) and negative impact of care-giving (Lamura et al. 2008), and these are then assumed to be an indication of the extent to which the carer's life is restricted by care-giving duties. Implicit within these assumptions is the view that subjective appraisal of objective difficulties and the extent to which lifestyles might be perceived as having been altered would be affected by all types of experience involved in care-giving (Horowitz 1985a). Whilst this might be true, it does little to advance our knowledge in helping to determine precisely which aspects of the care-giving situation are important in affecting outcomes and remains purely descriptive in its achievements. The lack of clarity surrounding these issues is disappointing in view of the duration and intensity of research on caring, which has provided few empirically-based solutions to highlight predictors of unsustainable carer strain and provide a rationale to guide interventions.

One reason for this is that for too long, deliberations on the nature of care-giving have occurred in a theoretical vacuum, without the recognition that employing a construct such as burden, implicitly assumes a theoretical model. The fact that answers in relation to questions of how best to help carers remain obscure, reflects the lack of methodological clarity in the way in which the concept of burden has been used. It is only in recent years that the multidimensional structure of instruments for measuring care-giving strain or burden, that have survived the test of time, has been demonstrated (e.g. Greene et al. 1982; Longmire and Knight 2011; Siegert et al. 2010) in keeping with the growing consensus that the multidimensional nature of burden should be recognised if it is to be useful in predicting the outcome for any care-giving situation (Ankri et al. 2005). Equally, the notion of burden has been used both as a ***predictor*** and as an ***indicator*** of the outcome (at a given point in time) for the carer, sometimes without demonstrating an understanding of the distinction between the two. The former use of the term, although not always explicitly acknowledged, invokes a version of stress theory (Pearlin et al. 1990) by implying that burden represents an intermediate stage in the stress process, being the result of the operation of various stressors (e.g. background variables such as the carer's age and sex, contesting work and family commitments and care-recipient variables including indices of disease, duration and functioning) thus constituting a predictor of the outcome for the carer. In this case, carer outcome is measured according to the researcher's preferences in more global terms, such as quality of life, well-being or depression and burden is considered to be a narrower concept leading to these potential outcomes. Where burden is viewed as an outcome measure in itself (i.e. an indicator variable strictly associated with the effects of care-giving), it is often represented as a detraction from well-being or a diminution in quality of life, in the form of depression, anxiety, sleep disturbances or increased health problems, placing the terms "burden" and "well-being" in opposition to each other, at the same time, implying that they are opposite poles of the same construct (George and

Gwyther 1986). As already pointed out, this need not be the case. A further difficulty with these positions is the lack of clarity in separating components of burden from those arising out of care-giving *per se* and those associated with more general characteristics of the carer. Many measures of care-giving burden attempt to overcome this difficulty by employing check-lists of "symptoms" of carer distress and attempting to tie them down specifically to the situation of care-giving (e.g. Zarit et al. 1980). The validity of this approach may be questionable, as it depends on a subjective judgement from the carer in determining whether his/her state of mind is attributable to care-giving. For example, is it reasonable to expect a carer to be able to differentiate between being depressed as a result of care-giving or for other reasons? Thus although burden scales may have sensitivity in serving to make a useful distinction between carers reporting high versus low levels of burden, their specificity remains to be determined.

A strong argument has been made for separating the notion of "burden" from the final outcome measure for the carer, so that the former is considered to be a predictor of the latter, with the consequent theoretical implications for the care-giving model. This position was exemplified in Poulshock and Deimling's (1984, 231) article in which they argued that the term "carer impact" should replace "objective burden" in order to describe the outcome measure of interest. In this they included the "... more or less objective changes in caregivers' lives... These include the impact caregiving has on family relationships, social activities, health and employment changes." They argued that "burden" was a more appropriate term for the carer's subjective judgement relating to the extent to which the care recipient's impairments or behaviour are perceived as being problematic, distressing, embarrassing or exceeding the carer's ability to cope, thus imposing on the more subjective aspects of the carer's life, such as his/her emotional state or relationships. Thus the subjective judgement of burden is seen as an intervening variable between the care recipient's characteristics and different types of impact for the carer and within this conceptualisation, it has a mediating role. This was an extremely important theoretical modification as it made it possible to account for the fact that some carers might experience significant levels of burden, whilst preserving a sense of well-being. In separating the concepts of burden and well-being, it was possible to explain why not all carers suffer physical or psychiatric morbidity as the result of caring.

Poulshock and Deimling (1984) also argued that carer outcomes required better specification and more precise measurement. Different types of impairment or behavioural and cognitive disturbances could be expected to impinge not only on the carer's perceived burden but lead to a variety of carer impacts. In particular, they identified two main types of impact: one related to the effects on the carer's family relationships and the other to infringement on the carer's time and activities. In general, the impact on family relationships is measured by the same kinds of items that other researchers use to quantify subjective burden and restriction of carer activities is measured using items associated with objective burden in other scales. This was a major reconceptualisation of theoretical models of the care-giving process in separating burden from final outcome measures for the carer and stimulating interest in understanding the subjective impact of care-giving, especially in terms of interpersonal, family relationships.

Carer burden remains one of the most commonly used variables in care-giving research both as a predictor of other carer outcomes (Gallagher-Thompson and Powers 1997) and as an outcome measure in its own right (Kramer and Kipnis 1995; Ostwald et al. 1999). Indeed Stull et al. (1994) have argued that burden may represent a unique domain in the care-giving experience that is not captured by more generic indicators. In their study of older adults, burden measures were more highly correlated with care receiver characteristics such as ADLs and IADLs and cognitive measures than were measures of carer well-being, and were better predictors of the need for formal care (e.g. day care and consideration of nursing home placement). Many conceptual models of care-giving processes thus include burden as an independent variable for the prediction of other outcomes. However, the main way in which the term "burden" is now used is to refer only to carers' subjective perceptions and reactions related to their care-giving function and this is reflected in the construction of scales to measure these constructs (e.g. the Relatives' Stress Scale; Greene et al. 1982; the Screen for Caregiver Burden; Vitaliano et al. 1991; the Zarit Burden Interview; Zarit et al. 1980).

Few studies have measured the prevalence of subjective burden among carers and indeed, because individual instruments may be indices of somewhat arbitrarily selected items chosen to reflect the negative consequences of care-giving, their psychometric properties are often unknown and their scores present difficulties for interpretation. Most therefore, correlate measures of so-called emotional well-being in the carer (or rather lack of it) and measures of perceived strain with variables related to the care recipient's condition, such as the degree (stage) of dementia (Zarit et al. 1980). Those that have attempted to provide estimates of the degree of subjective burden have highlighted the diversity of responses among different samples of carers. Comparisons between studies are difficult to make owing to the wide range of instruments used to measure the carer's response. This potentiates the problem of knowing what exactly is being measured in these studies and thus being able to compare like with like. Nonetheless a summary of findings is presented in chapter 7.

Summing up, a number of serious problems have been identified relating to burden. The first relates to there being little common agreement as to the precise meaning embodied in the concept of carer burden. One cause of the lack of clarity is the failure to take account of the two meanings of burden and the fact that they need not necessarily be complementary (Montgomery 1989). The term has been used interchangeably to reflect both subjective and objective qualities, which not surprisingly, generates confusion. Secondly, the continuing shortcomings in the ability of the notion of carer burden to underpin a sound theoretical approach or at least to provide an explanatory concept for care-giving, despite a wealth of research in this area over many decades, is disappointing. The term itself not only lacks conceptual clarity, but as a result of variations in its usage, research questions and hypotheses have reflected the confusion, as have instruments designed to measure carer burden. A further consequence of this has been a difficulty in identifying what levels of burden might be considered unacceptably high for carers. There continues to be little empirically supported evidence as to which aspects of the caring experience may need to be modified in order to ease the task for carers, and therefore interventions cannot be theory-led, making their applicability somewhat dubious. Worse still, given the persistence of "atheoretical" approaches to analyzing caring, a controversial notion has crept into the literature. This would appear to contend that burden can and should be measured in an "objective" manner and that this "objectivity" is superior to other types of measurement. Hence certain studies emphasise more objective measures (e.g. hours devoted to care-giving etc.) at the expense of so-called "subjective" variables (measures of carer distress). There are many parallels between this situation and the argument which ran between Lazarus and the Dohrenwends, reaching a peak in the 1980s, in relation to the subjective evaluation of stressors (Cooper and Dewe 2004, 47).

Finally, probably because of this confusion, it has not been possible to demonstrate unambiguous associations between burden and other aspects of the care-giving situation, with any degree of consistency. This is problematic for the concept of burden, for if it cannot be shown which factors are determinants of burden, or which aspects of burden bring about ill-effects for the carer (depending on the theoretical model used), its utility is undoubtedly in question. Unfortunately, there are a great many inconsistencies in the reported correlates of burden; these will be discussed in greater detail chapter 7.

This situation led some researchers (e.g. George and Gwyther 1986) to the conclusion that the concept of carer burden was too problematic to warrant its continued use and others have raised questions about the utility of the concept for advancing knowledge in this area (Montgomery 1989). Essentially, the survival of the notion of carer burden rests on the ability to demonstrate that it: "adds significantly to an understanding of the caregiving situation" (Montgomery 1989, 204). In order to verify the usefulness of burden as a concept, Montgomery argues that it should be judged against its ability to meet three criteria: (i) increasing understanding, (ii) facilitating explanation of the care-giving experience, and (iii) predicting future outcomes (Montgomery 1989, 204). Furthermore, it needs to be demonstrated that the concept of burden is unique. This means that other concepts which may be used synonymously in the psychological literature pertaining to caring, such as the notion of stress, and which may be used in the same way as burden in theoretical models, would render the concept of carer burden redundant. It should also be parsimonious, i.e. providing a sufficient and circumscribed description of the caring situation or prediction of outcome.

6.4.2 The concept of carer well-being

The concept of 'well-being' was favoured by George and Gwyther (1986) as a means of describing the extent to which the caring process affected the carer: "caring for an impaired relative is synonymous with the expectation that caregivers will experience decrements in selected dimensions of well-being relative to their age peers who do not have caregiving responsibilities" (George and Gwyther 1986, 253). Well-being is generally understood as including aspects of a person's spirituality, health, activity level, social support, resources, satisfaction with personal accomplishments and life situations (Diener and Suh 1997). It is a more generic concept than burden, without the specific referent of care-giving, which George and Gwyther (1986) considered to be one of its main advantages (see below). Well-being is also a complex multi-dimensional construct, although as with burden, this has not always been reflected in its measurement (e.g. Headey, Holmstrom and Wearing 1985). George and Gwyther (1986) considered it to be the opposite of the notion of carer burden, assuming a two-way symmetry between burden and well-being: high levels of burden leading to low levels of well-being and vice versa.

But this is evidently not the case. For although high burden may be associated with diminished well-being and this is frequently reported, the reverse need not be true. Indeed there is empirical evidence to show that the well-being of the carer need not be compromised by high levels of burden (Chappell and Reid 2002; Stull et al. 1994), emphasizing the conceptual distinctiveness of the two concepts.

George and Gwyther (1986) felt that the concept of well-being had three methodological advantages over that of burden. Firstly it provided the opportunity for comparing carers with other relevant comparison groups, such as the age matched control group of non-carers in their definition. Controls could not be expected to experience carer burden as they were not involved in a care-giving situation and yet they might be expected to show some deterioration in well-being associated with age-related effects. This then, would be an appropriate control for age. However, it cannot be assumed that well-being is determined only by age and caring responsibilities. Indeed, there is a considerable literature to show that it is influenced by health, income and social interaction, as might be predicted from its definition above (e.g. Stull 1988). Therefore it is inappropriate to make the simple assumption that differences in well-being between groups of carers and non-carers, even when age is controlled, are due to the caring process. As Montgomery (1989) points out, a sounder approach methodologically, is to invoke the concept of burden as an intervening variable representing the carer's perception of his/her caring responsibilities, which contributes in part, to the overall well-being of the carer. Within this view, burden might be subsumed under the more general concept of well-being, but is only one aspect of it.

Secondly, according to George and Gwyther (1986), the notion of well-being provided for conceptual and empirical freedom from the specific situation of caring. But it is not clear why one would wish to take this approach. Indeed, separating the concept from the situation of caring is problematic, as demonstrated in the first point above, where the comparison of carers and non-carers was considered, and in the preceding discussion. It would be reasonable to expect that the effect of caring responsibilities might be overwhelmed by other factors if the more global concept of well-being is used as the outcome variable (Montgomery 1989). Numerous control groups would be necessary in order to examine the effects of other potential factors affecting well-being. A more useful comparison is between different caring situations in order to examine potential variations in the impact on the carer and to identify those factors that are predictive of poorer outcome. Knowledge of the specific antecedents that predict worse outcome is of particular interest to researchers seeking to identify more vulnerable individuals or points for intervention in the caring process to relieve the burden on carers. A lack of understanding of the cause and effect relationship as regards carer outcomes is likely to have been the reason for the disappointing results of many intervention programmes, as plausible interventions are not possible without this knowledge (Torti et al. 2004).

Thirdly, George and Gwyther (1986) considered it to be an advantage to measure the dimensions of well-being rather than what they appear to have considered to be the less differentiated concept of burden. However, there is nothing to suggest that burden is a unitary concept. To the contrary, the previous discussion has shown that carer burden can and should be conceptualized as being multidimensional, having constituent elements, such as the objective and subjective aspects discussed, and therefore, like well-being, it can be measured along multiple dimensions. Furthermore, as mentioned above, there is empirical evidence to suggest that burden may reflect a unique domain of care-giving outcome that is not encompassed by well-being (Stull et al. 1994).

6.4.3 The concept of quality of life for carers

Quality of life (QOL) is another term that has been applied in the measurement of care-giving outcomes, often it appears, with little consideration as to what is meant with regard to the underlying concept (Dijkers 2007). Moons, Budts and De Geest (2006) identified eight conceptualisations of QOL which emerge from the literature on the subject, revealing the lack of clarity with which the term is used and highlighting the lack of consensus as to its definition and how it should be measured. In particular, it has emerged as an important parameter for evaluating the quality and outcome of health care and specific QOL measures have been developed for use with specific forms of illness. In the main these have included long-term conditions such as PD, where the notion of QOL has particular significance in the context of the progressive nature of the neurodegenerative disorder (e.g. the Parkinson's Disease Questionnaire (PDQ-39), Jenkinson et al. 1997).

Thus while QOL has figured as a frequent means of evaluating the effects of illness and treatment, the ubiquitous use of the concept has also led to its being applied to carer outcomes in a more generic form. Broadly speaking, its use in this context is equivalent to the notion of well-being. It is however, also defined in narrower terms, which emphasize certain specific aspects of the concept, such as health-related quality of life. Nonetheless, most investigators' notions of "well-being" or "quality of life" include both affective and cognitive components (Lawton, Kleban and DiCarlo 1984), as well as physical disabilities (Schulz et al. 1995) and self-care (Gallant and Connell 1997). Few instruments have been designed specifically to measure the quality of life of carers; they typically include assessments of emotional and social well-being as well as the physical strain of care-giving and in this they closely resemble many of the earlier burden scales (e.g. Glozman 2004). Some include factors such as the carer's family situation and spiritual and financial needs (see Deeken et al. 2003 for a review).

The quality of life literature has never made the distinction between subjective and objective aspects of experience that was made in the earlier debate on burden. Rather, subjective perceptions have been accepted as the determinants of QOL (Deeken et al. 2003); indeed they are regarded by some as being crucial to measuring the concept (Moons 2004). This is in keeping with the later models of burden, that defined the construct in terms of subjective perceptions of the tasks, obligations and restrictions of care-giving, i.e. the stressors or objective load placed on the carer. Deeken et al. (2003) also point to the considerable overlap in domains from which items are drawn for both burden and quality of life measures.

6.4.4 The mental health of carers

A variety of mental health measures have been used in the care-giving literature, both as indicators of carer outcomes and as predictors of care-giving burden. As with the concept of burden, the variability in the use of the mental health status of the carer as both an independent and dependent variable adds confusion to the literature, as the underlying theoretical models are rarely made explicit. Essentially, two possibilities exist. Where carer mental status is treated as an independent variable in the care-giving situation, it is assumed to be a predictor of, or contributor to, the outcome variable, which is then usually measured in terms of care-giving burden (e.g. Vitaliano et al. 1991). The logic of this assumption is somewhat circular however, as it is unclear why the diminished mental health status of the carer, for example in the form of depression, should specifically affect the burden of care-giving, except in so far as depression is likely to affect the carer's perceptions in all aspects of functioning, as encompassed in Beck's cognitive triad, consisting of: the self, the world and the future (Beck et al. 1979). Thus it is reasonable to expect that depressed carers might report higher levels of burden, but this is not the issue that is at stake here. The question of interest relates to the origins of depression in the carer, a question that is essentially empirical in nature. Somewhat surprisingly, it does not appear to have been investigated in any systematic way in the care-giving literature. Perhaps the strongest evidence in support of a care-giving model in which carer mental health status is viewed as contributing to burden is the observation referred to above, that ostensibly similar care-giving situations are not consistently predictive of carer outcomes measured in terms of burden (Poulshock and Deimling 1984; Reinhard and Horowitz 1995), although this observation can also be accounted for by alternative models of the care-giving process.

The second possibility is that carer mental status is the ***result*** or outcome of care-giving. In this theoretical model, burden is seen as a mediating variable leading to carer outcomes in the form of mental health status. This latter model would appear to have a number of advantages over the former. Firstly, it fits an accepted paradigm in terms of the stress process model in which care-giving burden is viewed as the result of the appraisal of the care-giving situation by the carer (Pearlin et al. 1990). This model has the advantage of being able to account for the now well-established phenomenon, that in situations which appear to be characterised by equivalent levels of care-giving burden, carer outcomes may be radically different. The details of this model are discussed in greater detail below. Secondly, measures of mental health status are more meaningful ways of assessing carer outcomes for the following reasons: (i) they represent a better operationalisation of the underlying concept e.g. depression; (ii) they are based on assessment procedures which have a more rigorous and established methodology than, for example, measures of burden (Deeken et al. 2003); (iii) they enable comparisons to be made with other groups with mental health problems, thus providing a useful means of identifying individuals in need of support and intervention. Thirdly, from a theoretical perspective it would appear parsimonious to assume that the raised levels of psychiatric morbidity found among carers are due to the care-giving situation in which they find themselves, with all of its repercussions. Otherwise, the logic of the argument would have to assume that those taking on the care-giving role would be more likely to have a predisposition for becoming depressed – a situation that would seem most unlikely. Nevertheless it might still be argued that carer vulnerability to depression is higher in those individuals who had experienced previous mental health problems and this is a question of empirical verification, although it is unlikely to be a full explanation, because of the raised prevalence of psychiatric morbidity among carers. It is for these reasons that this model of care-giving forms the basis of the theoretical approach adopted in the present work.

The majority of studies have demonstrated increased prevalence rates of psychiatric morbidity for carers, using a variety of different forms of measurement. Early studies, such as that of George and Gwyther (1986) reported increased levels of stress and negative affect using the Short Psychiatric Evaluation Schedule (Pfeiffer 1979) and the Affect Balance Scale (Bradburn 1969). Yet others employed measures of emotional distress, such as symptom checklists (Zarit et al. 1980), global ratings of mental health (Gilhooly 1984) or derived arbitrary indices of negative consequences or strain, based upon open-ended interviews (Hirschfield 1981; Johnson and Catalona 1982, cited in Gilleard 1984a). It is unlikely that these relatively unknown and mixed indices were measuring the same underlying concept, thus making comparisons between studies difficult. Greater sophistication in the development of standardised instruments for the measurement of psychiatric symptomatology provided some of the instruments that are still in use today, especially for the measurement of depression, such as the Beck Depression Inventory (BDI; Beck et al. 1961) and the Geriatric Depression Scale (GDS; Yesavage et al. 1983) which have increasingly been used with carers. In particular, the General Health Questionnaire (GHQ; Goldberg and Hillier 1979) provided a means of assessing probable psychiatric "caseness" (non psychotic conditions, mainly depression and anxiety) in non-psychiatric populations and so was especially suitable for use with carers.

From the earliest studies to use the GHQ, carers of people with dementia have, in the main, been shown to be at greater risk of developing a psychiatric disorder. Bergmann and Jacoby (1983) estimated that 33% of their sample of carers were at risk and Gilleard et al. (1984) found even higher rates: 68% exceeded the threshold value of 4/5 on the GHQ. The latter figure is considerably higher than the GHQ prevalence rates reported for other community samples (Benjamin, Decalmer and Haran 1982; Goldberg 1978; Tarnopolsky et al. 1979). More recent studies have confirmed these findings: 53% GHQ "caseness" was reported by Gonçalves-Pereira et al. (2010); 66% by Stirling et al. (2010); and Schneider et al. (1999) found rates of between 40-75% (the main difference being attributable to the country in the European community in which the assessments were conducted).

In contrast, Eagles et. al. (1987a,b) reported no differences in GHQ scores between co-resident carers of demented and non-demented elderly carers. They attributed the discrepancies between studies to a sampling bias, arguing that their families had been drawn from a community sample, whereas previous studies had examined the families of care recipients referred to psychiatric services. The latter are likely to represent a "selected" sample in whom the psychiatric referral may have been on account of the stresses and psychological disturbances arising in a family caring for someone with dementia and it may be that families that are better able to cope are less likely to come into contact with psychiatric services. Sampling bias is unlikely to be the whole explanation however, in view of the large number of studies that have yielded high rates of GHQ "caseness", whilst there is no reason to believe that their samples may have shown selection biases.

Numerous studies have also reported levels of depression higher than those expected for community samples, though prevalence rates vary widely among the groups of carers studied. Using the BDI, slightly increased rates of depression of 14% among carers have been reported by L.W. Morris, R.G. Morris and Britton (1988) and 12% by Watson et al. (2011). Other studies have reported significantly higher rates of carer depression on the BDI ranging from 20% (Mittelman et al. 2008) through 37% (Välimäki et al. 2009) to 53% (Garcia-Alberca et al. 2012).

Care needs to be taken in the interpretation of these findings, especially in terms of accounting for the widely discrepant results. One reason for the variation may be the sources from which samples are selected, making comparisons difficult. This and other reasons may be similar to those discussed in chapter 3 in relation to the discrepancies found in the literature concerning prevalence rates of depression in patients with PD, such as the idiosyncratic use of different threshold scores for determining clinically significant levels of symptoms. It should also be remembered that neither the BDI nor the GDS are diagnostic instruments for determining depression.

A final point concerning the choice of outcome measures for carers is worth making. Whilst the foregoing discussion has presented arguments in favour of a distinction between the concepts of care-giving burden and the mental health status of carers on the basis that they represent different underlying constructs, a curious tendency is to be observed in the literature. These have emerged in the context of attempts to validate measures of care-giving burden, such as the Zarit Burden Interview (Zarit et al. 1980), where the "gold standards" used for establishing the construct validity of the instrument were the GHQ and the HADS, both of which are established measures of psychiatric morbidity (Chattat et al. 2011; Seng et al. 2010). Moreover, there are also examples of attempts to provide threshold (cut-off) scores on burden scales, by comparing them to the GHQ and GDS (Ulstein, Wyller and Engedal 2007; Martin-Carrasco et al. 2010). Whilst it is understandable that both instrument validation and establishing cut-off thresholds is desirable and requires that the psychometric properties of the scales should be determined, the choice of "gold standards" is somewhat questionable if a distinction between care-giving burden and psychiatric morbidity is indeed valid. Many studies demonstrate high levels of correlation between measures of burden and levels of psychiatric morbidity for carers (e.g. Chattat et al. 2011; Miller et al. 1996; Ulstein et al. 2007) and so it remains to be established that the concept of burden is unique and that it does indeed make a specific contribution to understanding of the care-giving situation. Unfortunately, more than twenty years on from Montgomery's (1989) incisive analysis of the concept of care-giving burden, little progress appears to have been made.

6.4.5 The concept of carer stress/strain

Yet other theoretical approaches have viewed the care-giving experience as a specific form of stress or strain which might be amenable to modification, given an understanding of the factors that are associated with it (e.g. Pratt et al. 1985). Here too, however, there is a great deal of confusion relating to terminology and the concepts used, and this poses one of the greatest difficulties to evaluating research which has used stress theory to account for carers' experiences. Use of the terms "stress" and "strain" are inconsistent and definitions vary widely. In spite of, or perhaps because of this, the notion of stress in particular, has gained general acceptance and entered everyday speech. The elasticity of meaning associated with it may have had an advantage in allowing stress to be considered from a range of perspectives, and this has led to the development of more coherent, theoretical frameworks from which the concept may be analysed (Cooper and Dewe 2004). On the other hand, any attempt to understand a specific area of stress research, such as that of care-giving, requires a careful analysis of the way that the terminology is used in particular studies. This is especially important in studies which refer to a theoretical model of stress in attempting to identify those components of the stress process which are the most powerful determinants of outcome for the carer.

The fact that the multifaceted reactions of carers to the care-giving task have generally been construed in terms of "stress" reactions makes it incumbent upon a piece of research of this kind, to examine the concept of stress more closely. The term first appeared in "Psychological Abstracts" in 1944 (Jones and Bright 2001) though its origins outside the field of psychology can be traced back to the seventeenth century, where interestingly, it had come to mean "hardship" (Hinkle 1973). Towards the end of that century it was adopted by Robert Hooke and used in a technical sense in an engineering analogy of stress (Lazarus 1993). Hooke's work was concerned with how man-made structures, such as bridges, could withstand heavy loads and led him to elaborate the "Law of Elasticity" in which the term "***load***" was used to define the demand placed on the structure, and "***stress***" referred to the pressure within a body reacting to the applied forces. The net result of the interaction between the load and the pressure exerted gave rise to "***strain***" embodied in the resultant changes in form undergone by the structure (Hinkle 1973). The parallel for the use of these terms in psychology is quite clear and thus stress has been conceptualised as an external demand that is placed on a biosociopsychological system with the consequent results defined in terms of strain (Lazarus 1993). The attraction of this model for describing the care-giving process can be seen immediately, and in effect, it is the model underpinning most research in this area, although its theoretical roots may not be acknowledged and different terminology used. However it can be seen from the earlier discussion on burden, that the notion of stress is broadly equivalent to that of objective burden, and strain to that of subjective burden or other forms of outcome for the carer, such as "carer impact" in Poulshock and Deimling's (1984) terms. In some models, stress is viewed as simply being the result of some antecedent event or stimulus, as is the case when burden is treated as an indicator or dependent variable. This stimulus-response (S-R) model would predict that stress in carers is the result of adverse events arising out of the care-giving situation, implicitly assuming a simple linear relationship between the two (Nolan et al. 1996).

There is however, a wealth of research experience from the field of health psychology to show that this is unlikely to be true (Cooper 2005). The complexity of carer reactions towards the various situations that they encounter during the frequently long course of care-giving, the variability in their responses and the range of different outcomes in terms of carer well-being cannot be reduced to a simple S-R response model. Folkman and Lazarus (1985) define stress as "a relationship between the person and the environment that is appraised by the person as relevant to his or her well-being and in which the person's resources are taxed or exceeded." This implies an interaction between the person and the environment in which the person "negotiates" for him/herself the meaning of the interaction. It forms the basis of the transactional stress model (Lazarus and Folkman 1984; Folkman and Lazarus 1985) which is fundamental to our present-day understanding of stress. Within this model, events in a person's life are not automatically assumed to be stress-provoking; they have to be attended to, evaluated or appraised and a conclusion drawn about their meaning to the individual. Thus the subjective interpretation of events is crucial to the evolution of stress in a given situation and not their objective characteristics (Kane and Penrod 1995). This helps to explain why stressors that are ambiguous (Boss, Caron and Horbal 1988) or unpredictable (Archbold et al. 1990) pose the greatest problems for carers.

6.5 Theoretical models of the caring experience

One of the greatest obstacles to gaining a better understanding of the caring process, despite the wealth of studies that have emerged in this area over the last few decades, has been the fact that the research has seldom been guided by an explicit theoretical framework. The limitations of this purely descriptive approach were noted by Zarit more than twenty years ago, when in an editorial in "The Gerontologist", he was prompted to ask: "Do we need another "stress and care-giving" study?" (Zarit 1989), a sentiment that was echoed by others, including George (1990) and Twigg and Atkin (1994). The message that these authors were trying to convey was quite simple: we know that caring can be extremely stressful – what we still don't understand is why different carers, under ostensibly similar circumstances, may experience care-giving in strikingly different ways, some with severely negative consequences, whilst others remain well and contented with their situation. It was clear that theoretical models were needed in order to take care-giving research beyond the merely descriptive stage.

Zarit (1989) himself and Kramer and Vitaliano (1994) following a review of the care-giving literature, acknowledged that the main analytical framework in care-giving research has been the Transactional Stress Theory developed by Lazarus and Folkman (1984). This model may have been used either explicitly or implicitly, but it lay at the heart of the majority of studies. The aim of studies formulated within this general framework has been to examine any potential correlations between chosen independent or predictor variables and the outcome for the carer (e.g. Cifu et al. 2006; George and Gwyther 1986; Montgomery et al. 1985; Poulshock and Deimling 1984).

A logical assumption, frequently made, was that variables drawn from three broad areas of the caring situation may influence the dependent variable representing carer outcome; these independent variables include:

i) Characteristics of the care recipient (e.g. age, gender, physical, emotional and cognitive impairments),

ii) Characteristics of the carer (e.g. age, gender, education, relationship to care recipient, carer health status)
iii) Characteristics of the care-giving situation (e.g. nature of tasks and duties, number of hours involved in caring duties per week, length of time providing care, financial situation, whether the carer and care recipient occupy the same household).

Within the context of the stress model, most of the published research was concerned with testing hypotheses using traditional analytic approaches in which the influence of a selected factor (e.g. level of care recipient disability, duration of caring) was related to outcome (e.g. carer burden), whilst controlling for other variables (e.g. age, gender, ethnicity). In other words, the effects of "independent" variables such as care recipient disability were examined in relation to "dependent" variables such as carer burden (see figure 6-1).

Figure 6-1. Basic model of care-giving: effects of independent variables on burden as the dependent variable.

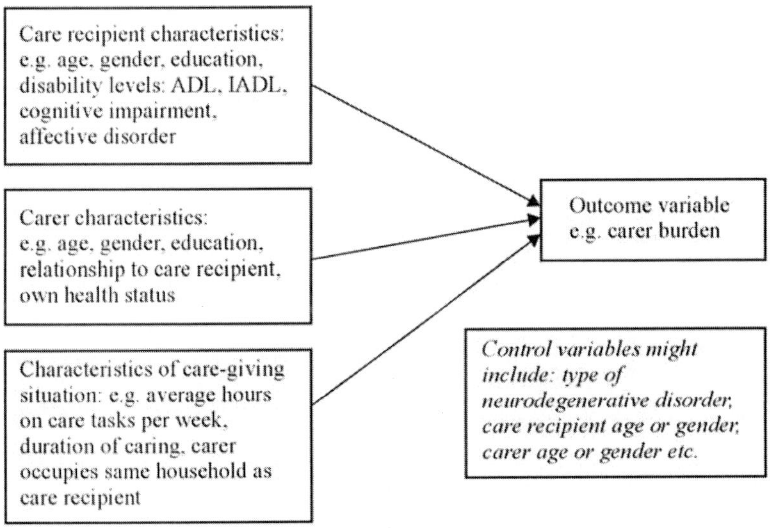

Studies of this kind were predicated on the assumption that an improved knowledge of the correlates of the outcome for the carer should provide a better understanding of the care-giving situation and the carer's needs, thus helping clinicians to prioritise treatment strategies and to plan intervention programmes.

However, these approaches are limited by a number of factors: first of all, their underlying models assume simple, linear and additive dependencies among the variables. None of these assumptions is likely to be true given the complexities of care-giving. Indeed the multidimensional nature of the concepts represented by both the independent and dependent variables and the complex relationship between them is well-established, if not fully understood. A second limitation is that early studies virtually ignored the possibility of interactions between independent variables in determining outcome for carers. Thus for example, drawing the conclusion that spouse carers experienced greater distress than adult children involved in caring for an elderly parent with dementia (e.g. George and Gwyther 1986; Gilhooly 1984) ignored the fact that spouses were living in the same household as the care recipient, often providing more "hands on" care and had fewer sources of external support. Taking account of these interactions involves recourse to the inclusion of moderator effects in the model (Baron and Kenny 1986), which in this case, may be conceptualised as that of sharing the same household (see figure 6-2). The effects of moderators versus mediators will be discussed in chapter 7.

Figure 6-2. Elaborated model of care-giving accounting for moderator effects among the independent variables.

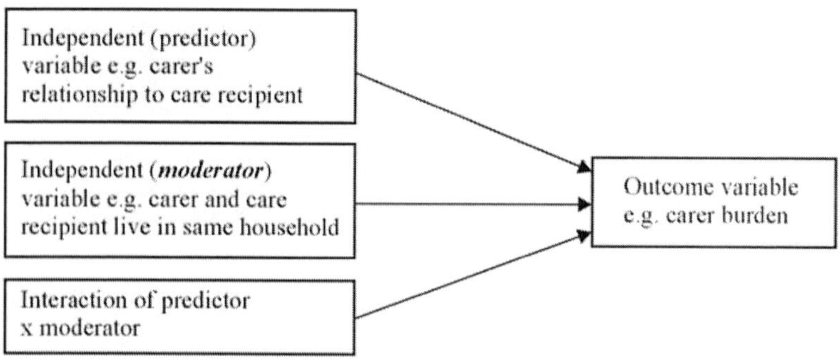

A third limitation of the original linear, essentially bivariate, model is that it failed to consider the role of intervening or mediating variables in their capacity to affect outcomes for carers. These considerations eventually led to a further modification of the basic stress model of caring, by reconceptualising certain aspects of care-giving in terms of their role as intervening variables (Montgomery 1989; see figure 6-3). For example, this view takes account of the fact that the types of tasks that are undertaken by the carer and the amount of time devoted to them, are a consequence not only of the care recipient's need for care, but also of the carer's characteristics (Davies et al. 1999). Eventually, other intervening variables such as carers' coping strategies, availability and reliance on social support, cultural factors and family relationships also came to be incorporated in the stress model (see chapter 7). It was eventually recognised that if these potential influences on care-giving are to be taken into account, research needs to be guided by models which specify the proposed inter-relations between the variables of interest from a conceptual point of view. The most influential of the models which accommodated this approach in attempting to account for care-giving has been the stress process model proposed by Pearlin et al. (1990).

Figure 6-3. Care-giving model accounting for effects of mediating variables.

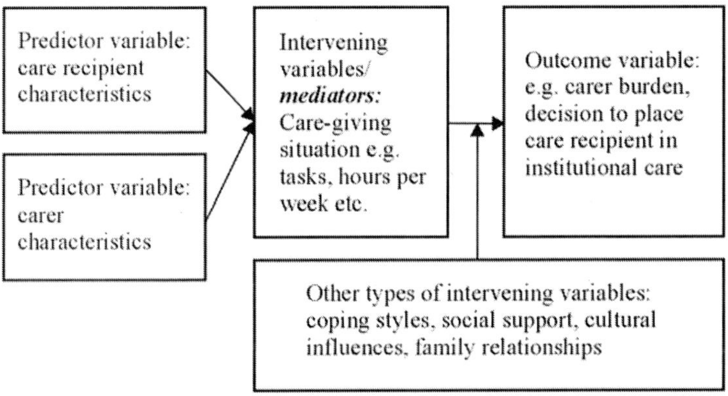

6.5.1 The choice of outcome indicators for carers

Before turning to an examination of the stress process model however, it is necessary to reconcile a further distinction that has been made in the literature in relation to ways of understanding and measuring carer outcomes. As we have seen, these have been conceptualised variously, sometimes as the "burden of care", reflecting the carer's subjective experience or appraisal of care-giving, sometimes in terms of Poulshock and Deimling's (1984) notion of care-giving impact, reflecting the effects on household routines, social activities, employment etc., and sometimes in terms of the carer's physical and mental health (Pinquart and Sorensen, 2003b; Vitaliano et al. 2003). In addition, a plethora of terms has been used to describe the effects of involvement in caring activities, many of which have been used interchangeably, as previously described. Apart from the obvious need for conceptual clarity, it is important to define these terms and to reach an understanding of the relationships among the constructs that they represent, in order to build logical, theoretical models.

When the outcome for the carer is depicted according to the variations of the model in figures 6-1 to 6-3, it is usually defined in terms of burden and is considered to be of interest in itself, because of its potentially detrimental effects for the carer. The theoretical assumption is that understanding the correlates of burden, its antecedents (i.e. predictor variables) and its consequences should provide an explanatory framework of the care-giving situation (Montgomery 1989). Care-giving burden is thus the outcome or dependent variable for the model, and its unique advantage is that it is a measure of hardship that has a specific referent, namely that of the care-giving role. The ability to identify specific factors in the antecedent conditions that might prove amenable to manipulation through appropriate interventions, thereby serving to reduce the undesirable impact on the carer, serves as the rationale for such models.

Essentially three types of antecedent variables have formed the subject of interest in these models. The first consisted of features defining the care-giving situation, namely the kinds of tasks that the carer helped with or had taken over responsibility for, the amount of time spent on these tasks, the length of time in the care-giving role, living arrangements and financial resources, i.e. the "objective" aspects of burden. The second related to the characteristics of the care recipient and included age, gender, marital status, physical and functional abilities, cognitive and latterly, affective and behavioural functioning. The third category included carer variables such as age, gender, relationship to the care recipient, education and health status. An analysis of the extent to which these three classes of variables predict carer outcomes is undertaken in chapter 7. They are enumerated here in order to draw attention to the fact that in the main, those in the first category, relating to the situation of care-giving, are the ones addressed by formal services and legislation conferring financial support and benefits. Apart from the availability of medical care, in the context of PD, far fewer resources are available in terms of helping to remediate the physical and functional limitations imposed by the illness (e.g. access to rehabilitation services, speech therapy etc.). However, it has been apparent, from the earliest work in this field, that carer characteristics have a significant role in determining outcome in the form of care-giving burden (e.g. Colerick and George 1986) but here, least progress has been made in identifying suitable interventions.

The early literature was witness to considerable debate over how the different aspects of burden should be measured. Essentially two positions emerged. The one most commonly held, was that only negative events resulting from the care-giving situation and the care recipient's illness should be included in the measurement of burden, in pursuit of greater objectivity. However, as Platt (1985) pointed out, this always included a subjective judgement on the part of the carer with respect to the origin of the events contributing to burden. Platt recommended that all negative events should be recorded, regardless of their perceived origin, as they are likely to be burdensome by their very nature. He argued that subjective attitudes on the part of the carer are likely to affect his/her decision relating to the causality of a given event. For example, carers who may be inclined to deny the extent of the care recipient's illness would be expected to understate its effects on their lives. Over-protective carers on the other hand, may exaggerate the effects. An alternative would be to ask the carer to make a judgement about the likely cause of an adverse event occurring in the household, and this could be confronted with a similar judgement made by an independent rater such as the interviewer; both ratings might then be used in analyses to check on differences in attributing specific components of burden to the care-recipient.

From a theoretical perspective, Platt's view was essentially in keeping with that of George and Gwyther (1986), who also argued that outcome measures in terms of general well-being were preferable to context sensitive measures such as care-giving burden. They held that use of general outcome measures allows for clearer conceptual and empirical separation from the specific care-giving factors that explain burden. Others have rejected the claim that care-giving burden is of secondary importance as an outcome variable. Stull et al. (1994) conclude there is room for both specific and general outcome measures because care-giving makes a unique contribution to understanding carer behaviour. This is because, although obviously related, the specific and more global measures of carer outcomes are conceptually and statistically distinct, as they have separate sets of correlates and have been shown to share little common variance (Montgomery et al. 1985).

An important variation to the stress model of caring came with the recognition that the concepts of carer burden, even if they were conceived of as subjective experiences, differed in significant ways from the concept of psychological distress (Brannan and Heflinger 2001), and this all the more so, if the latter are conceptualised in the form of psychological morbidity (Yates, Tennstedt and Chang 1999). This was first recognised by Poulshock and Deimling (1984) who recommended that subjective burden should be viewed as a form of stressor and seen as an intermediary stage in the stress process, leading eventually to the outcome for the carer or what they termed "caregiving impact". A significant theoretical development was achieved when studies began to include both measures of carer burden and of psychological morbidity in the carer. In some variations of this expanded model, psychological morbidity was conceptualised as the outcome variable, with carer burden seen as a risk factor for psychological disturbances. Hence burden was treated as another stressor that contributed to carer outcomes - a predictor of the effects for the carer, determining not only mental and physical health outcomes, but also the carer's willingness or ability to continue caring and maintain employment and social activities etc. (e.g. Son et al. 2007; Schulz and Sherwood 2008; see figure 6-4, path b). Other studies continued to treat burden, or strain, as the main outcome variable, using psychological morbidity in the carer as a predictor or explanatory variable; in these studies, for example, depression in carers was seen as contributing additionally to the strain of caring (e.g. Vitaliano et al. 1991; see figure 6-4, path a). There were also variations in how the antecedent conditions giving rise to burden were conceptualised.

Figure 6-4. Care-giving model showing different conceptualisations of burden.

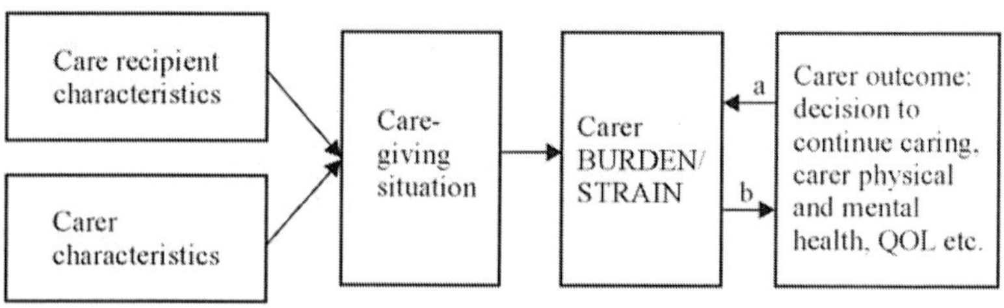

6.5.2 Burden as an independent versus dependent variable.

As has been described, much of the early literature in this field, treated care-giving burden as an outcome or dependent variable. Whilst this provided a measure of the hardship involved in caring from the carer's perspective, it was difficult to relate to any external criteria and therefore to understand precisely what it meant, in terms of the toll on the carer's health or willingness to continue caring. Measures of burden were unable to provide an indication of levels of strain that could reliably identify carers in intolerable situations or predict the risk of imminent breakdown in care. Furthermore a fairly consistent finding was that a significant proportion of carers reported only minimal burden, in circumstances demanding intensive levels of care and commitment (Cicirelli 1981; Zarit et al. 1980). This raised questions regarding the putative relationship between the obligations of care-giving and carer burden, highlighting the distinction that had earlier been made between the objective and subjective aspects of burden. However, from a theoretical perspective, it also challenged the utility of burden as a measure of outcome, given its poor correlation with independent variables, at least in the cases under consideration.

These findings confirmed that carers' reports of the effects of care-giving are coloured by their subjective appraisals and emphasised the need to take account of their judgements of the care-giving situation in the measurement of burden, as urged by Platt (1985). A corollary of this is that the subjective nature of burden, places it in more of a mediating role along the hypothesised pathway from care recipient impairments to any more global measures of the impact of care-giving on the carer (Poulshock and Deimling 1984). Alternatively, the added dimension resulting from carer characteristics means that burden could also be viewed as an independent variable in the care-giving process. Hence a model in which burden is treated either as an independent or as a mediating variable would seem to have clear advantages over one in which it constitutes the dependent or outcome variable. Such a model is able to provide an explanation for the observation that carer outcomes (e.g. in the form of psychological morbidity) do not correlate perfectly with levels of carer reported burden or strain. The same is true for other more generic measures of outcome, such as carer QOL, and their relationship to burden (e.g. Martinez-Martin et al. 2007).

Theoretical models in which carer burden is treated as an independent, predictor variable have increased in recent years. Outcomes examined have included elder abuse (Cooper et al. 2010; MacNeil et al. 2010; Wiglesworth et al. 2010; Yan and Kwok 2011), institutionalisation of the care recipient (Monini et al. 2001; Spitznagel et al. 2006) and long-term consequences for the carer such as poor physical health (Son et al. 2007), psychiatric morbidity (Schulz and Sherwood 2008) and death (Schulz and Beach 1999).

It is this model that has been at the heart of legislation aimed at providing appropriate services to support carers. The outcome for the carer of the care-giving situation (frequently defined as burden) is not only the result of a combination of care recipient and carer characteristics, but is a predictor of future status for the carer, in terms of his/her ability to continue in the care-giving role and of his/her physical and mental health.

The assumption is that the more onerous the care-giving situation (the greater the carer burden), the less willing or able the carer will be to provide care, thus precipitating the care recipient's entry into formal care (Montgomery 1989). However, a systematic finding of research in this area is that carer burden does not have a high correlation with the demands of care-giving and appears to be modified by a variety of intervening factors, including social support, carer coping strategies, family relationships, cultural factors and others. Thus burden may be ameliorated by supportive interactions with the care-giving environment; alternatively, the impact of negative events or the absence of support is likely to have an adverse effect on carer outcomes. An understanding of the factors that determine levels of burden and its relationship to other variables in the care-giving process is necessary in order to design and implement intervention procedures that may reduce the carer's experience of hardship and negative outcomes of care-giving.

6.6 The stress-process model

The central model upon which most of the care-giving literature is based is the care-giving stress-process model as described by Pearlin et al. (1990). The notion that care-giving stress is a dynamic process that evolves over the course of caring is strongly emphasised in this approach. The model focuses attention on the ways in which potentially stressful occurrences interact with each other and with intervening factors, such as personal or environmental resources, to intensify, and sometimes to reduce, stress effects and determine health outcomes for the carer. The primary interest is therefore not in identifying the conditions (stressors) which lead to difficulties for the carer, which was a major focus of early studies, but to understand how they arise and the relationships between them. The stress process as conceptualised within this model consists of four domains, each of which is made up of multiple components: background and contextual variables; the conditions giving rise to stress, i.e. the stressors; the intervening variables or mediators of stress; and the outcomes or manifestations of stress (Pearlin et al. 1990). The important features of this model lie in its recognition that multiple factors can affect carer outcomes, acknowledgement of individual differences and the use of multiple indicators to measure outcomes.

According to the stress-process model, burden is treated as a "primary" stressor and is made up of the difficult circumstances of care-giving. It is affected by background and contextual variables such as care-giving history and socioeconomic factors. Burden acts as an independent, predictive variable, directly affecting outcomes such as the physical and mental health of the carer. However, the situation is made more complicated by the fact that a serious life problem such as a chronic and progressive disease in a close family member does not exist in isolation from other problems. Stressors tend to produce other stressors which give rise to cascading effects affecting other areas of life. Thus a common problem for carers is that the demands of care-giving are time-consuming and tiring, a fact which inevitably has consequences in other areas of their lives such as work and family relationships, which may become strained and problematic in themselves. This expansion of stressors in areas outside the boundaries of care-giving has been termed "stress proliferation" and the original hardships associated with care-giving are referred to as "primary stressors", whilst those arising from them are known as "secondary stressors" (Aneshensel et al. 1995). Outcomes are affected indirectly by secondary stressors in the form of role strain, arising from negative repercussions on free time, social relations, family relationships and the employment or financial situation of the carer. The subjective assessment of these consequences can lead to secondary stressors in the form of mental or intrapsychic strains, such as diminished self-esteem and loss of feelings of competence. The term "primary" is intended to indicate that these stressors originate within the care-giving situation, while "secondary" refers to the difficulties that are consequent upon care-giving. They are not intended to signify that the stressors differ in their relative capacity to evoke stress in carers; their ability to do so is considered to be equally potent.

An important characteristic of the stress process model is that it attempts to account for the observation, referred to above, that seemingly similar situations are not experienced by carers in the same way. Earlier models had difficulty accounting for the fact that individuals perceive care-giving demands differently and have different thresholds at which events become onerous (Reinhard and Horowitz 1995). These considerations were embodied in the stress appraisal model proposed by Lawton et al. (1989;1991), which recognised the subjective elements in the care-giving process as reflecting the carer's appraisal of the situation and added this factor to the stress-process model. Appraisals were defined as "all cognitive and affectional appraisals and reappraisals of the potential stressor and the efficacy of one's coping efforts" (Lawton 1989, 61). Whether an event is perceived as stressful by the carer, depends on a multitude of intervening variables, such as their appraisal of it, ways of coping and social support, cultural factors and attitudes to family life and the quality of the carer's relationship with the care recipient, all of which may mitigate the undesirable effects of stress, thus protecting the carer from adverse consequences. Alternatively, other factors may magnify the effects of stress and render the carer particularly vulnerable.

Although the stress-process theory has received widest application, it has been criticised because of its overriding focus on coping mechanisms, its failure to account for positive care-giving outcomes and its reduction of care recipient characteristics to little more than stressors, failing to recognise the importance of the dyadic relationship between the carer and the care recipient, as well as other family relationships (e.g. Lyons et al. 2002). These relationships form the context to the care-giving situation, are multidimensional in nature and reflect cultural, historical and present-day interactions (Yates et al. 1999). In particular, the quality of the relationship between the carer and the care-recipient appears to be an important factor in this respect (Hodgins, Wuest and Malcolm 2011; Lyonette and Yardley 2003; Quinn, Clare and Woods 2012; Zarit et al. 1980). The appraisal model attempted to remedy these shortfalls by emphasising the dynamic and transactional nature of caring processes. However it was also criticised because of its confounding appraisals with components of resources and coping strategies (Braithwaite 1996).

Yates et al. (1999) attempted to integrate both these models in an approach which evaluated carer outcomes in terms of their appraisals of stressful situations and their reactions to them, taking account of their coping resources. Their model comprised five components: primary stressors (need for care as a result of cognitive impairments, functional disability and problem behaviours), primary appraisal (the carer's assessment of care needs manifested in the care provided, defined as care-giving hours), resources (personal and social resources that mitigate the effect of stressors, such as formal services, emotional support, quality of the relationship with the care receiver, carer feelings of mastery), secondary appraisal (carer appraisal of the care-giving situation, manifested as burden or overload), and outcome (in terms of psychological well-being). These models have not been replaced and continue to guide care-giving research to the present day, albeit with some refinements which reflect the preferences of individual researchers (e.g. Casado and Sacco 2012). Pinquart and Sorensen (2005) have criticised the model proposed by Yates et al. (1999) on the basis that it categorizes the number of hours of care provision as a form of primary appraisal; they argue that although this is a plausible standpoint, there is not convincing evidence to depart from the basic stress-process model, which viewed this variable as a stressor. This would seem to be unduly restrictive, however, as the time spent in care activities is clearly a subjective judgement made by the carer and there is evidence to suggest that such interventions are not always related to the disability of the care recipient (Davies et al. 1999).

6.7 Chapter summary

A major contribution of the stress-process model and its elaborations is that it helped to encourage a view which began to take account of the intricate relationships between causal and outcome factors in care-giving – a move away from examining the relationships as simple, unitary interactions between illness or situational variables and carer outcomes. These models provide a way of estimating complex interactive relationships between variables. However one of the problems in the literature is that these complex relationships have been conceptualised and operationalised in an over-simplified manner and the interdependencies among them, are only just beginning to be evaluated with the use of multivariate statistics. Only in recent years have studies begun to be published which use path analyses to estimate the complex interactions among the factors influencing care-giving in dementia (e.g. Losada 2010; Savundranayagam et al. 2011;Yates et al. 1999; this level of sophistication has not yet been reached in studies on PD care-giving.

In summing up the context of care-giving research and the theoretical advances that have been made in this area, the following recommendations emerge, highlighting the needs for future research, especially in the context of PD. The latter consideration is important in order to provide much needed comparisons of different care-giving situations. This necessitates that clearly defined theoretical models be made explicit in future research, in order to move beyond a purely descriptive approach to care-giving, and requires:

1. clearer specification of the concepts underlying key terms used in care-giving research, such as those of carer burden and care-giving outcomes;
2. accounting for antecedent conditions in terms of their effects on burden or more global carer outcomes;
3. understanding that carer subjective factors are important determinants of outcome;
4. taking account of the complex interdependencies among variables, so that concepts such as burden are understood in terms of their potential moderating and/or mediating properties;
5. differentiating measures with the specific referent of care-giving (i.e. burden) and more global indices of consequences for carers

(i.e. psychological morbidity) in order to guide theoretical frameworks of care-giving processes;

6. ensuring that the research methodology based on the foregoing considerations is able to identify vulnerable carers or points of intervention in the caring process in order to provide effective relief from the burden of caring.

Awareness of these factors in the design of studies is likely to constitute an essential preliminary criterion to meeting their central aim, which is to determine which component aspects of the carer's situation are relatively more important in determining care-giving outcomes and providing a rationale for intervention. These considerations formed an important factor in planning the study that is reported in the following pages (see chapters 8-12).

CHAPTER SEVEN

FACTORS AFFECTING CARE-GIVING IN PARKINSON'S DISEASE

7.1 Introduction

Research concerned with the impact of caring for a close relative with PD is still in its infancy. Not surprisingly, the main focus of the care-giving literature to date has been on DAT, as this is the most common of the neurodegenerative diseases (Murrel and Meeks 1992). However, the study of PD offers the unique opportunity of examining the effects of impairment arising as the result of the underlying neurodegenerative condition in three main areas of functioning in relation to care-giving. These derive from care recipient symptoms in the areas of physical (motor), cognitive and neuropsychiatric functioning and allows comparisons to be made with regard to the relative impact of these symptoms for care-giving. Importantly, since they arise within the context of the same disease process, this enables contrasts to be made, which control for the potentially confounding effects that might occur if parallels were to be drawn across different illness groups. At the same time, DAT like PD is a chronic and progressive condition, in which later life onset is most common and the course of the illness is variable and unpredictable. These characteristics are likely to be stressful for both the patients and their carers. Although neither condition places the patient at imminent risk of death, the symptoms associated with both DAT and PD are highly intrusive, affecting most aspects of everyday life (Haahr et al. 2010; and see chapter 5) and influencing daily routines for carers. The apparent similarities between the two conditions suggests that many lessons can be learned from the extensive literature on care-giving in dementia and that comparisons may prove to be instructive. Thus, the dementia care literature provides a natural starting point for identifying factors that are thought to determine the quality of care-giving experiences and revealing some of the difficulties in unravelling the complex relationships between them. In the following section, the research concerning factors that are considered to be implicated in shaping the experience of care-giving are summarized and compared for both PD and DAT. Apparent differences are highlighted with the purpose of providing a background to the research study described in chapters 8-11. In the following discussion the terms "strain" and "burden" are used to refer to subjective carer judgements of the negative outcomes of care-giving. The carer's long-term adaptation to caring and its consequences is described in more generic terms including "psychiatric disturbances", "psychological morbidity", "mental health status", "affective disturbances" and "depression", all of which have been used in the literature relating to care-giving in PD. The notion of "distress" is used to convey the meaning of general upset and ill-effects for the carer, without implying their specific relatedness to the care-giving situation or that they have reached clinically significant proportions.

7.2 Determinants of care-giving outcomes

Various aspects of the care-giving situation will now be discussed in terms of their ability to predict outcomes of care-giving, with a particular focus on the mental health of the carer. These hypothesized predictors (independent variables) of the care-giving experience (dependent variables) are considered under the headings of (i) characteristics of the care situation, (ii) care recipient, and (iii) carer characteristics.

7.2.1 Characteristics of the care situation

Characteristics of the care-giving situation (e.g. nature of tasks and duties, number of hours involved in caring duties per week, length of time providing care, financial situation) are generally considered to be the "objective" aspects of carer burden (see previous discussion, chapter 6) and their effects on the outcomes of caring are considered below.

7.2.1.1 Family income

Not surprisingly, low income has been found to disadvantage carers, both in dementia (Montgomery, Gonyea et al. 1985; Scott, Roberto and Hutton 1986) and in PD (Edwards and Scheetz 2002). In general however, finances do not appear to be a major concern for those involved in caring for people with PD (Davies et al. 1999), but this does not mean of course, that individual situations of hardship do not exist or that financial situations remain static.

7.2.1.2 Time spent in care activities

Few studies have attempted to measure the time spent in delivering care to the care recipient in PD. An exception is a study by Martinez-Martin et al. (2007) which found that the time spent on helping care recipients with the activities of daily living (ADL and IADL) and supervision required in order to avoid potentially dangerous situations such as falls, was related to carer burden, but not to depression. Davies et al. (1999) found that the time spent on care-giving activities was related to disease severity in PD and increased as the condition progressed, but they did not attempt to relate this to outcome for the carer. In their study, time spent on care activities averaged 35 hours per week and, as the authors point out, was equivalent to that of a full-time job. For patients with milder symptom severity, care demands were relatively low and carers were mostly able to continue working; in some instances the situation was better than that prior to the diagnosis, as medication produced a beneficial effect. Patients with moderate disease severity received an average of 21 hours of informal care per week, but this was strongly dependent on the care recipients' self-care abilities and involvement of formal services. Help was mainly needed in getting out of bed, rising from chairs and in bathing and dressing. This was also the point at which adaptations to the physical environment were made, for example raising toilet seats and adding rails. Care recipients required most help in the morning and this was particularly so for those who suffered from early morning dystonia. Some were unable to do anything for themselves until the effects of medication came into play, and then the amount of assistance required decreased considerably. Many carers had adapted by arranging household routines around the vicissitudes of the illness. Although it was unusual for carers to be disturbed at night, extra vigilance was required if the care recipient was prone to falls and problems also arose if s/he was unwilling to be left alone, if the carer needed to go out. Delivery of care in advanced PD required around the clock interventions and averaged 56 hours per week. Nevertheless, the picture remained quite mixed; some patients were able to live alone with adequate provision of formal support, but in general, carers were engaged in all aspects of care provision.

Perhaps the most important conclusion from the Davies et al. (1999) study however, is that time spent in care provision is not as objective a measure of hardship for the carer as at first it may seem. Particularly striking is the broad range in hours of care provided on a weekly basis (0-119 hours) and there are considerable variations at each of the levels of disease severity. Time spent in caring is clearly not just related to disease severity but to individual characteristics of carers and care recipients, which are probably associated with previous habits and routines established in the relationship, possibly reflecting attitudes and conventions assimilated by the couple.

It is also important to note that despite the similarities described at the beginning of this chapter, PD clearly differs from DAT with respect to the dynamics of care provision over the course of the illness. Although for both conditions carer involvement is probably greatest mid-course in disease progression, in DAT demands on the carer generally diminish as the patient becomes less capable of independent action (Dura et al. 1990). In PD however, the physical impairment means that demands on the carer increase as the disease progresses.

7.2.2 The impact of care recipient characteristics

There is a common-sense view that the impact on the carer is, to a considerable extent, likely to be determined by care-recipient characteristics. The dementia care literature has however, provided little evidence in support of this view. An examination of these relationships is particularly apposite in PD, because of the clinical presentation of the illness in three important areas of functioning: physical, emotional and cognitive performance, thus providing the opportunity to evaluate the relative contribution of each to the impact on the carer. In the following section, each of these will be examined in turn, in relation to the existing literature on the subject; demographic and clinical variables will also be considered.

7.2.2.1 Demographic and clinical variables

Relatively few studies of care-giving in PD, have attempted to demonstrate links between demographic variables such as the care-recipient's age and gender and the outcome for the carer. Negative carer outcomes appear to be associated, albeit weakly, with the care recipient's age at onset of the disease (Martinez-Martin et al. 2007) and this association is particularly evident for PD patients with dementia (Stella et al. 2009). However, the care recipient's age at the time of examination is more controversial as a predictor of carer strain: Martinez-Martin et al. (2007) found an association with carer burden, whilst Schrag et al. 2006) did not. The dementia care literature has been equally unclear in this regard, despite many more studies having addressed these questions. Little is known about whether the gender of the care recipient makes a difference to the experience of burden for the carer. This may be because the majority of carers are women and the question of gender is usually examined from the point of view of the carer rather than the care recipient. Alternatively, a large proportion of carers are caring for spouses, so a number of variables are potentially confounded with gender i.e. relationship and proximity to the care recipient.

It would be reasonable to expect that clinical variables such as the duration of illness and treatment effectiveness or complications are also potentially likely to contribute to carer burden or distress. Although disease duration appears to be a better predictor of carer outcome than the age of disease onset (Fernandez et al. 2001), here too, the findings are somewhat inconclusive. Some studies have found strong, positive associations between the duration of PD and both carer strain (Miller et al. 1996; Schrag, Hovris et al. 2006) and some measures of carer depression (GDS, GHQ, Miller et al. 1996; HAM-D, Fernandez et al. 2001), whilst others have reported only weak associations for carer strain (e.g. Aarsland, Larsen, Karlsen et al. 1999; Carter et al. 1998; Martinez-Martin et al. 2007; 2008; Meara, Mitchelmore et al. 1999; McRae et al. 2009; Stella et al. 2009) and depression as measured on the BDI (Aarsland, Larsen, Karlsen et al. 1999; Miller et al. 1996; Schrag, Hovris et al. 2006). One reason for the discrepancies in the results may be connected with the instruments used to measure depression or with the characteristics of the samples studied. For example, it is unlikely to be a coincidence that correlations between the BDI and duration of illness are consistently low in comparison to other measures of depression. Moreover, illness duration is inevitably confounded with age of disease onset and age at examination for the care recipient, severity of illness and concomitant complications such as the presence of dementia, making any potential relationships with carer outcomes difficult to disentangle. Interpretation of these findings is made more difficult by the fact that associations with duration of illness are not always reported and at least one study has failed to demonstrate a link between carer distress and disease duration in PD (McRae, Sherry and Roper 1999). In the dementia care research, by contrast, most studies do not demonstrate any relationship between duration of illness and carer distress (e.g. George and Gwyther 1986; Montgomery 1989).

The relationship with treatment variables does not appear to have been addressed in PD and is not applicable to the same extent in dementia care.

7.2.2.2 The physical and functional impairment of PD

The carer's involvement in providing assistance is likely to increase as the care recipient deteriorates in various areas of physical functioning and the activities of daily living become more of an effort, taking longer to achieve. The view that carer burden is related to the severity of the care recipient's disabilities in PD has received some support, both in relation to the amount of care provided (O'Reilly et al. 1996) and the time spent in providing it (Martinez-Martin 2007). The severity and stage of PD as measured on the Hoehn and Yahr scale (Hoehn and Yahr 1967) have been related to carer role strain (Carter et al. 1998), to carer burden (D'Amelio et al. 2009; Martinez-Martin et al. 2007; 2008) and to carer distress (Leiknes et al. 2010), although the association is not a strong one. It is more robust in demented PD patients, who are likely to have more advanced PD, but again dementia is a confounding factor (Stella et al. 2009). Nevertheless, a number of studies have not found any association between carer outcomes and motor impairment as measured on the Hoehn and Yahr scale (Aarsland, Larsen, Karlsen et al. 1999; McRae et al. 2009; Miller et al. 1996; Schrag, Hovris et al. 2006). Very few studies have reported any associations between carer difficulties and other measures of motor performance in PD, the exceptions being: Leiknes et al. (2010), Martinez-Martin et al. (2008) and Tanji et al. (2008). Thus the relationship between carer burden and disease severity/motor impairment is far from being a foregone conclusion; indeed there is little empirical evidence in support of it in the dementia care literature either (Zarit et al. 1980; Montgomery 1989).

Equally, attempts to relate care recipient functional performance (ADL) with outcomes for the carer have met with mixed results. Studies finding a positive association with carer burden include: Cifu et al. (2006), Martinez-Martin et al. (2007), Leiknes et al. (2010) and for both demented and depressed PD patients (Stella et al. 2009). Some authors have argued that ADL is the strongest single predictor of carer burden (Edwards and Scheetz 2002) and quality of life (Goldsworthy and Knowles 2008; Martinez-Martin et al. 2005) and an association has also been reported with the spouse carer's assessment of mutuality in the relationship with the care recipient (Tanji et al. 2008). On the other hand, at least one study was not able to establish any relationship between functional impairment and carer outcome in PD (D'Amelio et al. 2009). Attempts to correlate carer burden with ADL in DAT have also only been partially successful (Annerstedt et al. 2000; Gonyea et al. 2005; Price and Levy 1990; Zarit et al. 1986).

7.2.2.3 Cognitive impairment

The analysis of carer burden in relation to care recipient characteristics so far has revealed few substantive differences between care-giving in PD and DAT. However, indications are beginning to emerge, which suggest that not all findings may be generalized from DAT to other care situations. For example, a comparison of spousal carers of people with Alzheimer's disease and fronto-temporal dementia has shown that the latter condition is associated with higher levels of burden and diminished feelings of competency on the part of the carer (De Vugt et al. 2006). The main reason for these differences would appear to lie in the behavioural disturbances shown by the care recipient, which are known to be associated with greater carer distress in DAT (e.g. Savundranaygam, Hummert and Montgomery 2005), but which are more pronounced in patients with fronto-temporal dementia.

Of particular relevance to the present study is the finding that cognitive functioning in people with PD may adversely affect the experience of burden in carers of these patients (Aarsland, Larsen, Karlsen et al. 1999; Leroi, McDonald et al. 2012; Meara, Mitchelmore et al. 1999; Shin, Youn et al. 2012;Thommessen et al. 2002). Conversely, numerous studies have shown that there is only a weak association between severity of dementia and distress in the carers of people with DAT (e.g. Annerstedt et al. 2000; Bergvall et al. 2011; Gonyea et al. 2005; Rinaldi et al. 2005). These variations between groups of sufferers with different aetiologies highlights the need to understand the experience of caring in different situations.

Stella et al. (2009) reported that the highest level of burden for carers of people with PD was associated with a subgroup of patients with dementia as compared to those with depression or neither dementia or depression. The greatest contribution to burden appeared to be the neuropsychological disturbances, although this group also had the highest motor and functional impairment.

Nevertheless, the majority of studies, in keeping with the dementia care research, do not demonstrate any relationships between cognitive impairments in PD and carer outcomes (e.g. Cifu et al. 2006; D'Amelio et al. 2009; Fernandez et al. 2001; Martinez-Martin et al. 2005; 2008; Miller et al. 1996; O'Reilly et al. 1996; Stella et al. 2009; Tanji et al. 2008). This may be the result of patient sampling biases in some studies; for example, selection of younger PD patients, in the earlier stages of the disease (e.g. D'Amelio et al. 2009; O'Reilly et al. 1996) and specifically excluding those with evidence of dementia (Miller et al. 1996).

7.2.2.4 Behavioural disturbances

A well established finding in the dementia care literature is that behavioural disturbances have a major impact on carer outcomes

(Aneshensel et al. 1995; Baumgarten 1989; Beeri et al. 2002; Chappell and Penning 1996; Ingersoll-Dayton and Raschick 2004; Jarrott et al. 2000; Machin 1980; L.W. Morris, R.G. Morris et al. 1988; Sanford 1975; Savundranaygam et al. 2005; Schulz, Visintainer and Williamson 1990; Sink, Holden and Yaffe 2005; Yates et al. 1999; see also Pinquart and Sörensen 2003 for a meta-analysis), although this has not inevitably been the case (e.g. Fitting et al. 1986; Zarit et al. 1980).

Certain behaviours such as aggression, agitation and night-time wandering are especially problematic (Gallicchio et al. 2002; Gaugler, R.L. Kane, R.A. Kane, Clay et al. 2005) and others such as aimlessness, forgetfulness, withdrawal and a lack of interest in daily activities have also been found to contribute to carer feelings of burden and depression (Chappell and Penning 1996; Thomas et al. 2004). Behaviours which result in the need for constant supervision and a proneness to falls on the part of the care recipient are of particular difficulty for carers (Gilleard 1984b; Thomas et al. 2004). Behaviour problems have been identified as the leading cause for emergency hospital admissions of people with DAT (Nourhashemi et al. 2001) and care recipient behaviours that place considerable physical demands on carers, such as incontinence, immobility, difficulty in walking and increased night-time activity are predictive of institutionalization across different cultural groups (Asada, Kinoshita and Kakuma 2000; Bond and Clark 2002; Dunkin and Anderson-Hanley 1998; Gort et al. 2007; Haupt and Kurz 1993; Hope et al. 1998; Jerrom et al. 1993; Monini et al. 2001; Thomas et al. 2004). However, it is not only the aversive, over-demanding or intolerable behaviours that cause the greatest stress to carers, but the unrelenting "daily grind" that many carers find it most difficult to cope with (Gilhooly 1986).

Although behavioural problems have received very little attention in the care-giving literature on PD, there is some evidence that they may also be highly predictive of carer distress (Aarsland, Larsen, Karlsen et al. 1999; Goldsworthy and Knowles 2008).

7.2.2.5 Neuropsychiatric symptoms

Sparse attention has been focused on the neuropsychiatric symptoms of PD and their contribution to distress in carers. One of the earliest studies to show that depression in PD was strongly associated with emotional distress in carers was that of Miller et al. (1996). A number of studies have since added support to these findings (Aarsland, Larsen, Karlsen et al. 1999; Carter et al. 2008; Marsh et al. 2004; Meara, Mitchelmore et al. 1999; Schrag, Hovris et al. 2006; Thommessen et al. 2002) although some report that the association is only weak (Martinez-Martin et al. 2007; 2008). Stella et al. (2009) suggest the relationship between neuropsychiatric symptoms and carer outcome holds only for non-depressed and non-demented PD patients and D'Amelio et al. (2009) confirmed the association for neuropsychiatric symptoms more generally, but not for depression. Further evidence for the significance of the neuropsychiatric symptoms of PD, in determining carer outcomes, comes from a study by Leiknes et al. (2010), who found that carers of people with PD reported three-fold higher rates of distress associated with the neuropsychiatric symptoms compared to controls. This result is particularly striking, as patients and their carers were examined at the time of diagnosis, i.e. in the early stages of the disease. Carer distress was found to be most strongly associated with apathy and then depression, anxiety and irritability in the care recipient. Less common neuropsychiatric symptoms, but ones always associated with carer distress in PD include delusions, hallucinations, agitation, disinhibition and confusion (Aarsland, Larsen, Karlsen et al. 1999; Aarsland, Bronnick et al. 2007; Davies et al. 1999; Leiknes et al. 2010; Schrag, Hovris et al. 2006). Broadly speaking, these findings are in keeping with those of the dementia care literature (e.g. De Vugt et al. 2003; Greene et al. 1982; Landes et al. 2001).

Clearly, a number of factors are likely to influence the relationship between neuropsychiatric symptoms and carer outcomes and they may follow a hierarchy of importance. For example, in the presence of psychotic symptoms such as hallucinations and delusions, other symptoms such as depression may have lesser significance in determining carer distress. Some studies employ exclusion criteria which mean that PD patients with specific neuropsychiatric symptoms cannot participate (e.g. Miller et al. 1996), whilst others may focus on sub-groups of patients with certain symptoms such as dementia (e.g. Aarsland, Bronnick et al. 2007), thus giving rise to some of the variability in the findings from different research. This is not a problem when the exclusion criteria are explicit, but is more so, when they are not. Age and duration of illness may also be relevant factors from the point of view of the carer. With time, carers attitudes to different symptoms and behaviours in the care recipient are likely to change, as they become more skilled in managing them or simply do not attribute particular significance to them. Thus Zarit et al. (1986) found that carers' ability to tolerate difficult symptoms increased over the course of care-giving. This is also likely to be the case for caring in PD, as carers grow accustomed to dealing with different situations and adapt their routines accordingly to minimise difficulties.

Other factors contributing to the diversity in these findings are the measurement instruments used. Carer outcomes are measured by different instruments purporting to measure a variety of concepts, including quality of life (e.g. Goldsworthy and Knowles 2008; Martinez-Martin et al. 2005; 2007; 2008), depression (e.g. Aarsland, Larsen, Karlsen et al. 1999; Carter et al. 2008; Fernandez et al. 2001; Miller et al. 1996; Schrag, Hovris et al. 2006), burden (e.g. Cifu et al. 2006; D'Amelio et al. 2009; Edwards and Scheetz 2002; Goldsworthy and Knowles 2008; Martinez-Martin et al. 2007; 2008; Schrag, Hovris et al. 2006), role strain (Carter et al. 1998), strain in general (e.g. Aarsland, Larsen, Karlsen et al. 1999; Miller et al. 1996; Thommessen et al. 2002) and carer distress in relation to the care recipient's performance on the Neuropsychiatric Inventory (e.g. Aarsland, Bronnick et al. 2007; Stella et al. 2009) as well as several less well defined outcome variables. It is not unreasonable to expect that this wide range of variables is likely to contribute to the variance in these outcomes measures for the carer and thus to the diversity of results reported. In order to clarify these issues, studies need to specify their aims very precisely and select instruments for the measurement of the concepts studied, very carefully.

In summary, it remains controversial as to whether care recipient characteristics such as age and gender, length of illness, its severity and the disability that it causes, have a major impact on the carer. Studies from the dementia care and PD literature suggest that the effects of these variables, if they exist, are only minimal. However, there is some evidence that cognitive impairment may be more significant for carer burden in PD compared to DAT. On the other hand, behavioural and emotional disturbances in the care recipient seem to be closely related to carer distress and burden for both DAT and PD.

7.2.3 The impact of carer characteristics on the outcomes of care-giving

It is important to remember however, that it may not be certain characteristics of the care recipient, such as the behavioural and neuropsychiatric disturbances in themselves, but carers' perceptions of these symptoms and the meaning they attribute to them, that have the greatest impact on carer outcomes. Before turning to examine this question, more general characteristics of carers, and how they are associated with the outcomes of care-giving, will be discussed.

7.2.3.1 Carer age

Surprisingly, the age of the carer has received relatively little attention in the care-giving literature in general. The majority of carers of people with neurodegenerative conditions are older, frequently by virtue of being spouse carers of people with age-related chronic conditions. Older carers are likely to have more illness themselves, to be less fit in general and to have the kind of problems that accompany old age and thus one possibility is that the responsibilities of caring for a sick relative or spouse is especially burdensome. On the other hand, although younger carers may be more fit and have fewer health problems, they are likely to have young children still living at home, to be in full-time employment and possibly to have greater expectations with regard to fulfilling their own plans and expectations. Care-giving may interfere with the realisation of these plans and may even mean that they have to give up employment, with the consequent financial implications and restriction of social activities. As an illustration of this, resentment among carers was found to be highest in women with fewer roles i.e. those who had given up work in order to take on caring duties and who were without a partner (Murphy et al. 1997).

Moreover, depending on the closeness of their relationship with the care receiver, carers may experience the transition to care-giving as a major life event (Holmes and Rahe 1967), with the accompanying strains and emotional consequences that the diagnosis of a long-term neuro-degenerative illness brings for them and their families. Despite the different conditions that may be associated with age, it is not a variable that has been systematically explored in the care-giving literature. Only one study appears to have taken account of carer age with regard to care-giving in PD, with the finding that younger carers reported greater strain in the early stages of the disease process than older carers (Carter et al. 2010).

7.2.3.2 Carer gender

A very common finding in the dementia care literature is that female carers report worse outcomes than male carers (Almberg et al. 1998; Cantor 1983; Fitting et al. 1986; Gallicchio et al. 2002; George and Gwyther 1986; Morris et al. 1991; Noelker and Poulshock 1984; Pinquart and Sorensen 2006; Pruchno and Potasnik 1989; Schulz et al. 1995; Thompson et al. 2004; Yee and Schulz 2000; Zarit et al. 1980; 1986), although it is a relationship that has not always been found to hold (e.g. Annerstedt et al. 2000; Baker, Robertson and Connelly 2010). Female carer outcomes are worse both in terms of burden (Barush and Spaid 1989;

Gold et al. 1994; Pruchno and Resch 1989a) and depression (Dura, Haywood-Niler and Keicolt-Glaser 1990; Fitting et al. 1986).

Women carers of spouses with PD also appear to be more distressed than men (Edwards and Scheetz 2002; Lyons et al. 2009). However, a study by Hooker et al. (2000) found that gender differentiated Alzheimer and PD spouses, the latter showing no differences between men and women with respect to health and coping styles. Little is known about gender differences in carer outcomes over time in PD (Pinquart and Sorensen 2006).

There is some evidence to suggest that male and female carers respond to the demands of caring in different ways and this may account for the findings that women are more distressed (Ingersoll-Dayton and Raschick 2004). Specifically, male carers were found to develop a negative outlook and to experience a need for social support, whilst for female carers, problems lay in the fact that their relationships with other family members suffered, along with their own health (Almberg et al. 1998).

However, these gender differences might also be explained by methodological considerations. Most studies recruit a greater proportion of women carers in comparison to men (e.g. Miller et al. 1996) and although the prevalence of PD is slightly higher among males (Van Den Eeden et al. 2003), the proportion of female carers of people with PD reported in the literature is much higher than would be predicted on this basis. There is evidence that more women with PD either live alone or in institutions (Jones et al. 1999). The predominance of female carers may thus bias the results, as it is well established that women suffer from depression more frequently than men (Weissman et al. 1996) and the observed gender differences in care-giving may simply be a reflection of the pattern in the general population. Nevertheless, Yee and Schulz (2000) after reviewing 31 empirical studies on gender differences in care-giving, concluded that the levels of psychiatric morbidity among female carers exceeded that of male carers when compared with non care-giving community samples.

7.2.3.3 Relationship to the care recipient

It is well-established in the dementia care literature, that the carer's relationship to the care recipient is a significant factor in the carer's experience of care-giving. It was originally noted by Zarit et al. (1980) that wives tend to experience higher levels of distress in comparison to other family members and this finding has since been replicated by many authors (e.g. Almberg, Grafstrom and Winblad 1997a; Barusch and Spaid, 1989; Fitting et al. 1986; George and Gwyther 1986; Ingersoll-Dayton and

Raschick 2004; Miller and Montgomery 1990; Pruchno and Resch 1989a; Yee and Schulz 2000; Zarit et al. 1986). Daughters are also highly vulnerable and this is thought to be because of their close emotional involvement with the care recipient, although in general, they report less negative impact than wives (e.g. Coen et al. 2002; Horowitz 1985b). However, there are also studies that have not found any differences between adult children and spouses (Chumbler et al. 2003; Montgomery and Borgatta 1985; 1987, cited in Montgomery 1989).

Perhaps not surprisingly, there is evidence from the literature to show that the involvement of carers in care-giving tasks differs considerably according to their relationship with the care recipient (Colerick and George 1986; Horowitz 1985a). Spouses provide more personal care for longer periods of time than children, and women do so more than men and with less input from formal services (Horowitz 1985b). These differences in responsibilities may partially account for the differences observed.

In general, the closer the familial distance, the worse the carer's mental health (Annerstedt et al. 2000; Cantor 1983; George and Gwyther 1986; Gilhooly 1984). Nevertheless, it needs to be borne in mind, that these relationships are more complex than is often recognized in the literature. For example, the differences between male and female carers may be confounded with the relationship of the carer to the care recipient and kinship ties are frequently confounded with the fact that both the carer and the care recipient are living in the same household and as a result, the carer is "on call" for twenty-four hours a day. Under these circumstances it is difficult to determine objectively, how much time is spent directly on care-giving tasks and the responsibilities of caring. Related to this is the fact that the care recipient is less likely to be institutionalised if being cared for by a spouse than by other relatives or nonrelatives (Colerick and George 1986; Gilhooly 1986; Scott et al. 1997) and this may in fact be due to greater emotional and practical involvement of the carer. In a sense it is precisely because of the carer's special relationship with the care recipient, that s/he suffers so specifically in this role, yet is unwilling to relinquish it.

7.2.3.4 Carer's coping strategies

The ways in which carers cope with their responsibilities is also likely to influence their view of the situation in which they find themselves and their response to it. This aspect of caring in PD has been given less attention than might be expected, particularly in view of the fact, that if any theoretical approach can be seen as underpinning the majority of work in this area, it is the stress process theory (Pearlin et al. 1990) which places considerable emphasis on coping as a mediating factor in the experience of stressful situations.

Various coping strategies exist, but they can be seen as falling into one of two categories: that of emotion-focused coping and problem-focused coping (Monat and Lazarus 1985, 5). Emotion-focused coping is a way of dealing with the emotions associated with the strain arising out of the caring process, whilst problem-focused coping aims to confront the reality of stressful care-giving conditions by dealing with the tangible consequences. People are considered to choose one or other of these coping styles, but mixed patterns also exist. It is alleged that female carers engage predominantly in emotion-focused coping, whilst male carers opt for more problem-focused strategies (Almberg, Grafstrom and Winblad 1997b). The most effective strategies are problem-focused and mixed strategies (Monat and Lazarus 1985, 6-7), but dysfunctional coping strategies are also recognised. In one study, avoidant coping styles on the part of carers were found to be associated with more problem behaviours in the care recipient and hence greater depression in the carer (Mausbach et al. 2006).

Another way of examining coping strategies is to consider self-efficacy. Gonyea et al. (2005) found that levels of self-efficacy in the domain of symptom management for the care recipient, had a significant independent effect on the experience of care-giving. Carers reporting stronger feelings of self-efficacy and those who were effective in reserving time for themselves had lower levels of burden and better quality of life (Coen et al. 2002; Gonyea et al. 2005).

7.2.3.5 Social support

Social support, like coping strategies, has been strongly emphasised as an important modifier of the stress process (Pearlin et al. 1990; Yates et al. 1999). It is usually defined as an interaction that provides physical assistance, social contact, or emotional support for the carer. The concept of social support and its relationship to care-giving strain is complex, but in particular, three dimensions have been distinguished as being important. The first of these emphasises the subjective nature of social support by drawing attention to the fact that it is the carer's perceived satisfaction with the quality of support that is associated with less burden, diminished levels of depression, and fewer health problems (Schulz et al. 1995). This relationship is more important for informal social support networks, such as family and friends, than for formal sources of support or paid providers. However, this distinction reflects a confounding of variables that represent the second dimension that has been highlighted as of importance in social support, namely, the kind of support that is available (emotional versus physical assistance). The third aspect relates to the structure of the support network: the number and relationship between the people of which it is comprised (O'Reilly et al. 1996). Generally speaking, the larger the number in the network and the greater the differentiation of groups within it, the better the quality of social support, as different groups are able to meet the carer's needs in a variety of areas. A further factor that is recognised as being important is the extent to which support is maintained over the course of the illness, as care-giving demands increase.

There has been comparatively little research on the effects of social support in caring for a person with PD. One study by Monahan and Hooker (1997) found that although the availability of mainly physical support (IADL, ADL, help in a crisis) from family members was greater in a sample of spouse carers of people with PD compared to those caring for a spouse with DAT, there were no differences between groups in their appraisal of the social support received. Some caution is required in the interpretation of these findings, as the groups of carers differed on some critical variables, such as carer age, education, the time for which they had been involved in caring, number of children and financial resources, as well as the severity of the care recipient's functional disabilities, all of which, as we have seen, may potentially influence the outcomes of care-giving. Nevertheless, these results emphasise the subjective nature of social support and provide additional evidence in support of the view that the carer's appraisals of the care-giving situation may be critical in determining outcomes.

Social support in care-giving was the focus of much research in the 1980s and for the most part, its beneficial effects were emphasised (for reviews see Chappell 1992; Pearlin 1985). In particular, the subjective perception of social support was identified as having a major role in bestowing benefits for carers and leading to better physical and mental health (Chappell and Funk 2011). Research in relation to PD, however, has not always replicated these findings. For example, a study by Miller et al. (1996) was not able to demonstrate any beneficial effects of social support in relieving the burden or emotional distress for carers of spouses with PD. One reason for this may have been their significantly diminished social networks in relation to a control group of older people, so availability of support may have been the key determinant of these findings. There is also evidence that the social support of non-family members may be less important for spouse carers, but that it plays a more significant role in the lives of children caring for a parent with PD (Shin, Lee et al. 2012). It is now more generally accepted that social support has a crucial role in determining health outcomes, not only in care-giving, and the special role of spouses, partners and children is recognised in this (for a review see Chappell and Funk 2011). These aspects of social support will be discussed below in the context of dyadic approaches to caring, the influence of family relationships, the role of cultural factors and the importance of attachment relationships in determining attitudes to care-giving and the consequent implications for the health of carers.

7.2.3.6 Positive affect in carers

Although carers' affective status is often conceptualised as an outcome of care-giving, it is clear that both positive and negative dispositional qualities in carers may affect their reactions to caring. Whilst it may be difficult to determine the causal order of these effects, it is almost certainly the case that a feedback loop exists between the two, whereby carers who have a greater inclination to put a more favourable construction on their lives more generally, also have a greater tendency to make positive reappraisals of the care-giving situation and this leads to their experiencing more positive affect in their caring role. This is essentially the position described by Beck et al. (1979) in their conceptualisation of depression from a cognitive point of view. Hence certain predispositions of the carer, which have been variously conceptualised as "personality" (Hooker et al 1992; 1994; 1998), "optimism" (Lyons et al. 2004; 2009), "purposefulness", defined as a sense of direction in life (Konstam et al. 2003), "preparedness", which is the self-perception of carers with regard to how well they are carrying out their care-giving role (Archbold et al. 1990) and "mastery", which refers to how well carers feel that they are able to control and manage events (Lawton et al. 1989) are thought to determine feelings of strain in the carers of people with PD. Studies specific to care-giving in DAT equally suggest that positive affect is related to the use of positive reappraisal (Haley et al. 1987; Stephens et al. 1988), problem focused coping (Haley et al. 1996; Vitaliano et al. 1990) and receiving satisfaction from care-giving (Haley et al. 1987; Lawton et al. 1991). Folkman (1997) suggests that in the context of intense carer distress, positive affect serves multiple functions: (i) as a "breather and distractor" from everyday stressors; (ii) a "sustainer to enhance self-esteem and feelings of effectiveness; and (iii) a "restorer" that is, assisting individuals to feel connected and cared about.

7.3 Factors that modify the consequences of care-giving

The discussion so far cannot have left the reader in any doubt as to the hardships involved in caring for a dependant, close family member at home. However, despite the heavy demands placed upon carers by the care-giving situation, the majority manage very well and are committed to their role as carers. The foregoing discussion has attempted to provide a theoretically grounded explanation for the fact that carer outcome (i.e. in terms of general and psychological health) is not related in a simple, linear fashion to the weight of responsibilities carried by the carer and his/her appraisal of the difficulties and hardships they impose (i.e. burden or strain). Although levels of burden among carers are generally speaking, quite high, this does not translate into the conclusion that there is an imminent risk of breakdown in informal care, with carers themselves being in need of at least as much support as those they care for. On the contrary, experience shows that breakdown in family care is a relatively rare occurrence and most families express the wish to look after their older and infirm relatives at home. Despite the dominant view that carers are under high levels of strain, there is considerable variability in their reactions to the demands of care-giving (Farran and Kuhn 1998) and research studies show that most carers seem to cope fairly well (e.g. Chappell 2001) although this is not emphasized in the literature. In a number of reports in unselected samples, little or no evidence of increased carer strain or burden has been identified even though carers were dealing with apparently difficult circumstances (Aneshensel et al. 1995, 34; Eagles, Beattie et al. 1987; Eagles, Walker et al. 1987; Zarit et al. 1980). This is not to deny the widely held view, supported by empirical findings, that carers are subject to considerable hardships, but merely to qualify it, by adding that some appear to cope well and function normally (Zarit, Johansson and Jarrott 1998). Nor should it lead to the conclusion that since carers by and large remain committed to caring, this means that their situation cannot be so bad after all. Little is understood about why some carers respond well to the demands of the caring situation whereas others do not (Farran et al. 1999).

This qualification is important for a number of reasons. First of all, it is support for the view, that providing care for a family member is not just a tiring and burdensome duty, but that it has positive aspects for the carer, which may outweigh any negative experiences of caring (Cohen, Colantonio and Vernich 2002; George and Gwyther 1986; Lawton et al. 1991; Nolan et al. 1996). Secondly, the fact that the majority of carers manage well, means that we can look to them to understand how they cope and find ways of helping those carers who are in less favourable positions. Finally, accepting that there is considerable diversity in the way in which people cope in the care-giving role may help to explain why, despite the wealth of research in this area, we still do not understand a great deal about the psychological well-being, or otherwise, of carers. There has been a tendency to view all care-giving roles in the same light, differentiating only those aspects of the task which are relatively easy to measure, such as the number of hours a week spent in direct care activities or whether both carer and cared-for person live in the same household. Little attention has been given to formal comparisons between carers involved in supporting people with different long-term conditions, although, as referred to above, there is some evidence of differential effects on care-giving, emphasizing the need to broaden research to include conditions other than DAT.

In addition, as discussed in chapter 6, the application of stress process theories to the field of care-giving serves as a reminder, that a variety of situational factors may determine the vulnerability of carers to poorer outcomes, especially in terms of psychological morbidity. Where these factors interact with the hypothesised predictor or independent variables, changing their potency, they are termed ***moderators.*** Alternatively where they are intervening variables, that serve to alter the effects of the independent variables on carer outcomes, they are termed ***mediators*** (Baron and Kenny 1986). Mediators may also modify the effects of burden on carer outcomes, where burden is seen as an intermediary stage in the care-giving process.

The influence of moderators on the care-giving process, which in effect concerns the confounding effects of various situational factors that have been highlighted above, are of less interest to a neuropsychological analysis of caring in PD than the influence of mediators, and it is to these that attention is now turned, as they have been the primary focus of research in connection with care-giving. There is one important exception to this, namely in the consideration of burden. According to the stress process model of Pearlin et al. (1990) burden is viewed as a primary stressor in the care-giving process, and as such it may be open to both the effects of moderators and mediators (see section 7.4.2).

Before embarking on an analysis of the mediational effects of different variables that may shape the course of the care-giving process, thereby determining the consequences for the carer, it is necessary to take a brief departure in order to acknowledge an important source for the work on these effects in stress theory. In what is now a classic piece of research examining the influence of life events on stress processes, Brown and Harris (1978) highlighted a number of vulnerability factors for increased susceptibility to stress, ultimately leading to poorer mental health. Certain of these factors are likely to be context dependent and so may not be applicable to situations such as care-giving, but one in particular appears to be a potent determinant of whether exposure to stress results in affective disturbances, namely, the lack of a close, confiding relationship, and this has been systematically replicated by subsequent studies (see Miller and Morley 1986 for discussion). In so far as caring for someone with a neurodegenerative condition can be considered to be a life event (see chapter 5), albeit extended in time, the effects of family functioning and in particular, of mutuality in the relationship between the carer and the care recipient have been shown to be predictive of less carer strain in DAT (Archbold et al. 1990) and to mediate the relationship between burden and distress in carers of people with PD, helping to alleviate the stressful effects of burden (e.g. Mitrani et al. 2006). The mediating effects of family relationships on care-giving outcomes are discussed below in section 7.3.3.

Research into how life events may provide the trigger for depressive disorders also identified a number of potentially beneficial elements as intervening in stress processes to modify their outcome. These included involvement in a close-knit community and being participating members of a church, which seemed to have a protective effect against the development of depression (Brown and Prudo 1981). Thus social support and having religious beliefs would appear to have important implications for guarding against the effects of stress. It is of course possible, that the two are interconnected i.e. having religious beliefs may lead to being integrated into part of a larger community such as a church and engender feelings of support. The possibility also exists, that religious beliefs are important in themselves, as they may give meaning to one's experiences by placing them in a greater context.

These and other types of mediational effects which help to mitigate the burden of care-giving will be considered in more detail in relation to neurodegenerative diseases in the following sections of this chapter.

7.3.1 A sense of meaning in care-giving

Having strong religious beliefs or a commitment to a positivist philosophy of some kind appears to bestow a sense of meaning on individuals, which guides their behaviour in a variety of situations including care-giving. Irrespective of its origins, a number of authors have recognised that a sense of meaningfulness in care-giving is important to the well-being of carers (e.g. Pearlin et al. 1990; Farran et al. 1991; Farran et al. 1997; Lawton et al. 1991; Noonan and Tennstedt 1997) although in general, it is a theme that has received very little attention in the literature. Only one study appears to have considered the impact of finding meaning on the lives of carers of people with PD and has confirmed that it is an important explanatory variable in predicting well-being (Konstam et al. 2003).

Guiliano et al. (1990; cited in Chan et al. 2003, 4) defined the construct of meaning in care-giving as: "positive beliefs one holds about one's self and one's care-giving experience such that some benefits or gainful outcomes are construed from it". In a qualitative analysis of the concept, Farran et al. (1991) proposed that meaning in care-giving is a construct consisting of 3 dimensions: feelings of loss or powerlessness, provisional meaning (making sense of the experience through day to day events and attitudes), which is specific to the context of care-giving, and ultimate meaning (finding meaning through connections with a higher power or sense of purpose. The utility of the concept in explaining outcomes for carers was investigated in a later study (Farran et al. 1997) in which the relationship between race, finding meaning, and carer depression and global role strain among African American and white spouse carers of persons with dementia was evaluated. The notion of provisional meaning was found to increase the explained variance in depression, with high levels of provisional (care-related) meaning being associated with lower levels of depression. However, ultimate meaning did not significantly contribute to the model. There were no race differences with respect to the process by which stressors were associated with care-giving nor the way in which finding meaning influenced carer depression.

These findings in relation to care-related meaning were replicated by Noonan and Tennstedt (1997) who examined the relationship between meaning in care-giving and psychological well-being (defined in terms of depression, self-esteem, mastery, role captivity and loss of self) in informal carers of frail elders. Finding meaning in care-giving was negatively associated with depressive symptoms and positively with self-esteem. None of the objective care-giving stressors such as the variety of care tasks performed, the frequency of care delivery, care-recipient cognitive impairment or problem behaviours were associated with finding meaning in the caring process; nor were the carer variables of mastery, role captivity or loss of self.

The results of these investigations seem to suggest that attributing meaning directly to the care-giving situation is more relevant to the welfare of the carer, than a more global notion of meaning and these effects appear to be independent of culture. However, the study by

Konstam et al. (2003) which evaluated the contribution of finding meaning in general and finding meaning specific to care-giving as potentially important explanatory variables in predicting the well-being of carers of individuals with PD, failed to demonstrate any effects on well-being, of meaning connected with the specific situation of care-giving. On the contrary, they found that general meaning, which was defined as having a purpose, or a sense of direction in life, was central to carer well-being. The quality of purposefulness was found to predict positive carer affect, while an existential vacuum, which was connected with lack of meaning and direction in life was associated with negative carer affect. Reasons for the disparity in findings between studies are unclear, but may be due to a number of different factors. Firstly, in each of the studies, carers were providing care for individuals with different types of chronic disability: dementia (Farran et al. 1997), the frail elderly (Noonan and Tennstedt 1997) and PD (Konstam et al. 2003) and the variability in conditions might have affected the results differentially. Secondly, although the Farran et al. (1997) and the Konstam et al. (2003) studies involved mainly spouse carers, the Noonan and Tennstedt (1997) study included a greater proportion of adult children as carers. Determinants of meaning in care-giving may be significantly different for these two groups of carers. Finally, age effects may have contributed to the meaning ascribed to caring: spouses were more likely to have been caring for younger care recipients than children caring for parents, and although the data are incomplete in the publications, there is some evidence to suggest that this may have been true and these differences may have affected the meaning that carers attributed to their task.

7.3.2 Cultural factors affecting care-giving

Since informal care is deeply rooted in the home and family, cultural factors are likely to play a significant role in determining various aspects of the process, including the carer's experience. Until quite recently, this aspect of care-giving had not received a great deal of attention, although significant cultural differences have been recognized for some time. Perhaps the most important of these relates to willingness to place the care recipient in formal care. In the USA white people in need of care have been twice as likely to be institutionalized as African Americans (Greene and Ondrich 1990; Wolinsky et al. 1992). The South Asian population in the UK (Lawrence et al. 2008) and the Chinese in the USA (McBride, Morioka-Douglas and Yeo 1996) are also less willing to place their elderly dependent relatives in care homes.

In keeping with the results of care-giving studies more generally, female carers from different cultures caring for a close relative at home, tend to report the greatest levels of strain (Torti et al. 2004; Rinaldi et al. 2005). Comparisons between different cultural groups show that Caucasian carers tend to report greater depression and appraise caring as being more stressful than African Americans (see Janevic and Connell 2001 for a review). There is some evidence to suggest that the two groups do not differ in the amount of burden, but that African Americans express their reactions to it differently (Calderon and Tennstedt 1998; Haley et al. 2004). Differences have also been reported in Australia between Anglo-Celtic and Italian carers, with Italians reporting less trait anxiety than Anglo-Celts. The Italians were found to use more community support systems, were often employed full-time and had lower levels of education, but reported better levels of general health than the Anglo-Celtic carers (Carrafa et al. 1997). Asian cultures are renowned for their immensely strong sense of familial responsibility and their respect for older family members (Torti et al. 2004). Their feelings of self-sufficiency in this respect mean that they are unwilling to discuss family problems and hence family carers may feel isolated and their social and emotional support may be limited. In a comparative study of carers in the USA and China, whose relatives had similar care needs and levels of ADL, it was found that carers in both countries reported more depressive and physical symptoms than controls, but that there were no significant differences between the carers themselves, suggesting that both US and Chinese carers report being under similar amounts of pressure in their caring roles (Patterson et al. 1998). However, a study of Chinese and Korean carers of people with dementia, found higher levels of depression and increased scores on measures of burden in comparison to carers in Western societies (Torti et al. 2004). The reason for these differences are not clear, but as diversity in the older population increases, especially in multicultural societies such as the UK and USA, it is evident that cultural factors affecting carers need to be taken into account. Recent reviews have highlighted the necessity to measure and evaluate the effect that cultural values have on care-giving experiences (Janevic and Connell 2001; Dilworth-Anderson, Williams and Gibson 2002).

7.3.3 Family relationships and their effects on care-giving

Family relationships form a clear background to virtually all care-giving activities in the community and thus inevitably exert an influence on the well-being of carers. They are also probably the closest and most influential relationships throughout a person's lifespan and are therefore all the more relevant in situations of spousal care-giving, which are most commonly encountered for people with DAT and PD. An awareness of the importance of family relationships in the care-giving process as either protective or aggravating (Fisher and Lieberman 1994) has been accumulating in the literature, demonstrating that family factors such as marital cohesion (Rankin, Haut and Keefover 2001), couple identity (Badr, Acitelli and Carmack Taylor 2007), closeness (Norton et al. 2009), communication patterns (Braun et al. 2010), levels of intimacy (L.W. Morris, R.G. Morris et al. 1988), mutuality (Mitrani et al. 2006; Tanji et al. 2008) conflict (Semple 1992), boundary ambiguity (Boss et al. 1990) and adaptability (Deimling, Smerglia and Schaefer 2001; Majerovitz 1995) appear to influence the psychological well-being of carers. There is also evidence that the decision to institutionalise a family member with dementia is partly determined by levels of dysfunction in the care-giving family (Spitznagel et al. 2006).

Very few data exist specifically for PD, but high levels of stress in carers have also been associated with family functioning in the form of less cohesion and support and fewer opportunities to discuss feelings (McRae et al. 1999). The research in question also found an interesting age effect for both patients and carers in relation to family functioning, with older participants reporting lower levels of family conflict and stronger positive values in the variables mentioned. The suggestion from this research, that younger families with a person suffering from PD may fare worse in terms of functioning, has been confirmed by Schrag et al. (2004). These authors studied the well-being of patients' adolescent and adult children aged 12-48 years. They found higher levels of depression and lower quality of life among the participants. The greatest impact was found on family functioning and level of burden in the daily help provided, the latter being especially problematic for younger children (i.e. under 25 years old), possibly exacerbated by the fact that they were living in the same household as the parent with PD. Younger children also reported that their friends' reactions were more of a problem and that they felt more embarrassed about their parents' illness than older children. This may be because the older children were better able to explain about the illness and their friends had more experience and understanding of ill-health. Children over the age of 24 years reported greater disturbances in family functioning, which were also associated with longer disease duration. Schrag et al. (2004) interpreted these findings as reflecting that greater dependence of the ill parent on the child and impact of the disease on the whole family have considerable implications for the lives of those living with chronic illnesses such as PD and their families.

Family relationships are an obvious factor in providing the motivation to continue caring in spite of the hardships involved, although they are often overlooked. A quite natural state of affairs would seem to be that where the carer values the quality of the relationship with the care-recipient, this appears to offset the effects of the difficulties encountered in caring. Cultural and religious traditions which have established family care-giving as the norm, undoubtedly generate expectations of care provision and whilst these are stronger in some societies than others, they engender feelings of obligation with regard to care-giving. Some evidence exists to show that where the motivation is related to relationship factors rather than obligation, care-giving is longer lasting and more extensive (Cicirelli 1986).

Disturbances in family functioning affecting communication and roles has been found to be associated with carer burden (e.g. Tremont, Duncan Davis and Bishop 2006). However, only a few studies have attempted to provide theoretical models to explain the mechanisms by which the family affects the process of care-giving in DAT. Heru, Ryan and Iqbal (2004) elicited accounts of family functioning in terms of problem-solving, communication, affective involvement, affective responsiveness and control of roles and behaviour within a family systems approach. They found that whilst the majority of carers reported greater levels of reward compared to burden as a result of their care-giving activities, those with poor family functioning had higher ratings of burden and strain. For these carers, family functioning was weakest in the areas of affective responsiveness, problem solving and communication, but affective involvement and roles were also impaired. Moreover a study by Mitrani et al. (2006) attempted to test the hypothesis that family functioning partly mediated the relationship between objective burden and distress in carers of people with dementia. They used a structural family approach based on the work of Minuchin (1974) to explore the role of family functioning and found evidence in support of their prediction. Thus the quality of family relationships appears to be central not only to the motivation for care-giving, but also in terms of its outcomes for the carer, and probably also for the care recipient and other members of the family. Indeed, research has indicated that marital relationships and external social support are important to psychosocial functioning for people living with chronic illness (for review see: O'Connor, McCabe and Firth 2008).

Most studies related to care-giving have however concentrated on the relationship between the carer and the care recipient. Arriving at an estimation of the quality of the relationship involves an appraisal of the affective ties with the care recipient, which consist of feelings of emotional closeness, positive sentiment and similarities in values and beliefs (Lawrence, Tennstedt and Assman 1998). Relationship quality is however dynamic and may change in adversity of the kind wrought by the process of care-giving, especially if the carer attributes any negative consequences of the experience directly to the care recipient. Thus relationship quality has two aspects: one relating to its past characteristics which form part of the care-giving history and the other, to its current status. Although there may be continuity in relationship quality, and this has been shown to be associated with better adjustment to care-giving (Walters, Oyebode and Riley 2010), it is also possible that relational exchanges with the care recipient become increasingly imbalanced, losing the potential for reciprocity and shared meaning, as the couple enter deeper into the care-giving process (Pearlin et al. 1990). This may also explain gender differences in care-giving outcomes, as women have been shown to be more distressed in unequal interactions, than men (Sprecher 1992).

7.4 The effects of chronic illness on spousal relationships

In view of the fact that caring for a person with a chronic disease such as DAT or PD is typically carried out by their spouse, the impact of the condition upon the spousal relationship deserves particular attention. The chronic and progressive nature of neurodegenerative conditions means that both members of the couple have to make adjustments to their situation and this process of adaptation needs to take into account the long-term nature of the changes and the uncertainty and unpredictability with which the situation may develop (see chapter 5). It is not surprising therefore, that spousal relationships and communication can be altered by chronic illness (Druley, Stephens and Coyne 1997; Druley et al. 2003) and marital satisfaction may be eroded by declining physical and mental health (see Gagnon et al. 1999 for a review). This is likely to be particularly so for PD, which apart from the classical motor symptoms and the neuropsychological and neuropsychiatric features described in previous chapters, is also recognised as frequently giving rise to additional problems in areas such as sleep, sexual activity and speech communication, all of which provide difficulties for the care recipient and the carer (Brown et al. 1990; Miller et al. 2008; Pal et al. 2004).

Once again, most of the research in this area has concerned itself with DAT and is mostly based on carer perceptions of the marital relationship.

Overall, the impression gained is that among the difficulties faced by spouse carers, reduction in relationship quality and satisfaction, together with diminished emotional and physical intimacy, feature very strongly (e.g. Fearon et al. 1998; L.W. Morris, R.G. Morris et al. 1988; Wright 1991; de Vugt et al. 2003).

Another consistent finding in the literature on caring in Alzheimer's disease is that the neuropsychiatric and behavioural disturbances are foremost in contributing to the subjective experience of carer burden (e.g. Torti et al. 2004) and diminishing relationship satisfaction (e.g. de Vugt et al. 2003). The specific impact of behavioural changes has been demonstrated in a study comparing carer-patient couples in two types of dementia: fronto-temporal and DAT. Whilst patients with DAT demonstrate primarily cognitive impairments, those with fronto-temporal dementia are primarily behaviourally disturbed, with evident emotional, social and personality changes (e.g. Perry and Hodges 2000). The study found that carers of patients with fronto-temporal dementia demonstrated greater negativity in their discourse relative to carers of people with DAT and reported significantly lower levels of marital satisfaction (Ascher et al. 2010). The authors interpret these findings as demonstrating the specific challenge of behavioural changes to maintaining healthy marital bonds.

Since behavioural disturbances appear much later in the course of DAT, their effects might be expected to be less destructive of the marital relationship, or at least, that the quality of the relationship might be preserved for longer. Whilst this may be so, a study of carers of people with mild cognitive impairment found that carers reported the occurrence of distressing behaviours even in the early stages of the condition, which negatively affected the quality of their marital relationship (Garand et al. 2007).

Although behavioural disturbances are less common for people with PD than for DAT and fronto-temporal dementia, they nonetheless do occur and are intensified when the dementia of PD is present (Leroi, Harbishettar et al. 2012). It is therefore reasonable to expect that changes of a behavioural nature will also impact on the couples' relationship in PD. There do not appear to be any studies that have addressed this question directly, but indirect evidence does exist.

First of all, there is agreement in the research on DAT that cognitive deficits do not have a significant effect on carer distress (e.g. Pinquart and Sorensen 2003; also see section 7.2.2.3. above) and the same appears true for PD, although some studies have challenged this conclusion (e.g. Shin, Youn et al. 2012; Thommessen et al. 2002). Other research has also found that wives of patients with greater cognitive impairment experienced more burden (Hooker et al. 2000) and relational deprivation when compared to wives of patients with higher mental status (Bauer et al. 2001). Nevertheless, it does appear that under most circumstances, it is the behavioural manifestations of the neuropsychological impairment that are distressing to the carer. Interestingly, there is evidence too, that for DAT at least, it is not so much the excessive and inappropriate behaviour of care recipients that has a deleterious effect on the marital relationship, but behaviour that is extremely passive, such as apathy and withdrawal (deVugt et al. 2003). From the carer's perspective, it can be understood why such behaviours, although eliciting sympathy, might in the long-term, also change the carer's feelings about the marital relationship, as the expectation of reciprocity is gradually eroded (L.W. Morris, R.G. Morris et al. 1988; Wright 1991; Fearon et al. 1998).

The gradual loss of support from the care recipient is another theme running through the literature concerning the effects of chronic illness (DAT) on marital relationships. Apart from the economic and practical consequences for many marriages (Zarit et al. 1986), communication suffers (George and Gwyther 1986), companionship and the solace of having a close confidant is lost (Fitting et al. 1986), the sexual relationship may wane and become problematic (Quayhagen and Quayhagen 1988) and loneliness result (McRae et al. 2009). A study of female patients with PD (Fleming et al. 2004) explored how the condition had affected their perception of their own womanhood and the effect this had had on their relationships with close partners. For some, it seemed that PD had strengthened their marital relationships, while for others it had taken a heavy toll, resulting in the breakdown of these relationships. Other research has shown that for couples whose relationships had deteriorated since the onset of PD, more than half were suffering from significant levels of depression (Seiler et al. 1992). Furthermore, Schrag, Hovris et al. (2006) found that two-thirds of carers felt that both their close and more distant relationships had suffered as a result of PD and carer burden correlated significantly with carers' satisfaction with their marital and sexual relationships. The importance of social support and satisfaction with sex life to the marital relationship has also been confirmed for patients with PD in a study by O'Connor et al. (2008). These studies suggest that social support, both from the marital partner and from a wider network of family and friends, may help to sustain the well-being of people with PD and their carers, although as mentioned previously, not all research is in agreement with this premise (see section 7.2.3.5).They also confirm that there are important links between satisfaction with the marital and sexual relationship and the welfare of the carer. Finally, disturbances in sexual functioning following the onset of symptoms of PD are frequent; between 39% and 80% of people with the condition report dissatisfaction with their sex lives (Bronner et al. 2004; Brown et al. 1990; Macht, Schwarz and Ellgring 2005; Yu et al. 2004). Most studies report that the problem is worse for men (e.g. Macht et al. 2005). In view of the previously reported findings and the association of sexual functioning with the quality of the marital relationship, this is an area that may have important implications for the well-being of both the carer and the care recipient.

The apparent improvement in relationship quality for women with PD and their partners noted by Fleming et al. (2004) has been echoed by a number of studies in DAT which show similar effects for at least a portion of the participants interviewed (Fearon et al. 1998; Gilhooly et al. 1984; Nolan, Grant and Keady 1996). These studies contradict the notion that caring invariably has negative consequences and provide evidence for more rewarding effects as far as relationships are concerned. They also have theoretical implications for the role of relationship quality in the care-giving process. When the detrimental effects of illness on care relationships are evaluated, the concept of relationship quality is treated as an outcome in itself, and this may be an appropriate course of action in the context of neurodegenerative diseases, as has been demonstrated in the previous discussion. However, the fact that in some instances, relationship quality has been found to improve, suggests that alternative explanations of the role of relationships in caring may be appropriate. Equally, although the direction of the effect for the association between a deterioration in the marital relationship and spouse-carer depression cannot be determined (Seiler et al. 1992), it does raise the possibility that the marital relationship may be having a mediating effect on caring experiences. This possibility is examined in the next section.

7.4.1 Quality of the marital relationship between carers and care recipients

The quality of the relationship between the carer and the care recipient, is an important element in the carer's appraisal of the care-giving situation, at least for some carers (Lewis et al. 2005). Carers taking this perspective, interpret their experiences of the care-giving situation in the context of their relationship with their spouse, past, present and future. Viewed from this position, marital relationships are seen as intervening variables, which can attenuate or potentiate various effects emerging from the caring process. Whilst not all carers seem to have the relationship as their primary focus, this is not to say that it does not influence their experience of caring.

Research examining the role of the marital relationship in spouse care-giving has found that good quality relationships are associated with significant reductions in role captivity (i.e. strain from the subjectively experienced difficulties of providing care to a spouse) and decreased feelings of being "overloaded" with care responsibilities (Lawrence et al. 1998; Yates et al. 1999). Other types of strain related to more global concerns and tension, together with feelings of being manipulated are also reduced in good quality relationships (Archbold et al. 1990; Schumacher et al. 2008) although strain from worry is not (Archbold et al. 1990). Older studies had already paved the way for the viewpoint that satisfying marital relationships could ameliorate care-giving difficulties in demonstrating an inverse association between emotional closeness in couples and carer strain (Tobin and Kulys 1981). On the reverse side of the argument, interpersonal conflicts and difficulties in marital relationships are closely related to increased strain for the carer (Gilleard et al. 1982; Bookwala and Franks 2005). Taken together, these findings suggest that relationship quality may prevent resentments otherwise associated with care-giving from building up, but that it is not a buffer against more general concerns such as the partner's health and the day-to-day pre-occupations of life.

Different studies have conceptualised the quality of the marital relationship in different ways, for example, in terms of mutuality and intimacy, as referred to above, or closeness and couple identity. However, all of these definitions appear to have something in common, namely what Tanji et al. (2008, 1843), using the notion of "mutuality", refer to as: "the quality of interaction or reciprocity of sentiment in a relationship." This quality of mutuality is believed by some to be the key to understanding why carers remain steadfast, despite difficult care circumstances (Archbold et al. 1990). It is also associated with decreased role strain for the carer (Tanji et al. 2008; Lyons et al. 2009) and better mental health for both partners (Tanji et al. 2008). However, whilst high levels of mutuality can be protective, there is evidence that low mutuality may be a crucial risk factor for greater levels of subjective burden and higher levels of depression in the carer (Lyons et al. 2007), especially when the care-giving situation demands high levels of involvement (Schumacher, Stewart and Archbold 2007). Although mutuality appears to be a fairly stable variable, it does change over time, and has been shown to decline over the course of the care-giving period (Archbold et al. 1990) in the presence of DAT (Aneshensel et al. 1995) and in late stage PD (Carter et al. 1998).

Earlier studies, using constructs such as intimacy to describe the quality of the marital relationship, found that low levels of current intimacy were related to higher levels of depression, but not strain in carers of people with DAT (L.W. Morris, R.G. Morris et al. 1988). Thus it would seem that however onerous the caring task, carers could tolerate even high levels of resultant strain, so long as they continued to experience an intimacy with the cared for person and this did not appear to have adverse effects for their mental health. This might suggest that the quality encompassed in the notion of intimacy has either moderating or mediating effects on the carers' perceptions of the strain resulting from care-giving, helping to ameliorate any negative affective reactions. It is difficult to know whether notions of intimacy and mutuality differentiate the results for the carer in terms of potentially different outcomes for strain (moderator effects) versus mood disturbances (mediator effects), but work in this area still lacks the sophistication to have addressed these issues.

The quality of the past relationship is also important as it is strongly related to mental health in the carer (Gilleard et. al. 1984a): low levels of past intimacy are related to increased levels of perceived strain and depression in carers of people with DAT (L.W. Morris, R.G. Morris et. al. 1988; Steadman, Tremont and Duncan Davis 2007) to carer levels of criticism and hostility (Gilhooly and Whittick 1989) and to less reactivity to memory and behaviour problems in the care recipient (Steadman et al. 2007). Moreover, long-term unhappiness in marriage leads to feelings of entrapment in the carer role (Murray and Livingston, 1998). Carers with high levels of pre-morbid relationship satisfaction have been shown to have better problem solving skills and more effective communication with the care recipient, irrespective of disease severity and duration and care recipient functioning (Steadman et al. 2007).

7.4.2 The role of relationship quality in care-giving

The importance of relationships has been recognised for a long time, but only recently have they been investigated in terms of their potential to act as moderators or mediators in the care-giving process.

The quality of the relationship can thus be viewed either as (i) a protective factor which modifies the way in which the carer interprets or appraises the stressors of caring (including behavioural disturbances or other changes perceived in the care recipient, as well as care-giving burden), or (ii) modifying the relationship between these independent variables and carer outcomes. This leads to two main ways of understanding the interrelationships among stressors, quality of relationship and outcomes in the care-giving process. The first interpretation reflects a moderator hypothesis, treating quality of relationship as a moderating variable, which modifies the association between stressors and negative consequences of care-giving. Hence strong positive feelings and emotional proximity to the care receiver, allow the carer to make allowances for any negative results of his/her behaviour or to accept any limitations imposed by care-giving. This is essentially a "buffering" hypothesis, which supposes that a good quality of relationship with the care recipient helps to protect the carer against negative consequences by allowing him/her to evaluate the situation in a less strain-inducing manner. This is in contrast to the appraisal of a carer who does not feel strong commonality with the care recipient. Relationship quality in this case would not be expected to offset the effects associated with care-giving stressors and may in fact contribute to an increased sense of burden. The carer with a strong quality relationship may feel less burdened or stressed relative to someone with a poorer relationship quality, despite similarity of the care-giving situations.

The second conceptualisation is one in which relationship quality is seen as the product of stressors in the care-giving situation, and reflects a mediation hypothesis. In this case, as the burden of caring increases, so the quality of the relationship suffers, which in turn leads to increasing, costly negative consequences. In a pure mediational model, the relationship between the stressor and the consequences is completely explained by the deterioration in relationship quality (Lawrence et al. 1998).

In practice, it is likely that both the moderation and mediation processes play a role in care-giving (Pruchno and Resch 1989b). Quality of the relationship may suffer from increasing stress from the care-giving situation and may also buffer the consequences. Whilst a number of studies have included the quality of the relationships as a mediator (Yates et al. 1999) they have not attempted to measure its influence.

7.4.3 Interactions between relationship effects and gender

Loss of shared meaning and reciprocity in the marital relationship may affect overall psychological well-being more significantly for women than for men as suggested in section 7.3.3. above. Married women appear more conscious of the quality of their marriage and more sensitive to the emotional experiences of their spouse than men. They spend more time reflecting on their marital relationship and are more engaged in, and affected by, the condition of their spouse in the context of chronic illness (for review see Berg and Upchurch 2007). However, this may be less true for younger cohorts in whom these gender differences may be less significant, due to societal changes having affected the role of women over the last fifty years (Twenge 2001, cited in Berg and Upchurch 2007). Research on long-term marriages has found that wives' physical and psychological health is more highly correlated with marital satisfaction than that of husbands (Levenson, Cartensen and Gottman 1993). Further support for this idea comes from the work of Acitelli and Antonucci (1994) who found that perceptions of social support in marriage were more strongly related to the marital satisfaction and general well-being of wives than of husbands. This does not mean that men are unaffected by the experience of losing the reciprocity of social support in their long-term marital partner. The studies cited above suggest that men are better able to come to terms with the loss, by not allowing it to permeate all aspects of their lives, so that the negative effect on their overall well-being is not as damaging as it is for women. However, care-giving husbands have also been found less likely to consider their care-recipient wives as sources of social support and thus reported feeling lonely more often and were significantly more distressed than controls (Dura and Haywood-Niler 1990).

In conclusion it seems that in so far as the quality of the marital relationship is reflected in such concepts as mutuality, shared intimacy, closeness and couple identity, it may reflect the couple's journey towards a shared meaning in the experience of their relationship. Much of the research described above rests on a hypothesis which proposes that it is the loss of this shared meaning that attenuates the problems for couples living with chronic illnesses. In view of women's allegedly greater preoccupation with the meaning of relationships, this provides a plausible explanation for the gender differences among spouse carers.

7.4.4 Dyadic approaches to care-giving

Dyadic approaches to relationships serve to refocus attention on both members of the couple and have long been promoted by family researchers as being more valid approaches to the study of relationships (Pruchno, Burant and Peters 1997). These approaches realign the emphasis in the care-giving literature to include the perspective of the care receiver in addition to that of the carer (Lyons et al. 2002). Their departure point is the reasonable assumption that each member of the dyad has an influence on the well-being of the other member, rather than the unidirectional influence from care recipient to carer assumed by traditional stress-process models. In a study of care-giving dyads where the care recipients were older people with a wide range of both physical and mental impairments, Lyons et al. (2002) examined how members of the dyad viewed their interactions within the context of the care-giving relationship. They hypothesised that certain indicators such as the use of formal services or strain in care-giving relationships would predict incongruent judgements within the dyad relating to the level of the care recipients' impairment and appraisals of the care-giving situation. They found that relationship strain in the carer predicted his or her own depression and negative health outcomes, but that it was not associated with care recipient outcomes. Dyads showed little disagreement over the care recipient's needs, but there was a significant amount of variation in how much they agreed in their appraisals of care-giving difficulties. Relationship strain perceived by the carer, but not the care recipient, was significantly associated with this disagreement.

Studies taking this dyadic perspective are still few and far between, but they hold interesting potential for developing the care-giving literature. However, the study described above, though providing directions for the research on care-giving, needs to be treated with a certain amount of caution as far as drawing conclusions from the results is concerned. This is because respondents represented different disease aetiologies, and those who agreed to participate in the study were drawn from a larger sample and were younger, less impaired and more satisfied with their care arrangements (in their carers' estimation) than their counterparts who refused to participate. Although there were fewer differences between those carers who agreed to participate and those who did not, the authors acknowledge the potential bias in the sample studied and its consequent limitations for generalising to a larger population of carers. It is inevitable that dyadic work will be limited by the exclusion of more severely impaired care recipients who are unable to participate in the research interview for various reasons. Nevertheless, the dyadic approach serves to remind researchers of the necessity to take into account the perspective of both members of the dyad involved in care-giving.

7.4.5 The effects of familism on carers

Families' willingness to care for their elderly and disabled relatives, despite the consequent price that is often paid in terms of damage to family carers' health and well-being, is self-evident. This willingness to undertake care-giving has been conceptualised as resulting from a value system, that is thought to be particularly strong for certain cultures, which develops normative feelings in individuals, with an imperative for what has come to be called "familism". Sayegh and Knight (2011, 3) define this notion as follows:

> Familism refers to the strong normative feelings of loyalty, dedication, reciprocity and attachment of family members to their family and familial relationships, both nuclear and extended, as well as strong identification and solidarity with their family members.

Thus familism is seen as a duty or an obligation to care for family members, but one which comes from an inner need to do the right thing, rather than being imposed by the external pressures of society. The important distinction here seems to be the motivation with which caring is undertaken: with an emotionally positive approach, rooted in strong kinship ties. As such, it would be expected to have protective effects against any detrimental effects of care-giving and should be negatively associated with burden (Kim, Knight et al. 2007). It was proposed that these effects might be mediated by coping style, the expectation being that familism would be associated with active coping. Contrary to the hypothesised outcomes, the authors found that familism was associated with avoidant coping, resulting in poorer health outcomes for carers. Burden led to these poorer health outcomes through its association with avoidant coping.

These results were somewhat unexpected and appeared to suggest that familism may not have protective effects on carers' health, indeed actually leading to worse outcomes. Kim, Knight et al. (2007) interpreted their results as suggesting that the instrument used to measure familism was inadequate, as it may have reflected more the obligation to care rather than the positive motivation to do so. This possibility was explored by Sayegh and Knight (2011) who chose a different measure of familism, consisting of two main factors, "familial obligations" and "expected support from the family" as being more appropriate. They found that only the "familial obligations" factor of familism affected (detrimentally) the mental and physical health of carers of individuals with DAT, thus replicating the findings of Kim, Knight et al. (2007) and supporting their view that familism scales are tapping the imperative to provide care rather than more positive feelings about family support.

The "expected support from the family" factor did not have any effect on the carers' outcome, despite the appeal of the concept of familial support as providing protection against poor health outcomes. The expectation that social support should lessen the distress experienced by carers, all the more so if it comes from the family, would appear to be self-evident (Zarit et al. 1985) and has received some support in connection with reducing the detrimental effects of care-giving on physical health outcomes (e.g. Pinquart and Sorensen 2007). However, it has not always proved possible to demonstrate any protective effects for social support (e.g. Miller et al. 1996). One reason for this may be that there is a shortfall between the expectation of social support and its provision, leading to poorer outcomes for carers (Sayegh and Knight 2011). These considerations have so far only been explored in the dementia care research. Clearly, there is need for further investigation of carers' attitudes in terms of their preparedness and commitment to care-giving in all situations.

7.5 Attachment and the relationship to care-giving

The positive influence of close relationships has also been examined from the point of view of attachment theory, a lifespan theory of human bonding, which contends that patterns of emotional interaction in close relationships are determined by the attachment behavioural system and are established during the first year of life (Bowlby 1969/1982; 1973). Attachment behaviours are seen in the tendency of human beings to seek physical proximity and to form close relationships with an attachment figure, usually their mother, in order to gain comfort and security during times of difficulty. Such behaviours are considered to serve vital functions in promoting survival, protection, nurturing and learning. Bowlby's work focused on exploratory studies of the mother-child dyad and emphasized that, in order to manage their need for emotional security, children depend upon a close and continuing care-giving relationship, which is usually provided by their mother. They accumulate experiences of the responses of their carers, which help them to build up a mental representation or "internal working model" (Bowlby 1988) in terms of the immediacy, consistency, reliability and positive nature of the interaction. This in turn determines their expectations regarding the responsiveness of the carer and in time, is generalised to others. Naturally, carers are variable in their response patterns, some more than others, and children's understanding of what to expect, varies accordingly. During the course of development, repeated experiences are internalised in a working model reflecting these expectations and consequent beliefs about the self and others, which is termed an "attachment style". Different styles of attachment lead to responses with different behavioural manifestations. Seminal work by Ainsworth (Ainsworth et al. 1978) has provided a classification of these styles, differentiating secure versus insecure attachments. Responsive and nurturing experiences in early childhood are thought to produce greater attachment security, whilst less reliable non-nurturing experiences are associated with insecure attachment (Fiori, Consedine and Magai 2009).

The quality of the initial attachment has been shown to have implications well beyond the first social bonds formed in childhood and to influence subsequent interpersonal relationships, both in early adulthood (Hazan and Shaver 1987) and in later life (Andersson and Stevens 1993; Skolnick 1986). Attachment style also affects personality development and emotional regulation in later in life (Feeney and Noller 1996; Rothbard and Shaver 1994).

7.5.1 Attachment styles

Theoretical models have differentiated three (Hazan and Shaver 1987) and sometimes four attachment styles (Bartholomew and Horowitz 1991) although a dimensional view of attachment is gaining ground (Fiori et al. 2009). Reasonably robust characteristic profiles are associated with the different categories of attachment style. Thus, individuals with high levels of attachment security have positive internal working models of both self and others and this is reflected in their ability to value themselves and others, to feel comfortable with intimacy and to be willing to seek support when needed (Collins and Feeney 2000). Research indicates that individuals with secure attachments are cheerful and likeable, are high in trait joy and trait interest and are characterised by the absence of psychopathology (Magai, Distel and Liker 1993; Magai and Passman 1997).

Three types of insecure attachment have been differentiated: pre-occupied (or ambivalent), dismissive and fearful avoidant; in some classifications the last two are grouped together as avoidant styles (Collins and Feeney 2000; Fiori et al. 2009). Individuals with high levels of pre-occupied attachment have a positive internal model of others, but a negative model of self. They are high in anxiety, demonstrating high levels of personal distress, but low in avoidance and have a low sense of self-worth, tending also to have doubts about the reliability of others. A pre-occupied attachment style leads to an exaggerated desire for closeness and high dependency, combined with a heightened fear of rejection. Such individuals are constantly concerned that significant others in their lives do not really care about them and they tend to be perceived as clinging and "neurotic". The pre-occupied style is associated with heightened anxiety and depression (Magai and McFadden 1995; Magai and Passman 1997).

By contrast, individuals who have a dismissive style of attachment, hold a positive model of self, but a negative model of others. They are low in attachment-related anxiety and high in avoidance. They report high levels of self-esteem, view close relationships as relatively unimportant, have difficulty trusting others and place high value on independence and self reliance.

Finally, fearful avoidant adults represent an attachment style that is negative in respect of both self and others. They are high in both anxiety and avoidance and despite their desire for close relationships and approval from others, they eschew intimacy for fear of being rejected. The avoidant attachment style is associated with defensiveness, compulsive self-reliance, inhibited expressive behaviour and hostility (Magai and Passman 1997).

The internal working model, which determines attachment styles, was considered by Bowlby (1973) to remain consistent throughout the lifespan and early experiences with the attachment figure were thought to provide the basis for stable and enduring personality traits. The internal working model was thus seen as guiding experiences with others throughout the lifespan and being fundamental to the way in which a person's expectations and behaviour are formed and expressed in social relationships. A contrastive view is that of Bretherton and Munholland (1999) who viewed working models as largely unconscious mechanisms used to ".....(interpret) perceptions and emotions, appraise and shape expectations and influence beliefs and attitudes, which are continuously revised and updated throughout development" (Segal, Needham and Coolidge 2009, 120). Within this view, attachment behaviours are modified according to experience in different types of relationship (e.g. relationships with parents versus relationships with spouses). There is empirical support for both sides of the controversy regarding the stability versus variability in working models.

7.5.2 Attachment in adulthood and later life

Research with younger adults has shown that attachment styles are disproportionately distributed in the population with approximately 56% showing a secure pattern, 25% avoidant and 19% ambivalent (Hazan and Shaver 1987; 1990) and broadly similar figures have been obtained from other studies (e.g. Kirkpatrick and Davis 1994; Davila, Burge and Hammen 1997; Cassidy and Shaver 1999). These proportions correspond to those for the distribution of attachment styles found in childhood (e.g. Van Ijzendoorn and Kroonenberg 1988) and are seen as confirmation of the fact that the nature of early emotional bonds influences relationships in later life. Indeed, a meta analysis of studies has shown that attachment styles appear to be moderately stable over the first 19 years of life (Fraley 2002) and if anything, this stability increases across adulthood (Fraley and Brumbaugh 2004). As reflected above, this is not to say that they are permanently fixed in stone and research also shows that a variety of experiences may bring about shifts in attachment styles. During childhood, negative life events such as the death of a parent, parental divorce or abuse by adults may drive changes from secure to insecure attachment patterns (Waters et al. 2000; Weinfield, Sroufe and Egeland 2000). Later life experiences have also been shown to lead to undesirable changes in attachment (Kirkpatrick and Hazan 1994; Davila and Cobb 2003; Davila and Sergeant 2003). The implications of this for care-giving have not been explored, but to the extent that caring for a close relative may be seen as a life event (or a series of life events drawn out in time), carers' attachment patterns might also be expected to undergo modification over the course of the care-giving experience. However, there are encouraging results from short-term psychotherapy to indicate that attachment patterns may also be modified from insecure to secure in adults across the lifespan (e.g. Travis et al. 2001). Although interventions of this kind have not been attempted with carers, there does not seem to be any reason to doubt their potential effectiveness in this area.

However, the pattern of attachment for older populations has been found to be at variance with that of younger adults in some important respects. Although relatively few studies have evaluated attachment styles in older respondents, those that have, produced broadly consistent results. Insecure patterns of attachment, specifically dismissive styles, were more prominent with age while secure patterns were inversely related to age (Webster 1997; Diehl et al. 1998; Magai and Cohen 1998). In other studies dismissive styles were found to increase at the cost of preoccupied styles (Magai et al. 2000; Zhang and Labouvie-Vief 2004; Kafetsios and Sideridis 2006). In addition, economically disadvantaged older people living in urban communities were found to demonstrate very high levels of avoidant attachment (Magai et al. 2001). The conclusion drawn from this research is that dismissive avoidant attachment styles would be expected to be higher among older people than other attachment styles (Fiori et al. 2009) and that anxious attachments appear to diminish with age (Mickelson, Kessler and Shaver 1997; Segal et al. 2009).

Apart from the influence of economic conditions, the greater proportion of insecure attachments among older people has been explained in terms of their having suffered losses across the life span (Diehl et al. 1998), cohort (Consedine et al. 2002) and maturation effects (Kafetsios and Sideridis 2006). In order to test the hypothesis conceptualising changes in attachment as a reaction to losses, Magai and co-workers (1999; cited in Magai 2001) divided their sample of older respondents into a young cohort (born 1922-32) and an older cohort (born 1911-21). The younger cohort was found to have significantly fewer secure attachments, but there were no differences between the two cohorts in terms of the number of deaths of close relatives over the last 5 years. Having dispensed with the potential effect of life events to account for these differences, the authors proposed an interesting explanation in keeping with the essence of attachment theory, namely the effects of parental influences in determining attachment styles. They suggest that the younger cohort was exposed to the influences of behaviourism, which reached its peak in the 1920s and 1930s, in determining how infants were brought up. In emphasizing the importance of encouraging early independence and using strategies such as the withholding of affection to modify the child's behaviour, behaviourism may have determined the attachment styles that this generation of infants developed. If it is true, this explanation of attachment patterns seen in older people is in keeping with a cohort effect, rather than the view that attachment styles are significantly altered in later life as the result of experience. Longitudinal studies addressing these issues would be required to distinguish between the hypotheses. One such study of individuals across a wide age span (15-87 years) found that, for people who were older at time 1, both secure and dismissive attachment styles increased to time 2, whereas pre-occupied attachment declined (Zhang and Lobouvie-Vief 2004). This would appear to be further evidence in favour of a cohort effect in attachment patterns, but raises intriguing possibilities about the changes that occur. Whilst anxious attachment styles appear to decrease, both secure and avoidant styles increase. It would be interesting to know the directions in which these transitions are occurring in order to be able to relate them to later life experiences. However, as Fiori et al. (2009) point out, the increase in dismissive attachment in later life is disturbing, as it may indicate a lack of supportive relationships (Kafetsios and Sideridis 2006) and inability to come to terms with the increased dependency of old age (Magai 2008). This may explain some of the difficulties experienced by older people in accepting ill-health and its consequences, but also highlights the problems for carers, whose task it is to provide care to older people who may have become increasingly dismissive in later life.

7.5.3 Attachment and its relationship to care-giving

Attachment theory provides a useful framework for understanding care-giving and care-seeking processes in both normative adult relationships, and in the context of chronic, progressive disease, where one partner takes on the role of caring for the other, which is of particular interest to the present study. In the first place, attachment theory is specifically concerned with the provision of support in a dyadic relationship, and relies on two distinct behavioural systems: the attachment system and the care-giving system, which are closely interrelated (Bowlby 1982). Secondly, the theory provides an explanation for supportive and care-giving behaviours as a means of developing trust and security in intimate relationships. Care-giving behaviours are seen as being complementary to attachment behaviours; whilst the latter are part of a safety regulating system designed to ensure that no harm comes to the self, the former serve the function of ensuring that no harm comes to the other member of the dyad. Finally, important individual differences in attachment style may provide the basis for understanding differences in the quality of supportive exchanges within a relationship (Collins and Feeney 2000).

Thus the care-giving system, through its close association with the attachment system, serves to raise individuals' awareness of the needs of others and prompts them to provide emotional and instrumental support to those dependent on them. Attachment theory is thus able to provide an explanation of the motivation and importance of care-giving, not only in childhood, but also in adult relationships. Indeed relationship satisfaction in adulthood appears to be closely associated with perceptions of the partner's care-giving ability to provide a "safe haven of comfort and security" akin to Bowlby's parental "secure base" (Collins and Feeney 2000, 1055). In the context of neurodegenerative diseases, care-giving behaviours may be seen as responding to the needs of a partner faced with the fear and uncertainty of a chronic illness. Moreover, the carer's attachment style may not only dictate the quality of the care provided, but also affect perceptions of care-giving burden and the variety of subsequent consequences for the carer.

The notion of individual differences among carers is of course, not a new one. It goes without saying that carers vary in their motivation and responsiveness to the person they care for. Much in the same way that there are individual differences in attachment styles, so too, differences exist in the propensity for care-giving. The reasons for this can be accounted for by attachment theory which contends that, since individuals' awareness of care-giving responses arise in large part, from their own attachment experiences, their resultant understanding of when and how caring behaviours are triggered, influences their own beliefs and attitudes to providing care for others (Kunce and Shaver 1994). Collins and Feeney (2000, 1055) argue that the complementarities between attachment and care-giving mean that they can be conceptualised in the form of a single working model from which rules may be derived, not only with respect to patterns of attachment and regulation of personal distress, but also to patterns of care-giving and the regulation of a "significant other's" distress. They conclude that "individual differences in attachment style should influence care-giving behaviour."

Indeed, a number of studies have demonstrated that attachment styles are linked to patterns of care-giving in a systematic way in intimate adult relationships (e.g. Kunce and Shaver 1994; Carnelley, Pietromonaco and Jaffe 1996; Feeney 1996). Individuals with secure attachment styles seem to engage in more responsive forms of care-giving and are at ease with providing more physical and intimate forms of care; they are less likely to engage in controlling or over-involved care. Simpson, Rholes and Nelligan (1992) demonstrated that secure men showed more support as their wives displayed greater anxiety. On the other hand, preoccupied individuals who demonstrate high levels of anxiety show less sensitivity and co-operation in care-giving, but maintain high levels of proximity and compulsive attitudes to caring. As a result, their care-giving behaviours are likely to be inconsistent, intrusive and not in keeping with the needs of their partner (Feeney and Collins 2001). It is not surprising therefore that anxious attachment has been found to predict less supportive reactions and insensitive care-giving (Collins and Feeney 2000). Dismissive individuals are probably the least engaged in caring processes, as they report low levels of sensitivity, proximity and compulsivity with regard to care-giving. Individuals with a fearful avoidant style are low on sensitivity and proximity, but report high levels of compulsive care-giving. Thus anxious wives elicited less support (rather anger) from avoidant husbands (Simpson et al. 1992) and avoidant women displayed less care-giving behaviour to their partners during airport separations (Fraley and Shaver 1997).

The conclusion that emerges on the basis of these studies is that secure individuals (low anxiety, low avoidance) fulfil the criteria for sensitive and responsive carers. Individuals with insecure attachment styles tend to perform more poorly in the care-giving role, but for different reasons, depending on the nature of their insecurities. However, one problem with these studies is that they are based on self-report measures and are therefore subject to all the attendant difficulties in interpretation. Observational studies have been very few, and those that exist have yielded inconsistent results. Thus Simpson et al. (1992) identified avoidant individuals as particularly unresponsive carers, whereas anxious individuals appeared to be especially ineffective carers in a study by Collins and Feeney (2000). The question that arises is, to what extent are these patterns, based on normative adult relationships also characteristic of care-giving relationships in chronic illness such as DAT and PD?

7.5.4 Attachment and care-giving in chronic illness in later life

Having examined the contribution of attachment theory to our understanding of what happens to attachment style in later life and to the process of care-giving in adult relationships, it is now possible to evaluate its contribution to care-giving in situations of chronic illness in later life. The literature reviewed above in connection with attachment supports the premise that care-giving is a natural extension of attachment in adulthood (Cicirelli 1993) and hence would be expected to extend to spouses and close significant others. It also provides a basis for understanding care-giving as a form of protective behaviour in relation to the attachment figure (parents). The function of protective behaviour in the form of care-giving is to resist the threat of harm coming to the attachment figure (Cicirelli 1983). With increasing age, as the vulnerability of the parent (or other attachment figure) to ill-health and death is perceived as becoming ever greater, the adult child seeks to delay the loss of the person who has been the mainstay of his/her emotional security, through engagement in care-giving. Care-giving is thus seen as a form of protective behaviour in response to the challenge to attachment, presented by the parent's increasing dependency. It is motivated by a desire to sustain the attached figure for as long as possible and therefore explains the long-term commitment of many children to care for their elderly and sick parents (Cicirelli 1993). Similar patterns may be expected to apply to spousal care-giving.

If these premises are correct, care-giving behaviours in both spouses and adult children would be expected to be related to their attachment style. Furthermore, the experience of caring might also be modified by the carer's style of attachment. Specifically, individuals with a secure style of attachment would be expected to experience lower subjective burden and to adapt better in both mental and physical terms to the task of caring, because their warmth, sensitivity and cooperativeness predisposes them to actively seek to help others.

In keeping with theoretical expectations, early empirical studies in this area showed that stronger attachments to elderly parents generated a greater degree of care-giving behaviour (e.g. Cicirelli 1983; Finley, Roberts and Banahan 1988). Although these studies did not use theory-related measures of adult attachment, but concepts such as affection, enjoyment, love, expressed closeness, these are in any case considered to be components of attachment and therefore should be indicative of the relationships sought. Later work with care-giving daughters, which used formal measures of attachment was to confirm these initial findings, showing that stronger attachment bonds were associated with greater levels of care, independent of their mothers' level of functional dependency (Cicirelli 1993) and the commitment to future care (Cicirelli 1991). These relationships were further clarified in another study of daughters caring for their older, community-dwelling mothers, which found that whilst attachment style was unrelated to instrumental care provided, high scores on the secure dimension and low scores on anxiety were associated with the provision of more emotional care (Carpenter 2001). Similar results were found for secure female spouses caring for partners with cancer, although female carers with anxious attachments were also found to provide more frequent instrumental care (Kim and Carver 2007), possibly reflecting their expected tendency to more compulsive care-giving.

As expected, studies also show that high levels of attachment may decrease the subjective burden of care-giving (Cicirelli 1983; Horowitz and Shindelman 1983; Horowitz 1985; Pratt et al. 1985; Daire 2002) and this has been specifically related to the secure style of attachment (Carpenter 2001; Kim and Carver 2007). Secure carers also appear to be more sensitive than insecure carers to interventions targeting burden, as their perceptions of burden decreased following the intervention, whilst those of insecure carers did not (Dupart 2005).

In contrast, carer burden is higher for insecurely attached carers (Magai and Cohen 1998). Avoidant attachment styles are associated with greater burden in carers and declared unwillingness to provide future care (Karantzas, Evans and Foddy 2010). Moreover, avoidant carers are more likely to institutionalise frail parents than to provide care (Markiewicz, Reis and Gold 1997). Avoidant carers are also unresponsive to the needs of the care recipient (Feeney and Collins 2001) and find it more difficult to provide emotional care (Kim and Carver 2007). Unlike practical assistance, providing emotional care involves the carer in engaging with the care recipient in an emotional way, that is uncomfortable to people with high attachment avoidance. In order to protect themselves against exposure to a potentially distressing situation, they engage in avoidance strategies that include denying their own and their partner's attachment needs, eschewing emotional involvement, intimacy and dependence (Kim and Carver 2007).

Contrary to expectations, attachment anxiety is somewhat inconsistent in predicting difficulties in situations where care is being provided for frail elderly or individuals in poor health. Karantzas et al. (2010) did not find any effects of attachment anxiety on adult children's willingness to provide current or future care to their elderly parents. And in their study of caring in cancer, Kim and Carver (2007) did not find that attachment anxiety was a predictor of care-giving difficulty. The exception to this were younger carers with patterns of anxious attachments for whom levels of care-giving stress were significantly increased (Kim, Kashy and Evans 2007). However, in a study on dementia care, Perren et al. (2007) found that anxious attachments in carers were associated with lower levels of well-being. The lack of an association between attachment anxiety and care-giving is somewhat surprising, as attachment perspectives would anticipate an association of this kind. The results may be due to an age effect and the fact that in the Karantzas et al. (2010) study, the older care recipients (parents) were generally in good health, or it may be that issues of fear and rejection, characteristic of preoccupied patterns of anxiety are less important in predicting care-giving behaviour (Sorensen, Pinquart et al. 2002).

Most studies have addressed the potential influence of attachment on the extent and willingness of carers to engage in care-giving for their elderly and sick relatives and have considered the modifying effects of attachment patterns on carer burden, as described above; very few appear to have evaluated the possible link to the psychopathology associated with care-giving in chronic illness. In the main, positive associations with depression and anxiety have been found for ambivalent or anxious patterns of attachment as might be expected (e.g. Kuscu et al. 2009). The influence of avoidant patterns is less clear: a study of spouse carers in cancer confirmed the association between anxious and avoidant attachment styles in carers and their levels of depression (Braun et al. 2007). On the other hand, neither Kuscu et al. (2009) nor Kim et al. (2008) were able to find evidence for a connection between depression and anxiety in carers of cancer patients and avoidant attachment styles. A study of dementia care found that both anxious and ambivalent attachment styles in carers were associated with lower levels of carers' well-being (Perren et al. 2007).

The studies reported so far have been based on measurements of current attachment style for carers and this begs the question of whether attachment patterns may change as a result of the care-giving experience. It may be that the history of the couples' relationship is more important in determining attitudes and commitment to care. Some evidence for this comes from an older study by Horowitz and Shindelman (1981) which examined the association between closeness in the couples' relationships and the effects for care-giving. A measure of "reciprocity", which might be translated into "credits" gained by the dementia sufferer in the context of the relationship prior to the onset of the illness, did not affect the subjective burden of the spouse carer, but did determine the extent of involvement in caring. This suggests that the quality of the previous relationship does not provide much buffering against the levels of strain experienced, but that the commitment to care-giving is positively affected. A few studies have explored the question of how previous attachments between patients and their carers may affect their relationship at a later time when care is required. Cicirelli (1993) found that among patients with a history of strong attachment, carers reported less subjective burden. A close relationship with the care recipient before the onset of the illness appears to predict less burden (Williamson and Schulz 1990) and lower stress and depression with higher subjective feelings of self-efficacy for carers (Townsend and Franks 1995) than when the pre-morbid relationship was less close or characterised by conflict. Equally, Crispi, Schiaffino and Berman (1997) found that a small, but significant proportion of the variance in care-giving difficulty was accounted for by the carer's pre-morbid attachment style, with insecure (preoccupied) carers reporting higher levels of burden. Attachment style also predicted psychological symptomatology with insecure carers reporting greater levels of psychological symptoms than secure carers. Moreover, Magai and Cohen (1998) found that patterns of pre-morbid attachment were a better predictor of carer burden than demographic variables and care recipient variables such as the presence of a chronic illness, cognitive impairment and behavioural symptoms. Only depression in the care recipient added to the explained variance in a regression analysis of carer burden.

Although these findings are in keeping with the care-giving literature which suggests that carer outcomes are more to do with the characteristics of the carer than those of the care-recipient or the care-giving situation (Pearlin et al. 1990; Yates et al. 1999), as Cicirelli (1993) points out, without the dependency of the care recipient there would be no carer and no care-giving behaviour. Care-giving is a dyadic process which involves both carer and care recipient and the interaction between them, which is determined by their attachment styles. Although the major focus in the attachment literature, even in relation to adult relationships has been on the person seeking care, the reverse is true for the care-giving literature, where carers have been the main focus of investigations. Few studies have examined the role of differential attachment style in care recipients, although the implications for the care-giving process are immense.

7.5.5 Attachment style in care recipients and care-seeking

In so far as attachment can be considered to be a reasonably stable characteristic of human beings from infancy to advanced old age, and more importantly, attachment behaviours can be observed throughout the lifespan, it is valid to consider the role of differential attachment style in care recipients and the implications for care-giving. Attachment theory would predict that effects should be observed in relation to emotional and behavioural symptoms of care recipients and to carers' subjective experiences of burden and emotional outcomes.

Attachment style does not regulate behaviour all of the time; it is activated when the individual feels under threat or anticipates danger of some kind, either physical or psychological. The neurological, cognitive and psychiatric impairments that are characteristic of neurodegenerative diseases may be conceptualised as presenting the patient with the subjective experience of threat, thereby triggering attachment behaviour. Attachment theory has thus found application in dementia care and has guided research in this area (e.g. Miesen 1992; Ingebretsen and Solem 1997). The confusion and uncertainty experienced by the person with dementia is viewed as being extremely threatening, causing him/her to seek the safety that closeness to the trusted attachment figure brings. All behaviour which has the goal of maintaining a desired proximity with another person, in this case the carer, is seen as attachment behaviour (Bowlby 1969). Many of the behaviours commonly seen in dementia such as agitation, aggression, crying, clinging and wandering can be understood as attachment (care-seeking) behaviours (Miesen 1992). Moreover, organised forms of attachment behaviour are sustained in dementia patients well into the disease and, it is argued, only diminish in the advanced stages when orientation to the external world has become severely restricted by the cognitive impairment (Miesen 1992). However, some authors have claimed that attachment behaviours are unrelated to the severity of dementia (Steele, Phibbs and Woods 2004) and persist even when higher cognitive activity is severely compromised, as in the later stages of dementia (Browne and Shlosberg 2005) or even in comatose states (Flannery 2002).

There is no reason to believe that dementia patients would not also display differential styles of attachment related to pre-morbid personality, but evidence for this appears to be limited to the study of Magai and Cohen (1998), which found that the distribution of attachment styles did not resemble those typically found for younger individuals, the proportion of ambivalent to securely attached patients being lower than expected. This however, is congruent with the distributions of attachment styles reported by Crispi et al. (1997) for carers of dementia patients and broadly in keeping with the finding for older adults, that anxious attachments diminish with age (Mickelson et al. 1997; Segal et al. 2009).

Care recipient attachment style also seems to predict behavioural symptoms in patients with dementia (Magai and Cohen1998; Perren et al. 2007). Patients with a pre-morbid ambivalent attachment style were found to have higher levels of anxiety and depression than those with secure and avoidant attachments (Magai and Cohen 1998); they also displayed greater dementia-related problem behaviours (Perren et al. 2007; Magai and Cohen 1998). On the other hand, pre-morbid avoidant styles were associated with more frequent expressions of anger and contempt (Magai, Cohen et al. 1997) and with paranoid symptomatology; they were also predictive of greater activity and disturbances in diurnal rhythm (Magai and Cohen 1998).

The Magai and Cohen (1998) study appears to be the only one that has investigated the effect of care-recipient attachment style on carer burden. As might be predicted carer burden was found to be higher for carers of insecurely attached patients. The lack of studies in this area represents a surprising gap in the literature; indeed, the last decade has not produced the level of interest that might have been expected in furthering understanding of care-giving relationships in chronic illness with the help of insights from attachment theory. Rather, researchers turned towards examining cultural variations in attachment and the promise of these early studies in providing answers to the complex riddle of dependencies, seen in the care-giving relationships that sustain the elderly and chronically sick, has not been fulfilled.

The results of the studies described in this chapter in relation to attachment need to be replicated and investigated further, as small sample sizes mean that the results and interpretations need to be treated with caution. Other methodological problems also exist, such as the use of retrospective informant ratings of attachment style which may be potentially biased by factors such as the informant's own attachment style and the influence of the current situation on historical judgements. Nevertheless the studies reported provide convincing evidence of the utility of attachment theory in helping to understand some of the puzzles still extant in the care-giving literature. Among these, first and foremost, is the question of why some carers seem to cope relatively well in circumstances that appear to cause others considerable difficulty.

7.6 Chapter summary and conclusions

The findings of the studies reviewed in this chapter strongly suggest that attachment provides the basis for relationships throughout the lifespan and is important to the psychological well-being of older adults. However research concerning the application of attachment theory to later life, and in particular to care-giving in long-term, degenerative illness, is still in its infancy. Whilst attachment research involving children and younger adults has verified that attachment styles are related to qualities of emotion regulation, mental health, marital satisfaction and psychological well being (Magai and McFadden 1995), these issues have only recently begun to be examined for older people (e.g. Karantzas et al. 2010) and those with DAT (e.g. Perren et al. 2007), and there appears to be no research of this kind for other neurodegenerative diseases, such as PD. There is still a need to provide normative data regarding the distribution of attachment styles among different generations and questions relating to the influence of attachment styles, especially for care recipients, in relation to the care-giving process also need to be explored.

It would be reasonable to expect that attachment relationships become increasingly important in later life, as social networks gradually diminish (Lang and Carstensen 1994), especially for people with long-term illnesses and their carers (Lubkin and Larsen 2006, 125). The increasing dependence on a care-giving spouse or other close relative that ensues with the progression of various neurodegenerative diseases, probably means that the qualitative aspects of attachment relationships, such as comfort with dependency and trust in others on the one hand, or defensiveness, hostility and anxiety on the other, become more salient. In theory, patients who demonstrate secure patterns of attachment (past or present) should be easier to care for, because their sense of inner security has been soundly established through appropriate attachment bonds and they are more comfortable with dependence on others (Collins and Read 1990). They are also less likely to have a history of psychopathology (Magai and Passman 1997), the symptoms of which might be expected to re-emerge under the stressful circumstances of chronic illness. Insecurely attached individuals, who are characterised as having poor emotion regulation skills, might be expected to present greater care-giving difficulties during the course of neurodegenerative disease. Specifically, avoidant individuals in whom instinctive attachment behaviours are suppressed, should be more difficult to care for because of their basic mistrust and greater hostility, causing them to avoid carers at times of distress (Ainsworth et al. 1978). Ambivalent individuals, in whom attachment behaviours are heightened and intensified (Cassidy 1994) are prone to depression and anxiety, and thereby pose a different kind of care-giving problem. Both insecure types of attachment should place greater strain on the care-giving relationship. Some preliminary research shows that insecure attachment styles in care recipients are associated with dementia-related problem behaviours and that these have a direct effect on the carer's well-being (Perren et al. 2007).

Pre-morbid attachment style may help to better understand the behaviours of people with neurodegenerative diseases, thereby informing the development of interventions to manage such behaviours. However, the occurrence and significance of attachment behaviours of people who live at home with a carer are not well understood and merit further research (Browne and Shlosberg 2006).

Whilst the description of the expected effects of care recipient attachment styles in relation to the caring process is largely hypothetical, based on theoretical assumptions and observations of older adults in normative settings, there is empirical evidence to support expectations regarding the attachment styles of carers. It is evident that effective care-giving requires sensitivity and responsiveness to the needs of the care recipient which, according to attachment theory, should be reflected in his/her attachment behaviour (Kunce and Shaver 1994). In turn, the carer's ability to respond effectively is dependent on his/her own attachment orientation. The interdependency of the attachment and care-giving systems determines a person's motivation for caring, since responsiveness to the needs of a sick relative arises from his/her own attachment experiences. Thus attachment style is responsible for the quality of care provided, affects the carer's perceptions of burden and ultimately determines his/her psychological well-being. Little is known about quality of care, but there is empirical evidence to show that perceptions of carer burden are related to attachment style. Carers with secure patterns of attachment systematically report lower levels of burden, whilst those with insecure avoidant patterns are unwilling to take on care-giving responsibilities and demonstrate a greater tendency to institutionalise their relatives. Avoidant attachment styles are associated with unresponsive patterns of care delivery, marked by a tendency to denigrate the expressed needs of the patient. Ambivalent or anxious attachment styles are less predictable with regard to care-giving outcomes. Such carers have been described as over-controlling and over-protective – a compulsive care-giving style, which is insensitive to the patient's needs. Unlike the avoidant style of caring, anxious carers are keen to deliver care, sometimes in prolific amounts, but are oblivious to the fact that their efforts may be in conflict with the actual needs of the patient. The extent to which over-indulgent care-giving activities are harmful is a matter of degree and may be less relevant to the concerns of caring for someone with a neurodegenerative condition, where issues of preserving independence are being eroded by the disease process itself. Moreover, the concerns of anxious individuals with diminished self worth, may be allayed to some extent in these carers, by the fact that they are seen to be providing help in a situation where it is needed and this may elicit appreciation and approval from the care recipient and significant others from whom it is sought. In any case, as Sörensen, Webster and Roggman (2002) point out, worries regarding self-worth, may be more of an issue for care-seeking rather than care-giving behaviours. This may explain why some studies have not reported an association between anxious attachments in carers and increases in perceived burden.

In summary, the literature indicates that the characteristic patterns of attachment that carers bring to the care-giving relationship are associated with their experience of burden and psychological symptoms such as depression. This realisation is an important step forward in accounting for the findings reported in the first part of this chapter, which demonstrate that care-giving outcomes often appear to be primarily influenced by the characteristics of the carer, rather than the care recipient. Carers who have maintained secure attachments with their dependent relative (who is a spouse or parental attachment figure) are characterised by positive affect and a realistic sense of self-efficacy (Magai and Passman 1997) and generally speaking report higher levels of well-being than those with insecure attachments, who report greater levels of carer burden and stress. The potential impact of adult attachment patterns has implications for both family interventions and public policy, given the high level of family engagement in care activities.

In line with the conclusions drawn from the literature reviewed in chapter 6, care-giving burden was conceptualised not as an outcome variable, but as a putative stressor in the process, with care-giving outcomes being measured in more generic terms, i.e. including aspects of mental health, such as dysphoria, potential affective disorders and minor cognitive lapses in memory and concentration. Additionally, the following conclusions, based on the preceding discussion, determined the theoretical model of care-giving that was adopted for the present study:

1. characteristics of the care-giving situation and those associated with the care recipient are more likely to influence feelings of carer burden, rather than carer mental and physical health;

2. characteristics associated with the carer, in particular, his/her appraisal of the care-giving situation appear to be the main determinants of care-giving outcomes in terms of carer mental health;
3. since they appear to be influenced by somewhat different antecedent factors, feelings of burden and mental health outcomes for carers may represent distinct categories of hardship in caring;
4. a variety of interpersonal factors appear to affect the care-giving process, the most important of which seems to be the quality of the carer's relationship (past and present) with the care recipient, especially if the latter is a spouse or partner. Relationship quality may be conceptualised as buffering the effects of burden or mediating the connection between carer burden and mental health outcomes for the carer.

These considerations were instrumental to forming the view of the care-giving process in PD that was adopted for the purposes of the study that is described next.

CHAPTER EIGHT

THE RESEARCH STUDY

8.1 Introduction: justification for the study

The research undertaken in the present study employs a neuropsychological approach to care-giving in PD, in order to understand the problems faced by people suffering from neurodegenerative disorders and their spouse carers in everyday life. Rapidly ageing populations, particularly in the developed countries, and expectations that the number of people suffering from disorders of this kind is likely to increase dramatically by the middle of the twenty-first century, makes the need for a better understanding of these problems particularly acute. This is all the more so, in view of the fact that the majority of people with these conditions continue to live in their own homes, and despite considerable levels of disability, make relatively few demands on formal services. The main burden of care, especially in the more advanced stages of neurodegenerative conditions, is borne by families, whose engagement and frequently devoted support, is instrumental in helping to maintain their sick relative at home. Neurodegenerative disorders and the ensuing problems are thus the concern, not only of the afflicted person, but also of those family members providing care. Indeed, the nature and course of neurodegenerative disorders is such, that the patient's immediate family, and in particular his/her spouse, (referred to here as the carer) is closely involved in the experience and day to day management of the illness. The assumption on which the present research is built, is that it is not possible to gain an understanding of the problems faced by people with a neurodegenerative condition over the course of their illness, without taking full account of the perspectives of both of the people involved in the care situation, i.e. the person with the condition and the person who usually "evolves" to become their main carer.

Although a fundamental aim of the neuropsychological approach is to systematically explore both preserved and impaired functions in clinical populations and to relate them to different types of brain damage (Herzyk 2000b), it is also recognised that far from being purely theoretical, or restricted to that of a diagnostic exercise, neuropsychology may serve our understanding of the impact that the resulting disability may have on the individual (Miller 1984). This approach is especially important in the field of neuropsychological rehabilitation (Pąchalska 2007; Wilson et al. 2009). Thus traditionally, neuropsychology, even in its more applied forms, has always had the patient at the centre of its focus. A basic aim of the present study is to provide support for the view that in clinical neuropsychology, there is usually another dimension to be considered, namely that of the carer. Carers and those afflicted with neurodegenerative disease, who become recipients of their care, form an integral unit as the result of close, intimate relationship ties that are often long-standing, but become even more significant in the context of long-term illness. Research has shown that the well-being of one spouse is significantly related to that of the other (Bookwala & Schulz 1996). Any attempt to understand how carers and care recipients cope with the problems of chronic illness must take cognizance of the relationship between them and of the fact that this relationship is dynamic, with a past history, an ongoing reconstruction challenged by the necessity of coming to terms with the demands of the illness, and a future course, likely to be shaped by both past and present features. This necessitates a dyadic approach to care-giving, taking both the perspective of the carer and the care recipient into account (Lyons et al. 2002).

8.2 Parkinson's disease as the model of a neuro-degenerative disorder for the study

There were a number of reasons for the choice of PD as a specific model of a neurodegenerative disorder for the purposes of the present study. Firstly, PD is the second most common neurodegenerative disorder after DAT (Choonara et al. 2009), but has been less extensively researched with regard to the effects of neuropsychological and neuropsychiatric impairments for the everyday lives of both care recipients and their carers. The majority of family care studies in DAT involve samples of older adults in middle-to-late stages of the disease, resulting in limited knowledge about transitions in family care from the early to later stages of the disease process and associated changes that may occur, causing strain for carers and often resulting in deterioration in health. PD provides a noteworthy opportunity to study family care over time, as diagnosis is often made when the person with the disease does not require assistance from family members. However, disease progression is often accompanied by loss of physical function and increased need for care. Secondly, evidence is beginning to emerge, that research addressing the difficulties faced by carers in looking after a close relative with DAT cannot be generalized across diagnostic categories in a straightforward manner (Shin, Youn et al. 2012; Thommessen et al. 2002). In a study comparing spouse carers of older people with stroke, DAT and PD, these authors found that cognitive impairment contributed to the burden of caring in stroke and PD to a greater extent than it did in dementia. Thus PD may have to be examined separately, in order to take into account the specific conditions that pertain in different illnesses. Over the last two decades it has increasingly been recognized that PD presents not only with the physical symptoms that are so characteristic of the disorder, but also in the manifestation of neuropsychological and neuropsychiatric changes, which are crucial to determining the clinical picture and the successful management of the condition. It would be surprising if these changes did not contribute to the problems wrought by the illness-process for the care-recipient, as well as to the burden of the disease experienced by carers. Indeed, the third and most important reason for choosing to study PD is in terms of the rare opportunity that it presents for examining the three different and distinctive aspects of the characteristic symptom constellation associated with the disorder (i.e. motor, cognitive and affective) and the possible inter-relationships between them, in the same group of patients, thus improving the internal validity of the study by eliminating the threat posed by the use of multiple groups for comparisons. Moreover, this symptom complex, occurring in the same patient, made it possible to test the proposition outlined above, that different symptom constellations may engender different effects for the carer-care recipient relationship, thus shaping both the illness and the care-giving experience for the dyad.

8.3 Theoretical background to the study

The present work derives its theoretical grounding from three main sources. It is primarily embedded in a mainstream of research on care-giving, which has centred around the problems of caring for someone with a neurodegenerative disorder. Although the main impulse in the care-giving research has not come directly from neuropsychology, but rather from a variety of different disciplines involved in caring for the elderly with acquired brain disorders, it seems inevitable that the field should become a point of interest for clinical neuropsychologists for the reasons stated in the preceding section. Thus, clinical neuropsychology provides the second theoretical approach underpinning the current research. This drawing together of the two fields is particularly important in terms of the third theoretical component, which is that of a dyadic approach to understanding the illness and care-giving experience in neurodegenerative disorders.

8.3.1 Stress-process models of care-giving

The failure to adopt an explicit theoretical standpoint has continued to be a major weakness of much of the research on care-giving, especially in relation to PD. As described in chapter 6, the main theoretical model that can be identified as underpinning research in the area of care-giving is the stress-process model (Pearlin et al. 1990) which derives from the Transactional Stress Theory of Lazarus and Folkman (1984). An early modification in the form of the appraisal model (Lawton et al. 1989;1991) provided a means of accounting for the perplexing fact, that carers facing similar care-giving demands may react to their situation very differently, one person taking things in their stride, while another may prove to be completely unable to cope (Poulshock & Deimling 1984). Expanded versions of the model have also allowed mediating factors affecting the stress process to be taken into account, including ways of coping, social support, relationship factors, and most recently, cultural differences (e.g. Yates et al. 1999).

There is now a wealth of literature on the impact of caring for people suffering from neurodegenerative conditions, the most common of which is Alzheimer's disease and, as a result, has received most attention (see chapter 7). An unfortunate consequence of this focus, and that of adopting a theoretical model derived from the stress literature, has been to virtually ignore the perspective of the care recipient. This may have been conditioned by the fact that most studies have focused on the middle to late stages of Alzheimer's disease, when care-giving is most in evidence, but when the care recipient is already unable to express views regarding his/her experience of the illness and care-giving situation. Furthermore, adopting the nomenclature of stress theories has meant that the care recipient has been reduced to little more than a "potential stressor" and the carer is considered in terms of "outcomes" such as burden or depression or some other chosen variable, depending on the study (Lyons et al. 2002; Yates et al. 1999). It is understandable that constructs need to operationalised for the purposes of research, but if key characteristics of the situation being examined are lost in the process, knowledge is unlikely to be advanced. This unfortunately, has been a feature of the care-giving research. Both patient and carer are conceived of in a non-interactive way and whilst the stress models of care-giving have provided a powerful theoretical conceptualisation, they have also been instrumental in potentiating a static view of the main protagonists. While admitting the mediational effects of, for example, social support and coping for the carer, the models have nonetheless recognised mainly a uni-directional flow in the stress process from the patient variables to those of the carer. This failure to recognise the dynamic processes in the interaction between the carer and care recipient is likely to be a major obstacle to understanding the process of illness experience and care-giving in neurodegenerative disease.

Clinical observation and work with couples in which one person suffers from a neurodegenerative illness, clearly shows the limitations of the stress model in its oversimplification of the relationship between carer and care recipient. There can be no doubt that carers play a substantial role in the way in which a person with a neurodegenerative disorder is able to adjust and adapt to the condition. Nevertheless, scant attention has been given to this in evaluating the psychosocial impact of chronic illness. Moreover, a carer's presence might be expected to affect the course of the disease, or at least, its impact, by for example, influencing the care recipient's affective and motivational state and aspects of the management of the disorder. However, there do not appear to have been any studies which have attempted to examine this issue. But above all, the dynamic nature of the exchange that occurs between the carer and the care recipient over the course of the illness demands a dyadic approach to understanding their situation. This is not to detract from the importance of either the patient or the carer's narrative, but aims to foster an understanding of the dynamic relationship that exists between them, shaping both the illness and the care-giving experience and how they are received by both parties. In addition, it ensures that the care recipient's perspective is taken into consideration, along with that of the carer. This is something that has often been neglected by the care-giving research.

Despite advances in both the theoretical and empirical approaches to care-giving, the most valued objective of research in this area has not been achieved. As Pearlin et al. (1990) pointed out, what we would really like to know, is which aspects of care-giving are most burdensome for carers and are most likely to result in severe distress and other forms of psychological morbidity. It is somewhat surprising that after twenty years of intensive research, this has still not been achieved. A possible reason for this is that the adherence to a stress model, and the consequent implications, has not allowed other avenues to be sufficiently explored.

8.3.2 A neuropsychological and dyadic perspective on care-giving

A tenet of the present study is that important features of the care-giving situation have not, so far, been sufficiently taken into consideration. These include the dynamic and adaptive aspects of the relationship between the carer and the care recipient, as described above. It is proposed that care-giving outcomes are not solely determined by the carer's ability or otherwise to make effective use of mediating variables such as the social support or coping strategies invoked by stress models. Indeed, previous work has shown that these mediational hypotheses have only limited explanatory potential, as in the study by Miller et al. (1996) which did not find any effects of social support in a study of carers of people with PD.

Neuropsychological approaches are not without their difficulties either. For example, individuals with impaired cognitive functioning, such as that which occurs in PD, may be unaware of, or may under-report their own failures as a result of forgetting (Hickox & Sunderland 1992; Rabbit & Abson 1990). Whilst formal testing can help to resolve these problems, there are others that are more complex. Neuropsychological tests appear to lack ecological validity (Hickox & Sunderland 1992) and test performance does not correlate with problems in everyday life (Mahoney, Dalby & King 1998; Pollina et al. 1993). The carer's assessment of cognition and mood for the care-recipient may therefore be a more accurate reflection of the couples' experience of the illness and its impact on care-giving.

The proposition examined in the present study is that carers actively participate in making their own evaluations of the care recipient's condition and tailor their responses to their perceptions of the care recipient's needs accordingly. This would help to explain the variability in carers' responses to apparently similar situations and the differences in coping with them. Whilst such judgements conform to the notion of appraisal recognised in stress theories as having a major impact on carer outcomes, studies of care-giving have tended to conceptualise carer appraisals in terms of care-giving burden, particularly in terms of its more subjective aspects (Lawton et al. 1989; Yates et al.1999) which is reflected in the properties of the scales used to measure burden. This means that a more fundamental type of appraisal that is likely to be made by the carer has been neglected. Carers are likely to be sensitive to changes in the care recipient's functioning in all spheres of activity, but spouse carers, whose relationships with their partners have lasted for many years, are especially likely to notice psychological changes. This sensitivity appears to be particularly acute in PD, perhaps precisely because the changes are less severe than in DAT and from the point of view of carers, more unexpected and unaccountable (Aarsland, Larsen, Karlsen et al. 1999; Carter et al. 2008; Miller et al. 1996). It is thus postulated that carers' perceptions of the affective and cognitive status of the care recipient may be more important than objective measures of physical and neuropsychological functioning in determining their own psychological well-being. Because PD is still seen primarily as a motor disorder, many of the neuropsychiatric and neuropsychological symptoms of the condition may be baffling to carers, who may interpret them as changes in personality or straightforward awkwardness on the part of the care recipient. This situation may be inadvertently potentiated by clinicians, who may wish to spare both patients and their carers the stigmatising connotations associated with the neuropsychological presentation of the disorder, and fail to inform them about these symptoms and discuss their implications. Thus differences in carers' interpretation and understanding of such symptoms may be the key to understanding their patterns of engagement in care activities and their affective responses. Finally, in keeping with the dyadic approach, it may be possible to explain how the expression and reception of neuropsychiatric and neuropsychological (as well as other) deficits is regulated, at least in part, by the nature of the interaction between the carer and care recipient.

8.4 The neuropsychology of Parkinson's disease

From the point of view of neuropsychology as an applied clinical science, the symptom complex associated with PD (described in previous chapters) is that of a neurodegenerative disorder arising from brain function that has been compromised by acquired structural damage leading to disturbances at the neurochemical level. These abnormalities are considered to be reflective of damage to different brain systems which bring about the specific disintegration of brain function and result in the impairment of both psychological and motor functions, which present in terms of the specific symptom constellation of the disorder. Thus PD can be described at three levels of disturbance:

1. As a disorder consisting of a specific symptom pattern giving rise to difficulties in cognitive, affective, behavioural and motor functioning, which result in a range of secondary effects for the patient and the carer.
2. As a neurological, neuropsychological and neuropsychiatric disorder, giving rise to: (i) deficits in motor functioning, (ii)

impairments in higher level cognitive functions, including attention, memory, visuo-spatial and executive functions, and (iii) primarily affective and anxiety disorders, although other disturbances also exist.

3. At a neurobiological level i.e. at the level of disruption of brain systems which give rise to the neurological, neuropsychological and neuropsychiatric deficits referred to in (2) above.

In terms of the neuropsychology of PD, two main kinds of change occur, which have been described as depression and cognitive impairment. The clinical picture regarding the depression of PD remains poorly understood. Controversies surround its rate of presentation, the nature and profile of the symptoms and the extent to which they resemble the symptom pattern characteristic for MDD (see chapter 3). The cognitive decline of PD is somewhat better understood. It appears that the milder cognitive deficits, characterised by impairments in executive functions, arise as a result of dopaminergic deficits and are thought to share a common neurobiological substrate with the disturbances of motor function. Memory and visuospatial disturbances, however, are associated with Lewy body pathology and cholinergic deficits in more posterior cortical areas, involving the temporal and parietal lobes and the hippocampus (see chapter 4). In this respect, they resemble the neuropathological changes associated with DAT and a pattern of neuropsychological impairment involving memory and visuospatial deficits appears to be predictive of dementia in patients with PD. For this reason, in the investigations described here, greater emphasis has been placed on gaining a better understanding of the affective symptomatology of PD, than on the well-characterised picture of cognitive deficits. In order to meet the requirements of the study design, patients with MDD were also examined, along with normal, healthy age-matched people and older people with limited mobility living in their own homes in the community.

8.4.1 The depression of Parkinson's disease

Whilst there is general agreement that affective changes are a frequent concomitant of PD, considerable controversy still surrounds estimates of the prevalence of depressive disorder in PD. Prevalence rates of between 30% and 50% based on literature reviews have been reported (see chapter 3) and there appears to be an emerging consensus that the rate of depression is higher in PD than might be expected for the general population, matched for age (Reijnders et al. 2008). There are also reports suggesting that the nature of the depressive symptomatology may be different in PD, but only two previous studies have directly compared patients with MDD and PD along relevant dimensions (Merschdorf et al. 2003; Ehrt et al. 2006). A number of authors have also drawn attention to the fact that people who go on to develop PD are more likely to have suffered from MDD prior to the onset of their Parkinsonian symptoms (e.g. Nilsson et al. 2002).

A major focus in the present study was on the affective disorder in PD. Whilst not a case register study, patients were carefully selected from as many sources as was practicable in and around a chosen geographical area, so as not to bias selection procedures. Thus it was possible to attempt an estimate of depression rates in the sample examined. Furthermore, a measure of depression was developed especially for the purposes of this study, which was designed both to place less dependence on the somatic features of depression, such as psychomotor retardation, in order to minimise the overlap between the symptoms of MDD and PD, and to be more sensitive than alternative scales, to less severe degrees of depression. The question of appropriate sensitivity to the expression of affective change in PD is particularly important, as patients with PD demonstrate higher levels of milder depression as compared to MDD and it was postulated that this may account for the alleged differences in symptom profile in PD. Having established the psychometric properties of the new measure it was then possible to test this hypothesis. In addition, patients with PD were compared with patients meeting DSM-IV-TR criteria for MDD in order to determine whether their symptom profiles differed. An important consideration, was making sure that the patients from both groups were equated for severity of illness, so that alleged differences in symptomatology were not simply a reflection of differences in the severity of the affective disorder. As far as it has been possible to establish, a comparison of this kind has never been made in the literature, as patients were individually matched for severity of depressive symptoms and not on a group mean basis, as in the two previous studies to have attempted a similar comparison (Merschdorf et al. 2003; Ehrt et al. 2006). Both of these studies admitted to inadequacies in their matching procedures. Another aspect of the affective disorder in PD examined in the present study was its relationship to the other symptoms of PD and the extent to which it might contribute to the psychosocial functioning of the patient. Equally, the effects of the depressive disorder in the patient were investigated with regard to their influence on the well-being of the carer. As discussed in chapter 4, it was postulated that affective changes may be misinterpreted by the carer as indicative of the patient's withdrawal from, or rejection of, the former relationship with the carer, thus potentiating difficulties for care-giving.

8.4.2 The cognitive impairment of Parkinson's disease

Various estimates have been made of the proportion of patients with PD who develop dementia (see chapter 4), ranging from around 20-50%, but Aarsland et al. (2003) have argued that the majority do. Increasing sophistication in sampling and measurement techniques over the last twenty years have helped to clarify the nature of the cognitive disturbances, lending support to a dual syndrome hypothesis as described above (Kehagia et al. 2013). Essentially, executive deficits are thought to arise as a result of fronto-striatal dysfunction, while distinctive prodromal memory and visuospatial deficits are predictive of dementia.

A full investigation of all aspects of the cognitive impairment in PD was beyond the scope of this research, bearing in mind its principal objectives and the resources available. However it was considered important to gain an indication of cognitive performance in the patients examined for a number of reasons. Firstly, assessment of cognitive function was necessary in order to obtain a complete clinical picture of the patients with PD. Secondly, it was essential in order to evaluate the extent to which deficits in cognitive functioning may interact with other functions (e.g. motor and affective) to exacerbate functional impairment and affect the psychosocial functioning of the patient. Thirdly, a question examined in the present study was whether the cognitive dysfunction seen in PD might contribute to the strain experienced by the carer, perhaps mediated by detrimental changes to the carer – care recipient relationship. And finally, the carer's perceptions of cognitive changes in the patient were of interest, in order to determine the extent to which they might be recognised and the subsequent effects of this awareness for the carer. In order to understand the carer's perspective, it was necessary to match his/her evaluation to an objective measure of cognitive dysfunction. These considerations together with an understanding of the cognitive disturbances that occur in PD led to defining those aspects of neuropsychological performance, which it was expected, would be most sensitive to disruption in PD. The cognitive assessment was thus based on selected simple and easy to administer tests, known to be sensitive to the dementia-like changes and which could be carried out within the constraints of this study i.e. in the person's home, without specialised equipment, and within a limited time frame. Other considerations included the physical discomfort and fatigue produced by the illness which might limit the person's tolerance of extended neuropsychological testing, together with the fact that other aspects of functioning were also to be assessed.

It was thus decided to focus on memory and visuospatial impairments for two reasons. Firstly, deficits in these areas form part of the pattern of neuropsychological disturbances that has been established in PD. Secondly, according to current definitions (e.g. DSM-IV-TR) memory impairments are a *sine qua non* of any form of dementia, and they are also very often the first of the higher cognitive functions to show disruption. Many studies have reported memory impairments in people with PD (e.g. Wilson et al. 1980; Tweedy, Langer & McDowell 1982; Jacobs et al. 1995; Aarsland et al. 2003), especially when performance is measured on spontaneous free recall, which is generally a more difficult task.

In view of the limitations imposed by the study, which prevented use of a full neuropsychological test battery for the assessment of patients, it was decided to employ a measure of visuospatial function as part of the cognitive assessment, since deficits in visuospatial skills are among the most frequently reported cognitive changes accompanying idiopathic PD (Bentin et al. 1981; Montse et al. 2001; Thanvi et al. 2003). In view of the allegedly high risk of dementia in PD (Aarsland et al. 2003; Miller & Morris 1993), an estimate of IQ known to be sensitive to organic impairments, was also obtained (Nelson & McKenna 1975).

A major assumption of research concerning the welfare of carers of people with long-term neurodegenerative disorders has been that the nature and effects of the symptoms of the condition in question, are likely to affect the well-being of carers. This is not an unreasonable assumption, but as the preceding chapters have shown, it has only been verified in part. Research with the carers of people with DAT has shown that neither the physical nor cognitive disturbances appear to be closely associated with the burden of care-giving. The impact of affective disturbances in the care recipient is less well understood, because it has been less frequently studied, probably because the assessment of depression in a dementing disorder is fraught with much greater difficulties than the physical and cognitive dysfunctions. The present study undertook the evaluation of all three symptom domains, which characteristically occur in PD, in order to evaluate the impact on the carer. This concern with causal relationships in relation to understanding outcomes for carers, necessitated a conceptual framework within which to study the care-giving situation. This is illustrated in figure 8-1.

Figure 8-1. Hypothetical causal relationships in the care-giving pathway.

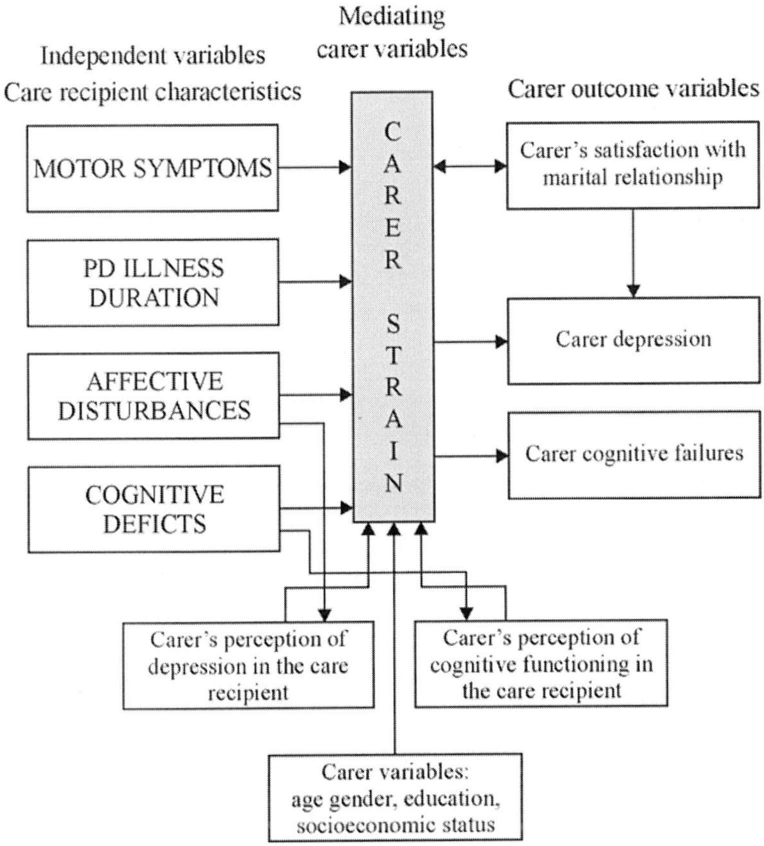

8.5 Aims of the research

As has been shown in the preceding chapters, PD is a complex disorder that presents a number of problems. One of these is the nature of the underlying pathophysiology of the disorder and much work has gone into gaining an understanding of these aspects of the condition. As discussed in chapter 2, pharmacological and surgical treatments have been developed, many of which have been shown to be of value, and advances have been made in the understanding of the basic mechanisms at the heart of the disease process. Despite continuing progress along these lines, and the understandable desire of patients and their families for "a cure", the possibility of this remains remote as regards the foreseeable future and even the likelihood of being able to reverse the disease process or to halt its effects before significant handicap has occurred is still a distant prospect. Given this state of affairs, questions arise which are of practical importance in understanding and managing the problems associated with PD. These questions have two main points of focus. The first concerns the person suffering from the disorder and the extent to which the triad of motor, affective and cognitive symptoms in PD, combines to produce the overall handicap. Of interest is the extent to which the non-motor symptoms affect the clinical picture in PD and are reflected in the patient's psychosocial functioning. The second point of focus is on the carer. Since PD produces significant handicaps increasing the dependency of the afflicted individual, the consequences for those who live with and care for the person with PD are likely to be considerable. The general aim of the research presented here was to explore aspects of these two focal areas, which are closely interlinked, and was formulated as follows:

> **To explore aspects of the neuropsychological impairment in PD and determine how the deficits in affective and cognitive functioning, characteristic of the disorder, may affect the patient and his/her carer in everyday life.**

The specific requirements for meeting this general aim determined the stages in which the research was carried out. The purpose of each stage was defined in terms of the hypotheses being examined and operationalised in the form of tasks designed to verify them. There were three stages to the research, each designed with the aim of contributing to a greater understanding of key issues raised in the preceding literature review, which remain controversial or where gaps in knowledge still exist.

8.5.1 Stage I of the research

Stage I of the research focused on the affective disorder of PD with a view to adding to the current debate on the nature of depressive symptoms in PD, in particular, their prevalence, the clinical profile of symptoms and appropriate ways of measuring depression in PD. A secondary aim of this stage of the research was to provide an estimate of the rates of depression in an unselected sample of patients with PD living in the community. Although not a case register study, the recruitment of patients ensured that they were not pre-selected in such a way as to potentially bias the results of the study. In general terms the aim of stage I was defined as follows:

I To achieve a better understanding of the nature of the affective symptomatology of Parkinson's disease;

and the specific aims of the research for stage I, arising from these considerations, were threefold:

I (i) to devise a research instrument for the measurement of depressive symptoms which would meet the special requirements for such an instrument in PD, and would allow specific hypotheses about the nature of the depressive disorder in PD to be tested.

I (ii) to determine how estimates of the prevalence of affective disorder in PD are affected by the use of different measurement instruments.

I (iii) to define the characteristics of the symptom constellation for depression in PD and to compare it to that of MDD.

8.5.2 Stage II of the research

Apart from addressing unresolved issues concerning the nature of the affective disorder in PD, important in their own right, stage I of the research also provided a foundation for the questions examined in the subsequent stages of the research. Building upon the findings of the first stage in relation to depression, stage II was concerned with reaching a clearer understanding of how the different symptom domains relate to one another in PD. The nature of the clinical and temporal relationship between the cognitive impairment and depression of PD and the motor symptoms remains unclear. Most studies to date have addressed specific hypotheses and have not tackled this general issue. In order to investigate the way in which the different manifestations of the disorder relate to one another, it is necessary to use longitudinal studies, or cross sectional studies which employ pattern recognition analyses, for example, factor or cluster analysis. Furthermore, measures covering all features of the disorder (i.e. motor, affective and cognitive) as well as demographic and clinical variables such as age, length of illness and treatment parameters should be included and they should give a reasonable degree of discrimination within the population examined. Studies published to date have followed this research design only partially: Zetusky, Jankovic and Pirrozzolo (1985) and others (e.g. Reynolds & Montgomery1987; van Rooden et al. 2009a) have only included measures of motor functioning or exclusively neuropsychiatric symptoms (Lloret et al. 2011) in their analyses. As far as can be ascertained, only one previously published study has included variables from all three symptom domains (van Rooden et al. 2009b).

Understanding the relationship between the different symptom domains and disease parameters is important for a number of reasons. Firstly, finding a way of determining whether the neuropsychological manifestations of disrupted affective and cognitive functioning in PD are primary or secondary symptoms in the disorder, would help to resolve a long-standing controversy in this area, which has never been entirely satisfactorily laid to rest. Although over the last twenty years or so the biological explanation, that neuropsychological symptoms are primary symptoms intrinsic to the disease has become the established view, this is due more to the emerging strength of the neurosciences as a discipline, and the powerful weight of evidence that they have generated in support of brain-behaviour relationships, than to the resolution of specific issues such as this. The notion that affective symptoms may be secondary to having a progressive neurological condition such as PD which produces significant motor impairment and functional handicap is nowadays more rarely entertained by researchers, except as a second-order mechanism, although it still appears as a question in the literature (Farabaugh et al. 2011; Frisina et al. 2009). That cognitive deficits are an integral part of PD is also now well established and their biological substratum reasonably well-defined, as has been shown in chapter 4. At one time, they too might have been seen as secondary to the affective disorder in PD or attributed to a concomitant degenerative illness such as DAT (e.g Boller et al. 1980). However, there is still some advantage in attempting to provide empirical evidence to differentiate the "primary" versus "secondary" hypotheses of neuropsychological symptoms, if only because the latter remains the popular view, often holding an intuitive logic for patients and their families (Oehlberg et al. 2008). Being able to provide them with better information in this respect might help in the process of long-term adaptation to living with the illness.

Secondly, the statistical relationships between symptom domains have been taken as evidence to enable the different positions regarding their aetiology to be discriminated. In the present study it was postulated that if the affective disorder is of "secondary" or "reactive" origin, that is, consequent upon the disability wrought by PD, then depressive symptoms should be correlated with motor symptoms, but more importantly, they would be associated within a single "illness" construct. If however, the depression of PD is not merely reactive to the condition, but may be a manifestation of the disease in its own right, independence of psychological and motor symptoms would be predicted. This latter position may at first appear confusing. If both affective and motor symptoms share the same underlying substrate in PD, then it would be reasonable to expect them to be related (a position indistinguishable in terms of the relationship between symptoms from the "reactive" hypothesis). In practice, this is not necessarily the case, as the expression of the separate symptom domains may be subject to the influence of intervening variables which could enhance or attenuate their manifestation. Moreover, the logic of this presumption would be that all patients with PD should demonstrate clinically significant depression. Clearly, as the foregoing discussion has shown, they do not. Although the pathophysiology of depression in PD remains unknown, hypotheses exist implicating specific diminution in dopamine and noradrenaline innervation in the limbic system (Remy et al. 2005) and cortical cholinergic denervation (Bohnen et al. 2007), but not damage to the main nigro-striatal pathways, responsible for the motor symptoms of PD. A similar logic pertains to the cognitive deterioration in PD. If the cognitive deficits (or at least some of them) are conceptualised as being dopamine dependent and associated with damage to fronto-striatal circuits in PD, they too should correlate with motor symptoms forming part of a single "illness" construct. If on the other hand, they are considered to be an expression of the illness, but dependent on other neurotransmitter systems, they should be independent. As described in chapter 4, evidence is emerging that in fact, both possibilities pertain, executive deficits being associated with the former, and memory and visuo-spatial deficits, predicitive of dementia with the latter, in the dual syndrome hypothesis described by Kehagia et al. 2013.

Thirdly, there arises the possibility that different patient subgroups may exist in PD, which may be identified on the basis of neuropsychological variables, either affective or cognitive. This may help to explain why some patients with PD are depressed or experience cognitive deterioration, whilst others do not. Finally, any inter-dependencies among symptoms, or indeed the lack of them, are likely to have significant treatment implications for patients with PD. On the basis of these considerations, the aim of stage II of the research was formulated with the purpose of:

II Evaluating the relationships among the main symptom domains of Parkinson's disease;

with the purpose of meeting the following aims:

II (i) to describe how the main symptom domains relate to one another and to the general illness and background variables in PD.

II (ii) to examine the evidence for the origin of the neuropsychological (affective and cognitive) symptoms in PD.

II (iii) to determine whether it is possible to identify patient subgroups within the sample studied on the basis of psychological variables, either affective or cognitive.

8.5.3 Stage III of the research

The guiding principle for stage III of the research was the awareness that PD is usually experienced, albeit in different ways, by two people in a close, dyadic relationship. As a result of the condition, their former roles in relation to each other and their closest family may be modified over time, with the patient assuming a care recipient role and his/her spouse, taking on the role of carer. These transitions may be unwelcome and adaptation to them achieved at considerable cost in psychological terms as described in earlier chapters.

The fact that the care-giving role is extremely taxing and takes its toll on the physical and mental health of carers is well documented in the literature and is described in chapters 6 and 7 of the present volume. Despite the wealth of literature that has accumulated in this area over the last forty years, relatively little is still known about the problems faced by carers, except for a general consensus that care-giving is "potentially a fertile ground for persistent stress" (Pearlin et al. 1990, 583). There is no commonly accepted or comprehensive model to assess the needs of carers (Cousins et al. 2002) which derives in part from the fact that there is little agreement as to the conceptualization and measurement of care-giving outcomes. Consequently, little progress has been made in identifying distressed carers and targeting strategies for intervention so as to optimise ways of relieving carer distress. These insufficiencies in the knowledge base on care-giving, which emerge from the foregoing analysis of the literature, led to the design of the study carried out in the third stage of the research, whose main aim was to provide:

III An analysis of the conditions influencing care-giving in PD.

The realisation of this general aim was approached by investigating a range of factors which might be expected to have an impact on the care-giving experience. Whilst stages I and II of the research were designed to address the specific aims outlined above, they also formed an important foundation for stage III of the research. Having a clearer understanding of how the different symptom domains relate to one another in PD, provided a starting point for building a theoretical framework in which to identify and describe the characteristic conditions and experiences of caring for someone with PD, which are associated with poorer outcomes in terms of health and well-being for carers. Of particular importance here, was the extent to which the main symptom domains of PD were inter-correlated or independent of one another, as this would have implications for the way in which they might act as potential predictor variables of carer outcomes. This was considered to be a factor of considerable importance in further investigating the influence of the disease parameters on the care-giving situation, and so a replication, in a different sample of patients with PD was judged to be apposite in order to confirm the reliability of the findings. Thus the first aim of this stage of the research was:

III (i) to replicate the findings in study II (i) showing how the main symptom domains relate to one another and to the general illness and background variables in PD.

A logical prediction made in the literature on caring for people with neurodegenerative diseases is that difficulties for the carer arise in connection with the main symptoms of the condition affecting the care recipient, which make him/her more dependent on physical care, such as assistance with self-care activities. This approach however, has had only limited success as described in chapter 7, and attempts to correlate carer burden with the physical aspects of the disease have been only partially successful. One reason for this in the existing literature, which in the main, has focused on DAT, is that the condition does not provide the opportunity to examine the effects of all three symptom domains – physical, affective and cognitive – at all stages of the disease process. Physical symptoms, for example, are a late manifestation of the disorder and their occurrence may be confounded with temporal and other factors, such as disease severity. As has already been mentioned, PD disease was the model of choice for this research, as it provides the possibility of examining the effects of all three symptom domains in the same patient at any point over the course of the development of the illness, from the time of initial diagnosis. This was an important control procedure for eliminating sources of experimental error and one which was particularly important in helping to ensure that the second aim of the research in stage III might be met. The second aim was formulated as follows:

III (ii) to determine whether any of the symptom domains of PD may be specifically associated with poorer outcomes for carers in terms of the strain they experience as a result of care-giving and to examine the consequent effects on their mental health.

Whilst it may be logical to expect that disease characteristics might be associated with carer burden, limitations to this approach have emerged from the literature review presented in chapter 7. One reason for this may be that objective measures of the care recipient's functioning, in both physical and neuropsychological terms, are not good indicators for either the carer or the care recipient, of the latter's level of dependency. Levels of functional disability in the care recipient may be related more to neuropsychological impairments than to physical ones. Equally the carer's view of the demands of the care-giving situation and the amount of care provided, may be more to do with his/her own perception of the care recipient's level of dependency, than with so-called "objective" measures of disability. Furthermore, understanding how carer reports of the carer recipient's condition may vary in relation to clinically derived information is important towards understanding the role of carers as proxy informants on behalf of the care recipient, both for clinical and research purposes. Hence determining the possible role of perceptual factors or appraisals of the neuropsychological functioning of the care recipient in mediating outcomes for carers was the third aim of the study:

III (iii) to determine whether carers' perceptions of specific aspects of the disability in PD, in particular neuropsychological and neuro-psychiatric aspects of the care recipient's functioning, may be instrumental in determining their own psychological health.

The burden on the carer may, at least in part, be attributable to the indirect consequences of the disease, such as the care-recipient's reduced mobility, which may mean that the carer's activities and movements also become restricted and additional problems are frequently encountered. These are the so-called "secondary stressors" as defined by Pearlin et al. (1990) which arise as a result of the mechanism known as stress proliferation (Aneshensel et al. 1995), whereby problems have the tendency to bring others in their wake. These additional problems are likely to be more complex in their evolution, but appear to be related to the carer's relationship with the care recipient and to ways in which the relationship becomes transformed as a result of the couple's having to adapt to and live with a long-term, progressive illness such as PD. It is postulated here, that factors which disturb or distort the relationship between the carer and the care-recipient are a particular source of distress for the carer. Changes brought about by the neuropsychological manifestations of the illness in the form of the patient's lowered mood, lack of interest or apathy, and general failure to interact with the carer as previously, are often a significant cause for concern in this respect. These effects do not occur in all cases, but they appear in a significant proportion. Almost paradoxically, it is the mild degree of such effects that makes them more difficult to recognise and to accept as being illness-related. Because the changes in mood and cognitive dysfunction are often relatively contained, they are perceived by the carer as changes in the "personality" or behaviour of the care recipient and are not seen as being part of the disease process. As such, they become something that additionally endangers the bond between the carer and the care recipient.

A proposition considered in stage III of the research was that the quality of the relationship between the carer and the care-recipient is likely to be an important factor in modifying the carer's experience of care-giving and may explain why so many carers continue to care for their spouse or close family member in spite of cumulative strains over many years. Indeed, this fact has initiated an approach to caring which emphasizes the positive aspects of the experience as opposed to the simple burden-account that has dominated the literature (Nolan et al. 2003). These considerations led to the fourth and final aim, which was:

III (iv) to gain a better understanding of how the relationship between the care recipient and the carer may help to mitigate the adverse effects of caring.

An important final goal in research of this kind is to provide clinical applications by helping to inform the way in which intervention strategies may be devised and implemented in order to be effective in helping to support the care-recipient and the carer in the community. A major long-term aim of the present work is to gain sufficient understanding of the care-giving situation in order to provide a knowledge base upon which intervention programmes can be devised and evaluated. The fourth general aim of the study was thus formulated as follows:

IV. to determine how the knowledge gained from the results of this research may be applied to clinical practice to help devise appropriately targeted neuropsychological assessment procedures and evidenced-based clinical intervention strategies in order to meet the needs of patients with PD and their carers.

8.6 Research questions

The research aims thus formulated were examined in the three stages of the study: stage 1, which was concerned with obtaining a better understanding of the affective disorder in PD, stage 2, which focused on establishing the relationship between the main symptom domains in PD and identifying any patterns in the symptom complex and stage 3, which was designed to explore how characteristic aspects of the disease presentation in the care recipient shape the care-giving situation and the extent to which other factors may modify the experience of looking after someone with PD for the carer. These aims were operationalised in terms of the following research questions:

1. What is the nature of the affective disorder in PD?

    1.1. What are the psychometric properties of the research instrument (ADQ) devised to measure the symptoms of depression in PD?
    1.2. What is the estimate of the prevalence for affective disorders in the sample of patients with PD studied and how do prevalence estimates differ according to different instruments?
    1.3. What is the profile of depressive symptoms in PD and how does it differ from that in MDD?
    1.4. Are patients with PD more consistent than those with MDD in their pattern of responses on instruments measuring depression?

2. Is it possible to identify characteristic patterns of symptom alignment in PD?

    2.1. What is the symptom profile arising out of the physical and neuropsychological impairments associated with PD, for the sample of patients studied?
    2.2. What is the relationship between the motor, affective and cognitive symptoms in PD and how is this related to their origin?

2.3. Is it possible to identify sub-groups of patients with PD, which might be characterised by different symptom clusters, e.g. a specific patterns of affective or cognitive impairments? and,

3. How do the characteristic aspects of the disease presentation in PD shape the care-giving situation and what additional factors modify the experience of caring from the point of view of the carer?

   3.1. What is the evidence that the carers of people with PD are under considerable amounts of strain or at increased risk of psychological morbidity?
   3.2. What aspects of the care-giving situation are especially problematic for carers?
   3.3. Is the carer able to recognise changes in the care recipient's behaviour associated with affective dysfunction and cognitive impairment, and how do these perceptions shape his/her responses to the care-giving situation?
   3.4. What factors affect the quality of the relationship between the patient with PD and his/her carer and what bearing does this have on care-giving outcomes?
   3.5. What is the relationship between different measures of carer outcome in the form of care-giving strain and more generic measures of psychological morbidity in the form of depression?

The final and important practical goal of this research regarding clinical applications was conceptualized in terms of the following question:

Does taking into account a wide range of situational dimensions in reaching an understanding of the care-giving situation in PD provide opportunities for specifying areas to be targeted by intervention programmes in order to ameliorate distress for both the patient and the carer and help to improve their quality of life?

8.7 Research Design

The research presented followed an *ex post facto* or causal-comparative design, in which it is assumed (*ex post*) that the value of the dependent variable is determined by the independent variable, over which the researcher has no control, as it has already occurred (Brzeziński 1996). Research of this kind explores possible causes and effects within the data obtained. Thus it was postulated that the constellation of symptoms and the quality of the neuropsychological and neuropsychiatric deficits observed, were the result of PD in the patient group. Analogously, it was assumed that the manifestations of psychopathology in the carers were determined primarily by the strain that they experienced in their care-giving role. Three control groups were also recruited to the study in order to allow specific contrasts to be made concerning the nature of depression in PD. These included patients with MDD and two groups of age-matched older people, one of which consisted of people with mobility problems, the other, in good health with uncompromised mobility. A comparison with the former enabled the profile of depressive symptoms to be evaluated in the two conditions, whilst the latter provided a control for age effects and mobility problems unrelated to PD brain pathology. The research design was cross sectional and was carried out in three stages as outlined above.

The approach used in the study for the measuring key constructs of interest is in keeping with concepts that are well established, both in the literature on the neuropsychiatric and neuropsychological aspects of PD, and in care-giving in neurodegenerative disease. Examples of the former include conceptualisation of the mood disorder in PD as a form of depression and in the case of the latter, the use of the notion of carer burden, although the preferred term in the present study was care-giving strain, and indices of psychopathology to measure outcomes for the carer. However, the research design also included several features which emphasize the distinctive aspects of the conceptualisation adopted in the present study. In particular, these were aimed at clarifying the observation from previous studies that carer-related variables often appear to be better predictors of care-giving outcomes, than other variables. These considerations can only be accommodated within a dyadic view of caring, which was an overriding priority for the study. In addition, the carer's appraisal of psychological symptoms in the care recipient and the quality of their marital relationship were evaluated, these variables being conceptualised as possible mediators at different stages in the care-giving process. A description of the methods and procedures used in the study forms the subject of chapter 9.

CHAPTER NINE

THE RESEARCH STUDY: METHODS FOR STAGES I-III

9.1 Overview of the study methods

Meeting the aims of the current research, outlined in chapter 8, followed a natural sequential order that was undertaken in three main stages. In the first instance, an attempt was made to clarify the nature of the depression in PD. This required the development of a new instrument to measure PD depression, which was especially designed to make it possible to evaluate areas in which the mood disturbance allegedly differed from that seen in MDD. Thus the first task was to design a new scale to meet these requirements and to establish its psychometric properties. Prevalence rates for depression in the samples studied, using this measure, were compared to those obtained from established instruments. The instrument was then used to test hypotheses concerning the symptom profile for depression in PD. The tasks undertaken in stage I were seen as an important preliminary step in guiding the successive stages of the research. Clarification of the questions outlined above, provided the basis for a clearer conceptualisation of the mood disorder accompanying PD. This guided the selection of instruments for the measurement of depression in the later part of the work. More importantly, at a conceptual level, it raised questions that have not been satisfactorily resolved to date, regarding the relationship between the three main symptom domains (motor, cognitive and affective) in PD. A number of possible explanations for the co-occurrence of motor and psychological symptoms have been postulated, as described in chapter 3 (section 3.6) and 4, including a "reactive" hypothesis where depression is seen as being consequent upon the limitations imposed by the illness and its impact on everyday life. Even the cognitive deficits might represent a form of "pseudo-dementia" associated with depression in later life. These two possibilities would be predictive of associations between the motor, cognitive and affective symptom domains. However, if the depression of PD is of "organic" origin, resulting either from damage to parts of the basal ganglia and their projections, or is connected with brain structures not implicated in the "classic" symptoms of PD, an association with the motor and cognitive symptoms would be less clear, if indeed it were to be expected at all. These possibilities were investigated in stage II of the research and the possibility of subgroups of patients with PD, which might be differentiated according to the psychological symptoms, was explored.

Establishing whether these symptom domains are strongly inter-dependent was also important for another reason connected with the design of the study in part III. Here one of the main independent variables influencing care-giving was defined as the functional brain state associated with the neuropathology of PD and was assumed to be the principal clinical variable shaping the results of the physical, neuropsychological and neuropsychiatric assessment. If the three domains are to be treated as independent or predictor variables, it is important to understand whether or not they are inter-related. The existence of intercorrelations would undermine any putative effects that might be found for a particular symptom domain in relation to care-giving outcomes and require further evaluation of these variables in terms of their moderating effects on each other. These considerations formed the background to the questions studied in stage II of the research.

Thus in helping to clarify a number of important issues surrounding the nature and relationship of depression to the other symptoms of PD, stages I and II paved the way for stage III of the research. A clearer understanding of the manifestation of PD symptomatology made it possible to build an explanatory model to account for both patient and carer variables which interact in creating the care-giving situation and determining outcomes for both parties to the relationship. Stage III of the research thus conceptualised the care-giving situation as a dyadic relationship between the patient and carer, in which their perceptions of selected aspects of their situation and mutual relationship were considered crucial to determining outcomes, for both the carer and the care recipient.

The variables selected to represent the constructs examined in the research were chosen in accordance with the aims of the study, as defined in chapter 8, and operationalised in the measures used as a means of answering the research questions examined at different stages of the work.

9.2 Participants

Participants were allocated to the main groups examined in the study, according to their pre-existing status:

(i) patients with Parkinson's disease;

(ii) three groups of age-matched control subjects: patients with a major depressive disorder, people with limited mobility and healthy older people;
(iii) carers of people with Parkinson's disease.

9.2.1 Patients with Parkinson's disease

A total of 232 patients with a diagnosis of idiopathic PD were recruited to the study. Of these, 97 patients who are referred to as PD1, completed a postal survey and two additional, independent groups, consisting of 60 (PD2) and 75 patients (PD3) respectively, underwent a full clinical interview. Patients from the PD1 and PD2 groups took part in stage I of the research, PD2 were further examined in stage II and in stage III patients from PD3 and their spouse carers were studied.

Although not a case register study, the selection of patients ensured that they were not pre-selected in any way so as to potentially bias the results of the study. A wide range of sources was tapped in order to obtain as representative a sample as was feasible within the constraints in which the study had to be carried out. The 135 patients comprising groups PD2 and PD3 were identified from both in-patient and out-patient records held at Addenbrooke's Hospital in Cambridge, (U.K.) and included patients currently attending, or who had in the past, attended the Neurology Department for consultation. Others were recruited through the local Parkinson's Disease Society and with the assistance of General Practices in and around the geographical area of Cambridge. Of the patients approached with a request for participation in the study, only one refused for reasons they did not disclose. The diagnosis of PD was made by neurologists from the Department of Neurology at Addenbrooke's Hospital according to the U.K. Parkinson's Disease Society Brain Bank criteria (Litvan et al. 2003); the diagnosis was supported by a history of unilateral onset, a progressive disease course and responsiveness to anti-parkinsonian drug therapy, as recorded in the clinical notes. All of the patients had attended the outpatient Neurology Clinic at some time during the course of their illness, usually at the point of diagnosis, although many of them had since been discharged to the care of their General Practitioners.

The remaining 97 patients (PD1) were a sub-group of people with PD recruited to the study through an advertisement placed in the Parkinson's Disease Society (now Parkinson's U.K.) newsletter requesting volunteers. These patients were a sub-group of the respondents, who were matched for age and gender to the sample of patients identified through patient records and who were interviewed for the study. They were sent protocols to complete, with a stamped, addressed envelope for returning the study questionnaire. As the same control with regard to verifying the diagnosis of PD was not possible in this sub-group, only those respondents who reported taking an L-dopa medication (Madopar or Sinemet) were included in the study. It was assumed that if patients were being prescribed anti-parkinsonian drugs and taking them, there was a high likelihood of responsiveness to the medication, which could be taken as indirect confirmation of the diagnosis of uncomplicated PD.

Entry criteria to the study required:

1. that all patients should be living in their own homes in the community; fewer than 3% were living in sheltered housing, none in nursing homes or residential accommodation;
2. a duration of illness (operationally defined as time since diagnosis) of more than 3 years in stages I and II, and of 1 year in stage III;
3. age below 70 years (stages I and II) and below 80 years (stage III);
4. absence of other neurological or cardiovascular disease, and treatment with neuroleptic medication or stereotaxic surgery.

The requirement that patients should be living in their own homes was central to controlling the conditions in which the study was carried out. The focus on understanding how patients with PD and their carers adapt to and cope with a chronic and progressively debilitating condition, in which the support of the carer is crucial, required that the couple should be studied in as natural an environment as possible. The reason for placing a lower limit on disease duration was to ensure that the sample should consist of patients whose diagnosis was confirmed and in whom symptomatology and treatment had been stabilised. Moreover the focus of the study was on an established form of the condition and long-term effects were primarily of interest. The estimate of illness duration was determined from the patients' medical record, but it is likely to be conservative because of the insidious onset of symptoms in PD (Lees 1981). An upper cut-off age limit was chosen in order to minimise the influence of other age related diseases and other chronic conditions were excluded in order to ensure that results were not confounded by their possible effects. Treatments known to produce Parkinsonian-like symptoms and other iatrogenic effects were excluded for the same reasons.

All patients gave their informed consent to participation in the study and ethical permission for the research was obtained from the Local Ethical Committee at Addenbrooke's Hospital in Cambridge, U.K.

Informed consent for cognitively impaired patients was obtained from spouses, but this was required in only one case.

9.2.2 Age matched control subjects

Three normative control groups were also assessed for the purposes of comparison with the PD groups. The control subjects were matched to the index group of patients with PD on the criteria of age and gender. All were living in their own homes in the community. They included a group of patients with a DSM-IV-TR diagnosis of MDD (N=40), who were currently suffering from an acute episode of the disorder and had been admitted to hospital for treatment. The diagnosis had been established by a trained psychiatrist. They were chosen as a control group against which to evaluate the severity and pattern of symptoms in depression in PD.

The remaining age-matched control subjects constituted a group of older people with mobility problems and a group of healthy, older people. They were recruited from a volunteer panel of subjects at the University of Cambridge, non-PD friends and neighbours of the index sample, and various community agencies such as local churches and older peoples' recreational groups. Additionally subjects for the low mobility group were identified from the Neurology Department of Addenbrooke's Hospital in Cambridge. All the potential control subjects were screened for concomitant general medical conditions (e.g. arthritis, diabetes, hypertension and respiratory problems) and their presence was recorded. Those with major psychiatric disorders (e.g. schizophrenia, dementia) and intracerebral disease (e.g. stroke, brain tumours and head injury) were excluded from the study. Those with long-term mobility problems as the result of conditions such as arthritis, lumbar disc herniation, spinal trauma or complications arising from hip fractures, were assigned to the low mobility control group. The screening measures resulted in a control group of older people with mobility problems (N=27) who had similar levels of functional disability to the patients with PD. It was assumed that limited mobility of any kind may increase the risk for depression and hence this group of subjects was expected to have raised levels of depressive symptoms in comparison to the third (healthy) control group (N=30), which did not report any significant health problems and in whom mobility was not restricted.

Relatives and spouses of the patients with PD were not used as control subjects, as in previous studies (see chapter 3) for a number of reasons. Firstly, there is evidence to suggest that relatives living with a person who may be depressed appear to have an increased risk of depression themselves (Benazon and Coyne 2000). Secondly, research has shown that relatives of patients with PD have an increased risk of depression and anxiety disorders (Arabia et al. 2007). Finally, the spouses of patients in PD are examined in stage III of the study in their own right. Furthermore efforts were taken to exclude control subjects who had been involved in care-giving activities during the previous 24 months, in order to avoid the possibility that they might still be recovering from any ill-effects of a previous care-giving experience (Gold et al. 1995).

All of the control subjects gave their informed, written consent for participation in the study.

9.2.3 Carers of people with Parkinson's disease

Seventy-five spouse carers of people with PD participated in stage III of the research. The carer was someone who lived with the patient, sharing the same household and had contact with him/her on a daily basis. Carers also provided written, informed consent for their participation.

9.3 Assessment procedures

The procedure for examining the groups participating in the study was tailored to the aims outlined in chapter 8. The primary concern of stages I and II was to investigate the characteristics of the symptom pattern resulting from the neurodegenerative changes that accompany PD and that of stage III was to determine the extent to which these and carer-related variables influence the results of care-giving.

The patients with PD and their carers served as the index group, who were of primary interest to the study and the questions raised were principally addressed to them. The three remaining groups studied served as controls: the group of patients with MDD provided a comparison for the assessment of depressive symptoms in PD, the low mobility group enabled levels of functional disability to be controlled in order to evaluate depression in people whose mobility was restricted as a result of PD compared to other aetiologies, and the third was a healthy control group. The design of the assessment procedures for the control groups reflected the purpose for which they were chosen.

The majority of patients in groups PD2 and PD3 (N=135), and their carers were interviewed in their own homes, having first been contacted by letter. This was followed up by a telephone call to obtain consent for visiting the patient at home and to arrange for an appointment. Some patients were seen on the Neurology Ward of Addenbrooke's Hospital in

Cambridge, although arrangements were made to see their carers at home. The interview lasted 2 to 3 hours and included both the patient and his/her spouse, where one was available. The interview with patients and their carers and control subjects was conducted by the author. It was carried out at a leisurely, conversational pace, allowing the patient and carer to take as much time as they needed to complete the examination procedure.

All of the subjects participating in the study completed a research protocol which recorded demographic and, where relevant, background clinical information on their condition. For PD1, this information was obtained in self-report form by means of a postal questionnaire. Patients in groups PD2 and PD3 underwent a full clinical interview which took account of their motor and functional impairment, their cognitive performance and affective status; in addition, clinician-ratings of the symptoms from these domains were also obtained.

The control patients with a DSM-IV-TR diagnosis of MDD were seen on the acute admissions ward of Fulbourn Hospital in Cambridge. They underwent a semi-structured clinical interview and completed questionnaires focusing on their affective disorder, lasting about one and a half hours. Where possible, the remaining control subjects, who comprised the low mobility and healthy control groups, were also interviewed in order to obtain a full response set to the protocol. They were mostly seen in their own homes, although some were in-patients of the Neurology Department at Addenbrooke's Hospital. However, in view of considerable difficulties in recruiting age-matched controls to the study, in some cases the research protocol was sent to subjects either by post or electronic mail with an explanation of the purposes of the study and their particular role in it as controls. They were requested to fill in the appropriate questionnaires relating to their physical condition and functional abilities and an assessment was also made of their affective state, but in such instances it was not possible to gain their responses to clinician-rated instruments. The assessment procedure for the control groups lasted about one hour.

9.3.1 Case notes analysis

Pąchalska (2007) emphasizes that it is important for the clinician to prepare for the subsequent interview with the patient by first becoming acquainted with the patient's case notes. The following information was recorded from the PD patients' case notes prior to the interview: where possible this information was verified against data reported by the patient and his/her carer.

1. Year of diagnosis with PD
2. Number of hospital admissions for PD
3. History of treatment for PD – pharmacological and surgical
4. Current medication

The information gained from the hospital case notes was used in order to obtain a description of the clinical characteristics of the patient group.

9.3.2 The clinical interview and psychological assessment

The research procedure was carried out in the form of a semi-structured interview in which a number of specific questions were put to the respondents in standardised form. Some of these were items from the standardised questionnaires used in the study, which are described below. However, in view of the fact that this, albeit research encounter, was in many respects, essentially of a clinical nature from the point of view of the patients and their carers, they were permitted, and indeed encouraged, to provide any information that they might consider relevant to the discussion and to ask questions of the researcher. In so doing it was hoped to facilitate a pleasant and non-intrusive atmosphere in which patients and carers might be encouraged to talk freely about their problems and feel that they were being listened to with concern and understanding. A number of the couples in whom one person had PD commented that they were happy to do so, in the hope that their contribution might help to make life easier for other people with PD. This serves to emphasize the ethical responsibilities of clinical research in placing an onus on researchers to use the results of their studies to find practical solutions to the problems under examination.

All clinical neuropsychology assessment takes place in the context of the clinical interview, which is one of the most important qualitative methods for clinical enquiry (Pąchalska 2007). Pąchalska maintains that the interview is of central importance to gaining specific information about the physical and psychological functioning of the patient. In her view, it may be conducted directly with the patient or with his/her closest relatives or carers. Many patients, because of their brain dysfunctions, are unable to provide a full picture of their condition; indeed it is more likely that their description will be coloured by their particular deficits. Hence it is important for the clinician to be able to confront the information gained from the patient with that obtained from his/her spouse or nearest relatives or friends in order to clarify the clinical picture. From the point of view of the present study it was essential that both the patient and the carer participated in the interview in stage III of the research, as both were the focus of the investigation. The carer's participation also made it possible to evaluate the information provided in terms of the carer's accuracy as a proxy informant.

In the case of neurodegenerative conditions such as PD, the clinician-interviewer is faced with meeting the demands elicited by the disease process in the form of specific difficulties encountered by the patient. These include being prepared for the fact that the interview will inevitably proceed more slowly because of both the bradykinesia and bradyphrenia associated with PD. The clinician must be prepared for numerous interruptions such as the result of the "wearing off" effects of medication, the onset of dyskinesias, sudden appearance of the "off" syndrome, the appearance of tremor and a range of other physical disturbances which may be distressing or embarrassing to the patient. In addition, some patients develop somewhat idiosyncratic ways of dealing with these problems, which may involve the assessment procedure having to be carried out in unconventional situations, such as with the patient lying on the floor. Because of the likelihood of subtle, but specific affective and cognitive deficits resulting from the illness, it is necessary to be aware of the psychological difficulties with which the patient has to struggle in order to comply with the demands of the assessment. At the same time, the clinician's sensitivity to these issues, is likely to have a deciding effect on the nature of the relationship established with the patient and his family and ultimately on the quality of the information gained.

The clinical interview and assessment procedures undertaken for the purposes of the study were tailored to the requirements for meeting the aims set out in chapter 8. Particular attention was paid to modifications that might need to be made to the assessment procedures in order to accommodate patients' limitations resulting from the nature of PD.

Patients and their carers were both interviewed in stage III of the research programme. One purpose of the interview was to verify the information obtained from the patient's case notes, especially with regard to the onset of the illness and symptoms that had presented prior to the diagnosis being established. In view of the insidious onset of symptoms in PD this was considered important to establishing disease onset.

The psychological dialogue established with the patient was particularly important in three respects:

1. For establishing rapport in order to encourage the patient and his/her carer to engage in the assessment procedure and to allow it to be

carried out in full, in spite of its length and the lowered fatigue thresholds of the patients.

2. For creating an environment in which to carry out the assessment of cognitive functioning in patients who had not encountered this form of examination previously; many of the patients were not aware of having potential deficits in the area of neuropsychological function, nor indeed of the fact that PD carries an increased risk of such problems. It was therefore necessary to approach the neuropsychological assessment with particular sensitivity and to provide an explanation of the rationale for the procedure without causing the patient and his/her carer undue anxiety.
3. For providing encouragement to complete a detailed neuropsychiatric assessment in this sample of non-psychiatric patients, who were unlikely to have been exposed to this line of questioning previously, and for whom some of the questions were disturbing (e.g. those relating to suicidal intent).

The fact that good rapport was established overall is evidenced by the fact that only two (informal, telephone) complaints were received during the course of this research programme: one was made by a carer in respect of his wife who suffered from PD and who, for religious reasons, had been upset by being asked a question with regard to suicidal ideation in relation to the assessment of depression; this was however, quickly resolved, and the couple later happily contributed to further research. The other was from a male patient who had appeared somewhat suspicious about participating in the study, despite giving consent; his anxieties were allayed after being reassured by the Consultant Neurologist that this was in fact *bona fide* research being carried out from the local hospital.

Most patients and their carers contributed to the project with a willingness to co-operate that was remarkable. Many commented that for the first time they had been asked about symptoms that were particularly problematic, but that no-one had shown interest in before. It appeared that the psychological approach to the condition of PD found a special resonance in these cases. Carers were appreciative of the fact that their situation had been recognised and was being investigated. Patients frequently responded with a warmth and humour that facilitated the encounter and served to remind the author of the essential humanity of neuropsychology.

9.3.3 The research protocol

A research protocol was completed for each participant in the study. This consisted of a data sheet recording personal details such as age, gender, marital status, years of education, socio-economic status (as reflected in the nature of past or present employment), current employment status (working or retired), number of years in retirement and the number of people living in the same household as the respondent. Details of the person's past medical history and current medical complaints, along with prescribed medication, were also recorded.

For the index patients with PD, clinical data relating to disease and treatment variables were obtained including: estimated age at onset of the condition, duration of illness, family history of PD, number of admissions to a neurological unit and pharmacological treatment (recorded in terms of the daily dosage and the length of time for which the drugs had been prescribed and taken). Enquiries were also made into the patient's past psychiatric history and related medication, in order to exclude the possibility of psychotic illness and to identify a personal history of depressive illness. These background demographic and clinical variables were considered to be controlled independent variables, likely to exert an effect on outcomes for patients, carers and control participants respectively. An assessment was also made of the three main areas of functioning in which the illness manifests. These consisted of the motor (ratings of severity and functional disability or handicap), affective and cognitive functioning and symptoms were assessed with the aid of at least two scales covering each domain, in order to ensure that sampling of patient-related variables was as representative as possible. Patients were interviewed, as far as possible, in the "on" state as regards medication.

Carers of the patients with PD also completed a detailed protocol designed to cover as many of the aspects of care-giving as was practical. In this part of the study, the main independent variable was defined as being actively engaged in caring for a spouse with PD and it was assumed that the hardships and strain of care-giving were, to a significant extent, likely to be shaped by illness-related variables, including the physical, affective and cognitive symptoms of PD. Carers were assessed for levels of strain as a result of their involvement in care-giving and for different aspects of psychological morbidity in the form of anxiety, minor cognitive failures and depression, including the possibility of psychiatric "caseness". In the model of caring tested in the presented study, the strain related to care-giving was conceptualised as being the result of a subjective appraisal of the care-giving situation by the carer. Care-giving strain was thus treated as both an outcome variable for the carer, and as a primary stressor (independent variable) determining carer outcomes in terms of psychopathology. Carers also provided an evaluation of their marital relationship with the care-recipient and their own assessment of the patient's psychological functioning in the area of cognition and mood, appraisals which were conceptualised as mediating the relationships among variables in the care-giving process.

9.3.3.1 Assessment of physical symptoms

The physical aspects of PD symptomatology were examined using established scales emphasizing different aspects of the motor and autonomic impairment as well as the functional consequences of these symptoms.

In stages I-III of the research study, the severity of motor symptoms in the PD patients was assessed by the author[1] using:

1. The Hoehn and Yahr scale (Hoehn and Yahr 1967); this is a five level-stage scale that describes disability and impairment in PD. Lower stages are indicative of better function. The scale's stages combine elements of objective signs and functional disability, and are based on two different indices of severity: unilateral vs. bilateral signs, and absence or presence of gait and balance impairments. While the strength of this mix is its ability to capture the clinical picture in an easy-to-use form, its weakness is the inability to encompass the full range of variability of symptoms observed clinically, such as that which occurs in patients with severe unilateral tremor who are functionally disabled. A recent report has recommended that the Hoehn and Yahr is useful for the demographic description of groups of patients in clinical and research settings. It is used universally as an indicator of severity. Rather than trying to rate only that part of a patient's status due directly to PD, the authors suggest a "rate what you see," approach thus incorporating the effects of comorbidity in determining the Hoehn and Yahr stage (Goetz et al. 2004).

Additionally, in stage III, the following scale of motor impairment was also used:

---

[1] The author had previously received training in the assessment of the motor and autonomic symptoms in PD.

2. The Webster Scale for motor impairment, which is specific to PD (Webster 1968); this scale was developed as a simple rating scale that can be used to evaluate the degree of impairment in PD. It is considered to be a relatively "pure" measure of the physical symptoms including motor impairment and autonomic dysfunction, consisting of nine impairment items and one disability (self-care) item. The scale applies a gross clinical rating to each of the 10 listed items (bradykinesia, rigidity, posture, upper extremity swing, gait, tremor, facies, seborrhea, speech and self-care), assigning a value rating of 0-3 for each item, where 0=no involvement and 1, 2, and 3 are equated to early, moderate, and severe disease, respectively. Scores range from 0 to 30, and lower scores represent less severe signs of PD. Values of 1 to 10 indicate early illness; 11 to 20, moderate disability; and 21 to 30, severe or advanced disease. The scale has been shown to have adequate inter-rater reliability (Geminiani et al. 1991; Ginanneschi et al. 1988).

In stages I-III, functional disability in the patients with PD was examined using:

3. The Northwestern University Disability Scale (NUDS)(Canter, de la Torre and Meier 1961); clinical experience suggests that the symptoms of PD make themselves felt most frequently in the areas of walking, personal hygiene, dressing, eating and feeding, and speaking. These five areas constitute the range of this scale. A maximum of 20 points is assigned to each of the five sub-scales, in this way a total of 100 points is possible, so that the degree of disability may be expressed as a percentage. Lower scores represent greater functional disability. The NUDS has been found to have good construct validity (Henderson et al. 1991) and the final score correlates highly with the total Webster score which is a measure of motor impairment; it also has excellent inter-rater reliability (Canter et al. 1961). The NUDS is one the most widely used, best evaluated, valid and reliable scales for the measurement of disability in PD (Ramaker et al. 2002).

In order to have a means of comparing the patients with PD and the control subjects, physical and functional abilities were assessed in all of the participants (with the exception of the patients with MDD) using the following scales for activities of daily living:

4. The Barthel Index (ADL; Mahoney and Barthel 1965); the Barthel Index is the oldest and most commonly used instrument for the assessment of physical disability in older people, though not specifically in PD. It is rated as having excellent reliability, validity, sensitivity and clinical utility (Wade and Collin 1988). It consists of ten items which are rated by the patient in terms of the amount of help needed with each. Items assess the patient's independence or otherwise in the following areas of functioning: feeding, moving from chair to bed, personal hygiene, ability to use the toilet, bathing, walking on level surfaces, use of stairs, dressing, and bowel and bladder control. They are rated as being achieved "with" or "without" help and certain items are weighted. The modified scoring method of Collin et al. (1988) was used with scores ranging from 0-20, lower scores indicating greater independence in the activities of daily living. The Barthel Index takes 5 minutes to complete (Burns, Lawlor and Craig 2004).
5. Instrumental activities of daily living (IADL; adapted from Lawton and Brody 1969); this scale is used to assess the functional ability of older people in relation to the instrumental activities of daily living involving more complex daily tasks such as use of the telephone, housekeeping, shopping, food preparation, laundry, transportation and ability to manage own medication and finances. It has excellent inter-rater reliability and validity. Scores range from 0-16, lower scores indicating greater independence in the instrumental activities of daily living. The scale takes 5 minutes to complete (Burns et al. 2004).

In addition, in stage III, functional assessment of the patients with PD included:

6. The Karnofsky Performance Status Scale (Karnofsky and Burchenal 1949; Schag, Heinrich and Ganz 1984); this index allows patients to be classified according to their functional impairment, and emphasizes physical performance and dependency, although it was not specifically designed for the assessment of PD. The Karnofsky score ranges from 100 to 0, where 100 is "perfect" health and 0 is death; patients are assigned a category by a clinician or other health-care professional. It was designed for use in clinical settings and can be used to compare the effectiveness of different therapies and to assess the prognosis in individual patients. The lower the Karnofsky score, the worse the survival for most serious illnesses. The Karnofsky scale is considered to be a "gold standard" in the measurement of functional performance

and is widely used throughout the U.S.A. and Europe. The scale may be used as a quality of life measure, although it is heavily weighted towards the physical rather than social and psychological dimensions of QOL (Bowling 1997).

7. The WHO Scale, (WHO 1980) which is a modification of the Karnofsky Performance Index; this scale assigns a grade from 0 to 4 to patients, reflecting their functional impairment, where 0 is "able to carry out all normal activities" and 4 is "completely disabled; cannot carry on any self-care; totally confined to chair or bed".

9.3.3.2 Assessment of depressive symptoms

Depressive symptomatology was measured in three ways: (1) by means of the structured clinical interview for depression (SCID; First et al. 2002) carried out by the author, in order to provide a DSM-IV-TR diagnosis of depressive disorder; (2) with the aid of the Hamilton depression scale (HAM-D), an observer-rated assessment instrument recommended for use in PD (Schrag et al. 2007) and, (3) using self-reported data from patients obtained with the aid of standardised questionnaires. The instruments used in stages I and II of the study were as follows:

1. The structured clinical interview for DSM-IV-TR Axis I disorders (SCID), which is a semi-structured interview for making the major DSM-IV-TR Axis I diagnoses. Patients with PD were classified according to whether they met DSM-IV-TR criteria for major depression or other depressive disorders.
2. The Hamilton Depression Rating Scale (HAM-D) (Hamilton 1960); this is a 21-item scale that evaluates depressed mood, vegetative and cognitive symptoms of depression, symptoms of comorbid anxiety and psychotic symptoms. The 21-item (as opposed to the 17-item) version was chosen in order to accommodate the possibility of psychotic and obsessional symptoms, sometimes present in PD. The HAM-D was one of the first rating scales developed to quantify the severity of depressive symptomatology, although the last four items do not contribute to the measurement of severity and are commonly omitted to give the 17-item version (Burns et al. 2004, 6). It has since become the most widely used and accepted outcome measure for evaluating depression severity in people of all ages, has high reliability and is frequently used as a "gold standard" for research purposes. The scale provides ratings on current DSM-IV-TR symptoms of depression, with

the exception of hypersomnia, increased appetite, concentration and loss of enjoyment or anhedonia, but these items were included in the clinical interview for the purposes of the present research. The 21-items are rated on either a 5-point (0-4) or a 3-point (0-2) scale. Cut-off points have been established for mild depression at scores of 10/11 and above, and for severe depression at scores above 17. The assessment based on the HAM-D takes 20-30 minutes to administer. Schrag et al. (2007) recently recommended that the HAM-D meets the required psychometric standards for evaluation of depression in PD.

3. The Leeds Scales (for the self-assessment of anxiety and depression (Snaith, Bridge and Hamilton 1976) were designed as self-rating scales to mirror the Hamilton Depression Scale and the Hamilton Anxiety Scale (HAM-A, also described in this section), and were validated against these scales. A number of items are modified from the Zung (1965). They are considered to have diagnostic potential in the sense of distinguishing between anxiety and depressive disorders (Snaith et al. 1976). Although not especially designed for use with older people or for assessment in comorbid physical illness, these scales were considered particularly suitable for use in the present study for two reasons: firstly, because they were derived from the HAM-D and the HAM-A, they provide a means of comparing clinician ratings of depression against these self-report measures in the same patients, and secondly because the authors emphasize that the items were selected in order that they might be used with any age group (hence the omission of items such as loss of libido, which coincidentally, are confounded with the symptoms of PD).

   The scales consist of 22 statements which the patient is asked to rate on a four point scale, as "definitely" occurring (3) to not at all (0). Items for anxiety and depression are randomly intermingled throughout the scale and statements are designed to cover the somatic, cognitive and behavioural features of the disorders. An example of a statement measuring symptoms in the domain of anxiety is: " I feel scared or frightened" and of depression: "I feel miserable and sad". In order to reduce the influence of response set, the scoring for items 2,5, 7 and 13 is reversed. The minimum score is zero and the maximum, 66, (for both scales together), higher scores being indicative of a greater likelihood of depressive and anxiety disorders. Depression and anxiety subscales have been derived, each of which have a cut-off score of 7 or more (Forrest and Berg 1982). The present study also used the score obtained for the depression and anxiety scales jointly as the index of performance in statistical analysis, as appropriate.

4. The Addenbrooke's depression questionnaire (ADQ), which is a new instrument, especially designed for the purposes of this study. It was specifically constructed for the assessment of depression in people with PD, bearing in mind the limitations of existing scales, that have been discussed in chapter 3. The rationale for, and the procedures involved in the development of the instrument are discussed in more detail in section 9.4. below. The final version consisted of 14 items selected to represent the affective, cognitive, behavioural and to a very limited extent, somatic domains of depression, but it was attempted to phrase them in such a way as to avoid confounding with the physical symptoms of PD. They included: low mood, crying, diminished feelings for other people, inability to maintain interest in and enjoy previous activities (anhedonia), worried preoccupation, concentration difficulties, self-blame and guilt, pessimism regarding the future, suicidal ideation, health concerns, appetite loss, sleep disturbance (initial insomnia and early morning wakening) and diurnal variation. The range of possible scores is from 14 to 56, with higher scores indicating more severe depression. The questionnaire takes 10-15 minutes to complete.

The following self-rating scale was used in stage III of the research for both PD patients and their carers:

5. The Geriatric Depression Scale (GDS; Yesavage et al. 1983), which is a brief 30-item self-report assessment instrument designed specifically to identify depression in the elderly. It is designed to be simple to administer and unlike the HAM-D, does not require the skills of a trained interviewer. Participants are asked to respond by answering 'yes' or 'no' in reference to statements about how they have felt over the past week. The straightforward forced choice between the two possibilities makes the task cognitively simpler and easier to complete than scales using response sets with a greater number of categories. One point is assigned to each answer in which the subject endorses a symptom of depression. A cut off score of 10/11 is the threshold for mild depression and scores of 20 or above are indicative of moderate to severe depression. The maximum score is 30. The GDS was considered to be a particularly appropriate instrument in this research, as it was devised to avoid items tapping physically related features of depression which could be confounded with the features of other disorders, such as PD or stroke, commonly experienced by older people. It has been tested and used extensively with older people, in whom it has been shown to be able to discriminate among normal and

mildly and severely depressed individuals. It is considered to be the "gold standard" for the assessment of depression in older people (Burns et al. 2004).

Additionally, in stage III, anxiety was measured on the basis of a structured clinical interview, using clinician-observed ratings on the:

6. Hamilton Anxiety Scale, (HAM-A; Hamilton 1959); this widely used interview scale measures the severity of a patient's anxiety, based on 14 parameters, including anxious mood, tension, fears, insomnia, somatic complaints and behaviour at the interview. Seven of the items are specifically in relation to psychic anxiety and the remaining seven items focus on somatic anxiety. For example, the third item specifically addresses fears related to anxiety, the fifth item, insomnia and sleeping difficulties, and the tenth item addresses respiratory symptoms. According to Hamilton (1959), examples of psychic symptoms (mental agitation and psychological distress) elicited by the HAM-A interview include a generally anxious mood, heightened fears, feelings of tension, and difficulty concentrating. Examples of somatic symptoms (physical complaints related to anxiety) include muscular pain, feelings of weakness, cardiovascular problems, and restlessness. Each of the 14 items is assigned a score from zero (not present) to four (severe). The total anxiety score ranges from 0 to 56. A psychic anxiety score (based on the psychic items) is derived, ranging from 0 to 28 as is a somatic anxiety score (based on somatic items) with the same range of scores. The HAM-A is widely used because reliability studies have shown that it measures anxiety symptoms in a consistent way and research has also confirmed the validity of the scale (Maier et al. 1988). There is also support for its use with older adults. The scale predates the current definition of generalized anxiety disorder (GAD); however, it covers many of the features of GAD and can also be helpful in assessing its severity. It takes 15-20 minutes to complete the interview and scoring. Relatively little attention has been given to anxiety in PD, but the HAM-A has been used to measure anxiety in PD in a number of previous studies, although its psychometric properties in this population are not known (Leentjens et al. 2008).

9.3.3.3 Assessment of cognitive dysfunction

In a study of this kind, which is concerned with evaluating specific aspects of the neuropsychological and neuropsychiatric symptoms in PD and their effects on the care-giving process, it would be impossible to include an in-depth assessment of all the cognitive functions that might be impaired in PD. The aim in selecting appropriate measures for the study was to focus on representative functions that are acknowledged as giving rise to the characteristic cognitive deficits of PD. Memory (verbal free recall) and visuospatial functions were chosen; an estimate of pre-morbid intelligence for the patients was also derived, significantly lowered scores, serving as an indicator of dementia.

The tests used in stages II and III of the study were:

1. The Schonell Graded Word Reading Test, which is reported to correlate with premorbid levels of intelligence and to be more sensitive at the lower ranges, (Nelson and McKenna 1975); the patients' task was to read the words included in the test, which were progressively graded from less to more difficult to read, in English. The final (error) score was represented by the number of words incorrectly read. There is an algorithm for converting the score to an estimate of pre-morbid IQ: the present study used the raw error score for the analyses. The test also served as a screening measure for dementia.
2. A Free Recall Test of immediate memory for words (Miller 1971). Patients received auditory presentation of 10 lists, each of 12 common, monosyllabic English words. At the end of each list, they were required to recall as many words as they could from that list in any order. The score was the total number of words correctly recalled; a cut-off point for impairment has been established at 30 words correctly recalled across all lists (Miller 1971).
3. The Benton Spatial Relations Test, (adapted from Benton, Hannay and Varney 1975). Patients were presented with a target card on which lines of equal length, numbered 1-11 were drawn in an arrangement resembling the rays of the sun against a flat horizon. The vertical line, occurring in the middle of the arrangement was numbered 6; to its left were equally spaced, angled lines, numbered 1 to 5 with line No 1 placed in a horizontal position. Lines 7 to 11 were arranged in similar symmetrical fashion to the right of the vertical, with line No 11 placed horizontally. The stimulus cards contained two lines placed in two of the orientations represented on the target card, but of shorter length. The patients' task was to identify these orientations by assigning them the numbers from the positions on the target card. There was a total of fourteen stimulus cards, giving rise to two responses; the score was the

total number of errors (possible range from zero to twenty-eight) and the cut-off for impairment was 8 errors.

9.3.3.4 Carer-related assessment

Carers were formally assessed only in stage III of the study. Information was obtained covering the following areas:

1. Carers' experience of strain was evaluated using the Machin Strain Scale (MSS; Machin 1980); carers were asked to answer 13 questions dealing with situations that may occur in the course of care-giving and are considered likely to cause increased strain for the carer. Items are intended to reflect the emotional (e.g. "Do you ever get depressed about the situation?") and social distress (e.g. "Do you ever feel embarrassed by your spouse in any way?") that carers may experience, as well as concerns they may have in relation to changes in the care recipient's behaviour (e.g. "Do you fear accidents or dangers concerning your spouse (e.g. fire, gas, falling over)?" and other factors that may have had a detrimental effect on their daily lives (e.g. "Has your household routine/standard of living been affected in any way due to the necessity of caring for your spouse?"). These were rated according to their frequency of occurrence from "never" (score 0) to "a great deal of the time" (score 2). One item, concerning pleasure derived from care-giving, required reverse scoring. The maximum possible score is 26 and the scale takes between five to ten minutes to complete. Higher scores indicate greater levels of perceived strain on the part of the carer. The version of the scale used was that provided by Gilleard (1984a) in which responses were reduced from 5 to 3 options and some items deleted (Gilleard 1984a, 123). Other versions also exist, which have been adapted under the name of the "Relatives' Strain Scale" (Greene et al. 1982). The scale has good internal consistency and established construct validity (Van Durme et al. 2012).
2. The General Health Questionnaire (GHQ; Goldberg and Hillier 1979) has established a place for itself in old age psychiatry as a measure of carer burden (Burns, Lawlor and Craig 2002). It is a self-administered screening instrument developed for the detection of psychiatric morbidity in community settings and with non-psychiatric populations, which focuses on two major areas of psychopathology – the inability to carry out normal functions and the appearance of new and distressing psychological phenomena (Goldberg and Williams 1988). It is not usually employed as a screening instrument with older people, but has

been used as a measure of psychological distress and psychiatric morbidity in carers of people with dementia (Marriott et al. 2000) and shown to be sensitive to change under these conditions. The 30-item version used in the present study consists of items tapping the cognitive and behavioural symptoms of depression and anxiety; it was developed from the GHQ-60 by removing all questions related to somatic symptoms and so is of particular value in the assessment of older people. It is the most widely validated version and is recommended as a screening tool for detecting caseness. The 30 items are rated according to a four point scale which describes the occurrence of the item being probed, at different levels, e.g.: "not at all", "no more than usual", "rather more than usual" or "much more than usual". In order to reduce the influence of response set, half of the items are illness statements, e.g. "have you recently lost much sleep over worry?" and half are positive health statements, e.g. "have you recently felt that you are playing a useful part in things?".

The GHQ-30 yields only an overall score, the minimum being zero and the maximum 30, for the GHQ scoring method employed in this study, with a threshold score of 4/5 for determining probable "caseness" (GHQ manual; Goldberg 1978). Higher scores are indicative of a greater likelihood of depressive and anxiety disorders.

3. The 30-item version of the Geriatric Depression Scale, (GDS; Yesavage et al. 1983) was used as a screening measure of depression for the carers. Details of the scale have been given above in connection with assessment of the care recipient.
4. The Beck Depression Inventory (BDI; Beck et al. 1961) is not a scale specifically designed for older people, but has gained extremely widespread use. It is a gold standard for self-rated depression scales and has frequently been used for assessing depression in carers of people with dementia (Burns et al. 2004) and in the carers of people with PD (e.g. Schrag et al. 2006). The BDI is a 21 item scale designed to measure the severity of depressive symptoms. The items are designed to assess feelings of sadness, concerns about the future, suicidal ideation, tearfulness, sleep disturbance, fatigue, interests, worries about health, sexual interest, appetite, weight loss and general enjoyment. Each item consists of a series of statements which are scored 0-3 and denote increasing severity. The carer's task was to read the group of statements associated with each item and to pick the one that best describes the way that they had felt over the preceding week. The final score, used as an index of performance on this scale, is the sum of the scores obtained on the individual items. Scores range from

0-63, with higher scores indicating greater levels of depression. A total score from 0-9 denotes the absence of depression and scores of 10-18 indicate mild to moderate, scores of 19-29, moderate to severe and scores of 30-63, severe depression. The BDI has excellent external consistency and validity as measured against independent clinical ratings made by psychiatrists (Beck et al. 1961). Some authors (Burns et al. 2004) recommend a general cut-off score of 12/13 to indicate the presence of depression.

5. An evaluation of the carer's marital relationship with his/her spouse (the care recipient) was made using the Marital Adjustment Scale (Locke and Wallace 1959); the carer was asked to rate the degree of happiness of his/her present marriage on a visual analogue scale, where a score of 0 represented "very unhappy", a score of 15 was "happy" and a score of 35 represented "perfectly happy". The carer was then asked to rate his/her perceived agreement with his/her partner on eight questions related to matters such as handling family finances, matters of recreation, demonstrations of affection, friends, sex relations, conventionality, outlook on life and ways of dealing with in-laws. These were assessed on a six-point scale from "always agree" to "always disagree". The remaining six questions required the carer to report on items relating to how disagreements between the couple are resolved, the extent to which they engage in outside interests together, confide in their spouse and a hypothetical question about whether they would choose to marry the same person, if they were able to live their lives again. The scoring system is weighted for the items related to intimacy and possible scores range from 2-158, with higher scores indicating greater levels of satisfaction with the marital relationship. The instrument has been widely used in marital therapy and research to distinguish distressed from non-distressed couples, and a cut-off score of 100 is recommended for these purposes (e.g. Birchler and Webb 1977; Williams 1979; Crane et al. 1990; Whiting and Crane 2003). It has good reliability (Locke and Wallace 1959) and validity (Gottman 1979), being a self-report measure for marital adjustment whose psychometric properties have been most extensively examined in the literature (Cohen 1985).
6. The carer's perception of his or her own cognitive status was assessed using a meta-memory evaluation in the form of the "Cognitive Failures Questionnaire" (CFQ; Broadbent et al. 1982). Cognitive failures are defined as cognitive-based mistakes on simple tasks that a person would normally be capable of completing without error (Martin 1983). The CFQ was designed as a self-report measure of failures in

perception, memory and motor lapses in everyday life. It consists of 25 items relating to minor mistakes which are commonly made by normal people, but which allegedly increase in frequency as individuals become more stressed (Wagle, Berrios and Ho 1999). The items included questions of the following kind: "do you read something and find you haven't been thinking about it and must read it again?" or "do you have trouble making up your mind?". Responses rated frequency of occurrence on a five point Likert scale from "never=0" to "very often=4". The minimum score was zero and the maximum score 100. The questionnaire takes about 10 minutes to complete. Its putative ecological validity is considered to be a major clinical advantage.

9.3.3.5 Carer's assessment of psychological functioning in the care-recipient

7. The carer was also asked to provide an assessment of the care-recipient's psychological function over the previous six months with the aid of a scale related to the Cognitive Failures Questionnaire and especially designed to provide such proxy measurements: the Cognitive Failures Questionnaire-for-Others (CFQ-Other; Broadbent et al. 1982). The questions tapped both cognitive function e.g. "during the last six months has your partner seemed to be: finding it difficult to concentrate on anything because his/her attention tends to wander from one thing to another?" and mood e.g. "low in spirits, sad or depressed, without there being a specific reason e.g. the death of someone very close?" This scale provided a score for the carer's perception of both cognitive (perceived cognitive) and affective (perceived affective) functioning in the care-recipient.

9.3.3.6 Methods of assessment for the control participants

A standard protocol was administered to all control participants from both the clinical (MDD) and non-clinical samples consisting of healthy age-matched control subjects and those with mobility problems. This consisted of a data sheet recording personal details such as age, gender, marital status, nature of past or present employment, current employment status (working or retired) and details of the person's past medical history and current medical complaints. The control subjects were evaluated using the same instruments as the patients with PD, but the choice of scales was tailored to the specific purposes served by the relevant control group.

Patients with MDD underwent a structured interview with the aid of the SCID, in order to verify their diagnosis. Their symptoms were also rated on the HAM-D and they completed the Leeds scales for the assessment of anxiety and depression and the ADQ.

Apart from the patients with a diagnosis of MDD, all control subjects were screened for the so-called "geriatric giants" (Isaacs 1992) which include: falls, a deterioration in mobility, memory and control of bladder and bowels, behavioural disturbances and any other significant deterioration in health requiring medical attention. They also completed the Barthel Index for the activities of daily living (ADL; Mahoney and Barthel 1965) and the instrumental activities of daily living (IADL; Lawton and Brody 1969). In addition, they completed the self-report measures of depression, consisting of the Leeds scales, the GDS and the ADQ; with a few exceptions, they were also rated on the HAM-D.

In the interests of clarity, the clinical and non-clinical samples and the type of assessment procedures which they completed are presented in table 9-1.

Table 9-1. Study design and measures used to operationalise constructs of interest.

Clinical variables			
Measures:	Physical impairment	Affective impairment	Cognitive impairment
Stage I Groups	Measures used: indices of performance are scale scores		
PD 1 (N=97)	*Motor*: H&Y *Functional:* NUDS; ADL; IADL	ADQ Leeds scales GDS	---
PD 2 (N=60)	*Motor:* H&Y *Functional:* NUDS; ADL; IADL	DSM-IV-TR HAM-D; ADQ Leeds scales	---
MDD controls (N=40)	---	DSM-IV-TR HAM-D; ADQ Leeds scales	---
Low mobility controls (N=27)	ADL; IADL	HAM-D ADQ; GDS	---
Healthy controls (N=30)	ADL; IADL	HAM-D ADQ; GDS	---
Stage II Groups	Independent variables	Dependent variables	Dependent variables
PD 2 (N=60)	*Motor:* H&Y *Functional:* NUDS; ADL; IADL	HAM-D ADQ Leeds scales	Free recall test Benton test Schonell test

Stage III Groups	Independent variables		
PD 3 (N=75)	*Motor:* H&Y; Webster *Functional:*NUDS; WHO; Karnofsky; ADL; IADL	HAM-D HAM-A GDS	Free recall test Benton test Schonell test
Stage III Groups	Independent variables	Mediating variables	Dependent variables
Carers (N=75)	PD illness-related variables	MSS CFQ-Others MAS	GHQ; BDI GDS CFQ-Self

MDD–hospitalized patients with major depressive disorder; H&Y–Hoehn & Yahr scale; NUDS–Northwestern University Disability Scale; ADL–Activities of daily living; IADL–Instrumental activities of daily living; ADQ–Addenbrooke's Depression Questionnaire; GDS–Geriatric Depression Scale; HAM-D–Hamilton Depression Scale; HAM-A–Hamilton Anxiety Scale BDI–Beck Depression Inventory; MSS–Machin Strain Scale; MAS–Marital Adjustment Scale; CFQ–Cognitive Failures Questionnaire (for self or others).

9.4 Stage I: procedures

In order to answer the research questions surrounding the nature of the affective disorder in PD, specified as questions 1.1 to 1.4 (see section 8.6) it was first necessary to construct a new instrument for the measurement of depression in PD and to establish its psychometric properties (1.1). This was accomplished in the initial phase of the research in stage I. The instrument was then used to estimate the prevalence of depression in PD in comparison to the other scales used (1.2), to compare the profiles of depressive symptoms in PD and MDD using item analysis (1.3) and to determine the consistency of responding among patients with PD and MDD (1.4).

Stage I of the research was thus focused around the development and testing of the Addenbrooke's Depression Questionnaire (ADQ), which was especially designed for the purposes outlined above. It was specifically constructed for the assessment of depression in people with PD, bearing in mind the limitations of existing scales, that have been discussed in chapter 3.

The ADQ was designed with three main aims in mind. The first of these was to overcome the problems of overlapping somatic symptoms occurring in both affective disorders and PD, hence the items chosen to be representative of depressive symptomatology were carefully selected to avoid this possibility. The second aim was to take account of the fact that, many older people may endorse items (such as withdrawal from social activities) on established depression scales, for reasons other than being depressed. The third was to provide a means of determining patients' levels of consistency (reliability) in responding to the items of which the questionnaire is composed. Stage I of the research was divided into three phases: (i) development of the questionnaire, (ii) its validation, and (iii) its use to test specific hypotheses regarding depression in PD.

9.4.1 Questionnaire development

The questionnaire was constructed according to a methodology described by Shapiro (1961). The technique consists of an ideographic approach, which Shapiro called the "Personal Questionnaire", and was designed as a means of monitoring an individual patient's symptoms over time, forming part of a whole family of techniques based upon the same principles (see Miller and Morley 1986). The technique used in the present study was adapted from Shapiro's original version of the Personal Questionnaire and the author is indebted to Professor Edgar Miller (personal communication) for drawing attention to the particular advantages of this method as a means of exploring aspects of the depressive disorder seen in PD.

Shapiro's (1961) original approach was to start with a structured interview covering most aspects of psychopathology. From this he derived a set of "illness statements" which consist of things actually said by the patient, describing his/her subjective feelings about the problem. In cases of depression, these might be something like: "I sometimes feel low and sad" or "I often feel that I have done something wrong" (Miller and Morley 1986, 74). The procedure typically yields fifteen to twenty statements of this kind, but there is no definitive rule to guide this extraction. The aim is to obtain a set of statements that adequately represent the range of the patient's problems and the actual number of statements needed to do this may be quite variable. There is no algorithm to determine the adequacy of the statements and the decision is based on clinical judgement. The main advantage of this approach is that it allows an individual and subjective approach to a patient's symptoms (enabling them to be scaled for severity) and provides a means of monitoring change in symptoms over time. As Miller and Morley (1986, 73) point out: "... it is useful to have some form of scale that can be used to measure the individual subject's own particular symptoms or worries."

However, whilst the original approach represented by the Personal Questionnaire is valuable in single-case research and routine clinical practice, it has clear limitations which make it unsuitable for use with groups of subjects without essential modification. The main adaptation to the technique applied in the present study was in the selection of items for the instrument and in the formulation of the illness statements. These were not derived, as in Shapiro's (1961) original work, from individual patients and were thus not personalised in the same way as in the original version of the questionnaire.

The areas of depressive symptomatology included in the questionnaire were selected on the basis of DSM-IV-TR criteria for a diagnosis of major depression (MDD), on clinical experience of patients with PD and MDD and against a background of knowledge derived from the literature on depression in PD. They were chosen to represent the affective, cognitive, behavioural and to a limited extent, somatic domains of depression. Initially twelve areas of symptomatology were tapped, including: low mood, crying, diminished feelings for other people, inability to maintain interest in and enjoy activities (anhedonia), worried preoccupation, concentration difficulties, self-blame and guilt, pessimism regarding the future, suicidal ideation, appetite loss, sleep disturbance and diurnal variation. A set of three illness statements was then prepared for each of the twelve symptom areas; these were formulated so as to provide a gradation in the level of severity with which symptoms occurred. Thus, one statement reflected absence of the symptom, whilst a second was associated with intermediate, and a third with high levels of endorsement of the symptom in question. The intermediate statement is intended to represent a mid-point on a subjective scale between the two extremes of a given symptom, such as low mood, and represented in the other two statements. For example:

A) I feel low and sad a lot of the time (high symptom intensity).
B) I sometimes feel low and sad (intermediate symptom intensity).
C) I do not feel low or sad (absence of symptom).

The same procedure was followed in order to create illness statements for the other symptom areas. In formulating the statements, effort was taken to phrase them in such a way as to avoid confounding with the physical symptoms of PD.

Having arrived at the three illness statements for each of the twelve symptom areas, it was possible to construct the final version of the questionnaire. Each illness statement, in combination with one other from the same symptom category, formed the basis for a binary choice item on the questionnaire. The pair of statements thus differed only with respect to the severity of the symptom that they probed. The three statements for each symptom category yield three possible arrangements of the paired statement combinations: high levels with intermediate levels of symptomatology (A with B); intermediate levels with the absence of symptoms (B with C); and high symptom levels with symptom absence (A and C). Each pair of statements was printed on cards, with one statement appearing above the other as shown in figure 9-1.

The order of the statements on the cards was randomised and balanced so that the stronger and weaker versions occurred in the upper and lower positions with equal frequency. This procedure was applied to all 12 items so that a total of 36 cards (12x3) containing the pairs of statements was generated. The cards were then shuffled to provide a random order of presentation for individual patients. The patient's task was to select one of the pair of statements, which s/he felt best described her/his current situation. Patients were instructed, that on occasions when they felt that neither statement applied to them, they should *reject* the most unsuitable one and *accept* the least unsuitable.

Figure 9-1. Sample card from the Addenbrooke's Depression Questionnaire showing layout of statements C & A for mood symptoms.

I do not feel low or sad I feel low and sad a lot of the time

Patients sorted the cards into two separate piles according to whether it was the "top" statement on the card or the "bottom" statement that best described how they were feeling. Their decisions (36 in all) were recorded and scored according to a four-point scale, on which a higher score indicated greater severity of symptoms. A total score could also be derived by adding the scores from each item; the range of possible scores was from 12 to 48. The task of sorting the cards took 15-20 minutes to complete.

A major advantage of this technique is that it contains an in-built system for monitoring the consistency of the patient's responses – a form of reliability known as internal consistency. The three cards from each item on the questionnaire can be sorted in eight possible ways as shown in table 9-2, of which four (response patterns i-iv) are consistent with each other (in normal type) and four (response patterns v-viii) are inconsistent (in bold type). Patients' responses are consistent when their choices are made in a systematic way e.g. someone with severe depression always choosing the statement reflecting high levels of low mood in preference to the intermediate one, and the intermediate level rather than the statement associated with absence of low mood, such that A>B>C. Inconsistent responses occur when this hierarchy of severity is not preserved in the response pattern. Nevertheless, final and hence total scores in cases of inconsistent responding may still be calculated as the inconsistent patterns of responses may be converted to the best approximation for a logical pattern of responses, as shown for response patterns v-viii in table 9-2.

Table 9-2. The scoring system for responses to the ADQ.

	Statement combinations appearing on cards			
Pattern of statements selected	A/B	B/C	A/C	score
(i)	B	C	C	1
(ii)	B	B	C	2
(iii)	B	B	A	3
(iv)	A	B	A	4
(v)	**A**	**C**	**C**	1
(vi)	**B**	**C**	**A**	2
(vii)	**A**	**B**	**C**	3
(viii)	**A**	**C**	**A**	4

Note: inconsistent response patterns are shown in bold type.

Patterns of inconsistent responding were of special interest to this study and thus the special feature of this methodology, which allowed them to be evaluated was especially attractive and useful in helping to answer the research question relating to the consistency of patients' response patterns on depression tests. Although it is recognised that a common feature of the clinical picture in depression is patients' tendency to show inconsistencies in their response patterns when describing their symptoms, little is known in this respect as regards patients with PD. In attempting to provide a fuller description of the nature of depression in PD, it was considered important to determine the extent to which PD patients resemble those with a MDD with regard to these features of the clinical presentation in PD.

However, response consistency may also be a feature of the procedures used in the assessment of depressive symptoms (i.e. the distance between items may have been inappropriately scaled by the constructor of the questionnaire – in this case the author) giving the instrument low internal consistency. It is possible to identify such deficits in the wording of statements during pilot trials and to make appropriate adjustments in order to achieve the correct relationships among the statements, thus improving the internal consistency of the measure. Experience with this methodology in the form of the Personal Questionnaire (Shapiro 1961) shows that inconsistent patterns of responses are very low (of the order of 2%-3% and even less) which suggests that the task is a meaningful one and does not cause patients undue difficulties (Miller and Morley 1986). However, in order to ensure that any potential differences in the consistency of response patterns in the present study were not due to the poor internal consistency of the questionnaire, its performance in this regard was also tested with a control group of age-matched (with respect to the PD sample), normal, healthy subjects.

Before turning to an analysis of these results however it is necessary to mention that initial piloting of the ADQ in four patients with PD, not included in the main study, revealed that two further items might usefully be added to the instrument. The first of these was related to sleep: patients' responses made it evident that it would be helpful to distinguish problems of initial insomnia from early morning wakening, and as this has established validity in the phenomenology of depressive symptoms, a distinction of this kind was introduced with the elimination of a general sleep item in favour of two separate items relating to these two aspects of sleep disturbance. The second item added at this stage was that of exacerbated concerns with health (hypochondriasis). It had originally not been included because of difficulties in choosing appropriate wording that would differentiate this symptom from the somatic symptoms of PD. However, the item was eventually worded in such a way (it was felt) as to avoid this confusion. This was achieved by weighting the question towards the possibility of having a serious illness that had not yet been detected, rather than incidental somatic symptoms, which in any case would be difficult to accommodate in a questionnaire of this kind.

The final questionnaire therefore consisted of fourteen items including (additionally) initial insomnia, early morning wakening and undetermined health concerns. This resulted in a total of 42 cards to be sorted (14x3) and a possible total score in the range between 14 and 56. It did not take significantly longer to complete than the shorter 12-item version. Although the card version of the questionnaire is convenient to use in face to face interviews with clinical samples, an alternative version consisting of binary forced choice options in the form of a more traditional questionnaire was also created for use with people who were not available to be interviewed. In this case, the 42 pairs of statements were written on paper, with one statement above the other, as in the original card version. Respondents were similarly asked to choose the statement which best applied to them. Appropriate instructions were included for the task.

The ADQ was then subjected to a series of psychometric evaluations in order to establish its properties in terms of reliability and validity for use in patients with PD. These are described in the following section on the validation of the ADQ.

9.4.2 Validation Procedure

All the patients in the MDD and PD2 groups underwent a standardised clinical interview based on the depression section of the Structured Clinical Interview for DSM-IV-TR (SCID; First et al. 2002) for the purposes of establishing a DSM-IV-TR diagnosis of major depressive disorder and severity of depression was assessed using the HAM-D. Patients were diagnosed as having MDD if they had at least one core symptom (i.e. depressed mood or anhedonia) and at least four other symptoms of depression that had lasted at least two weeks. In the case of the psychiatric in-patients with MDD this was essentially a verification of the diagnosis made on admission to hospital by the psychiatric team. In two patients the original diagnosis of MDD was not confirmed at the time of examination because their symptoms had resolved sufficiently to suggest that they were in remission. Nonetheless, because of the original diagnosis and their continued hospitalisation, they were still included in the study. Additionally, for the PD patients, a diagnosis of "minor depression" was made if patients had at least one core symptom and at least two, but fewer than five symptoms of depression in total, as defined in DSM-IV-TR. All interviews were carried out by the author who was trained in the use of these instruments. The patients also completed the Leeds anxiety and depression scales and the ADQ in the same session, along with other items in the extended protocol which formed part of the larger study reported in this volume.

In order to determine whether the scores on the ADQ were biased by errors or inconsistent patterns of responding, internal consistency, as measured by Cronbach's alpha was computed for both clinical and control samples. The split half reliability for the ADQ was also calculated.

To assess the optimum cut-off points for the PD sample, receiver operating characteristic curves were plotted for the scales used. The "area under the curve" (AUC) was calculated as a measure of overall accuracy of the scale. Additionally the positive predictive value and the negative predictive value were calculated for different cut-off scores in the central range of these scales (Baird and Noma 1978).

As might have been expected, a number of patients and control subjects reported difficulties in completing the self-rating scales for depression. For those patients (PD and MDD) who received a full clinical interview, inevitably contact with the interviewer, meant that they were able to seek clarification and additional explanations about filling in items on the scales. Although the interviewer attempted not to influence patients' decisions, in a clinical setting it is impossible not to offer advice when asked to do so, and difficult to refrain from encouraging patients to complete all items on the scales. It is thus likely that the interviewer's presence may have led to higher completion rates in the two clinical samples compared to the other groups. From the point of view of the hypotheses tested in this study, however, this bias is unlikely to render the interpretation of results invalid, as the main comparisons are made between the PD and MDD groups, who were treated in the same way and thus not open to differential influences.

Examination of responses in PD3 and the two normal control groups (low mobility and healthy groups) revealed that greatest difficulty on the ADQ arose with respect to having to make a choice between two items, each of which the respondents considered to be untrue in terms of describing their situation. The cognitive complexity of the choice under these circumstance is greater than for other, more straightforward choices, and requires that the respondent adhere closely to the instructions, placing an additional load on memory and understanding what to do under potentially confusing circumstances. In the PD and MDD groups, the presence of the interviewer served to clarify and remind the respondents of the instructions for the questionnaire, which stated that in such circumstances, the least inappropriate statement should be selected. However, it is apparent from the responses, that a number of subjects who were not interviewed, found the dissonance in being required to "accept" a statement that was not true for them, unacceptable and they left these items blank. This was especially so, for the statements regarding suicidal intent, where both were considered untrue; for example, the statement combinations: "I do not want to live any longer"- (C) and "I sometimes feel as if I do not want to live any longer"- (B) were among those that respondents were frequently unable to accept in either form. Such responses were scored "B" as it was evident that the respondents were rejecting both statements; indeed they frequently annotated these items to say that neither was true. It is also possible that these choices were more difficult for non-depressed subjects, who may have never experienced thoughts or feelings of this kind and thus find the task particularly inappropriate. The majority of blank responses were left in relation to this pair of statements on suicide intent and may reflect a different quality for this item in relation to others on the scale. Questioning patients and (all the more so) controls about suicidal intent requires very delicate handling, as it is a highly emotive subject, about which many people, especially the elderly, may be extremely sensitive for personal, moral and religious reasons. It is clearly easier in an interview, once rapport has been established, to put the patient at ease in this respect. Overall, if respondents did not reply to more than 80% of the items on a scale, their questionnaires were discarded. This resulted in the replies from 3 (5.3%) control subjects being excluded from the study.

9.4.3 Psychometric properties of the ADQ

In the development of the ADQ, item means and standard deviations were used to measure the relevance of the candidate items to the underlying construct of depression in PD, for which the questionnaire was designed. Item means and standard deviations were also used to determine whether adequate variability and symmetry in score distribution were achieved in the questionnaire.

9.4.3.1 Reliability estimates for the questionnaire

In order to rely on the measurement performance of the ADQ, the psychometric properties of the instrument need to be established. Specifically, it is necessary to determine the reliability of the questionnaire in terms of its internal consistency. Internal consistency is a measure of the extent to which the items within the ADQ are measuring the same characteristic, i.e. depression. However, Clark and Watson (1995) recommend that internal consistency as determined by alpha, should be viewed as a necessary, though insufficient condition for determining the homogeneity or unidimensionality of items on a scale and suggest that the average inter-item correlation is a better index of internal consistency. Inter-item correlations were thus examined against their recommended criterion range of 0.15 to 0.50.

The split-half reliability for the instrument was also calculated as a means of establishing whether the instrument has adequate consistency across items in measuring the construct of depression, for which it was designed. Since reliability is a property of the scores and not of the measure itself, it is sample-dependent. The measures of reliability were therefore calculated for each of the samples separately.

9.4.3.2 Questionnaire validity

The validity of the instrument also needs to be established and in the case of an instrument to measure depression, this is best done against the gold standard of a DSM-IV diagnosis of depressive illness or a well-established scale such as the HAM-D. Since the ADQ is a self-rating measure, its properties were also compared to that of an established self-rating measure of depression, derived from the HAM-D, in the form of the Leeds scales for depression and anxiety.

Mean item and total scores and their standard deviations for the ADQ were calculated to determine variability and symmetry in score distributions, which might indicate the discriminatory power of the instrument. The assessment of the psychometric properties of the ADQ in terms of its reliability and construct validity followed the guidelines for scale development and validation of results published by Clark and Watson (1995). An item analysis was conducted and the reliability of the questionnaire was assessed by determining Cronbach's alpha, inspecting the partial alphas for each item and calculating the corrected item to total correlations. A criterion for eliminating items with a corrected item-total correlation < 0.2 was adopted.

The construct validity of the questionnaire was assessed in a number of different ways. Firstly, convergent validity for the ADQ was assessed by examining the effect sizes of correlations between the new instrument and corresponding scales for the measurement of depression. These included the Hamilton Depression Scale, the Leeds depression scale and the Geriatric Depression Scale.

Secondly, construct validity was examined by identifying underlying constructs for the parent domain, defined as "depression in PD", by an exploratory factor analysis. Principal component analysis was initially performed to identify the eigenvalues of the components to calculate the communality estimates (proportion of multivariate variance explained) of the orthogonal vectors. A cumulative communality estimate that was greater than 80% was used to determine factors to be retained. Once the number of constructs had been initially defined, the factors were rotated in order to better isolate the item loadings on the factors. Items were considered to have loaded on a factor if the factor loading was 0.40. Items were considered for deletion from the questionnaire if the item had (i) an item-to-total correlation of less than 0.20; (ii) a partial alpha that indicated that Cronbach's alpha would increase substantially if the item were deleted; and (iii) loaded on more than one factor.

Third and finally, the criterion validity of the ADQ was assessed using DSM-IV-TR criteria for major and minor depression as the gold standard. Using the principles of signal detection theory (Baird and Noma 1978), a receiver operating curve (ROC) for the ADQ was plotted against the DSM-IV-TR diagnosis for depression. Positive predictive values and negative predictive values for different cut-off scores for the questionnaire were calculated and an optimal cut-off score for distinguishing between depressed and non-depressed respondents on the ADQ was determined. The usual a priori significance level of 0.05 was established for the statistical analyses.

9.4.4 Use of the ADQ to test hypotheses concerning the depression of PD

The ADQ was specifically designed to facilitate testing of the hypothesis that the depression observed in patients with PD differs in a number of significant ways from MDD as defined by DSM-IV-TR criteria. Moreover, the differences in symptomatology are held to be qualitative and not merely quantitative, as would result from a diagnosis of minor depression. Minor depression would appear to be more prevalent in PD, but should not, in itself, give rise to a qualitatively different symptom profile. It is alleged however, that the depression of PD differs from DSM-IV-TR depressive disorders in a number of ways which have been described in Chapter 3. In order to test this hypothesis, the characteristic presentation of the depression of PD was compared to DSM-IV-TR depressive disorders in both quantitative and qualitative terms. Further comparisons were also made with a healthy, elderly control group and a group of older people with mobility problems not arising from intracerebral damage.

9.5 Stage II procedures

The purpose of stage II of the study was to address research questions 2.1 to 2.3 (see section 8.6) pertaining to establishing characteristic patterns of motor, affective and cognitive symptoms in PD (2.1) and attempting to delineate the relationship among the various symptom domains in order to elucidate questions relating to the continuing debate on the origin of the psychological symptoms in the disorder (2.2). It also served in an attempt to identify subgroups of patients within the sample, whose pattern of symptoms might be characterised by either affective or cognitive symptoms (2.3). Question 2.1 was answered using zero-order correlations and question 2.2 using principal component factor analysis with varimax rotation. Components with eigenvalues greater than 1.5 and variables with loadings greater than 0.4 were accepted for interpretation. Multiple regression analyses were used to devise regression equations for the dependent variables. The question of potential subgroups within the sample (2.3) was addressed with the aid of cluster analysis and discriminant function analysis was then used to obtain an equation that might classify the subjects into the subgroups identified.

9.6 Stage III procedures

As far as was practicable, the same measures were used in stage III as in stage II of the study to evaluate patient characteristics, with the following exceptions:

1. In order to ensure that adequate account was taken of all aspects of motor performance, the Webster scale, the Karnofsky Performance Status Scale and the WHO scale were added to the evaluation. As no relationship between the motor and non-motor symptoms of PD had been established in stage II, it was considered important to determine whether this might have been due to limitations in the measures of motor performance used or whether similar results might be obtained using additional measures in an independent sample of patients.
2. The measures of depression for the patient in the form of the Leeds scales and the ADQ were substituted by the GDS and the HAM-A. The reasons for this were that although the Leeds scales were designed as self-rated versions of the HAM-D and the HAM-A, many of the items tapped are redundant as they do not contribute to the subscales of depression and anxiety that are derived from the instrument. The ADQ was not used as it was an experimental instrument designed for the specific purposes of stage I of the study and its use in routine clinical practice or as a research instrument for measuring depression in PD would not be justified, because of its lack of standardisation (other than for the purposes of the present study), its relative cognitive complexity and the fact that it is somewhat tedious for patients to complete, as it is extremely repetitive. Hence both of the self-rated measures of affective disorder used in stage II were considered unduly cumbersome for the patients with PD and the measure of depression was substituted by the

GDS, and that of anxiety by the HAM-A, both of which are widely used scales in PD research.

Stage III of the study focused on an evaluation of an independent sample of people with PD (PD3) and their carers in order to answer research questions 3.1 to 3.5. (see section 8.6). Levels of care-giving strain and psychological morbidity in carers were assessed using the standardised instruments described above, and levels of depression measured against existing norms, addressing question 3.1. A factor analysis of PD patient variables using the principal component method with varimax rotation was carried out, in an attempt to replicate the findings established in stage II of the research in this independent sample of patients with PD. The aim was to determine whether the underlying structure of the data was relatively stable and reflective of the earlier established relationships among the main symptom domains of PD.

The main focus of stage III however, as defined in question 3.2, was on carer outcomes and how these might be related to the disease variables of PD. Because of the relatively large number of variables that could potentially be used as predictors of carer outcome and problems with collinearity in the data, an exploratory factor analysis was carried out using the principal components method with varimax rotation, in order to achieve groupings among the variables of interest. The resulting factors were then used as independent variables for the prediction of carer outcomes using step-wise multiple regression analyses. The possibility that specific aspects of the care-giving situation, such as the carer's perceptions of his/her spouse's psychological functioning (addressed in question 3.3) and the quality of the relationship with the care recipient (question 3.4) might modify carer outcomes was explored with the aid of statistical comparisons specifically designed to evaluate the effects of potential mediating variables (Baron and Kenny 1986). Finally, the question of the relationship between carer strain and depression outcomes (3.5) was addressed using multiple regression analyses and possibilities for mediation were evaluated with causal steps analysis. Discriminant function analysis was used to confirm that the features identified as being the most difficult aspects of the care-giving situation distinguished between depressed and non-depressed carers.

9.7 Statistical Analyses

The statistical analyses referred to above were performed using the Statistical Package for the Social Sciences (SPSS version 14.0 PL for

Windows). In all cases, the distributions of the data were inspected for normality and where the data did not conform to a normal distribution, non-parametric tests were used (Brzeziński 1996; Howell 2002). Comparisons between groups for normatively distributed data were made with the aid of the Student's t-test, for categorical data using Chi-square tests and for non-normative or nonparametric data consisting of continuous variables using Mann-Whitney tests. Where more than two groups were compared, the Kruskal-Wallis ANOVA was used. Non-parametric tests were used for most of the analyses because of the categorical nature of much of the data. In order to examine the associations between the variables, Spearman's rank correlations were obtained. All tests were two tailed. The accepted significance level was $p<0.05$, but the Bonferroni correction (Howell 2002) was applied to adjust for multiple comparisons in the correlation analyses. The *a priori* significance level of 0.05 for each set of tests was divided by the number of separate statistical tests. Specific hypothesis were tested using the forms of statistical analysis detailed in the previous section.

CHAPTER TEN

THE RESEARCH STUDY: RESULTS

10.1 Stage I: analysis of results

Stage I of the study was concerned with gaining a better understanding of the affective disorder in PD. A scale with specific properties especially designed to measure the symptoms of depression in PD was constructed and its psychometric properties evaluated. It was then used to determine whether the depression of PD differs in several important respects from MDD defined according to DSM-IV-TR criteria.

10.1.1 Descriptive statistics: demographic data for the PD samples

The demographic characteristics for the three independent patient samples suffering from idiopathic PD are presented in table 10-1. Samples PD1 and PD2 participated in stage I of the study, sample PD2 in stage II and PD3 in stage III. None of the patients took part in both stages II and III, in order to avoid the participants' responses being influenced by prior exposure to the interview questions or any of the materials used in the study. Stage I of the study was concerned with establishing the properties of the ADQ, and the results for PD2 were carried through to stage II, so that this group did not receive any additional exposure to study materials and their participation in stage I did not require additional engagement in terms of time or effort.

With the aid of the Kruskal-Wallis ANOVA,7 it was demonstrated that there were no significant differences between the three PD samples with respect to gender distribution (χ^2=2.9, df=2, p=0.23). Groups PD1 and PD2 did not differ with respect to age (Mann-Whitney U=2510.5; p=0.15), but the participants recruited to PD3 were older, reflecting the higher cut-off age of 80 in the selection criteria for the study (PD1&2 vs. PD3; Mann-Whitney U=3830.0; p=0.00). The extension of the cut-off age for

PD3 was necessitated by the difficulty in recruiting patients with carers to the research in stage III.

Table 10-1. Demographic characteristics of the PD patient samples.

Variable	Sample PD1	Sample PD2	Sample PD3
No. in sample:	N=97	N=60	N=75
Gender:	Female = 35 (36.1%) Male = 62 (63.9%)	Female = 29 (48.3%) Male = 31 (51.7%)	Female = 26 (34.7%) Male = 49 (65.3%)
Age at examination (years) mean ± SD:	62.1 ± 5.4 range: 50 - 70	63.2 ± 5.6 range: 47 - 70	66.1 ± 6.2 range: 52 - 79
Patient occupation: I Professional: lawyer, doctor II Intermediate: manager, teacher III Skilled non-manual: clerical, shop assistant IV Manual: factory worker, dressmaker V Unskilled: labourer, cleaner	I = 18 18.6% II = 21 21.6% III = 38 39.2% IV = 16 16.5% V = 4 4.1%	I = 5 8.3% II = 11 18.3% III = 16 26.7% IV = 18 30.0% V = 10 16.7%	I = 7 9.3% II = 15 20.0% III = 20 26.7% IV = 23 30.7% V = 10 13.3%
Age at retirement (years) mean ± SD: full sample: still working: women: men:	range: 45 - 70 56.3 ± 7.0 N=11 (11.3%) 50.8 ± 8.2 56.0 ± 5.5	range: 47 - 66 58.9 ± 3.8 N=9 (15.0%) 60.3 ± 1.6 57.3 ± 4.8	range: 46 - 74 59.1 ± 5.4 N=9 (12.0%) 58.6 ± 2.8 59.2 ± 6.0
No of people in household:	1 = 0 00.0% 2 = 72 74.2% 3 = 15 15.5% 4 = 5 5.2% 5 = 5 5.2%	1=13 21.7% 2+ = 47 78.3%	1 = 0 00.0% 2 = 61 81.3% 3 = 13 17.3% 5 = 1 1.3%

There were also differences between the groups with regard to socio-economic status as measured by the profession of the patient (Mann-Whitney U=1993.0; p=0.001). From table 10-1 it can be seen that there was a tendency for the participants in PD1 to be of higher socio-economic status as defined by occupation, than those in PD2. This is likely to be the result of sampling methods. PD1 were self-selected participants who had responded to an appeal to participate in the research, whereas PD2 were selected according to criteria carefully designed to be as unbiased as possible. This inequality between the two samples, however, was not considered to be an insurmountable hindrance to the research, as PD1 participated only in that part of the study used to establish the properties of the ADQ as a means of measuring depression. In view of the need to match the PD sample for severity of depressive symptoms with a sample of patients with MDD, and the difficulties of doing so using data from PD2 alone, it was considered a justifiable solution. It is unfortunately a reality of clinical research, that study participants cannot be matched with respect to all desirable criteria.

The Kruskal-Wallis ANOVA did not reveal any differences between the three PD samples with regard to age at retirement (χ^2=3.9, df=3, p=0.14). The distributions of the number of people living in the patient's household were equivalent across the samples, with the exception that PD2 also contained patients with PD living alone.

Further details of the PD samples examined, together with characteristics of the control groups and carers will be given below, as relevant to the stages of the study in which they took part. In the first instance, the development of the ADQ in stage I of the research will be presented.

10.1.2 Stage I: Development of the ADQ

10.1.2.1 Background characteristics of the samples

Table 10-2 presents the mean ages and gender distributions in the PD and normative samples studied in stage I. In addition, group size is shown, as well as the results of tests for establishing any potential differences between groups with respect to age and gender. Application of the Bonferroni correction for multiple comparisons between groups required a significance level of p=0.05/7=0.007.

Table 10-2. Background characteristics of the clinical and normative samples.

	Clinical and normative samples					
Characteristics	PD1 & PD2 (N=157)	PD1 (N=97)	PD2 (N=60)	MDD (N=40)	Low mobility controls (N=27)	Healthy controls (N=30)
Gender: Male (N)	93 (59.2%)	62 (63.9%)	31 (51.7%)	17 (42.5%)	12 (44.4%)	13 (43.3%)
Female (N)	64 (40.8%)	35 (36.1%)	29 (48.3%)	23 (57.5%)	15 (55.6%)	17 (56.7%)
K-W ANOVA	$\chi^2 = 8.34$ $df = 4$ $p = 0.08$ (NS)					
Mann-Whitney test: gender comparisons	PD1 *vs* PD2 U = 2553.5 $p = .13$ (NS)		PD1&2 *vs* MDD U = 2614.5 $p = .06$ (NS)	PD1&2 *vs* low mobility controls; U = 1806.0 $p = .15$ (NS)		MDD *vs* low mobility controls; U = 529.5 $p = .88$ (NS)
Mann-Whitney test: gender comparisons	PD1&2 *vs* healthy controls; U=1980.5 $p = .11$ (NS)		MDD *vs* healthy controls; U=595.0 $p = .94$ (NS)	Low mobility *vs* healthy controls; U = 400.5 $p = .93$ (NS)		
Age (mean years)	62.5	62.1	63.2	60.5	63.3	61.9
SD	5.5	5.4	5.6	9.7	8.2	9.0
Age range	47 - 70	50 - 70	47 - 70	39 - 78	39 - 70	47 – 79
K-W ANOVA (age)	$\chi^2 = 6.02$ $df = 4$ $p = 0.2$ (NS)					

Table 10-2 (cont'd). Background characteristics of the clinical and normative samples.

Mann-Whitney test: age comparisons	PD1 *vs* PD2 U = 2510.5 $p = .15$ (NS)		PD1&2 *vs* MDD U = 2835.5 $p = .34$ (NS)	PD1&2 *vs* low mobility controls U = 1671.00 $p = .08$ (NS)	MDD *vs* low mobility controls U = 431.00 $p = .16$ (NS)	
Mann-Whitney test: age comparisons	PD1&2 *vs* healthy controls U = 2058.0 $p = .27$ (NS)		MDD vs healthy controls U = 591.0 $p = .91$ (NS)	Low mobility *vs* healthy controls U = 337.5 $p = .28$ (NS)		
ADL (mean)	5.4	5.6	5.1	-	4.6	0.08
SD	3.3	3.1	4.1	-	5.0	0.27
range	0-18	0-18	0-16	-	0-16	0-1
Mann-Whitney test: ADL comparisons	PD1 *vs* PD2 U = 2686.0; $p = .40$ (NS)		PD1&2 *vs* low mobility controls U = 1596.0; $p = .07$ (NS)		PD1&2 *vs* healthy controls U = 843.0; $p = .00$	
IADL (mean)	4.3	4.2	4.4	-	2.8	0.04
SD	3.3	3.1	3.5	-	2.9	0.20
range	0-8	0-8	0-8	-	0-8	0-1
Mann-Whitney test: IADL comparisons	PD1 *vs* PD2 U = 2896.0; $p = .96$ (NS)		PD1&2 *vs* low mobility controls U = 1626.0; $p = .10$ (NS)		PD1&2 *vs* healthy controls U = 405.0; $p = .00$	

K-W ANOVA Kruskal-Wallis ANOVA

There were no significant differences in age or gender distribution among the groups as shown by the Kruskal-Wallis ANOVA for non-parametric distributions (χ^2=6.02, df=4, *p*=0.2 for age and χ^2=8.34, df=4, *p*=0.08 for gender). As the two groups of patients with PD were drawn from different samples, separate values are given for each subgroup: PD1 was the larger group which completed and returned the questionnaires by post; PD2 was the group of patients interviewed. Values for the combined group PD1&2 are also shown. Comparison of the characteristics of groups PD1 and PD2 did not reveal any differences in age (Mann-Whitney U= 2510.5; *p*=0.15) or gender distribution (Mann-Whitney U=2553.5; *p*=0.13) in the samples. Neither were there any differences in the planned comparisons between the PD samples and any of the control groups or among the control groups themselves, indicating that matching for age and sex had been successful across groups.

Equivalence on measures of ADL and IADL was established between the two PD groups (P1 & PD2) (for ADL, Mann-Whitney U=2686.0; *p*=0.4 and for IADL Mann-Whitney U=2896.0; *p*=0.96) and between the combined PD group and the low mobility control group (for ADL, U=1596.0; p=0.07) and (for IADL, U=1626.0; p=0.10) respectively. There was however, a significant difference between the PD groups and the healthy control group on these measures (for ADL, U=843.0; *p*=0.00 and for IADL, U= 405.0; *p*=0.00), as might be expected.

It should also be mentioned at this point, that the PD subgroups did not differ with respect to their mean total scores on the ADQ (U=2403.5; *p*=0.07), although PD1 had a slight tendency towards higher scores than PD2 (see table 10.4 below). The two PD groups were thus considered to be equivalent and all further analyses are based on the combined group, PD1&2, except where this is not possible, owing to appropriate data not being available.

10.1.2.2 The psychometric properties of the ADQ

Item means and standard deviations for the 14 items of the ADQ in the sample of 157 patients with PD (PD1&2) are shown in table 10-3. The score distribution of the 14 items achieved good variability (SD > 0.5) and symmetry (standardized means ranged from -1.7 to 1.7).

Table 10-3. Item means and standard deviations for the ADQ in the PD patients (N=157).

No	Item	Mean value (range: 1-4)	S.D.
1	Feeling low & sad	2.10	0.97
2	Self blame & guilt	1.89	1.18
3	Concentration problems	2.01	0.87
4	Feeling weepy	1.79	0.88
5	Difficulty in falling asleep	1.95	1.13
6	Pessimism about the future	1.86	1.01
7	Loss of interest	1.81	0.85
8	Diminished appetite	1.33	0.67
9	Suicidal ideation	1.21	0.57
10	Diminished feelings for others	1.23	0.54
11	Diurnal variation	1.90	1.15
12	Tendency to worry	1.90	1.11
13	Health concerns	1.51	0.92
14	Early morning waking	2.36	1.20

The possible range of total scores on the ADQ was from 14 to 56. The distribution of scores for the full PD sample (subgroups PD1&2) is shown in figure 10-1. The mean total score for the full sample was 24.9 (± 7.5) with a range from 14 to 44. The distribution of total scores was slightly positively skewed (skewness=0.57, S.E.=0.19), which is not surprising, as only a proportion of the patients were expected to be depressed.

10.1.2.3 Reliability estimates: internal consistency

Estimates of the internal consistency of the ADQ, based upon Cronbach's alpha coefficient for the standardised item variables, were determined as follows: 0.85 for the PD1&2 group as a whole, 0.85 for the PD1 group and 0.83 for the PD2 group, 0.78 for the MDD group, 0.80 for the low mobility control group, and 0.87 for the healthy control group, representing good levels of internal reliability (George & Mallery 2003; see table 10-4). This means that in the samples studied, at least 78% of the total within-test score variance was due to true score variance rather than to item content heterogeneity or poor item quality. The highest alphas (83-87%) were obtained for the PD samples, for whom the ADQ had been designed, and for the healthy control sample. Moreover, the inter-item correlations are only moderate, which is in keeping with the classic attenuation paradox in psychometric theory and means that the items comprising the questionnaire are not redundant.

Therefore it may be concluded that the ADQ has high internal consistency in both clinical and nonclinical samples.

Figure 10-1. Distribution of scores on the ADQ for the PD1&2 sample (N=157).

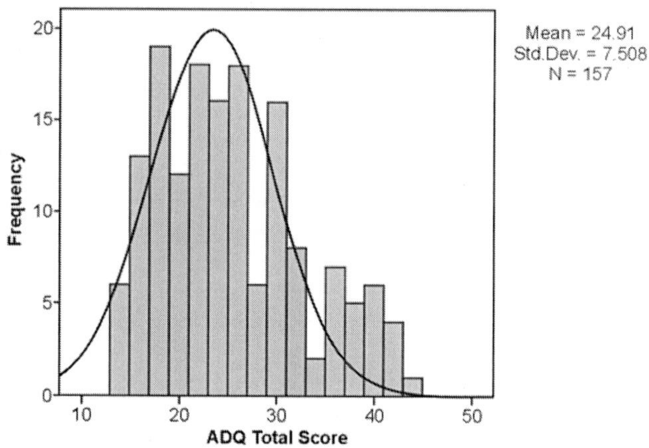

10.1.2.4 Split half reliability

In order to further examine the internal consistency of the 14-item questionnaire, the Spearman-Brown formula for split-half reliability of equal lengths was calculated and is shown is shown in table 10-4. Overall the questionnaire was found to have good split-half reliability with high correlations between the two halves in all of the groups, ranging from r=0.65 for the patient group with MDD to r=0.81 for PD2 and r=0.82 for the healthy control group. From these reliability coefficients it may be inferred that the test halves are highly correlated and the questionnaire has good internal consistency, especially for the healthy control and PD groups, for whom it was specifically designed. It is interesting to note that the least favourable parameters emerged for the MDD group and this may reflect certain features of their response pattern to be discussed later. Thus, from the point of view of the questionnaire's reliability, the ADQ meets the requirements for an instrument to measure depression in PD.

Table 10-4. The psychometric properties of the ADQ: internal consistency and split-half reliability.

ADQ	Clinical and normative samples					
	PD1& PD2	PD1	PD2	MDD	Low mobility control	Healthy control
N	157	97	60	40	27	30
Mean score ± SD	24.9 ± 7.5	26.0 ± 7.7	23.1 ± 6.9	31.9 ± 7.5	23.6 ± 6.4	18.7 ± 5.7
Score range (full scale)	14 - 44	14 - 42	14 - 44	21 - 45	14 - 37	14 – 36
Skewness of scores (S.E.)	0.57 (0.19)	0.41 (.24)	0.92 (.31)	0.13 (.43)	0.64 (.45)	1.67 (.43)
Full scale α-coefficient	.85	.85	.83	.78	.80	.87
Split-half reliability						
Spearman-Brown correlation *r*	.74	.72	.81	.65	.70	.82
Summary statistics for ADQ						
Mean score ± SD items 1-7	13.4 ± 4.5	14.3 ± 4.6	12.0 ± 4.0	17.3 ± 4.8	12.6 ± 3.6	9.7 ± 3.4
Mean score ± SD items 8-14	11.4 ± 3.5	11.7 ± 3.7	10.9 ± 3.1	14.5 ± 3.4	11.0 ± 3.3	8.9 ± 2.6

Cronbach's alpha coefficients are described as: unacceptable < 0.50; poor >0.50; questionable >0.60; acceptable >0.70; good >0.80; excellent: >0.90 (George & Mallery 2003)

10.1.2.5 Item analysis

An item analysis was carried out in order to determine the appropriateness of including all of the individual items in the questionnaire. With the aid of the scale reliability analysis of SPSS, Cronbach's alpha for the questionnaire, when individual items are removed, and the corrected correlation of individual items on the questionnaire with the total score for the patients with PD was calculated; the results are shown in table 10-5. Alpha did not increase above that for the full questionnaire when any of the items were removed, indicating that each of the items was contributing to the underlying construct of depression, which the instrument was designed to measure. The corrected item-total correlation is an indication of the contribution of individual items to the total score on the questionnaire. All of the corrected item-total correlations were positive demonstrating that each of the items makes a contribution to the overall score. Furthermore, none of the 14 items had a corrected item-total correlation below the criterion of 0.2 indicating that each item in the ADQ is making an adequate contribution to the underlying construct of depression.

The size of the individual correlations indicates that low mood, pessimism regarding the future, lack of interest in activities, feeling weepy, concern about health, worried pre-occupation and poor concentration are the items which contribute most to the overall score in patients with PD, whilst suicidal ideation, lack of feelings for others, diurnal variation, loss of appetite, sleep disturbance and guilt or self-blame contribute least to the total score for depression.

10.1.2.6 Convergent validity

The convergent validity of the ADQ was examined against established scales for measuring depression, including the HAM-D, the Leeds and the GDS. With the exception of the Leeds, these have been recommended as being appropriate for use in PD (Schrag et al. 2007). The Leeds scales however, are self-rating versions of the Hamilton Anxiety and Depression scales and have established psychometric properties (Snaith, Bridge and Hamilton 1976).

Table 10-5. Item analysis for the 14 items of the ADQ for PD1&2 (N=157)

No	ADQ Item content	Scale mean if item deleted	Scale variance if item deleted	Corrected item-total correltn.	Sq. multiple correlation	Cronbach α if item deleted
1	Feeling low and sad	22.76	44.97	.76	.65	.80
2	Self-blame and guilt	22.97	49.97	.27	.14	.83
3	Problems with concentration	22.84	48.96	.51	.36	.82
4	Feeling weepy	23.06	47.76	.60	.46	.81
5	Difficulty in falling asleep	22.90	49.64	.31	.34	.83
6	Pessimism regarding future	22.99	45.77	.67	.63	.80
7	Loss of interest and enjoyment	23.04	47.59	.65	.53	.81
8	Loss of appetite	23.53	52.29	.33	.26	.83
9	Suicidal ideation	23.64	51.75	.47	.41	.82
10	Change in feelings for other people	23.63	52.10	.45	.32	.82
11	Diurnal variation	22.96	49.14	.34	.23	.83
12	Worried preoccupation	22.97	46.30	.55	.48	.81
13	Health concerns	23.34	47.99	.55	.37	.81
14	Early morning wakening	22.49	49.72	.28	.30	.83

Table 10-6 shows the intercorrelations between subject data and performance on the depression measures for the full sample of patients with PD (PD1&2). The ADQ can be seen to have high correlations with the other instruments for measuring depression, confirming that it is likely to be measuring the same underlying construct as the other scales. The Spearman correlation coefficients for the ADQ with other depression scales ranges from 0.75 to 0.87 confirming that the convergent validity of the ADQ is good.

Table 10-6. Spearman correlations between the ADQ and other depression scales for PD(1&2).

variable	ADQ	HAM-D	GDS	Leeds-D	Leeds-A	Leeds-FS
Age	-0.08	-0.14	0.02	-0.02	-0.02	0.01
Gender	-0.02	-0.02	-0.08	-0.15	-0.09	-0.09
ADQ	1.00	0.75**	0.87**	0.86**	0.66**	0.86**
HAM-D		1.00	-	0.81**	0.79**	0.90**
GDS			1.00	-	-	0.84**
Leeds-D				1.00	0.68**	0.86**
Leeds-A					1.00	0.85**
Leeds-FS						1.00

** p=0.01 (2-tailed); * p=0.05 (2 tailed); correlations are for N=157 patients with PD
ADQ – Addenbrooke's Depression Questionnaire; HAM-D – Hamilton Depression Scale; GDS – Geriatric Depression Scale; Leeds-D – Leeds depression subscale; Leeds-A – Leeds anxiety subscale; Leeds-FS – Leeds full scale.

10.1.2.7 Dimensionality of the questionnaire

A principal component analysis of the scores on the ADQ for the full PD1&2 sample (N=157) was carried out, with the forced restriction that only one component be extracted. Item loadings of ≥ 0.3 were accepted as demonstrating a significant association with the component. The results showed that all of the items for the questionnaire loaded on this single component, indicating that the items of the ADQ are assessing a single construct (depression). The items with the weakest loadings are items: ADQ14-early morning wakening, ADQ2-guilt and self-blame and ADQ5-difficulties in falling asleep. Factor 1 accounted for 35.8% of the variance with an eigenvalue of 5.02. Factor loadings ranged from .30 to .84 as shown in table 10-7.

Table 10-7. Factor loadings for component 1.

ADQ	Questionnaire item	Component 1
ADQ1	Feeling low and sad	.84
ADQ6	Pessimism regarding the future	.80
ADQ7	Loss of interest and enjoyment	.74
ADQ4	Feeling weepy	.73
ADQ12	Worried preoccupation	.69
ADQ13	Health concerns	.65
ADQ3	Problems with concentration	.63
ADQ9	Suicidal ideation	.62
ADQ10	Loss of feelings for other people	.53
ADQ11	Diurnal variation	.40
ADQ8	Loss of appetite	.39
ADQ5	Difficulty in falling asleep	.33
ADQ2	Self-blame and guilt	.32
ADQ14	Early morning wakening	.30

In order to assess the structure of item-groupings within the ADQ, a full principal component analysis was carried out with varimax rotation, which produced three principal components for the questionnaire. The various indicators of factorability were good: Bartlett's test of sphericity gave an approximate χ^2 value of 714.25 (df=91, p=0.00) and the Kaiser-Meyer-Olkin (KMO) measure of sampling adequacy, which is a test of the amount of variance within the data that can be explained by the factors, was 0.85. There were three components with an eigenvalue greater than 1.0 and together these explained 55.1% of the variance in scores for the PD sample. Cattell's scree plot also suggested a final solution of three components above the break between the steep and shallow parts of the curve (see figure 10-2).

In the rotated component matrix (table 10-8) below, the heaviest loadings for each item are highlighted. Item loadings above 0.4 were considered significant. Nine of the fourteen items comprising the questionnaire loaded significantly on the first component, three on the second and the remaining two items loaded on the third component. The items loading on the first component would seem to represent the core symptoms of the depression that is typical of PD, insofar, at least, as these have been included in the questionnaire. The second component contains items relating to loss of feelings for other people, diurnal variation and self-blame and guilt. The third component represents sleep disturbance (initial and late). As these symptom groupings are aligned along different components of the principal components analysis, it would appear that they represent distinct clusters of symptoms, that are unrelated to each other. Thus sleep disturbance does not appear to be related to depressive symptoms in PD and change in feelings for other people, diurnal variation, and guilt also seem to be less strongly associated (if at all) with the other symptoms of depression loading on components 1 and 3.

Figure 10-2. Scree plot for the components of the ADQ.

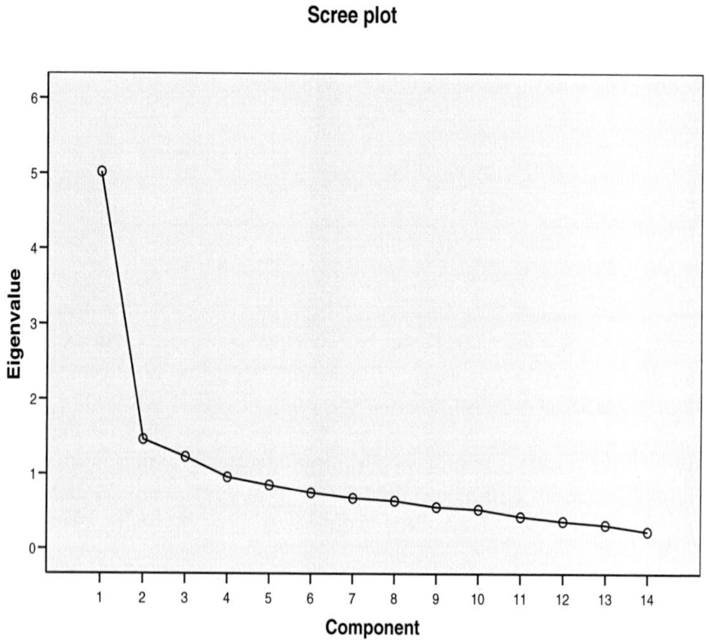

10.1.2.8 The discriminative validity of the ADQ

In order to determine the capacity of the ADQ to identify depression in PD, the discriminative validity of the questionnaire must be established. This may be evaluated using receiver operating characteristic (ROC) curves, a technique derived from signal detection theory (Baird & Noma 1978). This methodology, enables optimal cut-off points to be determined on instruments measuring depression, when the true diagnosis for the patients with PD has been established according to an external criterion. DSM-IV-TR criteria for depressive disorder are considered to be a gold standard for establishing the diagnosis.

Table 10-8. Rotated component matrix.

ADQ items		Component		
		Core symptoms 1	Distinguishing symptoms 2	Sleep disturbance 3
ADQ6	Pessimism regarding the future	**.780**	.228	.082
ADQ1	Feeling low and sad	**.766**	.270	.223
ADQ4	Feeling weepy	**.727**	.174	.054
ADQ12	Worried preoccupation	**.723**	.153	- .337
ADQ9	Suicidal ideation	**.707**	.092	- .184
ADQ7	Loss of interest and enjoyment	**.663**	.193	.309
ADQ3	Problems with concentration	**.647**	.048	.118
ADQ13	Health concerns	**.547**	.321	.162
ADQ8	Loss of appetite	**.496**	- .400	.359
ADQ10	Loss of feelings for other people	.304	**.687**	.055
ADQ11	Diurnal variation	.182	**.613**	.086
ADQ2	Self-blame and guilt	.104	**.567**	.088
ADQ5	Difficulty in falling asleep	.122	.017	**.838**
ADQ14	Early morning wakening	.007	.241	**.782**

The ROC curves are a plot of the true positive rates against false positive rates for a series of cut-off values. In other words, they are a graphical display of the trade-off between the sensitivity of the scale with respect to 1 minus the specificity for every possible cut-off point. Sensitivity refers to the likelihood that a person's score on the scale will be above the cut-off value for depression, when s/he is found to be depressed according to DSM-IV-TR criteria and specificity to the likelihood that a given score on the scale may misclassify the person as being depressed when s/he is not. An ideal cut-off point is one at which the instrument has the highest possible sensitivity with the lowest possible false positive rate (i.e. highest specificity). This is the point lying geometrically closest to the top-left corner of the graph (where the ideal cut-off value with 100% sensitivity and specificity would be plotted). The choice of the ideal cut-off score is, to some extent, dependent on the clinical context, that is, the purpose for which the tool is to be used. The area under an ROC curve (AUC) can be used as an overall estimate of the discriminating ability of the instrument and is sometimes expressed as its accuracy in determining (in this case) depression. The area under the ROC curve is equal to the probability that a test correctly classifies patients as true positives or true negatives with respect to the diagnosis i.e. its ability to discriminate depressed from non-depressed patients. The larger the AUC, the greater the accuracy of the instrument.

The sensitivity and specificity of the ADQ were thus evaluated using ROC curves and the AUC was calculated. The optimal cut-off point was determined visually by assessing which score combined maximum sensitivity with optimal specificity. For the purposes of comparing the performance of the ADQ with respect to other well-established measures of depression, ROC curves were plotted for the ADQ and the HAM-D. Optimal cut-off scores were determined for each of the instruments. In order to determine whether the ADQ could be used as a predictive test for patients with PD, the percentage of PD patients with a positive test result who met the DSM-IV-TR criteria for a depressive disorder (referred to as positive predictive values or PPV) and those who were correctly identified as not being depressed (negative predictive values or NPV) were calculated for different cut-off scores in the central range of the questionnaire. The DSM-IV-TR criteria for depression were used as the gold standard for determining the existence of depression in the PD2 sample examined at interview.

Mean scores on the ADQ, ranges and standard deviations are presented in table 10-9 for the group of patients with PD (PD2), subdivided according to whether they were classified as having major depression, minor depression or no depression according to DSM-IV-TR criteria. For comparison, summary data are also shown for the control group of patients with MDD. Frequency distribution analysis showed that there were no missing scores in the central score range of the ADQ in the two groups of patients.

Of the sixty patients comprising the PD2 group, who underwent a comprehensive clinical assessment, six (10%) were found to satisfy the DSM-IV-TR criteria for MDD and a further 18 (30%) met the criteria for minor depressive disorder giving an overall prevalence for depression in this group of 40%. Thirteen (56.5%) of the depressed patients were women. There was a significant difference in HAM-D scores between patients with both major and minor depression (mean=18.9 ± 5.3) and those who were not depressed (mean=8.9 ± 4.6) on the Mann-Whitney test (U=54.5, p=0.00). Of the control group with major depression, 38 (95%) met the DSM-IV-TR criteria for MDD at the time of testing. The remaining two patients were in remission.

Table 10-9. Means, standard deviations and ranges for the ADQ scores in PD2 and MDD samples.

Samples	DSM-IV-TR	ADQ		
	No. & %	Mean score	± SD	range
PD2 full sample	N=60	23.1	± 6.9	14 - 44
PD2 Non-depressed	N=36 (60%)	19.7	± 4.5	14 - 30
PD2 depressed	N=24 (40%)	28.5	± 6.9	16 - 44
PD2 major depression	N=6 (10%)	32.2	± 9.0	22 – 44
PD2 minor depression	N=18 (30%)	25.9	± 4.8	16 - 37
MDD full sample	N=40	31.9	± 7.5	21 - 45
MDD depressed	N=38 (95%)	32.5	± 7.3	21 - 45
MDD in remission	N=2 (5%)	23.0	± 2.8	21 - 25

Whilst the number of PD patients satisfying the DSM-IV-TR criteria for MDD is very small (N=6), it can be seen from table 10-9 that the mean ADQ score (32.2) for these patients is similar to that of the MDD control group (32.5); statistical analyses were not performed to confirm the lack of a significant difference between these groups, because of the small number of patients in the PD group with MDD. The AUC for both the depression instruments for which ROC curves were plotted was large: 0.94 for the HAM-D and 0.85 for the ADQ, and both were significant at p=0.00 thus rejecting the null hypothesis (true area = 0.5). This indicates that both the HAM-D scores and the ADQ scores have high concurrent validity with the DSM-IV-TR criteria for major and minor depressive disorder in PD. The performance of the HAM-D is better than that of the ADQ, as might be expected for a clinician rated versus a self-rating instrument.

Figure 10-3. ROC curve for the ADQ and HAM-D in PD2 patients.

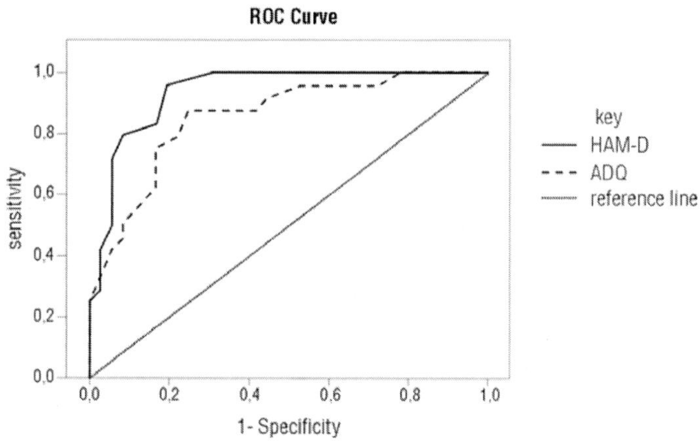

The sensitivities, specificities, PPVs and NPVs for different cut-off scores on the ADQ are shown in table 10-10 for the patients with PD. ROC curves for the PD2 patient group are shown in figure 10-3.

The cut-off score giving maximum discrimination (dichotomization) between depressed and non-depressed patients in the PD group was determined on visual inspection from the ROC curves, as the point at which the highest sum of sensitivity and specificity was achieved. As can be seen both from the ROC curves (figure 10-3) and table 10-10, this was achieved at a cut-off point of 22/23 (sensitivity 0.83, specificity 0.75) for the ADQ and at a cut-off point of 12/13 (sensitivity 0.83, specificity 0.75) for the HAM-D.

Optimal cut-off points were also determined both for diagnostic and screening purposes. In order to be useful for diagnostic purposes, cut-off points on an instrument should combine high specificity with high PPV and this leads to higher threshold scores than those for screening purposes.

Table 10-10. Sensitivity, specificity, positive and negative predictive values at different cut-off scores for the ADQ and HAM-D for patients with Parkinson's disease (N=60).

ADQ																	
Cut-off			16/ 17	17/ 18	18/ 19	19/ 20	20/ 21	21/ 22	22/ 23*	23/ 24	24/ 25	25/ 26	26/ 27	27/ 28	28/ 29	29/ 30	30/ 31
sensitivity			1.00	.96	.96	.92	.87	.87	.83	.75	.71	.58	.46	.42	.37	.29	.21
specificity			.22	.39	.47	.56	.58	.72	.75	.78	.83	.83	.92	.92	.94	.97	1.00
PPV			.46	.51	.55	.58	.58	.68	.69	.69	.74	.70	.79	.77	.82	.87	1.00
NPV			1.00	.93	.94	.91	.87	.89	.87	.82	.81	.75	.72	.70	.69	.67	.65
HAM-D																	
Cut-off value	5/6	6/7	7/8	8/9	9/ 10	10/ 11	11/ 12	12/ 13*	13/ 14	14/ 15	15/ 16	16/ 17	17/ 18	18/ 19	19/ 20	20/ 21	21/ 22
Sensit -ivity	1.00	.96	.96	.96	.96	.96	.96	.92	.79	.75	.67	.58	.46	.38	.29	.25	.21
Specif -icity	.22	.33	.44	.53	.56	.64	.69	.81	.83	.92	.94	.94	.94	.94	.97	.97	1.00
PPV	.46	.49	.53	.58	.59	.64	.68	.76	.76	.85	.89	.88	.85	.82	.88	.88	1.00
NPV	1.00	.92	.94	.95	.95	.96	.96	.94	.86	.85	.81	.77	.72	.69	.67	.66	.65

*Maximum sensitivity and specificity.
PPV = positive predictive value.
NPV = negative predictive value.

From table 10-10 it can be seen that the optimal cut-off point for diagnostic purposes was found to be a score of 30/31 on the ADQ at which point the sensitivity is 1.00 and the PPV is 1.00.

For screening purposes, however, an instrument requires a combination of high sensitivity and high NPV. These requirements are usually met at lower scores, as in this case, where a score of 16/17 (sensitivity 1.00, NPV 1.00) on the ADQ was established as a cut-off point for screening purposes.

10.1.3 Use of the ADQ to test hypotheses concerning the depression of PD

10.1.3.1 Characteristics of depression across the samples

The means and standard deviations of the scores on the respective instruments for measuring depression in the clinical and control samples are shown in table 10-11.

The distribution of total scores on the ADQ for the clinical and control samples is shown in figure 10-4. Because of skewness in the distribution of the mean scores among the samples, non-parametric analyses were used to make comparisons between groups. The Kruskal-Wallis ANOVA revealed differences between the groups for the HAM-D (χ^2=65.7, df=3, p=0.00), the Leeds (χ^2=32.55, df=3, p=0.00), the GDS (χ^2=24.09, df=2, p=0.00) and the ADQ (χ^2=44.02, df=3, p=0.00). A priori planned comparisons between the patients with PD (PD2) and those with MDD revealed a statistically significant difference between the groups on all of the measures used: Mann-Whitney test for the HAM-D, U=265.5, p=0.00; for the Leeds depression scale, U=428.5, p=0.00; for the ADQ, U=340.0, p=0.00. There was also a significant difference between the PD2 group and the healthy age-matched control group in relation to all of the depression measures: for the HAM-D, U=137.5, p=0.002; for the Leeds, U=130.5, p=0.004 and for the ADQ, U= 507.5, p=0.003. The PD2 and the low mobility groups demonstrated significant differences on the HAM-D, U=220.00, p=0.006 and the Leeds, U=241.00, p=0.013. These differences remained meaningful, even when the Bonferroni correction for multiple comparisons was applied (giving an equivalent p-value at the 5% level of p=0.016 for three and p=0.025 for two comparisons). However, neither the ADQ, nor the GDS differentiated between the patients with PD and the low mobility control group, indicating that both groups had similar levels of depression as measured by these two instruments (Mann-Whitney U=749.5, p=0.58 for ADQ; Mann-Whitney U=642.0, p=0.79 for GDS).

Table 10-11. Group mean scores and standard deviations on depression scales.

Group	ADQ Mean ± SD (range)	HAM-D Mean ± SD (range)	LEEDS Mean ± SD (range)	Leeds-D Mean ± SD (range)	Leeds-A Mean ± SD (range)	GDS Mean ± SD (range)
PD(1+2) (N=157)	24.9 ± 7.5 (14-44)	-	25.0 ± 11.4 (1-52)	5.8 ±4.1 (0-15)	6.5±3.9 (0-15)	-
PD(1) (N=97)	26.0 ± 7.7 (14-42)	-	25.9 ± 11.0 (1-48)	6.3 ± 4.2 (1-15)	6.8 ± 3.7 (0-15)	14.9 ± 7.8 (0-29)
PD(2) (N=60) 10% meet DSM-IV criteria for MDD	23.1 ± 6.9 (14-44)	12.0 ± 6.2 (1-27)	23.7 ± 11.9 (3-52)	5.5 ± 3.8 (0-15)	6.2 ± 4.0 (0-15)	-
MDD (N=40) 95% meet DSM-IV criteria for MDD	31.9 ± 7.5 (21-45)	24.6 ± 7.2 (10-37)	35.0 ± 11.8 (18-55)	11.0 ± 4.1 (3-18)	9.0 ± 4.9 (0-18)	-
Low mobility group (N=27)	23.6 ± 6.4 (14-37)	7.1 ± 4.2 (1-15)	15.5 ± 11.9 (4-43)	4.0 ± 3.9 (0-11)	3.1 ± 3.6 (0-12)	14.2 ± 8.8 (1-30)
Healthy controls (N=30)	18.7 ± 5.7 (14-36)	5.7 ± 5.5 (0-16)	10.9 ± 10.9 (0-32)	3.1 ± 3.7 (0-10)	1.8 ± 2.6 (0-7)	5.4 ± 5.3 (0-19)

Figure 10-4. Distribution of scores on the ADQ for the samples.

Patients with PD: sample PD2

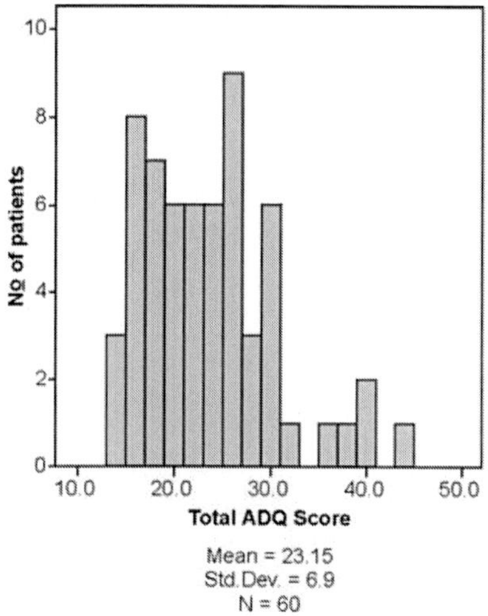

Patients with MDD

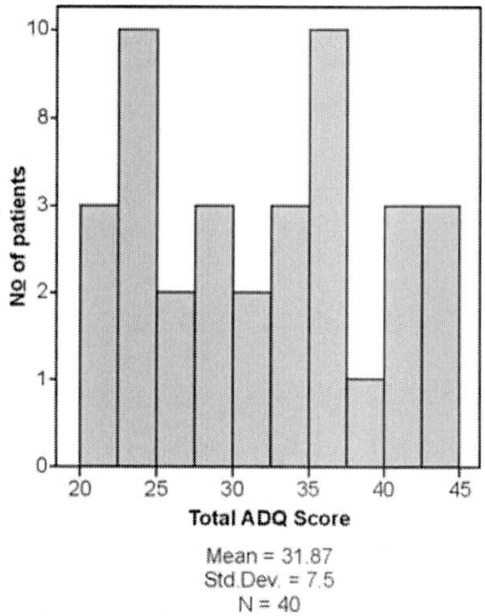

Age matched low mobility control group

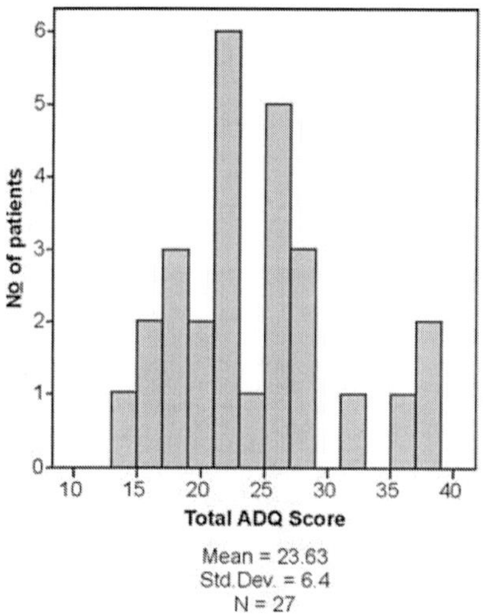

Age matched healthy control group

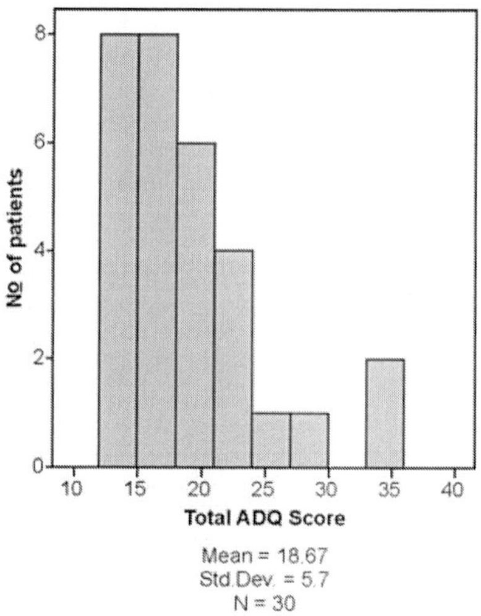

Table 10-12. Proportion of participants in the clinical and non-clinical samples classified as depressed according to different cut-off points on the depression scales.

	Cut-off stores						
Group	ADQ		HAM-D		Leeds-D	GDS	
	severe > 30	mild - moderate ≥ 23	severe > 17	mild - moderate ≥11	≥ 7	severe > 20	mild - moderate >10
PD(1)	27.8%	33.0%	-	-	51.5%	32.3%	31.2%
PD(2)	15.0%	35.0%	18.3%	38.3%	33.3%	-	-
	10% meet DSM-IV-TR criteria for MDD						
MDD	56.7%	33.3%	82.5%	17.5%	90.0%	-	-
	95% meet DSM-IV-TR criteria for MDD						
Low mobility	14.8%	33.3%	0.0%	12.3%	21.4%	14.3%	50.0%
Healthy controls	6.6%	10.0%	0.0%	6.6%	15.0%	0.0%	19.1%

The proportion of participants scoring above the standard cut-off points for depression on the individual scales is shown in table 10-12. 56.6% of the patients in sample PD2 were classified as having mild to severe depression on the HAM-D, but when the higher cut-off point of ≥13, established against DSM-IV-TR criteria using ROC curve methodology, was applied, the proportion of mildly depressed patients was 28.3% and together with those more severely depressed, amounted to 46.6% of the sample. 100% of the patients with MDD were classified as having mild to severe depressive symptomatology on the HAM-D. None of the patients in the low mobility or healthy control group fell within the class for severe depression and 12.3% and 6.6% respectively were found to have mild depression. As might be expected, the proportion of depressed patients with PD was less than those with MDD, but more than in the low mobility and healthy control groups.

For the patient groups, results on the ADQ closely followed the pattern for the HAM-D: 60.8% of patients in PD1 and 50% in PD2 were classified as having mild to severe depressive symptoms, compared to 90% of the group of patients with MDD. However, among the group of age-matched older people with low mobility, 48.1% met the criteria for depression according to the ADQ and in the healthy control group, the figure was 16.6%, both considerably higher than the estimates obtained with the clinician rated HAM-D. The pattern of classification according to the Leeds scale for depression was broadly similar to that of the ADQ, although at the standard cut-off values applied, it appeared to be less sensitive, especially in the group with low mobility; however, it revealed higher proportions above the cut-off value in the healthy control group than on any of the other scales, apart from the GDS. The highest estimates for depression were obtained with the GDS. Accordingly, depression was revealed in 63.5% of PD1, 64.3% of the low mobility group and 19.1% of the healthy controls.

In summary, the PD2 sample was significantly more depressed than the age-matched healthy controls, but showed lower levels of depression than the patients with MDD. A similar pattern was observed for PD1. With the exception of the healthy controls, about one-third of the respondents in all of the remaining samples fell within the mild to moderate levels of depression on the ADQ. These proportions showed greater variation on the other depression scales. The ADQ consistently differentiated between the groups in a similar way to the other self-completion measures of depression. As might be expected, higher levels of depressive symptoms were recorded on the self-rated scales than on the clinician rated assessments. This resulted in there being no differences between the PD groups and the low mobility control group on the ADQ and GDS, although differences were obtained on the HAM-D, PD patients demonstrating greater severity of depression.

The Mann-Whitney test did not reveal any differences between PD1 and PD2 for any of the variables on which they had been assessed in common: i.e. the Leeds depression scale ($U= 2522.5$; $p=0.16$), the ADQ ($U=2403.5$; $p=0.07$), measures of ADL ($U=2686.00$; $p=0.40$) and IADL ($U=2896.0$; $p=0.96$). The two PD groups were thus considered to be equivalent and all further analyses are based on the combined group, PD1 & 2, except where this is not possible, owing to appropriate data not being available.

Table 10-13 shows the zero-order correlations between the respondents' age and gender and their performance on measures of depression and manifestations of physical disability. Measures of ADL and IADL were obtained for the entire sample; in addition the patients with PD were assessed with the aid of two scales designed especially for use in PD for the motor (H&Y) and functional disability (NUDS). In the case of table 10-13, the results are reported with reference to both the uncorrected and corrected correlations, as some authorities have argued that the Bonferroni procedure is too conservative (Perneger 1998).

Table 10-13(i). Correlations on depression scales for patients with MDD (N=40).

Variable	ADQ	HAM-D	Leeds-D	Leeds-A	Leeds-FS
Age	- 0.27	- 0.22	0.03	0.19	-0.18
Gender	0.39*	0.30*	0.25	0.55*	0.45*
ADQ	1.00	0.35*	0.81***	0.71***	0.83***
HAM-D		1.00	0.43*	0.22	0.63**
Leeds-D			1.00	0.62**	0.77***
Leeds-A				1.00	0.86***
Leeds-FS					1.00

* $p= 0.05$; ** $p=0.01$; *** $p=0.00$
With the Bonferroni correction (0.05/20), $p=0.002$

It can be seen from the tables that high correlations were consistently obtained between the ADQ and the other instruments for measuring depression for all of the groups, confirming that it is likely to be measuring the same underlying construct as the other scales. The association continued to hold, even when the Bonferroni correction for multiple comparisons was applied, suggesting that it was a strong one. Age was not correlated with any of the depression measures in either the patients with PD, those with MDD or the healthy controls. In the low mobility control group however, there was a negative correlation between age and depression, such that older people were found to have lower depression scores. This association no longer held however, with the Bonferroni correction. The expected association between gender and depression was evident in the patients with MDD and both the low mobility and healthy control groups, although it was not present on all measures of depression, especially as far as the control groups were concerned. No such association emerged for the PD group, but this may have been because male patients were over-represented in this group. However, the association between depression and gender did not withstand application of the Bonferroni correction. Finally, depression was also correlated with impaired levels of ADL and IADL in the PD and low mobility control groups, although this association did not survive the multiple comparison correction. Furthermore, no association was found between depression and motor or functional disability for the patients with PD on scales specifically designed for the measurement of disease-related symptoms and consequent disability. This might indicate that performance as measured on ADL and IADL scales is influenced by factors other than physical ability, for example the patient's cognitive or affective state. These considerations are explored in greater detail in stage II of the research.

Table 10-13(ii). Correlations for age and gender, depression scores and physical abilities for PD1 & P2 (N=157).

variable	ADQ	HAM-D	Leeds-D	Leeds-A	Leeds-FS	GDS	H&Y	NUDS	IADL	ADL
Age	-0.07	-0.14	-0.01	-0.02	0.02	-0.19	0.11	-0.13	0.21*	0.19
Gender	-0.07	-0.02	-0.23	-0.14	-0.09	-0.05	-0.22	0.11	-0.09	-0.10
ADQ	1.00	0.76***	0.86***	0.66***	0.87***	0.87***	-0.01	-0.17	0.47***	0.46***
HAM-D		1.00	0.79***	0.76***	0.85***	-	0.16	-0.39**	-	-
Leeds-D			1.00	0.67***	0.86***	0.85***	-0.06	-0.15	0.50***	0.48***
Leeds-A				1.00	0.85***	0.69***	-0.03	-0.22	0.43**	0.41**
Leeds-FS					1.00	0.84***	-0.01	-0.22	0.52***	0.49***
GDS						1.00	-	-	0.53***	0.53***
H&Y							1.00	-.74***	-	-
NUDS								1.00	-	-
IADL									1.00	0.79***
ADL										1.00

* p= 0.05; ** p=0.01; *** p=0.00
With the Bonferroni correction (0.05/56), p=0.001

Table 10-13(iii). Correlations for age and gender, depression scores and physical abilities for low mobility control group (N=27).

variable	ADQ	HAM-D	Leeds-D	Leeds-A	Leeds-FS	GDS	IADL	ADL
Age	-0.17	-0.32*	-0.20	-0.49**	-0.27	0.26	0.26	0.34*
Gender	0.00	0.23	0.65**	0.78***	0.72**	-0.20	0.25	0.13
ADQ	1.00	0.88***	0.49**	0.22	0.46**	0.87***	0.35*	0.27
HAM-D		1.00	0.47**	0.33*	0.46**	0.77***	0.32*	0.12
Leeds-D			1.00	0.30*	0.91***	0.53**	0.56**	0.37*
Leeds-A				1.00	0.52**	0.31*	0.49**	0.43*
Leeds-FS					1.00	0.50**	0.50**	0.38*
GDS						1.00	0.50**	0.62**
IADL							1.00	0.92***
ADL								1.00

* $p= 0.05$; ** $p=0.01$; *** $p=0.00$
With the Bonferroni correction (0.05/40), $p=0.001$

Table 10-13(iv). Correlations for age and gender, depression scores and physical abilities for healthy control group (N=30).

variable	ADQ	HAM-D	Leeds-D	Leeds-A	Leeds-FS	GDS	IADL	ADL
Age	-0.26	-0.32	-0.43	-0.26	-0.23	0.07	-0.15	-0.05
Gender	-0.36	-0.61^{**}	-0.62^{**}	-0.42^{*}	-0.64^{**}	-0.15	-0.16	-0.29
ADQ	1.00	0.88^{***}	0.99^{***}	0.59^{**}	0.87^{***}	0.71^{***}	0.21	-0.01
HAM-D		1.00	0.83^{***}	0.51^{**}	0.78^{***}	0.81^{***}	0.23	0.19
Leeds-D			1.00	0.61^{**}	0.87^{***}	0.94^{***}	0.05	0.01
Leeds-A				1.00	0.83^{***}	0.57^{**}	-0.11	-0.03
Leeds					1.00	0.91^{***}	-0.18	-0.06
GDS						1.00	0.06	0.15
IADL							1.00	0.56^{**}
ADL								1.00

* $p= 0.05$; ** $p=0.01$; *** $p=0.00$
With the Bonferroni correction (0.05/40), $p=0.001$

10.1.4 A comparison of depressive symptoms between PD and MDD

In terms of the quantitative analysis of the data described above, it has been shown that the proportion of patients qualifying for a DSM-IV-TR diagnosis of MDD in the sample of patients studied (PD2) is 10%, with a larger proportion (30%) meeting the criteria for minor depression. The preceding analyses have also demonstrated that the severity of depressive symptoms in PD for the majority of patients is therefore not as great as that in MDD. It has also been alleged however, (for discussion, see chapter 3) that the pattern of symptoms in PD varies from that in MDD. The proposed qualitative differences in symptomatology between PD and MDD are examined in the following section.

10.1.4.1 Establishing equivalence for severity of depression in the examined groups

From the results of the principal component analysis of the scores for the ADQ, described above, it would seem that certain symptoms of depression such as sleep disturbance, feelings of guilt and self-blame, and possibly diurnal variation and appetite loss, are divergent from the main symptom cluster for depression in PD. These symptoms are among those that have been described by previous studies as occurring less frequently in the depression of PD compared to MDD.

In order to further examine the hypothesis that the profile of depressive symptomatology for PD patients differs from that of patients with MDD, appropriate comparisons are necessary between the two groups. Primarily, it is important to establish whether any alleged differences in the symptom profile for PD represent true differences in the phenomenology of PD depression, or whether they simply reflect differences in the severity of the depressive disorder. This is particularly important in view of the fact, that the prevalence of MDD in PD may not exceed that in the general population, but that milder forms of depression (minor depression) may be elevated. Furthermore, it would not be surprising if the profile of depressive symptoms were to differ between major and minor forms of the disorder, as suggested in the literature (see chapter 3, section 3.5.4). For example, certain symptoms such as weight loss, insomnia, psychomotor agitation, indecisiveness, psychotic features, suicidal ideation and increased levels of vegetative symptomatology are thought to be associated with greater severity of depressive illness (e.g. Gaudiano et al. 2008; Schrag et al. 2007). In order to test this possibility, comparisons were made between the control group with MDD and PD subgroups, selected for different levels of symptom severity.

The PD(1&2) (N=157) and MDD (N=40) samples were initially matched for severity of symptoms on the ADQ in order to ensure that patients with equivalent levels of symptomatology were being compared from both groups. Matching of total scores > 23 (the cut-off for depression established for dichotomization of groups on the ADQ) was done by hand and was achieved for a total of 30 patients from each of the PD and MDD groups. The mean ADQ score for the PD (severely depressed) subgroup was 31.9 (±7.2) and for the MDD subgroup was 31.8 (± 7.5); the differences in the ADQ scores between the two groups were not significant (Mann-Whitney U= 442.5, p=0.91), showing that the groups represented equivalent levels of severity of depressive symptoms. Two further groups were selected in order to meet the criterion for milder depression on the ADQ with a score within the range of 20-23. The first of these was a group of PD patients (N=29), with a mean ADQ score of 21.4 (±1.02) and the second was a non-PD control group (N=35) extracted from the low mobility and healthy control groups, with a mean ADQ score of 21.0 (±1.4). These groups did not differ from each other in terms of severity (Mann-Whitney U=418.5, p=0.22). Significant differences in severity of depression as measured on the ADQ were confirmed with the Kruskal-Wallis ANOVA for the mildly depressed groups in comparison to the group with MDD (χ^2=49,54, df=2, p=0.00). Post-hoc tests confirmed that the patients with MDD were more severely depressed than either the patients with PD (Mann-Whitney U=54.00, p=0.00) or the non-PD control group (Mann-Whitney U=54.00, p=0.00), who met the criteria for mild depression. Data from these participants were used to perform the subsequent analyses.

10.1.4.2 The profile of depressive symptoms in PD

A comparison of group mean scores for the individual items of the ADQ was made between the PD and MDD groups, and between PD patients with milder depression and the non-PD control group. Both pairs of groups were matched for severe and milder levels of depression respectively, as described in the previous section. The purpose was to determine whether any differences in their symptom profile could be established. A similar comparison was also made for PD patients with milder levels of depression and the patients with major depressive disorder (unmatched for severity). The results are shown in table 10-14. It can be seen from table 10-14 that there are significant differences between the PD and MDD patients matched for severity of symptoms on the following items of the ADQ: feeling weepy, loss of appetite and concerns regarding health.

The group of patients with PD was more likely to feel weepy and to have health concerns than the MDD group, but was less likely to report loss of appetite. There were no differences between the groups with regard to the cognitive symptoms of depression. However, on application of the Bonferroni correction for multiple comparisons to the results of the test of differences between the means, any differences between the PD and MDD groups disappeared. The application of the Bonferroni procedure has been criticised as being too conservative, increasing the risk of type II errors (Perneger 1998) and so it is possible that the differences found, may indeed be meaningful and reflect a different pattern of symptoms in PD. Indeed, the effect size (power) for the differences found to be significant between the PD and MDD groups are of medium strength: "feeling weepy" (Cohen's d=0.54), loss of appetite (Cohen's d=0.75), health concerns (Cohen's d=0.62) and therefore acceptable. Moreover, with the exception of item 14 (late insomnia), the effect size for the differences between the remaining ADQ items for the two groups, range from being acceptable to high, indicating that type II errors are unlikely to have arisen. This suggests that the failure to find differences with respect to the remaining items is likely to be a reliable finding and not due to lack of power in the analyses.

A similar comparison between the PD and the control group matched for severity of milder symptoms of depression, revealed differences between the groups with respect to only two items: diurnal variation and difficulties with concentration. The PD patients endorsed these symptoms to a greater extent than the controls. The effect size (power) for these differences is of at least medium strength, suggesting that they are statistically acceptable: "problems with concentration" (Cohen's d=0.66) and diurnal variation (Cohen's d=0.98). However, application of the Bonferroni procedure would eliminate the effect for concentration difficulties, but not diurnal variation.

The results demonstrate that different symptom clusters appear to differentiate the groups at different levels of symptom severity. Hence differences in symptom specificity between PD patients and control groups may indeed be a feature of the severity of depression, rather than true differences in symptom profile for PD.

Table 10-14. A comparison of scores on individual items of the ADQ for patients with PD and MDD matched for severity of depressive symptoms and differences between groups. Comparative results are also shown for a group of PD and control patients with milder depression.

ADQ item	PD (N=30) Severe depression mean (SD)	MDD (N=30) Severe depression mean (SD)	T-test PD vs MDD severe depression (df=58)		PD (N=29) Mild depression mean (SD)	Control (N=35) Mild depression mean (SD)	T-test PD vs controls matched for mild depression (df=62)		T-test PD with mild depression vs MDD group (df=57)		Effect size for PD mild vs MDD Cohen's d
			t	*p*			t	*p*	t	*p*	
Feeling low and sad	2.80 (1.00)	3.03 (0.93)	-0.94	0.35	1.79 (0.67)	1.80 (0.53)	-0.05	0.96	5.85	0.00**	1.55
Self-blame and guilt	2.37 (1.33)	2.43 (1.19)	-0.20	0.84	1.76 (1.06)	1.97 (1.20)	-0.74	0.46	2.29	0.02	0.60
Concentration problems	2.53 (0.90)	2.43 (0.93)	0.42	0.67	1.83 (0.71)	1.43 (0.50)	2.63	0.01	2.79	0.007	0.73
Feeling weepy	2.37 (0.85)	1.90 (0.88)	2.08	0.04	1.52 (0.63)	1.49 (0.56)	0.21	0.83	1.90	0.06	0.57
Difficulty in falling asleep	2.47 (1.22)	2.50 (1.28)	-0.10	0.92	1.79 (0.98)	2.29 (1.23)	-1.75	0.08	2.38	0.02	0.63
Pessimism regarding the future	2.70 (1.09)	2.20 (1.19)	1.70	0.09	1.65 (0.72)	1.37 (0.73)	1.55	0.12	2.12	0.04	0.58
Loss of interest and enjoyment	2.47 (0.86)	2.83 (0.98)	-1.53	0.13	1.31 (0.60)	1.17 (0.45)	1.05	0.30	7.13	0.00**	1.92

Table 10-14 (cont'd).

Loss of appetite	1.40 (0.67)	2.07 (1.11)	-2.81	0.007	1.14 (0.44)	1.26 (0.66)	-0.83	0.41	4.19	0.00**	1.20
Suicidal ideation	1.50 (0.73)	1.50 (0.82)	0.00	1.00	1.00 (0.00)	1.00 (0.00)	--	--	3.28	0.002*	0.61
Change in feelings for other people	1.53 (0.82)	1.43 (0.82)	0.47	0.64	1.03 (0.19)	1.14 (0.58)	-1.48	0.14	2.56	0.01	0.79
Diurnal variation	2.23 (1.25)	2.60(1.33)	-1.10	0.28	1.86 (1.12)	1.2 (0.88)	3.03	0.004*	2.30	0.02	0.60
Worried preoccupation	2.57 (1.04)	2.87 (1.19)	-1.04	0.30	1.38 (0.77)	1.60 (0.52)	-1.05	0.30	5.65	0.00**	1.52
Health concerns	2.23 (1.19)	1.57 (0.93)	2.41	0.02	1.17 (0.47)	1.29 (1.07)	-0.91	0.37	2.04	0.05	0.57
Early am wakening	2.73 (1.11)	2.47 (1.31)	0.85	0.40	2.17 (1.04)	1.97 (1.36)	0.76	0.45	0.96	0.34	0.25

p values are at the 95% confidence interval.

The effect size (power) for the differences found to be significant between the PD and MD groups equated for severe depression are of medium strength: "feeling weepy" (Cohen's d=0.54), loss of appetite (Cohen's d=0.75), health concerns (Cohen's d=0.62 and therefore acceptable.

The effect size (power) for the differences found to be significant between the PD and control groups equated for mild depression are of medium strength: "problems with concentration" (Cohen's d=0.66), diurnal variation (Cohen's d=0.98) and therefore acceptable.

*p is significant at 5% and **1% after application of the Bonferroni correction for multiple comparisons.

It might be instructive to the present analysis to observe what happens when the criterion for equal symptom severity between groups is not met. When a similar comparison is made between PD patients with a milder form of depression and the patients with MDD, a pattern of differences emerges which appears to differentiate the two groups of patients. In relation to the MDD group, the mildly depressed PD patients demonstrate diminished feelings of guilt and self-blame, fewer concentration difficulties, fewer problems with initial insomnia, a lesser tendency towards worrying, future pessimism and change in feelings towards other people, less diurnal variation, fewer health concerns, fewer feelings of loss of interest and enjoyment (anhedonia), less frequent suicidal ideation, little appetite loss and fewer feelings of sadness. All of these differences demonstrated an acceptable effect size, measured in terms of Cohen's d (see table 10-14). Items that do not show differences between the groups are also of interest as these are symptoms present in PD even in milder states of depressive disorder. No differences between groups were elicited for weepiness and early morning wakening, demonstrating that these symptoms are endorsed even in the mildly depressed PD patients. However, the effect size for the late sleep disturbance is somewhat low (Cohen's d=0.25), though for weepiness it is of medium strength (Cohen's d=0.57).

Application of the Bonferroni correction procedure for multiple comparisons would mean that only the differences between groups for low affect, appetite loss, suicidal ideation and worry remain significant. As the procedure applies very strict statistical criteria, it also draws a distinction between those relationships that are particularly strong and those that are not. It is worth noting that two of the symptoms allegedly differentiating PD depression, namely worry (anxiety) and suicidal ideation, survive this more rigorous test. These comparisons would seem to confirm that the different symptom patterns between PD and MDD patients are mainly due to variations in levels of depression severity. Such findings are crucial to clarification of the question examined. It might be expected that the differences in the symptom profile for depression in PD, especially with regard to symptoms that are allegedly more prominent, such as anxiety, suicidal ideation, future pessimism and problems with concentration, should already be established, even at levels of milder severity. The present data do not appear to support a prediction of this kind.

10.1.4.3 Methodological inadequacies in establishing symptom profile in PD

Although previous studies have used comparisons of this kind as evidence in support of the alleged differences in symptom profile between

PD and MDD groups, they are likely to be inadequate for a number of reasons. The method of comparing mean scores in order to establish differences between groups is limited by a number of factors. The most important of these is that in attempting to establish a profile of depressive symptoms for the two groups under consideration, more is required than establishing differences in the magnitude of the mean scores for one group with respect to the other on a range of symptoms. It is theoretically possible that both groups might achieve a similar score on a particular item, but that item might make a significantly different contribution to the overall profile of depressive symptoms in one group as compared to the other, depending on the contribution of the other items on the measurement scale. In other words, the sensitivity of the item in contributing to the diagnosis of depression may vary between different groups of patients. Comparison of individual mean scores is therefore problematic in determining differences in symptom profile, as it does not simultaneously take the other scale items into consideration.

Another difficulty, where the comparison of means is concerned, is that with a relatively small range for the scores (1-4), the validity of such comparisons is brought into question, as floor and ceiling effects are more likely when the range of scores is restricted. This is a particular problem at both high and low extremes of symptom severity. Although in general, this does not appear to have been a problem in the study, it is a point that needs to borne in mind.

Furthermore, mean differences between groups for individual items may be misleading if score distributions are skewed and especially if sample sizes are relatively small. Both of these factors are relevant in the present study. The distribution of scores on individual items of the questionnaire are clearly skewed for some items. To take an extreme example, scores on suicidal ideation are strongly positively skewed, because the majority of patients, even in samples with severe depression, do not endorse the highest levels of severity for this item. As regards sample size, two considerations apply. The first is that clinical samples in studies of this kind are of necessity restricted by the availability of patients meeting the study criteria and the patients' ability to complete the protocol in full, given the limitations imposed by their illness. The second concerns the requirement to match samples for severity of symptoms. The relatively small number of patients in the PD group when patients' scores are matched for severity with the group of patients with MDD reflects the fact that a relatively small proportion of the PD patients meet the DSM-IV-TR criteria for major depression. Since a larger proportion of the PD patients satisfy DSM-IV-TR criteria for minor depression, matching for severity of symptoms with the MDD group is problematic and yields a relatively small number of patients in the PD group. A more appropriate comparison would be with a group of patients suffering from minor depression, but this was not available for the present study.

In order to make a comparison of the PD and MDD patients on their symptom profile, a different approach was adopted, taking account of the scores on the individual items of the ADQ that contributed to a greater or lesser degree to the overall score on the questionnaire and determining any differences between the groups on the resultant profile. In order to accommodate these considerations, a form of data analysis is required that is not dependent to the same extent, as is the comparison of means, on the assumptions of normality for the distribution of scores. Thus, non-parametric (Spearman's rho) correlations were calculated for the scores on the individual items of the ADQ with the total scores for the questionnaire. The magnitude of the correlations indicate the degree to which the respective items contribute to the overall score on the scale, for each of the groups. The difference between the correlation coefficients for the PD and MDD groups for each of the items of the ADQ was then tested for significance. The item-total correlations, and the results of testing for differences between groups are presented in table 10-15.

Statistical testing of differences between the item-total correlations for the individual items of the ADQ revealed differential patterns of endorsement for only three items in the comparison for PD and MDD groups equated for severity of depressive symptoms. These included: loss of appetite, health concerns and a change in feelings for other people. A comparison of the mean scores on these items (see table 10-14) revealed that PD patients differ from those with MDD in not demonstrating loss of appetite, and, perhaps not surprisingly in view of this, appetite loss does not make as great a contribution to their overall depression score as it does for the MDD group. Health concerns, on the other hand, were higher for the PD patients and were more significant in their profile of depressive symptoms than in the MDD group. Interestingly, the feeling of being unable to respond with the same emotional engagement to other people was endorsed to the same extent by both PD and MDD groups, but it played a more significant role in the profile of depressive symptomatology for the PD patients compared to those with MDD. The effect size q ($q = zA - zB$, where z=Fisher's z; Cohen 1992), which is an index of the size of the differences between independent correlation coefficients, was large (> 0.5).

Table 10-15. Patterns of item endorsement on the ADQ for different groups compared to the MDD control group.

		PD (N=30) *vs* MDD (N=30)					PD (N=29) *vs* control (N=35)				
		Matched for severe depression ADQ score >23					Matched for mild depression ADQ score = 20-23				
	Item-total Spearman rho correlation, Fisher's *z*, significance (*p*) of difference between the correlation coefficients for different groups & the effect size (*q*)[1]										
	ADQ items	r^{MDD}	r^{PD}	*q*	$z^{PD/MDD}$	*p*	r^{PD}	$r^{control}$	*q*	$z^{PD/contr}$	*p*
1	Feeling low and sad	.60	.75	.28	1.03	NS	.05	.41	.39	1.46	NS
2	Self-blame and guilt	.54	.38	.20	0.75	NS	-.03	.41	.41	1.79	.07
3	Problems with concentration	.67	.39	.40	1.47	NS	.44	-.03	.44	1.92	.05
4	Feeling weepy	.51	.70	.30	1.12	NS	.26	.29	.03	0.12	NS
5	Difficulty in falling asleep	.62	.37	.34	1.24	NS	-.10	.23	.13	1.27	NS
6	Pessimism regarding the future	.62	.65	.05	0.18	NS	-.05	-.16	.11	0.41	NS
7	Loss of interest and enjoyment	.67	.62	.09	0.32	NS	.17	-.005	.17	0.68	NS
8	Loss of appetite	.65	.24	.53	1.96	.05	.27	-.02	.26	1.13	NS
9	Suicidal ideation	.52	.44	.10	0.38	NS	--	--	++	--	NS
10	Change in feelings for other people	.32	.74	.62	2.27	.05	-.08	.05	.03	0.50	NS
11	Diurnal variation	.30	.50	.24	0.88	NS	.13	.32	.20	0.74	NS
12	Worried preoccupation	.53	.54	.01	0.05	NS	.08	.21	.13	0.50	NS
13	Health concerns	.13	.63	.61	2.24	.05	.16	.17	.01	0.02	NS
14	Early morning wakening	.31	.22	.10	0.36	NS	.20	-.16	.04	1.40	NS

z = unit-normal-curve deviate. Values of 1.96 and 2.58 required for significance at 5% & 1% levels. q[1] is the index of effect size for differences between independent correlation coefficients; q = zA - zB where z = Fisher's z. Values for q: 0.1 – small, 0.3 – medium, 0.5 – large (Cohen 1992).

A comparison of the PD and control subjects with milder symptoms of depression revealed differences in the symptom profile for only two items: problems with concentration and a tendency towards self-blame and guilt (the latter fell just short of reaching significance). There was a medium effect size for these differences. The PD patients tended to report greater problems with concentration but fewer feelings of guilt. There were no differences between the groups with mild depressive symptoms on any of the other items of the ADQ.

The symptoms contributing most to the total ADQ score in the severely depressed patients with PD are low mood, a change in feelings for other people and feeling weepy, but only the change in feelings for other people differentiate them from the MDD group. For those PD patients with milder depression, the symptoms that influence the total score most are problems with concentration, loss of appetite and feeling weepy; but only concentration difficulties are significantly greater than for the control group. The fact that certain symptoms appear to be more important in contributing to the overall score at different levels of depression would suggest that differences in symptom profile are at least in part, determined by depression severity.

Taken together, these results seem to indicate that different symptoms contribute to any differences between the PD and MDD groups at milder and more severe levels of depressive symptoms. Specific symptom profiles are thus more likely to be a feature of symptom severity than to reflect differences between groups of patients.

10.1.4.4 Consistency of responses on the ADQ

A further dimension in which PD patients may be expected to differ from patients with MDD is the consistency of their responses on depression scales. Patients with MDD characteristically have difficulty in making decisions and this is reflected in their response pattern, which is frequently inconsistent. The ADQ, because of its specific structure, required participants to make a series of choices in relation to the same symptom of depression and thus precipitated a situation that was likely to be challenging for patients with MDD. The construction of the ADQ is such that each symptom statement is defined at three levels of severity, and is thus presented to patients three times, with pairs of statements at different levels of severity. It is thus possible to monitor any inconsistencies in response pattern on the part of the patients (see table 9-2 showing how inconsistent response patterns may arise). These inconsistencies are reflected in their scores on the ADQ, which contributed to the lowest levels of split-half reliability for the questionnaire, of all the groups examined. Patients with PD would not be expected to show similar difficulties in their response patterns, as confirmed in their scores on the ADQ, which generated high levels of split-half reliability.

In order to test the hypothesis that inconsistent responding is a feature of MDD, but not PD, the pattern of responses on the ADQ was analysed and inconsistent responses to individual items compared for the PD2 and MDD groups.

Fifteen (37.5%) patients with MDD (N=40) and 17 (28.3%) with PD (N=60) produced an inconsistent response pattern. Those with MDD produced a total of 44 inconsistent replies (a mean number of 2.9 per person for those producing a pattern of inconsistent responses) whilst those with PD disease produced a total of 20 inconsistent replies (a mean number of 1.2 per person for those producing inconsistencies). The likelihood of producing inconsistencies was thus almost two-and-a-half times greater for patients with MDD than for patients with PD. A comparison of the two groups with regard to the number of inconsistencies, gave a value of χ^2= 18.2 (df=1; p=0.0001, 95% confidence interval) indicating that the patients with MDD had significantly greater difficulty in providing consistent responses to the statements on the ADQ than the patients with PD.

10.2 Stage II: analysis of results

The focus of stage II of the study was to examine the relationship between motor, depressive and cognitive symptoms in PD.

10.2.1 Characteristics of the patients examined

Sixty patients with idiopathic PD (sample PD2), meeting the entry criteria to the study described in chapter 9 (section 9.1.1.) were examined further in stage II of the study. Table 10-1 above, shows the demographic characteristics of the patient sample.

10.2.2 Missing data

Sixty cases were entered into the analysis; some data were missing in four patients. For two of the patients, it was not possible to obtain scores for performance on the measures of cognition and depression used on account of their handicap (one was too severely demented, the other too depressed). Scores one standard deviation below the mean were used to substitute for the missing data. A third subject refused to perform on the cognitive instruments and a fourth was unable to complete the free recall test because of deafness. Here group means were entered (Afifi & Clark 1984). Running the statistical analyses, omitting the four cases with missing data, made no difference to the final results.

10.2.3 Demographic characteristics of the sample

All but one of the patients who were approached with a request to participate in the research gave their written agreement; the patient who declined did not give any reason for her refusal to participate in the study. 60 patients (31 men and 29 women) with idiopathic PD were enrolled in the study. All were living in their own homes in the community; three of the patients were living in sheltered housing. 21.7% (N=13) of the sample were living alone and 78.3% (N=47) were living with at least one other person, in households which usually consisted of the patient and their spouse; in a few instances there were also adult children living in the household and in one case the patient was living with a sibling. The majority of the sample (over 55%) were in social classes III and IV (skilled non-manual and manual).

The patients' mean age at retirement was 58.9±3.8 years, and for men (57.3±4.8 years) it was slightly lower than that for women (60.3±1.6 years). This would appear to support the assumption that patients' working lives had been foreshortened by the illness. 15% of the patient sample were still working, probably reflecting the fact that this was a relatively young sample of patients with PD.

10.2.4 Clinical characteristics of the sample

The clinical characteristics of the PD2 sample, who underwent a full clinical evaluation are presented in table 10-16.

The mean age for the onset of PD in this sample was 55.6 (± 7.1) years, indicating that it was a sample with a relatively early onset of PD. This focus on younger patients was brought about as a result of the exclusion criteria (age below 70) adopted in this sample in order to reduce the possibility of concomitant illnesses associated with age. Duration of illness was 7.6 (± 4.2) years, suggesting that this was a sample of patients in whom the disorder was well-established, and who might be expected to have a predominance of moderate to severe functional disability. 95% of the patients were taking a combination of L-dopa and carbidopa in the form of either Madopar or Sinemet and 46.6% were taking benzhexol. Only one patient remained unmedicated for PD.

Table 10-16. The clinical characteristics of the sample (PD2).

Variable		PD2 sample N=60	
Age at onset of PD (years±SD)		55.6	± 7.1
Age at examination (years±SD)		63.2	± 5.6
Duration of illness (years±SD)		7.6	± 4.2
Positive family history of PD (N)		4	6%
Positive personal history of depression (N)		14	23%
Taking anti-depressive medication (N)		11	18.3%
PD medication at time of examination:		N	%
L-dopa+carbidopa		31	51.7
L-dopa+carbidopa & benzhexol		26	43.3
Benzhexol		2	3.3
No medication for PD		1	1.7
Additional medication for PD		10	16.7
No. of admissions to Neurology Dept:	0	28	46.7
	1	22	36.7
	2-4	10	16.6
Hoehn and Yahr grade	1	5	8.3
	2	9	15.0
	3	24	40.0
	4	21	35.0
	5	1	1.7
Northwestern University	mean score±SD	38.3±6.9	
	mode	39.0	
	range	10-48	
Occurrence of tremor:		45	75.0
Occurrence of rigidity:		50	83.3

Over half of the sample (53.3%) had had at least one admission to the Neurology Department at Addenbrooke's Hospital in Cambridge. Four (6%) of the patients had a family history of PD and 14 (23%) reported a personal history of depression, of whom 11 (18.3%) were currently taking anti-depressive medication. In spite of the precautions taken to ensure that the patient sample would not be additionally burdened by the effects of other health complications, 45% of the sample reported having at least one other physical complaint and 65% were also taking medication for conditions other than PD (e.g. hypertension). This was deemed inevitable in a sample of older people.

The majority of patients (75%) were in stages 3 and 4 of the Hoehn and Yahr scale, indicating moderate to advanced impairment due to PD and in keeping with disease duration for this sample. Functional impairment was also considerable, the majority of scores on the NUDS (63%) occurring in the upper 25th percentile on the scale. 75% of patients had marked hand tremor and in 83.3% cog-wheeling rigidity could be elicited in the upper limbs. These results indicate that the sample represented a group of patients with moderate to severe symptoms of PD.

Table 10-17. Results of the neuropsychiatric and neuropsychological assessment for PD2 patients.

Variable	PD2 (N=60)			
Depression:	**Mean**	**SD**	**range**	**% depression**
DSM-IV-TR	-	-	-	10% (N=6) satisfy criteria for major depression 30% (N=18) satisfy criteria for minor depression
HAM-D	12.0	6.2	1-27	Severe (cut-off >17) 18.3% N=11 Mild (cut-off =11-17) 38.3% N=23
Leeds scales	23.7	11.9	3-2	-
Leeds depression	5.5	3.8	0-15	Depression (cut-off ≥7) 33.3% N=20
Leeds anxiety	6.2	4.0	0-15	Anxiety (cut-off ≥7) 46.6% N=28
ADQ	23.1	6.9	14- 4	Severe (cut-off ≥30) 15.0% N=9 Mild (cut-off =23-29) 35.0% N=30
Cognitive:				**% cognitive impairment**
Free recall	39.70	11.6	10-65	Cut-off =30; 20.0% N=12
Delayed recall	5.08	3.4	0-17	-
Benton errors	12.7	8.6	1-41	Cut-off=8; 30.0% N=18
Schonell (IQ)	105.2	12.0	72-117	Cut-off=70 IQ points; 0.0%

The results of the assessment for depression and cognitive impairment in PD2 are presented in table 10-17. The estimate for the prevalence of MDD based on DSM-IV-TR criteria for the sample was 10% and for minor depression, it was 30%. In comparison, using the cut-off score established for diagnostic purposes on the ADQ, 15.0% of the PD2 sample were found to meet the criteria for depressive disorder (i.e. severe depression). Using the less strict criterion for dichotomization of the PD2 group into patients who were depressed versus non-depressed (i.e. including patients characterised as having "minor" depression), 50% of the sample were found to be depressed on the ADQ. This compares with rates of 33.3% on the Leeds depression scale and 56.6% on the HAM-D, for this sample of patients with PD. 18.3% were depressed according to the cut-off score (17) for severe depression on the HAM-D. 46.6% of the sample presented with clinically relevant levels of anxiety as measured on the Leeds anxiety scale.

As regards cognitive function, only 20% of the sample were found to have impaired performance on the free recall task, which is a good screening instrument for dementia (Miller 1971), and 30% were impaired on the visuospatial task. The mean estimated IQ score from the Schonell reading test for the sample was 105; none of the patients had an estimated IQ score below 70 (two standard deviations below the population mean for IQ) indicating that their estimated pre-morbid IQ was within the normal range for the general population.

10.2.5. Correlation results

A Spearman correlation matrix for the main variables of interest in this part of the study was generated in order to examine the relationship between the symptom domains in PD. This is presented in table 10-18. The Bonferroni correction for multiple comparisons was applied in order to reduce the risk of type I errors. No significant correlations were consistently obtained between any of the three types of variables representing the main symptom domains of PD, which included physical, affective and cognitive manifestations of the illness.

10.2.6. Exploratory factor analysis

An exploratory factor analysis (principal components with varimax rotation) was carried out in order to ascertain patterns in the data.

Twenty variables, derived from the measures used, were entered into the analysis. The indicators of factorability were good: Bartlett's test of sphericity gave an approximate χ^2 value of 668.75(df=190, p=0.00) and the Kaiser-Meyer-Olkin (KMO) measure of sampling adequacy, which is a test of the amount of variance within the data that can be explained by the factors was 0.62.

The principal component analysis with varimax rotation yielded six components (table 10-19) and four of these, with an eigenvalue > 1.5 were interpreted. The four components accounted for nearly 58.7% of the variance in the sample. These components were considered to represent: "PD somatic symptoms", "depression", "chronicity" and "cognition"; their loadings are shown in table 10-20.

Table 10-18. Spearman correlation coefficients for the main motor, affective and cognitive variables.

	1	2	3	4	5	6	7	8	9	10
1. AGE	1.0	.8***	.11	-.13	-.14	-.007	-.06	-.27	.01	.07
2. ONSET		1.0	-.17	.11	-.15	.06	-.10	-.05	-.04	-.03
3. H&Y			1.0	-.74***	.12	-.01	-.01	-.28*	-.04	.24
4. NUDS				1.0	-.31*	-.22	-.17	.33*	-.11	-.38**
5. HAM-D					1.0	.87***	.81***	-.12	.34**	.08
6. LEEDS						1.0	.83***	-.15	.36**	.20
7. ADQ							1.0	-.26*	.27*	.20
8. FR								1.0	-.29*	-.55**
9. Benton									1.0	.26*
10.Schonell										1.0

* denotes significance at $p \leq 0.05$; ** $p \leq 0.01$, *** $p \leq 0.00$
For corrected significance (Bonferroni correction) items must have a p-value of 0.001.

Table 10-19. Factor structure.

Factor	Eigenvalue	% of variance	Cumulative % of variance
1	**4.61**	**23.06**	**23.1**
2	**2.86**	**14.31**	**37.4**
3	**2.25**	**11.26**	**48.6**
4	**2.02**	**10.08**	**58.7**
5	1.42	7.11	65.8
6	1.15	5.77	71.6

Table 10-20. Rotated factor matrix with loadings.

variables	Component loadings			
	PD somatic	**depression**	**chronicity**	**cognitive**
Age at examination	.196	.008	**-.857**	.165
Age at onset of PD	-.197	.036	**-.922**	-.067
No. of admissions to Neurology dept.	**.553**	.100	**.422**	.137
Duration of L-dopa	**.560**	.163	.387	.080
Duration of benzhexol	.217	.068	**.486**	.284
Current daily L-dopa dose	**.439**	.217	.111	-.077
Current daily benzhexol dose	.053	-.031	.351	**.488**
Other medication for PD	**.565**	-.021	.400	-.154
Antidepressive medication	.093	.131	.122	.158
H &Y (motor)	**.794**	.027	-.109	.121
NUDS (functional)	**-.648**	-.107	-.019	**-.526**
Tremor rating	.049	.183	.103	-.050
Rigidity rating	**.806**	.035	-.069	.101
Personal history of depression	.008	.210	.092	-.037
HAM-D score	.182	**.885**	.077	.107
Leeds full score	.019	**.933**	-.102	.104
ADQ depr. score	.024	**.933**	.033	.105
Free Recall score	-.234	-.092	.127	**-.820**
Schonell (IQ)	.012	.071	.016	**.828**
Benton test	.036	.381	.060	**.545**

10.2.7 Cluster Analysis

In order to explore the possibility that different sub-groups of patients might be identified in this patient sample, a cluster analysis was carried out. The following clustering variables were included: age at examination, age at onset, duration of illness, the NUDS for functional disability, levodopa dose, benzhexol dose, the HAM-D and the ADQ as measures of depression, and the free recall test, the Schonell reading test and the Benton test as measures of cognitive function. The complete linkage method was used and dendrograms plotted. The main clusters were identified with the single most important variable differentiating the two groups, being duration of illness. One group (n=17) was associated with relatively early onset of illness (49.8 years), long duration of illness (155.6 months); whilst the second (n=12) included subjects with later age of onset (61 years) and shorter duration of illness (49.2 months). Longer duration of illness was associated with poorer motor functioning, higher drug dosages and poorer performance on tests of free recall (immediate memory) and the Schonell (estimate of IQ). The short duration-late onset group was worst on the Benton test of visuospatial ability. This cluster may still involve some more generalised cognitive decline, since performance on free recall, although better than in the other cluster, was nonetheless at the lower end of the normal range. The two clusters did not differ on the depression measures used. The group profiles obtained from the cluster analysis are shown in table 10-21. For the purposes of comparison, the profiles for the whole sample are also presented.

Table 10-21. Mean values for selected variables according to obtained clusters (sample means included for comparison).

Variable	Cluster 1 (n=12)	Cluster 2 (n=17)	Full sample (n=60)
Age at examination (years)	64.9	62.8	63.2
Age at onset (years)	61.0	49.8	55.6
Duration of illness (months)	49.2	155.6	91.4
L-dopa dose (low vs high dose)	2.08	2.29	2.23
Benzhexol dose	.417	1.4	0.88
Northwestern scale (functional disability)	40.2	34.8	38.2
HAM-D (depression)	14.4	13.7	12.6
ADQ (depression)	25.2	24.0	22.8
Free Recall test (total correct)	40.0	35.6	39.4
Schonell test (errors)	11.8	16.3	12.7
Benton test (errors)	15.9	12.8	12.5

10.2.8 Discriminant function analysis

In order to determine which variables produce the best fitting equation for classifying patients into subgroups, a discriminant function analysis was carried out. The following discriminant variables were entered into the analysis: gender, age at onset, L-dopa dose, benzhexol dose, the NUDS (functional ability), the ADQ, and scores on the tests of free recall (immediate memory), Schonell (IQ) and Benton (visuospatial ability).

These were chosen as being representative of the three main domains of disease variables: physical illness, affective and cognitive. Multi-colinear variables were avoided. The grouping variables were: gender, age at onset, L-dopa dose and benzhexol dose and the latter three were dichotomised (see table 10-22). Gender was chosen in order to identify any possible differences relating to this variable; the other three, because of reports in the literature which have claimed associations with cognitive loss and depression.

Table 10-22. Results of discriminant analysis: numbers of subjects in chosen groups and percent classified correctly according to groups.

Variable	Group 1	Group 2	% correct classification
Gender	Female = 29	Male = 31	71.67%
Age at onset	> age 55 = 29	< age 55 = 31	71.67%
Benzhexol dose	No benzhexol = 32	Taking benzhexol = 28	70%
L-dopa dose	None or low dose = 33	High dose = 27	75%

Classification values for the best discriminant functions are shown in table 10-22. The results indicate that all four of the variables chosen have a reasonably high classification rate of over 70%. The classification values for the one variable-discriminant functions are shown in table 10-23. For ease of understanding the variables making a significant contribution to each of the discriminants are qualitatively described as "high" or "low/poor" in table 10-24.

Table 10-23. Contribution of individual variables to discriminant functions.

	Grouping variables			
variable	Gender	Onset age	L-dopa dose	Benzhexol dose
Gender	70.0%		60.0%	58.3%
Age at onset	70.0%		63.3%	58.3%
NUDS		53.3%	56.7%	
Free recall				65.0%
Benton			56.7%	
Schonell				66.7%

Table 10-24. Contribution of individual variables to discriminant functions.

Grouping variables			
Gender (male)	**Onset age**	**L-dopa dose**	**Benzhexol dose**
	Male patients	Male patients	
Early onset age		Early onset age	Early onset age
Lower functional ability	Lower functional ability	Lower functional ability	Lower functional ability
High L-dopa dose			
High benzhexol dose			
			Poor scores on free recall
		Poor scores on Benton	
			Lower IQ

10.3 Stage III: analysis of results

Stage III of the study was concerned with the evaluation of an independent sample of patients with PD (PD3) and their carers in order to determine how selected factors shaping the care-giving situation may determine outcomes for the carer.

10.3.1 Characteristics of the patients examined

Seventy-five patients with idiopathic PD (sample PD3), meeting the entry criteria to the study described in chapter 9 (section 9.1.1) and their carers were examined in stage III of the study. The background characteristics of the PD3 sample are presented in table 10-1 above.

10.3.2 Missing data

The amount of missing data was not substantial. Over 97% of carers (N=73) completed the study protocol without difficulty, frequently annotating their responses to add clarification. The remaining two carers returned incomplete protocols as they appeared to have missed part of a scale through oversight. In these cases, proportional estimates of the missing responses were made on the basis of responses within the scale or similar items on other scales. The patient protocols were completed in full, as information and responses were obtained during the course of the clinical interview with the patients. In fewer than 10% of cases, they were spread over more than one session in order to accommodate clinical symptoms and fatigue.

10.3.3 Demographic characteristics of the patients and carers examined

All the patient and spouse-carer dyads who were approached with a request to participate in the research gave their written agreement: there were no refusals. 75 patients (49 men and 26 women) with idiopathic PD were enrolled in the study. They were all living with their spouses in their own homes in the community. The spouse carers were, in the main, female (N=49; 65.3%) and the majority (N=61; 81.3%) of households consisted of the carer-patient couple alone, 17.3% (N=13) of couples were living with one child and in one case (1.3%) the couples' son, daughter-in-law and grandchild were living in the same household. All of the couples were living in accommodation of at least an adequate standard and none were in significant financial hardship.

Table 10-25 shows the demographic characteristics of the patient and carer samples.

No significant differences in mean age at interview (65.4±7.7 vs. 66.1±6.2 years; Mann-Whitney U=2217.0, p=0.84) were observed between the carers and the care-recipients respectively. The carers had received a mean of 10.5 years of education: 50.6% had left school at the age of 14 and only 8% had attended university, although another 17.3% had received further education of some kind. The majority of couples (57%) were in social classes III and IV (skilled non-manual and manual) and PD3 represented a sample of patients who were mostly retired from full-time employment (only 12% were still working). The patients' mean age at retirement was 59.1±5.4 years (see table 10-1) and as the majority of the patient sample were men, this strongly suggests that many of them had retired early as a result of ill-health. Indeed, as the mean retirement age for men (59.2±6.0 years) was only slightly higher than that for women (58.6±2.8 years), and in view of the different statutory retirement age for men and women, this would appear to support the assumption that their working lives had been foreshortened by the illness.

Table 10-25. Characteristics of the sample: carer and care recipient demographic variables.

Variable	Carer		Variable	Care recipient	
	N	%		N	%
Female	49	65.3	Female	26	34.7
Male	26	34.7	Male	49	65.3
Age 75+	5	6.7	Age 75+	6	8.0
Age 60 – 75	58	77.3	Age 60 - 75	60	80.0
Age < 60	12	16.0	Age < 60	9	12.0
Age range (years):	45 - 81		Age range:	52 - 79	
Higher education	19	25.3	Benefits		
< 11 years education	56	74.6	Mobility allowance	14	18.6
Relationship to care recipient:			Attendance allowance	13	17.3
Married/co-habiting	75	100.0	Invalidity pension	8	10.7
Carer illness:			Disabled car sticker	17	22.7
diabetes	1	1.3	Social class		
arthritis	6	8.0	I	7	9.3
hypertension	6	8.0	II	15	20.0
other cardiac	4	5.3	III	20	26.7
depression	4	5.3	IV	23	30.7
other illness	21	28.0	V	10	13.3
medication	20	26.7			

More than half of the carers (56%) reported having chronic health problems which affected them on a daily basis; these included hypertension (8.0%) and other cardiac problems (5.3%), arthritis (8%), diabetes (1.3%) and interestingly enough, 5.3% had received a diagnosis of depression. 26.7% were receiving medication for their medical problems. However, carers did not differ from the non-PD age-matched control groups in stage I of the study with respect to the prevalence of chronic health problems. Fewer than 20% of couples were receiving benefits in the form of mobility, attendance or other allowances.

10.3.4 Clinical characteristics of the patient sample

The clinical characteristics of the PD3 sample, who underwent a full clinical evaluation, are presented in table 10-26. The mean age of disease onset for this sample of PD patients was 57 (±7.1) years and the average

Table 10-26. PD3: care recipient disease related variables.

Variable	PD3 sample (N=75)		
Disease variables:	Mean	SD	Range
Age at onset of PD (years)	57.0	± 7.1	37-70
Age at examination (years)	66.1	± 6.2	52-79
Duration of illness (years)	9.3	± 5.0	1-26
***PD medication at examination*:**			
L-dopa dose (mg daily)	620	± 505	0-4000
Benzhexol dose (mg daily)	2.8	4.2	2-20
Physical:			
Webster Scale (motor disability)	14.9	±5.6	1-26
NUDS (functional disability)	36.4	±8.1	4-49

Rating of physical condition: proportions of patients according to scale stage								
Hoehn and Yahr			WHO scale:			Karnofsky		
Grade	N	%	grade	N	%	grade	N	%
1	10	13.3	0	4	5.3	20	0	0.0
2	5	6.7	1	21	28.0	30	1	1.3
3	31	41.3	2	25	33.3	40	6	8.0
4	27	36.0	3	21	28.0	50	9	12.0
5	2	2.7	4	4	5.3	60	19	25.3
						70	14	18.7
						80	11	14.7
						90	15	20.0

Proportions of patients taking:	N	%	
L-dopa+carbidopa	46	61.3	
L-dopa+carbidopa & benzhexol	27	36.0	
Benzhexol alone	2	2.6	
No medication for PD	0	0.0	
Additional medication for PD	26	34.7	
Anti-depressive medication	13	17.3	
Sedatives for sleep problems	14	18.7	
Non-PD medication	48	64	

duration of the illness to the time of examination was 9.3 (± 5.0) years. The median Hoehn and Yahr stage was 3 (range 1-5), with 77.3 % of patients being in stages 3 and 4, indicating that this was a sample of PD patients in whom the illness was well-established and who were classified as being in the moderate to severe stages of motor impairment. This was in keeping with the mean score of 14.9 (±5.6) on the Webster scale, indicative of moderate impairment. The Webster scale is considered to reflect a fairly "pure" measure of the physical symptoms of PD, in terms of both the motor and autonomic disturbances. Furthermore, scales designed to measure the functional disability consequent upon the somatic features of the illness revealed clear evidence of physical handicap; the mean score on the NUDS was 36.4 (±8.1), indicating on average, a two-thirds loss of functional ability. Decreased levels of functional performance were further confirmed by the results of assessment on the Karnofsky and WHO scales, which showed that over 60% of the PD patients fell in the moderate to severe range for functional disabilities. Hence, assessment of the physical features of PD in the sample clearly showed that both levels of impairment and functional disability were prominent among the patients.

Prescribed medication was in keeping with these levels of disability. At the time of examination, 46 patients were receiving L-dopa+ carbidopa; 2 were receiving benzhexol alone; and 27 were receiving both. Thus 97.3% (N=73) of the sample were receiving a combination of L-dopa+carbidopa in the form of Sinemet or Madopar. The mean daily dose for those taking L-dopa preparations was 620mg (± 505mg; range: 100-4000mg). 38.6% (N=29) of the sample were receiving benzhexol, an anticholinergic drug, which in all but two of the patients who were taking benzhexol alone, was an adjunct therapy, useful in the control of tremor in PD. The mean daily dose of benzhexol was 2.8mg (± 4.2mg; range: 2-20mg).

None of the patients were without medication for PD. 17.3% of the patients were receiving anti-depressant medication and 18.7% were taking medication to improve sleep. A further 64% of patients were receiving medication for problems unrelated to PD, indicating that this sample of patients was burdened by additional health problems, which may also have affected their level of functional performance.

The results of the assessment for depression and cognitive impairment in the PD3 sample are presented in table 10-27.

Table 10-27. Results of neuropsychiatric and neuropsychological assessment for PD3 patients.

Variable	PD3 (N=75)			
Affective:	**Mean**	**SD**	**Range**	**%**
HAM-D	12.9	±5.5	2 – 24	Severe (cut-off >17) 20.0% N=15 Mild (cut-off=11-17) 49.3% N=37
GDS	13.0	±6.0	2 – 28	Severe (cut-off >20) 18.6% N=14 Mild (cut-off=11-20) 38.6% N=29
HAM-A	15.5	±5.6	4 – 29	Severe (cut-off=25) 8.0% N=6 Mild to moderate (18-24) 25.3% N=19
Cognitive measure:				**% cognitive impairment**
Free recall score	34.7	±10.2	10 – 58	Cut-off = 30 30.7% N=23
Benton errors	7.5	±6.4	0 – 33	Cut-off = 8 33.3% N=25
Schonell IQ	106.5	±10.6	67- 117	Cut-off = 70 IQ points 1.3% N=1

Results from the clinician rated assessment on the HAM-D revealed that 20% (N=15) of the patient sample were severely depressed with another 49.3% (N=37) being mildly depressed. These results were broadly compatible with the patients' self-ratings for depression as measured on the GDS, especially as regards the category of severe depression (18.6%, N=14) with a further 38.6% (N=29) in the category of mild depression. In addition, 8% (N=6) of the patients were considered to have the symptoms of severe anxiety and 25.3% (N=19) as having milder levels of anxiety on the HAM-A.

Assessment of cognitive function revealed that 30.7% (N=23) of the patient sample was impaired on the test of verbal free recall and 33.3% demonstrated impairment on the Benton visuospatial relations test. The estimate of pre-morbid IQ obtained with the aid of the Schonell reading test gave a mean IQ for the sample of 106.5 (±10.6) and only one patient achieved a score below 70, possibly indicating the onset of dementia.

10.3.5 Clinical characteristics of the carer sample

Outcome measures for the spouse carers of the patients with PD were obtained in three main areas, including self-assessment of depression, care-giving strain (or burden) and cognitive performance. Carers were also asked to evaluate their level of satisfaction with their (marital) relationship with the care recipient and to assess the care recipient's functioning in the affective and cognitive domains. The latter were investigated as potential mediating variables for carer strain and depression outcomes. The results are presented in table 10-28.

Table 10-28. Outcome measures for carers of patients with PD.

Carer variables	**Mean**	**SD**	**range**	**% according to cut-off**
Carer age	65.4	7.7	45-81	-
General Health Questionnaire	4.7	6.9	0 - 32	Cut-off = 4 32.0% N=24
Beck Depression Inventory	7.2	6.1	0 - 26	Moderate (score =19-29) 5.3% N=4 Mild (score=10-18) 26.6% N=20
Geriatric Depression Scale	7.8	6.3	1 - 28	Severe (cut-off >20) 5.3% N=4 Mild (cut-off=11-20) 20.6% N=15
Machin Strain Scale	11.7	6.0	1 - 25	18.6% in upper 25th percentile
CFQ-carer	32.6	13.2	5 - 62	21.3% in upper 25th percentile
Marital Adjustment Scale (cut-off =100)	112.6	29.7	31-158	Distressed= 28.0%; N=21 Non-distressed=72.0%; N=54
CFQ-other-depression	13.7	6.3	2 - 25	18.6% in upper 25th percentile
CFQ-other-cognitive	16.4	8.2	1 - 31	22.7% in upper 25th percentile

As can be seen from the table, three measures of psychiatric morbidity were obtained for carers, all of which were broadly in keeping with one another. 32% of the sample (N=24) met the criterion score for probable "caseness" for psychiatric morbidity on the GHQ. Similarly, 32% (N=24) of the carers were found to be depressed according to the BDI whilst 26% (N=19) met the criteria for depression on the GDS. The mean score of 11.7 (±6.0) on the Machin Strain scale was in keeping with the results of other studies when differences in scoring are taken into account (e.g. Miller et al. 1996; Aarsland, Larsen, Karlsen et al. 1999; Thommessen et al. 2002). 18.6% of the scores were in the upper 25th percentile on the Machin scale, indicating the proportion of carers with higher levels of strain. Cut-off scores are not available for this scale.

According to the Marital Adjustment scale, 28% (N=21) of carers reported high levels of marital distress, above the cut-off point of 100, established for the scale. Of these 90.5% (N=19) were female and 9.5% (N=2) were male carers.

The CFQ does not have cut-off values intended to produce classifications according to established norms, but 21.3% of carers had scores in the upper 25th percentile of the score distribution on this instrument. Previous work with the CFQ (Poliakoff & Smith-Spark 2008) yielded mean scores for older control subjects (mean age 62.8±10.3 years) of 39.2 (±2.3) compared to the lower mean CFQ score of 32.6 (±13.2) obtained in the present study. The CFQ-other-cognitive which was used to gain the carer's perspective of the patient with PD, placed 22.7% of patients in the upper 25th of the score distribution and yielded a mean score of 16.4 (±8.2) compared to 11.0 (±1.4) in the Poliakoff and Smith-Spark (2008) study which also obtained an assessment of the cognitive functioning of their relative from the partners or close family members of people with PD. These figures suggest that carers in the present study viewed their partners as being more cognitively impaired. A similar comparison is unfortunately not available for the CFQ-other-depression measure, although in the present study, 18.6% of patients were placed in the upper 25th percentile of the distribution (indicating greater severity) by their carers.

10.3.6 Correlation results

10.3.6.1 Patient variables

Table 10-29 shows the Spearman correlation coefficients for the main motor, affective and cognitive variables measured in the patient with PD and the carer variables covering domains including affect, strain, marital satisfaction and perception of affective and cognitive functioning in the care recipient. The Bonferroni correction for multiple comparisons was applied in order to reduce the risk of type I errors. As with PD2, no significant correlations were consistently obtained between any of the three types of patient-related variables included, nor were these symptom domains related to either the patient's age or gender. Hence motor, affective and cognitive functioning appeared to be independent of one another. Measures of motor performance, however, were highly correlated with each other. Not surprisingly, illness duration was associated with increasingly severe motor symptoms (H&Y, Webster) and functional disability (NUDS), reflecting the progressive nature of PD. The correlation between clinician assessed (HAM-D) and patient-reported depression (GDS) was good, suggesting that self-reported measures such as the GDS are valuable as a screening tool for assessing depression in PD. Significant correlations were also found among the measures used to assess cognitive function in the patients; social class was related to the estimate of pre-morbid IQ for the patient as measured by the Schonell reading test, but not to any of the other measures of cognitive impairment (FR, Benton).

10.3.6.2 Carer variables

Carer measures of depression were highly correlated with one another (GDS, BDI, GHQ). They were, in turn, associated with carer strain (GSS) and marital satisfaction (MAS) and with the exception of the GHQ, with the generic measure of strain in the form of self-reported cognitive failures for the carer (CFQ). In addition, the carers' perception of both depression and cognitive failure in the care recipient was related to carer strain and depression, and to a lesser extent, to marital satisfaction.

Identifying potential relationships between patient and carer variables was of particular interest to this stage of the research in order to delineate possible predictors of carer outcome. Significant correlations were obtained between measures of depression in the patient (especially the GDS) and all three instruments used to identify carer depression. However, no significant relationships were found between psychiatric morbidity in the carer in the form of depression and either motor or cognitive functioning in the patient. The Machin strain scale for carers (MSS), on the other hand, was associated with both illness variables in the form of disease duration, motor and functional impairment, and measures of depression in the patients (HAM-D, GDS), but not with cognitive impairment. This is likely to reflect the multidimensional nature of a strain measure related to the care-giving situation. Neither marital satisfaction, nor the carers' assessment of their own cognitive failures (more generic strain) were associated with any of the patient illness-related variables.

Table 10-29. Spearman correlation coefficients for the main patient and carer variables.

	Patient variables											
	Age	Gen -der	Social class	illness durtn	H&Y	Web-ster	NUDS	HAM-D	GDS	FR	Bent	Schon
Patient variables:												
Age	1.00	-.32	-.27	.16	.16	.01	-.17	-.01	-.11	-.07	.19	-.04
Gender		1.00	-.14	-.04	-.10	.09	-.06	.18	.27	-.01	-.18	-.09
Social class			1.00	.11	.18	.22	-.17	.01	.07	-.26	.24	.55**
Illness durtn				1.00	.51**	.40**	-.54**	.03	.03	-.10	.12	.05
H &Y					1.00	.70**	-.83**	.22	.18	-.23	.14	.20
Webster						1.00	-.78**	.29	.28	-.28	.13	.23
NUDS							1.00	-.30	-.29	.22	-.14	-.26
HAM-D								1.00	.69**	-.06	-.12	.13
GDS-patient									1.00	-.23	.07	.27
Free Recall										1.00	-.52**	-.48**
Benton											1.00	.50**
Schonell												1.00

** denotes significance at the $p < 0.05$ level following application of the Bonferroni correction procedure for multiple comparisons; in order to meet corrected significance levels at $p < 0.05$ items must have an uncorrected p-value of 0.00.

Table 10-29 (cont'd). Spearman correlation coefficients for the main patient and carer variables.

	Carer variables									
	Age	gender	GDS	BDI	GHQ	MSS	MAS	CFQ	CFQ-depr.	CFQ-cog.
Patient variables										
Age	.66**	.30	.13	.06	-.17	.09	-.06	.18	.11	-.07
Gender	-.40**	-.97**	.10	.11	.19	.12	-.17	.07	.08	.25
Social class	-.05	.10	-.04	.01	.12	.05	-.10	-.18	-.17	.04
Illness durtn	.15	-.02	.20	.15	.08	.35**	-.02	.09	.13	.22
H &Y	.02	.02	.08	.09	.16	.48**	-.09	-.09	.23	.26
Webster	-.02	-.10	.15	.08	.21	.42**	-.13	-.03	.14	.16
NUDS	-.02	.07	-.16	-.14	-.17	-.56**	.10	.04	-.20	-.34**
HAM-D	-.19	-.21	.28	.20	.39**	.39**	-.09	.10	.49**	.21
GDS-patient	-.26	-.29	.44**	.37**	.50**	.55**	-.33	.02	.61**	.52**
Free Recall	.09	.10	-.11	-.17	-.12	-.23	.19	-.02	-.10	-.27
Benton	.16	.08	.02	-.02	-.03	.14	-.16	-.10	-.01	.12
Schonell	-.06	.05	.05	.15	.16	.10	-.09	-.17	-.01	.17
Carer variables										
Age	1.00	.43**	-.08	.04	-.31	-.16	.15	.14	-.32	-.36
Gender		1.00	-.13	-.15	-.22	-.15	.20	-.10	-.14	-.33
GDS-carer			1.00	.78**	.66**	.65**	-.57**	.43**	.41**	.50**
BDI				1.00	.66**	.53**	-.38**	.40**	.30	.52**
GHQ					1.00	.64**	-.47**	.22	.48**	.48**
MSS						1.00	-.53**	.17	.59**	.60**
MAS							1.00	-.25	.38**	.44**
CFQ-carer								1.00	.22	.25
CFQ-other-depr.									1.00	.63**
CFQ-other-cog.										1.00

Interestingly, significant correlations were obtained between the carers' perception of depression in the patient (CFQ-other-depression) and both clinician rated (HAM-D) and self-rated (GDS) depression in the patient. On the other hand, the carers' perception of cognitive difficulties for the patient (CFQ-other-cognition) was unrelated to objective measures of cognitive functioning in the patient (FR, Benton). The CFQ-other-cognition was however significantly related to the NUDS, which is a measure of functional performance in PD and to the GDS for the patient. This suggests that whilst the carers' perception of depression in the patient is accurate, they may have a tendency to confuse patient-depression with deficits in cognitive functioning and possibly to regard functional disabilities as reflecting cognitive dysfunctions in the patient.

10.3.6.3 Effects of disease stage on carer outcomes

As PD is a progressive disorder, it is reasonable to expect not only that the physical impairment and functional disability should increase with more advanced stages of the disease, as described above, but also that carer outcomes might suffer as a result. When the disability of the patients in PD3 was stratified according to the stages of the Hoehn and Yahr scale, a Kruskal-Wallis ANOVA revealed that carer strain as measured on the Machin Strain Scale increased as the disease progressed (χ^2 =14.6; df=4; $p \geq .006$). This relationship however, did not continue to hold when carer outcomes were measured in terms of depression; there was only a weak, insignificant association on the GDS (χ^2 = 9.13; df=4; $p \geq .06$) and the relationship did not hold for the BDI (χ^2 = 3.0; df=4; $p \geq .56$) or for the GHQ (χ^2 = 2.8; df=4; $p \geq .59$). Equally marital satisfaction did not appear to be affected by disease stage (χ^2 = 8.0; df=4; $p \geq .09$). These analyses, however are limited by the possibility that carer outcomes are unlikely to show a simple linear relationship to disease stage, as shown in figure 10-5. It can be seen that while carer strain progressively increases in relation to disease stage, other carer-related measures show a different dynamic pattern. Carer depression increases most from stage 1 to stage 2 of the Hoehn and Yahr and thereafter shows a gradual decline, despite the likelihood that the demands on the carer continue to increase systematically. The CFQ shows a similar pattern to depression measures. Carers' marital satisfaction on the other hand, followed an inverted Yerkes-Dodson curve, such that it dropped in the early stages of the illness, but improved towards the later stages. It should be remembered however, that these interpretations are limited by the fact that this was not a longitudinal study and so these observations refer to different patients and their carers at the respective stages of the disease.

Figure 10-5(i). Carer outcomes in relation to the stages of PD.

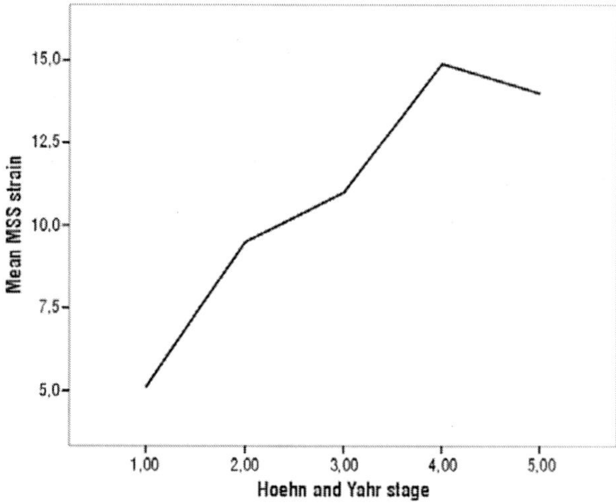

Figure 10-5(ii). Carer depression.

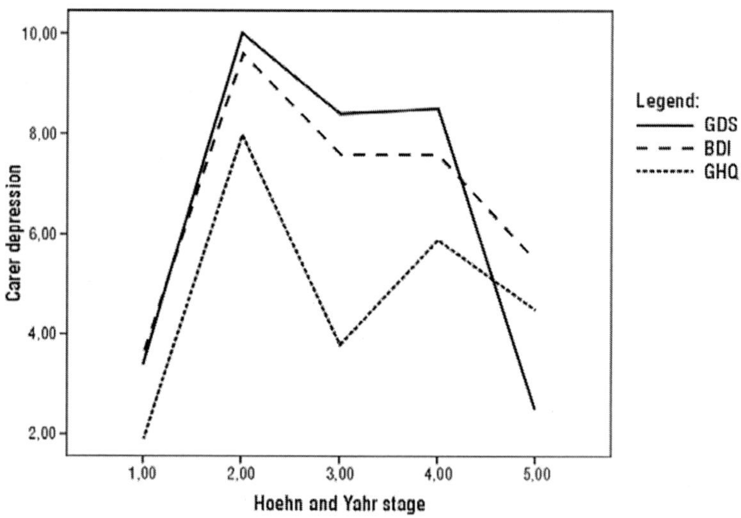

Figure 10-5(iii). Carer marital satisfaction.

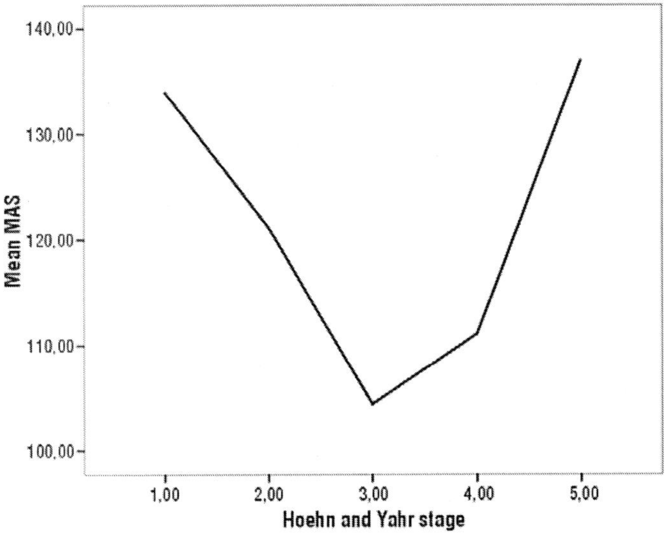

Figure 10-5(iv). Carer cognitive failures (non-specific strain).

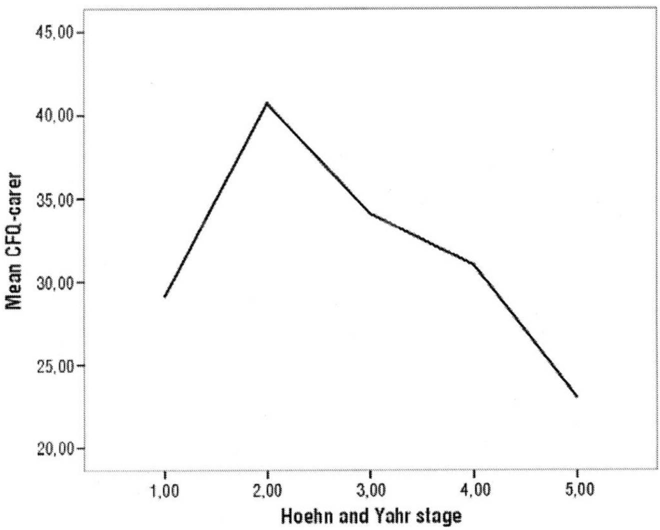

The stage of advancement of PD might also be expected to predict depression in the patient. However, a nonparametric analysis of variance, the Kruskal-Wallis ANOVA revealed that there was no significant relationship between the level of disease progression (H&Y) and depression in the PD patients as measured on both the HAM-D (χ^2 =5.5; df=4; $p \geq .24$) and the GDS (χ^2 =5.9; df=4; $p \geq .20$). Repeating these tests with other measures of motor performance yielded similar results. The same reservations apply to these results as to those reported above, although from figure 10-6 it can be seen that patient depression appears to increase slowly, albeit insignificantly across the stages of PD.

Figure 10-6. Patient depression in relation to the stages of PD.

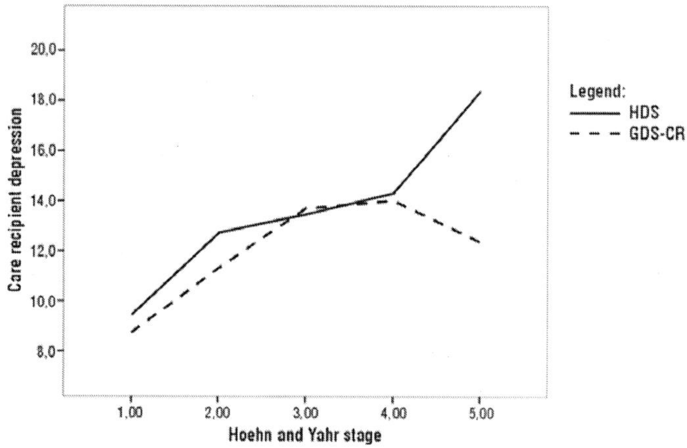

A further limitation of these analyses is that stratification according to the Hoehn and Yahr categories may be inappropriate, because of the relatively small number of patients in certain categories. The categories were therefore dichotomised to reflect early and late stages of the illness (stages I & II versus III, IV & V) and the resultant groups of patients with milder versus more advanced symptoms of PD were compared in relation to carer outcomes. The results are shown in table 10-30.

It appears that certain of the carer outcomes are sensitive to disease severity, in particular care-giving strain, which increases with severity, but also GDS-depression and marital satisfaction which decrease over the course of the illness. The carer's perceptions of psychological symptoms in the care-recipient also tend to increase with illness progression.

Furthermore, both patient depression (GDS) (Mann-Whitney U=197.00; $p \geq .02$) and anxiety (HAM-A) were related to carer (GDS) depression

(Mann-Whitney U=195.00; $p \geq .02$). Patient cognitive impairment, on the other hand, did not appear to result in greater marital dissatisfaction (MAS) (U=288.0; p=0.11) or GDS-depression in carers (U=350.0; p=0.73).

Table 10-30. Carer outcomes in relation to PD disease severity.

Carer outcome	Hoehn and Yahr stage					Mann-Whitney	Signif. level
Mean scores	1 N=10	2 N=5	3 N=31	4 N=27	5 N=2	U	p
Strain (MSS)	5.1	9.5	11.0	14.9	14.0	151.0	0.00
GDS	3.4	10.0	8.4	8.5	2.5	270.5	0.017
BDI	3.7	9.6	7.6	7.6	5.5	323.0	0.092
GHQ	1.9	8.0	3.8	5.9	4.5	321.5	0.086
MAS	134.0	121.2	104.4	111.1	137.0	220.0	0.002
CFQ-carer	29.1	40.7	34.1	31.0	23.0	410.0	0.596
CFQ- depr	9.3	12.8	13.7	15.7	10.0	282.5	0.026
CFQ-cog	9.9	14.8	16.7	18.7	16.0	234.0	0.004

Figures in the main body of the table represent mean scores for carer outcome measures according to H&Y stage. H&Y categories 1 and 2 combined vs H&Y categories 3,4 and 5 for the Mann-Whitney test.

These analyses, whilst providing some insight into the complex relationships in the data, are limited in so far as they do not account for multi-collinearity among variables. Before turning to the multivariate statistical analyses that are required for these purposes, a replication of the factor analysis of the variables representing the main symptom domains of PD will presented, in order to confirm that the underlying patterns in the data remain constant in an independent sample (PD3) of patients with PD.

As a preliminary step to attempting a replication of the factor structure obtained with sample PD2, a comparison of samples PD2 and PD3 was carried out, in order to determine whether the groups differed in any significant way from each other in relation to the demographic and clinical criteria examined. The results of this comparison are presented in table 10-31. It can be seen that there were no differences between PD2 and PD3 with respect to gender distribution, social class, the severity of PD (Hoehn & Yahr scale) or functional disability (NUDS). As a consequence of the age differences which occurred as a result of difficulties in recruiting patients to stage III, the mean age for PD3 was higher and duration of illness longer, than for PD2. There were no differences with regard to levels of depression, though PD3 had worse memory but better visuospatial performance than PD2. There were no differences between the groups on estimates of pre-morbid intelligence.

Table 10-31. Comparison of samples PD2 and PD3.

Patient variable	**PD2**	**PD3**	**Statistical comparison of PD2 & PD3**			
Nonparametric tests	**N**	**N**	**U**	***p***		
Gender	male N= 31 female N= 29	male N=49 female N=26	1942.50	0.11	*two-tailed*	
Social class	I=5; II=11 III=16 IV=18 V=10	I=7 II=15 III=20 IV=23 V=10	1816.00	0.27	*two-tailed*	
H&Y (grade)	median = 3	median = 3	2193.00	0.79	*two-tailed*	
Parametric tests	mean ± SD	mean ± SD	t df=133	*p*	95% confidence interval of the difference	
					Lower	Upper
Age (yrs)	63.2 ± 5.6	66.1 ± 6.2	2.84	0.005	-4.98	-0.89
PD duration (yrs)	7.6 ± 4.2	9.2 ± 5.0	2.06	0.04	-3.26	-0.07
NUDS	38.3 ± 6.9	36.4 ± 8.1	1.48	0.14	1.95	1.32
HAM-D	13.0 ± 6.9	13.4 ± 5.7	0.39	0.70	-0.42	1.08
FR (no. correct)	39.7 ± 11.6	34.7 ± 10.2	2.67	0.009	5.01	1.88
Benton (errors)	12.7 ± 8.6	7.49 ± 6.4	4.00	0.00	5.19	1.30
Schonell (IQ)	105.2 ± 12.0	106.5 ± 10.6	0.65	0.52	1.31	2.01

U = Mann Whitney U statistic; *p*= significance level.
Scales: H&Y – Hoehn & Yahr scale, NUDS – Northwestern University Disability Scale, HAM-D – Hamilton Depression Scale, FR – immediate free recall test of verbal memory, Benton – visuospatial test, Schonell – Schonell Reading Test (estimate of pre-morbid IQ).

10.3.7 Replication Factor Analysis

Sixteen variables, derived from the measures used, were entered into the replication factor analysis. The indicators of factorability were good: Bartlett's test of sphericity gave an approximate χ^2 value of 562.47 (df=120, p=0.00) and the Kaiser-Meyer-Olkin (KMO) measure of sampling adequacy, indicated that 0.78 of the variance is explained by the factors.

Table 10-32. Factor structure of PD-illness related variables.

Component	Eigenvalue	% of variance	Cumulative % of variance
1	**5.16**	**32.26**	**32.3**
2	**2.17**	**13.59**	**45.8**
3	**1.76**	**11.00**	**56.8**
4	1.26	7.9	64.7

Table 10-33. Rotated factor matrix with loadings.

Patient Variables	Component loadings		
	PD somatic	cognitive	depression
Patient age at examination	.233	-.032	- .019
Current daily L-dopa dose	.293	**-.591**	.184
Current daily benzhexol dose	.112	**-.631**	- .080
Other medication for PD	.362	-.108	- .400
Antidepressive medication	.042	-.041	.268
Duration of illness	**.680**	-.014	- .242
Hoehn &Yahr (motor) score	**.871**	.071	.129
WHO scale	**.868**	.177	.227
Karnofsky scale	**-.860**	-.188	- .207
Webster scale	**.798**	.104	.179
NUDS (functional)score	**-.860**	-.060	- .216
HAM-Depression score	.269	-.098	**.824**
GDS score	.201	.134	**.857**
Free Recall memory score	-.246	**-.732**	-.098
Schonell (IQ) score	.094	**.679**	.295
Benton: visuospatial abilities	.190	**.669**	.004

The replication factor analysis with varimax rotation yielded four components (see table 10-32) and three of these, with an eigenvalue > 1.5 were interpreted. The loadings for the factors are shown in table 10-33. The three factors accounted for nearly 56.8% of the variance in the sample. These factors were considered to represent: "PD somatic symptoms", "cognitive symptoms" and "depression"; the fourth factor, although not interpreted here, appeared to be a "chronicity" component. The factors are therefore the same as those identified in stage II of the research and replicate the findings of stage II in an independent sample of patients with PD.

10.3.8 Analysis of the care-giving situation in PD

10.3.8.1 Factor analysis

A principal components factor analysis was also used in order to examine patterns in the relationships between patient and carer variables. Twenty-four variables were entered into the exploratory factor analysis using varimax rotation. The analysis yielded five components accounting for over 70% of the total variance, which are shown in table 10-34. Bartlett's test of sphericity gave an approximate χ^2 value of 915.83 (df=253, p=0.00) indicating good factorability and the Kaiser-Meyer-Olkin (KMO) measure of sampling adequacy was 0.72. Cattell's scree plot suggested a final solution of four factors above the break between the steep and shallow parts of the curve (see figure 10-7). The first four components with an eigen value > 1.5 were interpreted and accounted for 66.2% of the total variance in the sample. These component factors were considered to represent: (1) "PD patient somatic symptoms", (2) "Carer well-being", (3) "PD patient cognitive symptoms", and (4) "PD patient neuropsychiatric symptoms". Their loadings are shown in table 10-35; variables with loadings $\geq$ 0.4 were interpreted.

Table 10-34. Factor structure of PD-illness and carer variables.

Component	Eigen value	% of variance	Cumulative % of variance
1	**7.62**	**33.1**	**33.1**
2	**3.44**	**15.0**	**48.1**
3	**2.23**	**9.7**	**57.8**
4	**1.93**	**8.4**	**66.2**
5	1.06	4.6	70.8

Figure 10-7. Cattell's scree plot of component factors.

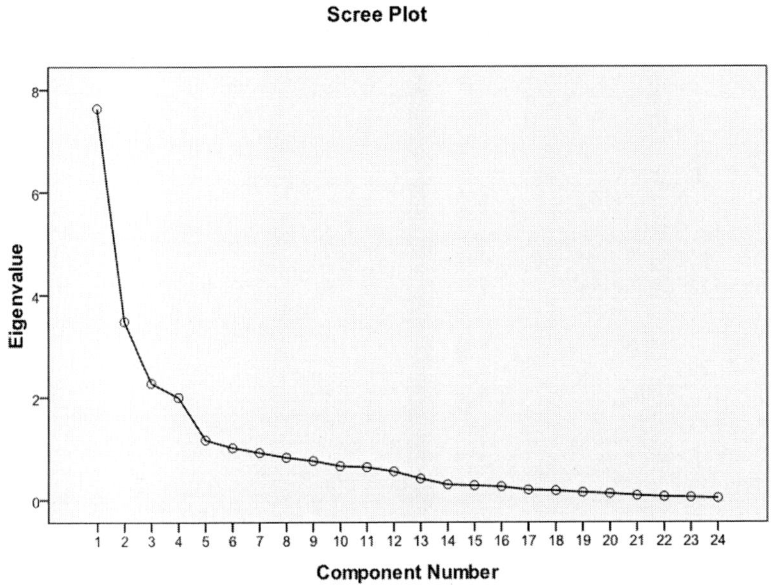

Of the carer variables only carer strain was associated with the physical measures of PD in component (1). This is not surprising, as the Machin Strain Scale is a measure of the strain associated with care-giving, and probably reflects additional tasks for the carer associated with the care recipient's deterioration in physical functioning. Carer variables, including measures of depression, strain and marital relationship satisfaction loading on component (2) are associated with the carer's perception of cognitive failure and depression in the care recipient and with the daily dose of L-dopa taken by the patient. Component (3) which represents cognitive function in the care recipient demonstrates that cognitive performance is associated with levels of medication taken by the patient in order to control the symptoms of PD. Component (4), comprises exclusively the measures of anxiety and depression for the patient, suggesting that depressive symptoms are independent of both the motor and cognitive symptoms of PD and of carer variables representing depression and the strain of care-giving. Neither do the neuropsychiatric symptoms in the patient appear to be associated with the carers' perceptions of these symptoms.

Table 10-35. Rotated factor matrix with loadings.

	Factor loadings			
	PD somatic	**Carer welfare**	**Patient cognitive**	**Patient neuro-psychiatric**
***Patient variables*:**				
Duration of illness	**.690**	.206	-.056	-.319
Daily L-dopa dose	.231	**.439**	**-.514**	.266
Daily benzhexol dose	.062	.103	**.727**	-.214
Other PD medication	.362	-.108	**- .400**	-.060
Antidepr. medication	-.059	-.165	-.134	.139
H &Y (motor) score	**.867**	.029	.057	.170
WHO scale	**.860**	.174	.190	.202
Karnofsky scale	**-.883**	-.087	-.151	-.205
Webster scale	**.850**	-.028	.153	.158
NUDS (functional)	**-.879**	-.018	-.104	-.200
HAM-Depression	.275	.129	.038	**.811**
GDS-patient	.186	.294	.186	**.607**
Hamilton Anxiety	**.451**	.154	.164	**.745**
Free Recall score	-.299	-.064	**-.748**	-.091
Schonell (IQ) score	.021	.116	**.725**	.328
Benton score	.207	-.028	**.699**	.158
Carer variables:				
GDS-carer	.097	**.920**	.006	.142
BDI	.026	**.879**	.080	.188
GHQ	.073	**.823**	-.159	.283
Machin Strain Scale	**.523**	**.570**	.054	.206
MAS	-.102	**- .651**	-.128	.039
CFQ-carer	-.056	**.504**	.042	-.267
CFQ-other-cognitive	.206	**.583**	.181	-.006
CFQ-other-depression	.146	**.400**	.019	.224

10.3.9 Testing models of carer outcome using multiple regression analyses

A difficulty in interpreting correlations in the data set is that many of the predictor variables are intercorrelated and not independent of one another. To overcome this complication and to identify which patient characteristics are predictive of carer outcomes, stepwise multiple regression was used. This procedure identifies the most significant predictor first and then eliminates the potential influence of this predictor from the remaining potential predictors before searching for a second significant predictor, and so on. Two main models of care-giving were examined, one based exclusively on PD-illness related variables, the other with the addition of carer variables. Each of these models was tested using four dependent variables reflecting carer outcomes: depression (GDS, BDI and GHQ), strain (MSS), cognitive failures for the carer (CFQ) and marital satisfaction (MAS). The choice of independent variables was guided by the results of the factor analysis and representative variables were chosen to reflect each of the four factors obtained. PD-illness related (independent) variables were chosen to represent the main illness domains and, as far as possible, to avoid collinearity. They included: disease duration, disease severity (H&Y), patient cognitive (FR) and affective symptoms (GDS). Although disease duration and severity are significantly correlated (see table 10-29), they were both included in the analyses because illness duration is also an indirect measure of the length of time devoted to care-giving and as such reflective of carer characteristics. The Hoehn and Yahr scale was selected as being representative of the motor disability in PD for two reasons. Firstly, perhaps more than any of the other measures used, it can be considered as more closely reflecting the motor symptoms without "contamination" from other variables. Secondly it has been used in previous studies, more frequently than other scales and therefore provides a basis for comparison. However, it should be remembered that PD is a singularly unpredictable illness, in which motor symptoms may sometimes fluctuate from hour to hour, and it is not uncommon for patients to describe themselves as having "good" and "bad" days. The extent to which these fluctuations affect patients' responses in any of the main symptom domains of PD at any given time is difficult to establish. Nevertheless, the Hoehn and Yahr, which provides a broad measure of disease severity in terms of the stage of advancement of the illness, appeared to provide an adequate measure of overall physical functioning for the purposes of the present study.

Using the stepwise method for multiple regression, a significant model was developed for each of the carer outcome variables for depression using, in the first instance, only PD-illness related variables. All three measures of carer depression were predicted by depression (GDS) in the care recipient: carer-BDI ($F(1,73)=10.26$, $p=.002$), where it accounted for 14% of the variance in scores; carer-GHQ ($F(1,73)=11.54$, $p=.001$), where it explained 15% of the variance; and carer-GDS ($F(2,72)=9.20$, $p<.00$), where together with duration of illness, the model explained 22% of the variance in carer depression.

Unstandardised (B) and standardised correlation coefficient (β) estimates and their significance values for predictors which reached the significance level of <0.05, with the proportion of the variance (R^2) in the carer outcomes accounted for by the six regression equations calculated are presented in table 10-36. Only those predictors which were included in the model derived from the analysis are shown, in the order in which they were extracted.

Table 10-36. Stepwise multiple regression analyses using PD illness-related variables to predict carer outcomes.

Carer outcome		Regression coefficients			t-value	Signif	95% confidence interval for B	
Step	Predictor Variables	B	SE B	β	t	*p* value	Lower Bound	Upper Bound
GDS		R^2=0.25 Adjusted R^2=0.22						
1	CR: GDS	0.42	0.11	0.43	3.68	0.001	0.19	0.66
2	Illness durtn	0.32	0.15	0.25	2.18	0.03	0.03	0.62
BDI		R^2=0.15 Adjusted R^2=0.14						
1	CR: GDS	0.38	0.12	0.39	3.20	0.002	0.14	0.61
GHQ		R^2=0.17 Adjusted R^2=0.15						
1	CR: GDS	0.45	0.13	0.41	3.40	0.001	0.18	0.71
MSS		R^2=0.25 Adjusted R^2=0.22						
1	CR: GDS	0.44	0.10	0.47	4.57	0.00	0.25	0.63
2	CR: H&Y	2.25	0.60	0.38	3.72	0.00	1.04	3.46
CFQ-carer		No relationships established for CFQ-carer.						
MAS		R^2=0.09 Adjusted R^2=0.07						
1	CR: GDS	-1.42	0.59	-0.30	-2.39	0.02	-2.60	-0.23

CR – care recipient, GDS – Geriatric Depression Scale, BDI – Beck Depression Inventory, GHQ – General Health Questionnaire, CFQ-carer – Cognitive Failures Questionnaire for carer, MSS – Machin Strain Scale, MAS – Marital Adjustment Scale, H&Y – Hoehn & Yahr stage.

Further, carer outcome in the form of strain as measured on the Machin scale was predicted by patient depression and motor stage but not by cognitive performance ($F(2,72)=23.13$, $p=.00$); these variables accounted for 22% of the variance in the strain measure. It should be noted that similar results were obtained when the clinician rated Hamilton Depression Scale (HAM-D) was used as the measure of depression for the patients ($F(2,72)=13.35$, $p=.00$; adjusted $R^2=0.30$), indicating that motor stage (H&Y) and the HAM-D accounted for 30% of the variance in carer strain. However, patient variables completely failed in significantly contributing to the variance in cognitive failures for the carer (CFQ-carer), which was treated as a potential measure of strain, though not with specific reference to care-giving. Finally marital satisfaction (MAS) was examined as a possible outcome variable for carers. The multiple regression analysis showed that of the patient variables, only depression made a significant contribution to marital satisfaction ($F(1,73)=5.70$, $p=.02$) and accounted for 7% of the variance.

A model of carer outcome was also developed in which carer characteristics were included with the PD-illness related variables described above. Using carer age and gender, perceptions of psychological symptoms in the care recipient, carer strain and marital satisfaction, quite different relationships with carer depression were identified through the regression analyses.

The results of the regression analyses are summarised in table 10-37. Carer depression (GDS) was associated with carer strain and marital satisfaction ($F(2,72)=20.77$, $p=.00$), which accounted for 44% of the variance in carer depression. Carer depression (BDI) was predicted by higher levels of carer strain and carers' heightened perceptions of cognitive dysfunction in the care recipient ($F(2,72)=19.97$, $p=.00$) accounting for 33% of the variance, and carer psychological morbidity (GHQ) by carer strain and carer age ($F(2,72)=25.33$, $p=.00$), accounting for 40% of the variance. Younger carers had a tendency to be more depressed. Here too, using a clinician measure of depression in the patient (HAM-D) rather than patient self-report measures in the form of the GDS did not alter the results. These results may reflect a different focus on symptoms in the depression scales and underlines the need to use a variety of instruments in order to capture the variance in the data. Of the regression models developed in the analyses, that using the Geriatric Depression Scale to estimate carer depression, allowed for the largest proportion of the variance (44%) to be explained by the independent variables for the main model of care-giving tested, which conceptualised carer outcomes in terms of psychological morbidity.

Treating care-giving strain (MSS) as an outcome variable in its own right revealed an association with the carer's perception of depression in the care recipient, more severe motor impairment, decreased marital satisfaction, increased patient depression and longer illness duration ($F(5,69)=19.70$, $p=.00$), which explained 65% of the variance in the strain measure. These findings underline the multidimensional nature of care-giving strain. Use of the HAM-D as the measure of patient depression produced broadly similar results to those obtained with the GDS. None of the independent variables entered into the regression equation proved to be

Table 10-37. Stepwise multiple regression analyses predicting carer outcomes.

Carer outcome		Regression coefficients			t-value	Signif	95% confidence interval for B	
Step	Predictor Variables	B	SE B	β	t	*p* value	Lower Bound	Upper Bound
GDS		R^2=0.46 Adjusted R^2=0.44						
1	MSS	0.50	0.13	0.46	3.72	0.001	0.23	0.77
2	MAS	-0.07	0.03	-0.32	-2.57	0.01	-0.12	-0.01
BDI		R^2=0.36 Adjusted R^2=0.33						
1	MSS	0.38	0.15	0.36	2.63	0.01	0.09	0.68
2	CFQ-other-cognitive	0.27	0.11	0.33	2.40	0.02	0.04	0.49
GHQ		R^2=0.43 Adjusted R^2=0.40						
1	MSS	0.67	0.14	0.54	4.91	0.00	0.39	0.94
2	Carer age	-0.30	0.11	-0.30	-2.78	0.01	-0.51	-0.08
MSS		R^2=0.68 Adjusted R^2=0.65						
1	CFQ-other-depression	0.24	0.10	0.25	2.30	0.02	0.03	0.45
2	CR: H&Y	1.30	0.54	0.23	2.40	0.02	0.21	2.40
3	MAS	-0.06	0.02	-0.30	-3.33	0.002	-0.09	-0.02
4	CR: GDS	0.28	0.10	0.31	2.88	0.006	0.08	0.47
5	Illness durtn	0.24	0.11	0.21	2.24	0.03	0.02	0.46
CFQ-carer		None of the variables were significant predictors of CFQ-carer.						
MAS		R^2=0.27 Adjusted R^2=0.25						
1	MSS	-2.62	0.61	-0.52	-4.28	0.00	-3.86	-1.39

Note: unstandardised (B) and standardised regression coefficients (β) for the variables entered into the model for each of the regression equations derived are shown. Predictor variables include carer characteristics. CR – care recipient, GDS–Geriatric Depression Scale, BDI – Beck Depression Inventory, GHQ – General Health Questionnaire, CFQ-carer – Cognitive Failures Questionnaire for the carer, MSS – Machin Strain Scale, MAS – Marital Adjustment Scale, CFQ-other-depression – carer perceptions of depression in the patient, CFQ-other-cognition – carer perceptions of cognitive dysfunction in the patient.

significant predictors of cognitive failures in the carer (CFQ). Evaluation of marital satisfaction as an outcome for carers demonstrated an association with care-giving strain ($F(1,73)=18.33$, $p=.00$), accounting for 25% of the variance in this measure. However from these results it is clear that there is a reciprocal relationship between care-giving strain and marital satisfaction, demonstrating that they have a mutual influence on each other.

In summary, it should be remembered that regression analyses are based on correlations and cannot be used to determine causality, unless it can be demonstrated that the independent variables preceded the dependent variables in time. Clearly in an analysis of the kind undertaken here, it is not possible to make this assumption and care needs to be taken in interpreting these results.

10.3.10 Classification of carers using discriminant function analysis

Discriminant function analysis was performed in order to generate functions which might correctly classify carers into two groups on key dependent variables. Recommended cut-off points for the standardised measures of carer depression were used to dichotomise the carers into groups defined as "depressed" versus "non-depressed" on these dependent outcome variables, which included the GDS, BDI and GHQ. For the remaining carer dependent variables, where cut-off points were not available, a dichotomous classification was derived from the standardised distributions of group scores (mean score + 2S.D.). This was the case for the Machin Strain Scale, the Marital Adjustment Scale and the Cognitive Failures Questionnaire. In addition carer age and gender were also used as grouping variables. The independent or predictor variables entered into the analysis included: duration and severity of illness (H&Y stage), patient depression (GDS) and cognitive function (FR), patient depression and cognition as perceived by the carer (CFQ-other), and as appropriate – measures of carer strain (MSS), marital satisfaction (MAS), and carer age and gender for analyses in which the results from these instruments were not treated as dependent variables in their own right. These variables were chosen as being representative of the main domains of disease variables, motor, affective and cognitive, and of the main carer variables. Multi-collinear variables were avoided. The stepwise method was used in the analysis. A single discriminant function was calculated for each of the dependent variables considered.

Classification values for the best discriminant functions are shown in table 10-38. The results indicate that all of the dependent carer variables chosen as outcome measures, with the exception of carer age and gender, have a correct classification rate in the region of 70% or higher. The analysis revealed that neither age nor gender discriminated carers with regard to the predictor variables used.

In each of the remaining cases, the value of the discriminant function was significantly different for the dichotomised groups (see χ^2 values shown in table 10-39). The predictor variables contributing to the functions differed in each case, but there were some commonalities. The Machin Strain Scale contributed to the discriminant function obtained for two of the measures of carer depression (both the GDS-carer and the GHQ) and to the measure of satisfaction with the relationship between the carer and the care recipient (MAS), lower levels of marital satisfaction being associated with greater depression and higher levels of strain in the carer.

Table 10-38. Results of discriminant analysis: proportions of carers classified correctly according to groups.

Carer Variables	Predicted Group Membership		% correctly classified	variables contributing to correct classification
	Group 1	Group 2		
Age	Not significant	Not significant	-	-
Gender	Not significant	Not significant	-	-
GDS	Non-depressed = 85.4%	Depressed = 80.0%	83.9%	MAS MSS
BDI	Non-depressed = 83.3%	Depressed = 66.7%	77.8%	CFQ-other-cognition Carer age
GHQ	Non-depressed = 92.3%	Depressed = 73.7%	86.2%	MSS Illness duration
MSS	Low strain= 80.6%	High strain = 85.7%	83.1%	Illness duration Patient GDS MAS
MAS	High marital satisfaction = 68.2%	Low marital satisfaction = 83.3%	77.6%	MSS Carer gender
CFQ-carer	Low perceived cognitive failure =80.0%	High perceived cognitive failure = 58.6%	69.5%	MAS Carer GDS

Table 10-39. Characteristics of the discriminant functions derived for the carer outcome variables.

Carer Outcome/ significant predictor variables	Level of difficulty on measure for groups (Mean score ± S.D.)		Discriminant Function			Test of function		
GDS-Carer/	Least	Most	Wilks' λ	Exact F	*p*	χ^2	df	*p*
MAS MSS	124.0±25.2 9.4 ± 5.0	90.1±27.2 16.8±4.5	.61	15.3	0.00	23.8	2	0.00
BDI-Carer/								
CFQ-other-cognition Carer age	13.3±6.7 65.1±7.5	22.6±5.4 66.0±7.3	.59	17.0	0.00	25.8	2	0.00
GHQ-Carer/								
MSS Illness duration	9.1±5.0 9.8±5.3	16.2±4.5 8.7±4.8	.57	18.7	0.00	27.8	2	0.00
Machin Strain Scale/								
Illness duration Patient GDS MAS	7.5±4.0 10.5±5.9 126.6±24.3	11.8±5.4 16.1±5.9 99.5±29.2	.52	15.1	0.00	32.5	3	0.00
MAS/								
MSS Carer gender	9.5±6.0 Female carers	14.6±4.1 Male carers	.73	8.8	0.001	15.0	2	0.001
CFQ/								
MAS	124.2±25.5	105.6±31.2	.90	5.5	0.02	5.2	1	0.02
Carer GDS	5.7±5.1	10.3±6.8	.87	7.7	0.008	7.1	1	0.008

However, the depressed versus non-depressed carers also differed significantly with respect to a number of predictor variables which are presented in table 10-38 for each of the outcome measures used. For example, the MAS was a significant predictor of carer GDS-depression and duration of illness, of the GHQ. Poorer relationship satisfaction and shorter illness duration were associated with greater depression on the respective outcome measures. The BDI for the carer was best predicted by the carer's age and his/her perception of cognitive decline in the care recipient. Older carers appeared to be more depressed on the BDI, as were those who reported higher levels of cognitive dysfunction in the care recipients.

The analysis also revealed that longer duration of illness and greater depression in the care recipient (GDS-patient), together with diminished satisfaction with the marital relationship (MAS), contributed to higher levels of carer strain (MSS).

Poor relationship satisfaction, appeared to be associated with high levels of care-giving strain and was greatest for male carers. Finally, higher scores on the CFQ-carer, which may be treated as a measure of more general strain, were predicted by low levels of marital satisfaction (MAS) and increased levels of depression in carers (GDS-carer).

10.3.11 Evaluation of potential mediation effects in the care-giving process

10.3.11.1 Testing the mediating effect of marital satisfaction in the relationship between carer strain and depression.

Regression equations were calculated according to the procedure recommended by Baron and Kenny (1986), in order to clarify whether marital satisfaction can be considered a mediating variable between carer subjective strain and depression. A variable is regarded as a mediator of the effect between a predictor or independent variable and a criterion or dependent variable, when it alters either the direction or the strength of the relationship between the two. A mediator effect is recognised as occurring, when the effect of the independent variable on the dependent variable changes, in keeping with changes in the mediator. Figure 10-8 illustrates the path model for the hypothesised relationship between the three variables.

Figure 10-8. Hypothesised path model with marital satisfaction acting as a mediating variable between carer strain and depression.

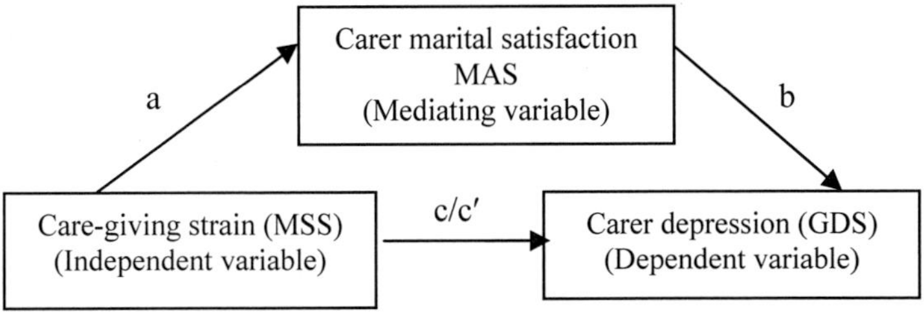

Path *ab* represents the mediated effect of carer strain on carer depression via the mediator. Path *c* represents the total effect of carer strain on carer depression; path *c′* is the direct effect.
Note: $c=c'+ab$

In order to demonstrate the mediating effects of marital satisfaction it is necessary to meet the following conditions: (1) variations in levels of the independent variable (MSS) should significantly account for variations in the presumed mediator (MAS), i.e. path a, (2) variations in the mediator (MAS) should significantly account for variations in the dependent variable (GDS), i.e. path b, and (3) when paths a and b are controlled, a previously significant relationship between the independent (MSS) and dependent variables (reflecting carer depression e.g. GDS), i.e. path c, should no longer exist, or at least should no longer be significant (Baron and Kenny 1986). Analysis of variance techniques are considered to provide only a limited test of mediation hypotheses (Fiske, Kenny and Taylor 1982) and it is recommended that a series of regression models should be estimated to test for any potential effects of mediators (Judd and Kenny 1981).

The following steps are necessary in order to establish the possible mediating role of marital satisfaction on carer outcome, using multiple regression analysis:

1. carer strain (the independent variable) has to be shown to be correlated with carer outcome. Carer depression (GDS-carer) was used as the criterion variable and carer strain (MSS) as the predictor variable in order to estimate and test path *c* in figure 10-8. This step establishes that there is an effect that may be mediated;
2. carer strain (the independent variable) must be correlated with marital satisfaction (the mediator). Marital satisfaction (MAS) was used as the criterion variable and carer strain as a predictor, in order

to estimate and test path *a* in figure 10-8. This step essentially involves treating the mediator as if it were an outcome variable in its own right;

3. marital satisfaction (the proposed mediating variable) has to be shown to affect carer outcome. Carer depression (GDS-carer) was used as the criterion variable and carer strain and marital satisfaction, as predictors in the regression equation in order to estimate and test path *b* in figure 10-8. Since the mediator and the outcome variables in this model may be correlated, because they are both caused by the same independent variable (carer strain), it is not sufficient to correlate just the mediator with the outcome. The independent variable must be controlled in establishing the effect of the mediator on the outcome;
4. if marital satisfaction were to completely mediate the relationship between carer strain and depression, then the effect of carer strain on carer depression, controlling for the mediator (marital satisfaction) i.e. path c' should be zero. The effects in both steps 3 and 4 are estimated in the same equation.

If all four of these steps are met, then the data are consistent with the hypothesis that the proposed mediating variable *completely* mediates the relationship between the independent and dependent variables, and if the first three steps are met, but step 4 is not, then *partial* mediation is indicated. Meeting these steps does not, however, conclusively establish that mediation has occurred because there are other (perhaps less plausible) models that may be consistent with the data. These three regression equations provide the tests of the linkages in the mediation model for marital satisfaction (after Baron and Kenny 1986). The results are shown in table 10-40.

In accordance with the steps outlined above for testing mediation, it was first established that carer strain (the independent or predictor variable) did indeed have an effect on carer outcome, by regressing carer depression (GDS-carer) on carer strain (MSS). The unstandardised regression coefficient (B=0.67) associated with the effect of carer strain on carer depression was significant (p=0.00). Thus, path *c* was significant and the requirement for establishing mediation in step 1 was met. In order to establish that carer strain was related to marital satisfaction (the hypothesised mediator), marital satisfaction (MAS) was regressed on carer strain (MSS). The unstandardised regression coefficient (B=-2.73) for this relationship was also significant at p=0.00 and so the conditions for step 2 were met, demonstrating that path *a* was significant.

Table 10-40. Regression equations for estimating the effect of marital satisfaction as a potential mediator of the relationship between carer strain and depression.

Test of steps in the mediation model	B	S.E.	t	*p*	R^2	β	Sobel test
Test of step 1 (path *c*)							
Dependent: Carer depression (GDS-C)	0.67	0.11	5.94	0.00	0.40	0.63	Z=2.53
Predictor: Carer strain (MSS)							SE=0.06
Test of step 2 (path *a*)							*p*=0.01
Dependent: Marital satisfaction (MAS)	-2.73	0.58	-4.73	0.00	0.29	-0.53	
Predictor: Carer strain (MSS)							ab/c=0.24
Test of step 3 (paths *b* and *c'*)							
Dependent: Carer depression (GDS-C)							
Mediator: Marital satisfaction (MAS) (Path *b*)	-0.06	0.02	-2.34	0.02	0.45	-0.28	
Predictor: Carer strain (MSS)	0.51	0.13	3.99	0.00		0.48	

Note: MAS – Marital Adjustment Scale; MSS – Machin Strain Scale; GDS-C – Geriatric Depression Scale for the carer.
B = unstandardised regression coefficient; S.E. = standard error term; R^2 = proportion of variance explained by the regression equation; β = standardised regression coefficient.

Further, to test whether marital satisfaction was related to carer depression, the GDS-carer was regressed simultaneously on both the predictor variable (carer strain) and on the mediator (marital satisfaction). The unstandardised regression coefficient (B=-0.06) associated with the relationship between marital satisfaction and carer depression (controlling for carer strain) was also significant (p=0.02), meeting the conditions for step 3 and indicating that path *b* was significant.

The third regression equation also provided an estimate of path *c'*, the relationship between carer strain and carer depression, controlling for marital satisfaction. Complete mediation is assumed when this path is zero. However, path *c'* as estimated by B=0.51 remained significant at *p*=0.00, although it was smaller than path *c* (B=0.67), suggesting that the mediation effects of marital satisfaction were only partial.

Given that the required conditions all hold in the predicted direction, it is likely that the analysis supports the hypothesis that marital satisfaction is indeed a partial mediator in the relationship between care strain and depression. However, since it is assumed that the mediator is caused by the independent variable, the two must be correlated, and this gives rise to multicollinearity when the effects of both variables on the dependent variable are estimated. In consequence, power is reduced in equation three, where the product of the mediator and the independent variable are added to the regression equation. A test of the significance for the indirect effect of the independent variable on the dependent variable, via the mediator is given by:

$$(b^2sa^2 + a^2sb^2 + sa^2sb^2)^{-1}$$

where sa and sb are the standard errors of a and b in the model illustrated in figure 10-8 (after Sobel 1982 cited in Baron and Kenny 1986). Following this procedure, the mediating effect of marital satisfaction (MAS) was found to be significant at *p*=0.01 (Sobel statistic Z= 2.53; S.E.= 0.05). Hence, it may be concluded that marital satisfaction does indeed demonstrate the hypothesised mediating role between carer strain and depression. The Sobel test is very conservative (MacKinnon, Warsi and Dwyer 1995) and so it can be assumed that the power of the analysis is adequate to support the conclusions.

According to Shrout and Bolger (2002) the effects of mediation may also be described in terms of the proportion of the total effect of the relationship, in this case between carer strain and depression, that is mediated by marital satisfaction. The proportion is given by ab/c; using the unstandardised regression coefficients for the model analysed in the present case, this is 0.164/0.67 = 24.4. Thus about 24% of the total effect of carer strain on carer depression is mediated by marital satisfaction. Estimates of this kind need to be treated with caution however, as sample sizes of at least 500 are needed for accurate estimation of the proportion of the total effect mediated (MacKinnon et al. 1995); such numbers are extremely difficult to achieve in clinical samples and more especially, in research conducted by one author, as in the kind of study reported here. It is therefore important, as Frazier, Tix and Barron (2004) point out, to be aware that this is merely a way of describing the amount of mediation, rather than being a formal test of the significance of the mediation effects. Figure 10-9 shows the standardised regression coefficients for the relationship between care-giving strain and carer depression as mediated by marital satisfaction.

Figure 10-9. Standardised regression coefficients (β) for the relationship between care-giving strain and carer depression as mediated by marital satisfaction. The standardised regression coefficient (c′) between carer strain and carer depression controlling for marital satisfaction with the care recipient is also shown.

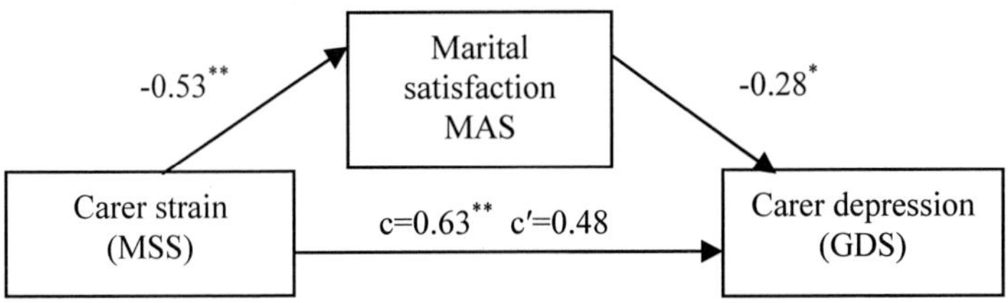

10.3.11.2 Evaluation of the role of potential mediators in the relationship between patient and carer variables

In the next stage of the analysis, the causal steps procedure recommended by Baron and Kenny (1986) was used to test linear mediator effects on the relationship between patient and carer variables. A path model was constructed for examining the potential mediating effects of carer strain and carers' perceptions of psychological functioning in the patient in the relationship between the independent (patient motor, affective and cognitive symptoms) and dependent variables (either carer depression or strain). In these analyses strain is treated alternately, as an intervening or mediating variable and as an outcome variable in its own right. The former assumption would appear reasonable, as strain is one of the strongest correlates of carer depression in the present study.

Furthermore, there are strong theoretical grounds based on stress process theory to expect a relationship of this kind. However, as described in chapter 6, carer strain is also frequently viewed as a dependent or outcome variable and to the extent that it is, at least partially, dependent on illness-related variables as the foregoing analyses have shown, it is treated as the outcome of these in the analysis that follows.

The nine sets of regression equations tested (three mediators x three patient symptom domains) for carer strain and depression are presented in tables 10-41 to 10-43. From table 10-41 it can be seen that neither motor nor cognitive symptoms of PD are associated with carer depression and thus, the conditions of step 1 for establishing mediation are not met. This however does not preclude mediation, but suggests that it is inconsistent (Kenny 2012). Only patient depressive symptoms are directly related to carer depression. The regression analysis (step 3) shows that the relationship between carer strain and depression, when patient depression is controlled (path *b*) is significant (B=0.62. p=0.00) and thus the conditions for step 3 of the analysis are met. Path c′ (B=0.08), the relationship between patient depressive symptoms and carer depression, is greatly reduced and statistically insignificant (p=0.56), suggesting that carer strain is a strong mediator in this relationship. This was confirmed using the Sobel equation to test for the significance of the difference between paths c and c′ in this model. The Sobel statistic was Z=2.77 (S.E.=0.09) and was significant at the p=0.005 level.

Thus mediation via strain appears to occur in the pathway from all three patient symptom domains to carer depression, but for both motor and cognitive symptoms, it is inconsistent. The proportion of the total effect of the relationship between patient depression and carer depression, that is mediated by strain is ab/c = (.53 x .62)/.43 = 76.4. Strain therefore, might be expected to mediate 76% of the effect of patient-related depression on carer depression. These relationships are shown in figure 10-10.

Figure 10-10. Standardised regression coefficients (β) for the relationship between PD-related affective symptomatology and carer depression as mediated by care-giving strain.

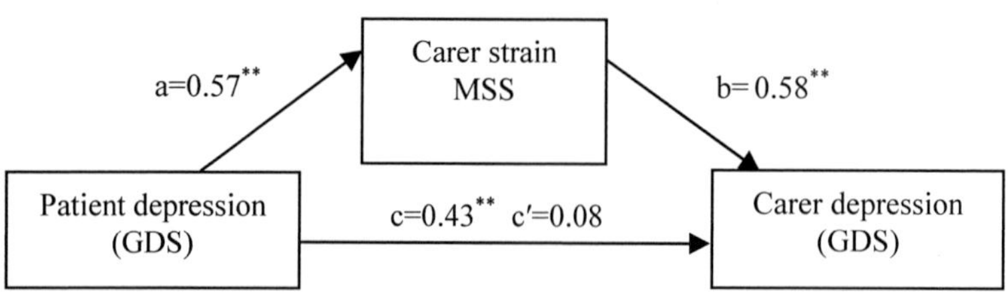

Table 10-41. Regression equations for estimating the effects of carer strain as a mediator of the relationship between patient (independent) variables relating to the main symptom domains of PD and carer depression (GDS-carer) as the dependent outcome variable.

Test of steps in the mediation model for PD *motor* symptoms:	B	S.E.	t	*p*	R^2	β	Sobel test
Test of step 1 (path *c*) Dependent: carer depr (GDS) Predictor: motor (H&Y)	0.72	0.82	0.88	.38	.01	0.12	path *c*=NS
Test of step 2 (path *a*) Dependent: carer strain (MSS) Predictor: motor (H&Y)	2.93	0.67	4.37	.00	.24	0.50	§*Z=3.67 SE=.65 *p*=.00
Test of step 3 (paths *b* and *c'*) Dependent: Carer depr (GDS) Mediator: Carer strain (MSS) (Path *b*) Predictor: motor (H&Y)	0.81 - 1.64	0.12 0.72	6.49 - 2.28	.00 .03	.45	0.76 - 0.27	
Test of steps in the mediation model for the ***depressive*** symptoms of Parkinson's disease:							
Test of step 1 (path *c*) Dependent: Carer depr (GDS) Predictor: Patient depr (GDS)	0.43	0.12	3.58	.001	.19	0.43	*Z=3.40 SE=.1 *p*=.001 ab/c=.76
Test of step 2 (path *a*) Dependent: Carer strain (MSS) Predictor: Patient depr (GDS)	0.53	0.10	5.18	.00	.32	0.57	
Test of step 3 (paths *b* and *c'*) Dependent: Carer depr (GDS) Mediator: Carer strain (MSS) (Path *b*) Predictor: Patient depr (GDS)	0.62 0.08	0.14 0.13	4.35 0.58	.00 .56	.40	0.58 0.08	
Test of steps in the mediation model for the ***cognitive*** symptoms of Parkinson's disease:							
Test of step 1 (path *c*) Dependent: Carer depr (GDS) Predictor: Patient free recall	-0.05	0.08	-.708	.48	.009	-0.09	path *c*=NS
Test of step 2 (path *a*) Dependent: Carer strain (MSS) Predictor: Patient free recall	-0.14	0.07	1.99	.05	.06	-0.25	§*Z=1.89 SE=0.05 *p*=0.05
Test of step 3 (paths *b* and *c'*) Dependent: Carer depr (GDS) Mediator: Carer strain (MSS) (Path *b*) Predictor: Patient free recall	0.69 0.04	0.12 0.06	5.91 0.68	.00 .50	0.40	0.65 0.07	
* Indicates that a set of regression equations meets the criteria for demonstrating the effects of the mediator; § indicates inconsistent mediation.							

Table 10-42. Regression equations for estimating the effects of carers' perceptions of depressive symptoms in the care recipient as mediators of the relationship between patient variables and carer strain.

Test of steps in the mediation model for PD *motor* symptoms:	**B**	**S.E.**	**t**	***p***	**R^2**	**β**	**Sobel test**
Test of step 1 (path *c*) Dependent: carer strain[1] Predictor: motor (H&Y)	2.93	0.67	4.36	.00	0.25	0.50	Z=1.82 SE=.41 *p*=.07 NS
Test of step 2 (path *a*) Dependent: CFQ-other-depr Predictor: motor (H&Y)	1.53	0.78	1.95	.05	0.06	0.25	
Test of step 3 (paths *b* & *c'*) Dependent: Carer strain[1] Mediator: CFQ-other-depr (Path *b*) Predictor: motor (H&Y)	0.49 2.39	0.10 0.57	4.97 4.15	.00 .00	0.51	0.49 0.41	
Test of steps in the mediation model for ***symptoms of depression*** in Parkinson's disease:							
Test of step 1 (path *c*) Dependent: Carer strain[1] Predictor: Patient GDS)	0.53	0.10	5.18	.00	0.32	0.57	[*]Z=2.68 SE=.09 *p*=.007 ab/c=.44
Test of step 2 (path *a*) Dependent: CFQ-other-depr Predictor: Patient GDS	0.60	0.10	5.78	.00	0.37	0.60	
Test of step 3 (paths *b* & *c'*) Dependent: Carer strain[1] Mediator: CFQ-other-depr (Path *b*) Predictor: Patient GDS	0.39 0.30	0.13 0.12	2.96 2.43	.005 .02	0.41	0.39 0.32	
Test of steps in the mediation model for ***cognitive symptoms*** in Parkinson's disease:							
Test of step 1 (path *c*) Dependent: Carer strain[1] Predictor: Patient free recall	-0.14	0.07	-1.99	.05	0.06	-.25	Z=-.86 SE=.05 *p*=.39 NS
Test of step 2 (path *a*) Dependent: CFQ-other-depr Predictor: Patient free recall	-0.07	0.08	-0.96	.34	0.02	-.12	
Test of step 3 (paths *b* & *c'*) Dependent: Carer strain[1] Mediator: CFQ-other-depr (Path *b*) Predictor: Patient free recall	0.57 -0.12	0.11 0.06	5.36 -1.97	.00 .05	0.39	.57 -.21	

[1] Machin Strain Scale
* Indicates that a set of regression equations meets the criteria for demonstrating the effects of the mediator.

Table 10-43. Regression equations for estimating the effects of carers' perceptions of cognitive function in the care recipient as mediators of the relationship between patient variables and carer strain.

Test of steps in the mediation model for *motor* symptoms of Parkinson's disease:	B	S.E.	t	*p*	R^2	β	Sobel test
Test of step 1 (path *c*) Dependent: Carer strain[1] Predictor: motor (H&Y)	2.93	0.67	4.36	.00	0.25	0.50	*Z=2.08 SE=.41 *p*=0.04 ab/c=.29
Test of step 2 (path *a*) Dependent: CFQ-other-cognition Predictor: motor (H&Y)	2.37	1.01	2.34	.02	0.09	0.29	
Test of step 3 (paths *b* & *c'*) Dependent: Carer strain[1] Mediator: CFQ-other-cog (Path *b*)	0.36	0.08	4.52	.00	0.48	0.46	
Predictor: motor (H&Y)	2.33	0.60	3.91	.00		0.40	
Test of steps in the mediation model for ***symptoms of depression*** in Parkinson's disease:							
Test of step 1 (path *c*) Dependent: Carer strain[1] Predictor: Patient GDS	0.53	0.10	5.18	.00	0.32	0.57	*Z=2.66 SE=.07 *p*=.008 ab/c=.37
Test of step 2 (path *a*) Dependent: CFQ-other-cognition Predictor: Patient GDS	0.63	0.15	4.25	.00	0.24	0.49	
Test of step 3 (paths *b* & *c'*) Dependent: Carer strain[1] Mediator: CFQ-other-cog (Path *b*)	0.31	0.09	3.33	.002	0.44	0.39	
Predictor: Patient GDS	0.35	0.11	3.15	.003		0.37	
Test of steps in the mediation model for ***cognitive symptoms*** in Parkinson's disease:							
Test of step 1 (path *c*) Dependent: Carer strain[1] Predictor: Patient free recall	-0.14	0.07	-1.99	.05	0.06	-0.25	*Z=-1.91 SE=.05 *p*=0.05 ab/c=.63
Test of step 2 (path *a*) Dependent: CFQ-other-cognition Predictor: Patient free recall	-0.21	0.10	-2.10	.04	0.07	-0.27	
Test of step 3 (paths *b* & *c'*) Dependent: Carer strain[1] Mediator: CFQ-other-cog (Path *b*)	0.42	0.09	4.84	.00	0.35	0.55	
Predictor: Patient free recall	-0.08	0.07	-1.29	.20		-0.15	

[1] Machin Strain Scale

* Indicates that a set of regression equations meets the criteria for demonstrating the effects of the mediator.

However, not all carers are depressed and it is clear from these analyses that the measure of carer strain does not mediate the effects of either the motor or cognitive symptoms of PD. It is therefore important to consider carer strain separately and to evaluate variables that may be influencing this measure.

With this purpose in mind, and using carer strain as the dependent or criterion variable in the analysis, the carers' perceptions of psychological symptoms in the care recipient were conceptualised as possible mediators of the relationship between patient variables and carer strain. The results of the evaluation for carers' perceptions of depressive symptoms in the care recipient are summarised in table 10-42.

Mediation occurred only in the case of PD-related depressive symptoms and not for cognitive or motor symptoms. The relationship between patient depression and carer strain was mediated by the carer's perceptions of depression in the patient. As figure 10-11 illustrates, the standardised regression co-efficient for the relationship between patient depression and carer strain decreased substantially when controlling for carer perceptions of depression in their spouse. The other conditions of mediation were also met: patient depression was a significant predictor of carer strain and of the carer's perceptions of patient depression, whilst the latter were also a significant predictor of carer strain, while controlling for patient depression. Carer perceptions of depression in the patient accounted for 44% of the mediated effect of patient depression on carer strain (ab/c = .60 x .39/ .53= 44.1).

Figure 10-11. Standardised regression coefficients for the relationship between patient affective symptoms and carer strain as mediated by carer perceptions of depression in the care recipient.

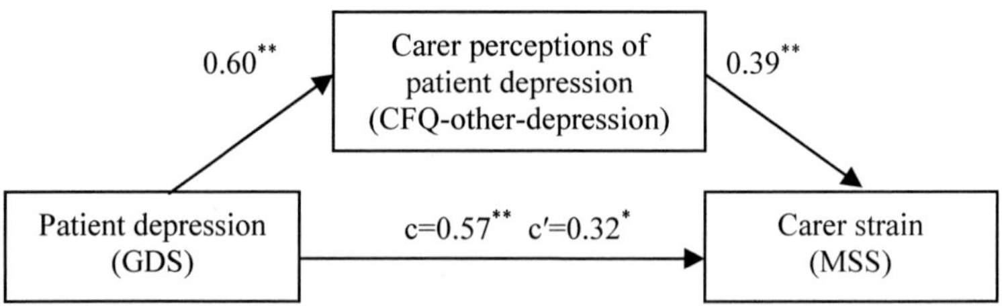

Results of the evaluation for carers' perceptions of cognitive symptoms in the care recipient are summarised in table 10-44. In this case, mediation occurred in all three symptoms domains associated with PD and accounted for 29% of the effect of patient motor (ab/c = 2.37 x .36/2.93= 29.1), 37% of affective (ab/c = .63 x .31/.53= 36.8) and 63% of cognitive (ab/c = -0.21 x 0.42/-0.14 = 63.0) symptoms on carer strain. These mediating effects are illustrated in figures 10-12 to 10-14.

Finally, a note of caution is also required regarding the power of these analyses. The relationships among the mediator, predictor and outcome can affect the power of tests of mediation. In particular, the power associated with the test of the relationship between the mediator and the outcome (path *b*) and between the predictor and outcome variables, when the mediator is controlled (path *c′*) decreases as the relationship between the predictor variable and the mediator (path *a*) increases (Kenny et al. 1998 in Kenny 2012). This is because as increasing amounts of variance in the mediator are explained by the predictor, less variance in the mediator is available to contribute to the prediction of the outcome. Thus as the relationship between the predictor and the mediator increases (path *a*), larger samples are needed to provide equivalent power levels to test the effects of path *b* (mediator-outcome) and path *c′* (predictor-outcome controlling for mediator) in comparison to situations in which the relationship between the predictor and mediator are smaller (Frazier et al. 2004). Furthermore, the requirement in the causal steps approach that the relationship between the predictor and the outcome (path *c*) be significant means that in order to obtain a power value of 0.8 with relatively small effect sizes for paths *a* and *b*, unrealistically high numbers of subjects would be required (Fritz and MacKinnon 2007).

Figure 10-12. Standardised regression coefficients for the relationship between patient motor symptoms and carer strain as mediated by carer perceptions of cognitive functioning in the care recipient.

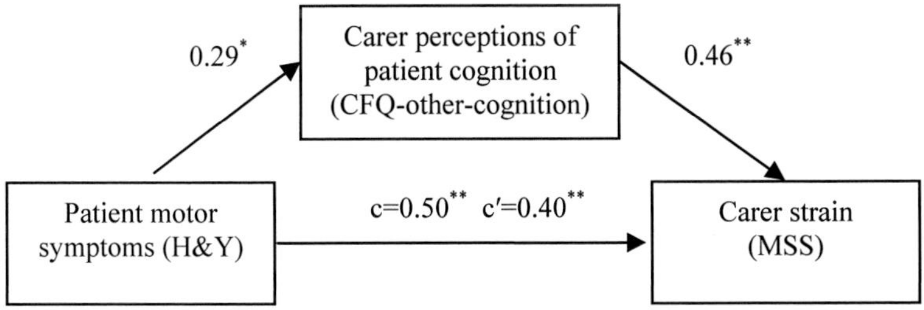

Figure 10-13. Standardised regression coefficients for the relationship between patient affective symptoms and carer strain as mediated by carer perceptions of cognitive functioning in the care recipient.

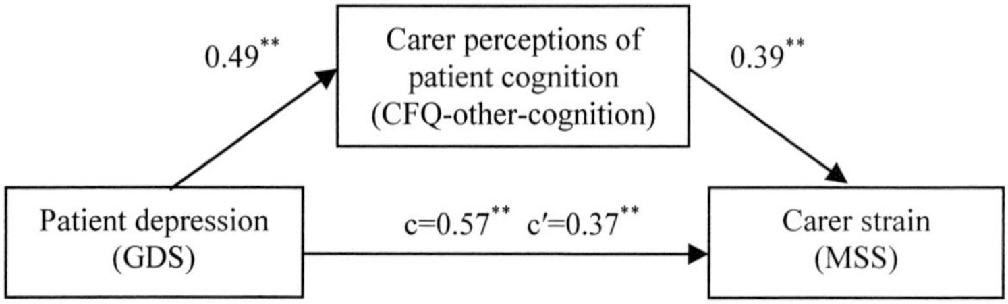

Figure 10-14. Standardised regression coefficients for the relationship between patient cognitive symptoms and carer strain as mediated by carer perceptions of cognitive functioning in the care recipient.

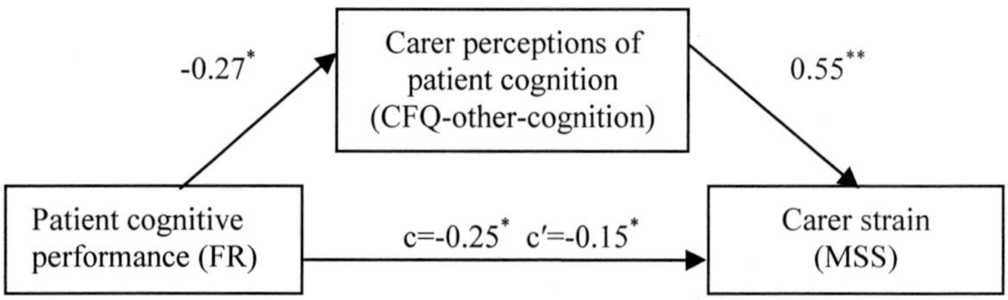

10.3.12 The accuracy of carers' perceptions of PD-related symptoms

Finally, in order to ascertain the accuracy of carers' judgements concerning the symptoms of PD, their evaluations were compared with more "objective" clinician-rated measures of motor, affective and cognitive functioning and with patients' self-rated affective symptoms. Raw scores from the instruments used were converted to standardised Z scores in order to make the comparison across different scales. Specifically, a test of the carers' perceptions of cognitive functioning in the care recipient versus the latter's performance on the free recall test of memory revealed significant differences (Wilcoxon's Z = -7.03, p= 0.00, N.S.) and similar results were obtained with the Benton visuospatial test (Wilcoxon's Z=-6.18, p=0.00). However, the carers' appraisal of the affective status of the patient compared to the patient's self-rated assessment of depressive symptoms on the GDS did not show any disparities (Wilcoxon's Z=-1.06, p=0.29, N.S.), nor were there any differences in relation to the clinician-rated HAM-D (Wilcoxon's Z=-0.23, p=0.82, N.S.). A comparison of clinician-rated functional performance for the patient (NUDS) and the carers' assessment of the activities of daily living in the patient revealed significant differences (Wilcoxon's Z=5.38, p=0.00). Hence carers' evaluation of affective symptoms in the care recipient do not differ significantly from either the patients' own reports or those of the clinician. However, their appraisals of the motor and cognitive symptoms show considerable divergence from clinician ratings of the patients' functioning in these areas.

The results of these analyses are discussed in relation to the questions posed for the study in chapters 11 and 12 that follow.

CHAPTER ELEVEN

THE RESEARCH STUDY: DISCUSSION - STAGES I-II

11.1 Introduction

The main focus of stage I of the research was the development and testing of a new instrument, the Addenbrooke's depression questionnaire, for measuring depressive symptomatology in patients with PD, with a view to determining whether their profile of depressive symptoms differs from that of DSM-IV-TR depressive disorders. Establishing the nature of depression in PD was an important preliminary step towards gaining a better understanding of the relationship between the main symptom areas in PD, which was the task of stage II of the research. Stage III of the study, which examined an independent sample of patients with PD, provided an opportunity to validate the results of stage II, in relation to the identification of characteristic symptom patterns in PD. The resultant findings, which helped to clarify relationships among the symptoms, were then used to investigate the outcomes of care-giving for spouse carers of the patients with PD studied in stage III of the research. The effects of potential mediating factors, such as the quality of the marital relationship for the couple in which one partner has PD, together with the carer's perceptions of the care recipient's disability, were also included in the assessment of carer outcomes. Relationship quality was identified from the literature as having potential significance to care-giving, but has hitherto been given little attention in the context of PD. Evaluation of carers' appraisals of the care-giving situation, and in particular, the way in which their subjective views of the non-motor symptoms of PD may affect the care-giving process, do not appear to have been examined previously.

11.1.1 Stage I: discussion of results

The assessment of depression in PD is fraught with difficulties, as described in chapter 3. Confusion arises from the overlap of motor and depressive symptoms in PD, causing difficulties in attributing symptoms to specific domains and because of the alleged differences in symptom profile for PD and DSM-defined depressive disorders. In addition, it seems that non-demented patients with PD may be more systematic in reporting their symptoms of depression than non-PD patients with MDD.

In order to investigate these questions, an instrument to measure depressive symptoms in PD was specifically designed for the purposes of this study. Items were chosen to reflect as broad a range of symptoms of depression as possible; they included mood and anhedonia, cognitive symptoms and certain of the somatic symptoms of depression such as diurnal variation, appetite and sleep problems. In so far as was possible, statements were worded in such a way as not to be confounded with the physical symptoms of PD. The structure of the instrument allowed a measure of the respondents' consistency in replying to the items to be determined. The properties of the instrument met established psychometric criteria to enable a comparison of symptom profiles for different groups of interest to be made. These are described in the following section.

11.1.1.1 Psychometric properties of the ADQ

Before the ADQ could be used for the purposes outlined above, it was necessary to establish its psychometric properties. In order to do so, it was important to ensure that certain key variables, such as age and gender, which are known to be associated with depression, were strictly controlled. This condition was achieved for the two groups of patients with PD (PD1 and PD2) that were examined and for the control subjects, there being no differences among the groups with respect to age and gender.

The study demonstrated that the ADQ had high internal consistency in both the clinical (PD and MDD) and nonclinical (control) samples studied. The split-half reliability of the ADQ was acceptable in all of the groups. It was lowest in the group of patients with MDD, probably reflecting the inconsistency of their responses to individual items. Good results were obtained for the PD groups indicating that from the point of view of reliability, the ADQ meets the requirements for an instrument to measure depression in PD.

Item analysis of the ADQ revealed that each of the component items of the questionnaire made an adequate contribution to the overall score. The corrected item-total correlations ranged within acceptable limits and in no instance did Cronbach's alpha for the full questionnaire increase when an item was removed, indicating that each of the items was contributing to the underlying construct of depression. The convergent validity of the

ADQ was found to be high in relation to established scales such as the HAM-D, the Leeds scales and the GDS for measuring depression, confirming that it is measuring the same underlying construct as these scales. Furthermore, principal component analysis of the ADQ with the forced restriction that only one factor be extracted, demonstrated that all the items loaded on this factor, with acceptable factor loadings. Thus it may be concluded that the questionnaire is indeed assessing a single construct, in the form of depression.

Finally, the discriminative validity of the ADQ was evaluated using ROC methodology and cut-off scores established for the instrument. The AUC for the ADQ was high (0.85) indicating that it has high concurrent validity with DSM-IV-TR criteria for depressive disorders in PD. The determination of an optimal cut-off point for any instrument depends upon the purpose for which it is to be used. For diagnostic purposes, an instrument requires a combination of high specificity and high PPV, which yields higher cut-off points than those used for screening purposes. For the ADQ this was established for a score of 30/31, which yields a specificity of 1.00 and a PPV of 1.00. At this cut-off point, patients are likely to be correctly classified as being depressed, but the likelihood that patients will also be correctly identified as not being depressed (NPV) is somewhat lower (0.65), i.e. cases of depression may be missed.

To be useful as a screening instrument, however, levels of high sensitivity and high NPV are required, i.e. minimising the risk of missing cases of depression. The cut-off for screening purposes was thus established at 16/17, with a sensitivity of 1.00 and an NPV of 1.00. Here the tendency is for cases to be falsely classified as being depressed. An optimal cut-off point for dichotomization of patients on the ADQ into depressed versus non-depressed individuals occurred at a score of 22/23 and this was used for the purposes of the present study.

11.1.1.2 Use of the ADQ to test hypotheses concerning depression in PD

The debate concerning the nature of depression in PD is characterised by a number of unresolved issues. These relate to (i) the true prevalence of depressive disorders in PD; (ii) the symptom profile for PD depression; and (iii) the origins of depression in PD.

(i) The prevalence of depression in the groups studied

A gold standard for the diagnosis of depression is the DSM-IV-TR (APA 2000). This classification however, precludes the diagnosis if depression is "due to a general medical condition" (diagnostic criteria: 293.83; APA

2000). In theory, this means that a diagnosis of depression cannot be made in PD, without a knowledge of its aetiology. Whilst this exclusion criterion serves to tighten up diagnostic procedures in psychiatric conditions, it is unhelpful in conditions such as PD, since the aetiology of certain symptoms, both physical and psychological, is usually unclear. Strict application of DSM-IV-TR diagnostic criteria would invalidate a diagnosis of depression in the majority of patients with PD. To a certain extent, this problem has been recognised with the introduction of a new category of "mood disorder due to Parkinson's disease", but whilst this overcomes a practical dilemma, it does little to resolve the theoretical need for clear diagnostic criteria in relation to the depressive symptoms of PD (Ehrt 2009). More recently, Starkstein et al. (2011) have argued that the full (DSM-IV-TR) criteria are appropriate for use in PD for diagnosis and research purposes.

Another problem for the diagnosis of depression in PD, as mentioned previously, is the difficulty of dealing with symptom overlap between depression and PD (Hoogendijk et al. 1998). Many of the somatic symptoms of affective disorder such as sleep disturbances, weight and energy loss, gastro-intestinal problems including constipation, sexual dysfunctions and psycho-motor retardation are also part of the presentation of PD. Thus their specificity for identifying depression in PD is considerably reduced. This means that a choice has to be made between what is called an "inclusive" or "exclusive" method of scoring in relation to these symptoms. The former method is based on the not unreasonable assumption that it is difficult to attribute individual symptoms to a particular source (affective disorder versus neurological disease process) and thus recommends that symptoms should be rated irrespective of their ambiguity. The latter method assumes that an experienced rater is able to make the crucial distinction regarding the alleged origin of the symptoms observed. Clearly, an inclusive approach to scoring inevitably results in higher rates of depressive symptomatology. Moreover, patients' responses based on self-rated depression scales are more likely to be based on an inclusive approach. The recent recommendations of an expert working group on setting provisional diagnostic criteria for depression in PD was to use an inclusive approach to symptom assessment in order to enhance the reliability of ratings and avoid the need for attributing symptoms to a specific cause (Marsh et al. 2006). In practice, neither of these solutions is satisfactory and the problem of symptom overlap remains a major obstacle to the diagnosis of depression in PD.

Bearing in mind these difficulties and the recommendations to ameliorate their consequences at least in part, the present study adopted an inclusive approach to scoring on the assessment instruments used to measure depression, and patients were instructed to record their symptoms on self-rating scales, as they were experienced, without attempting to identify their cause. In the sample of patients with PD who were interviewed (PD2) using the SCID, a standardised clinical assessment method for the diagnosis of depression, 10% were found to have a DSM-IV-TR diagnosis of major depression and a further 30% of minor depressive disorder. Although these prevalence rates are lower than those reported in the earlier literature on PD (see Cummings 1992), they are in keeping with those of a recent review (Reijnders et al. 2008), which controlled for the different settings from which patients were drawn and different diagnostic methods used, as well as using a quality assessment in order to select studies for inclusion in the review. By comparison, they found an average prevalence of 17% for MDD in PD, 13% of dysthymia, and 22% of minor depression, indicating that around 52% of patients might be expected to be suffering from depression at a given point in time. The results of the present study are also broadly in keeping with the recent study of Starkstein et al. (2011), using DSM-IV-TR criteria, which found that 11% of the sample of patients with PD were in the severe category for depression, 48% were moderately depressed and a further 41% did not meet the criteria for a depressive disorder.

As might be expected (see chapter 3) the estimates obtained for the prevalence of affective disorders on the instruments used in the present study were higher than when using DSM criteria, but they were still in keeping with those of the Reijnders et al. (2008) review. Overall, depression on the HAM-D was estimated to be 56.6% for the sample, with 18.3% of the patients obtaining a score in the range for severe depression, above the criterion score of 17. The prevalence of major depression on the ADQ was estimated to be 15.0% and 50% of the entire sample were found to have some kind of depression (either mild or severe). 33.3% of patients were found to be depressed according to the Leeds depression scale. These figures confirm that depression is a common concomitant of PD and are higher than for the general population (Boyd and Weissman 1982); they probably reflect a pre-existing vulnerability to depression in PD which may be associated with the same neurobiological substrate as the motor disorder. Furthermore, 23.0% of the patients interviewed had a personal history of unipolar depression, for which they had received treatment in the past, and the manifestation of which preceded the onset of the motor symptoms of PD. This is in keeping with other studies which have also reported that depression frequently predates PD (e.g. Looi et al. 2005).

Comparison of PD2 with the control groups, showed that a significantly higher proportion of the patients with MDD (82.5%) were above the criterion score for severe depression on the HAM-D, whilst none of the age-matched control group with impaired mobility or the healthy control group were depressed at this level. On the other hand, a considerable proportion of the PD2 group (35.0%) were within the mild to moderate range for depressive symptoms compared to the control groups, where only 12.3% of the low mobility control groups and 6.6% of the healthy control group were in this category. These figures confirm the greater prevalence of depression in PD reported in earlier studies (see Reijnders et al. 2008).

Broadly similar findings were obtained with the ADQ, in that the proportion of patients in the severe category was greatest (56.7%) for the MDD group, the PD2 group did not differ with respect to the control group with impaired mobility (15.0% versus 14.8%, respectively) and the healthy control group contained the fewest severely depressed people (6.6%).

A somewhat surprising finding was that although the PD groups studied (PD1 and PD2) had been matched for age, gender, physical disability and levels of depression on the two depression scales on which they had been assessed in common (Leeds and ADQ), the rate of severe depression in PD1 was almost twice that in PD2 as measured on the ADQ. The levels of milder depression in the two groups were similar. The reasons for this are unclear, but they may reflect sampling differences (self-selected respondents replying to a postal questionnaire versus an unselected sample chosen to be as representative as possible of people suffering from PD). The overall prevalence of depression for PD1 as measured on the GDS was comparable to that found on the ADQ, with similar proportions of patients in the severe and milder categories, so that the greater prevalence of patients in the severe category cannot be attributed to the measurement scales. It is unfortunate that the study design did not allow all of the groups to be examined with the same instruments, in particular with the observer rated HAM-D, as this may have helped to clarify these comparisons. However, the estimated prevalence for depression on the HAM-D (56.6%) for PD2 is slightly higher than that for the ADQ (50%). This pattern is a little unusual, in that observer ratings of depressive symptomatology are usually more conservative than self-rated reports. The possibility therefore arises that the ADQ has achieved its goal in minimising the problems of symptom overlap in PD, which it is contended, is a considerable problem for most depression rating scales (e.g. Koerts et al. 2008). It is recognised however, that further work with the ADQ is required in order to confirm this suggestion.

Overall, since this was not intended to be an epidemiological study, and was not designed as one, the estimate of depression prevalence was a secondary aim, and it is important not to over-interpret these results. The differences in the rates of depression found with the use of various assessment methods may simply reflect sample sizes that are not designed for epidemiological research. Equally however, they are reflective of differences reported in the literature associated with the use of diverse instruments (see Chapter 3). Suffice it to say that the prevalence rates for the PD samples are in keeping with the results of other studies evaluated for quality, and in which patients were drawn from a setting similar to that in this study and with comparable methods of assessment.

In addition the results of the present study confirm the picture that has emerged from the literature, suggesting that whilst around 50% of patients with PD are affected by depression, in the main, the depression is of a type characterised by milder symptoms than in MDD (Starkstein et al. 2011). Moreover, although no differences were found between the PD groups and the control group with impaired mobility when depression was assessed on self-rated instruments such as the ADQ and GDS, considerable differences emerged with observer rated evaluations using the HAM-D. As previously mentioned, this pattern for self-rated reports of symptoms to be elevated with respect to observer rated ones is a frequent finding in the literature (see Chapter 3). The age matched healthy control group reported significantly lower rates of depressive symptomatology than either the PD or the low mobility groups, but the same trend for self rated assessments to give higher levels of reported symptoms was observed.

Finally, the difference in the frequency of severe symptoms of depression between groups PD1 and PD2, is not a hindrance to the interpretation of the results of this study, as the questions of interest to the research are evaluated primarily in PD2, whose characteristics were established with the aid of interviews and therefore include the possibility of clinician-verification of the data obtained. Results from PD1 were used only to form the subgroup of patients with high scores for depression on the ADQ for comparison with an MDD sample with equivalent scores. Thus the higher rates of severe depression in this sample were of particular advantage to the hypotheses tested in this study.

(ii) The symptom profile for depression in PD

The possibility that differences in the psychopathological features of depression in PD may be distinctive and differ from DSM-IV-TR depressive disorders has been raised by several authors (e.g. Gotham et al. 1986; Pereira do Prado and Barbosa 2005; Ehrt et al. 2006). However, others have challenged this view, concluding that there are no significant differences between the features of depression in PD and MDD (e.g. Merschdorf et al. 2003). Clarification of these positions is important from the point of view of the conceptualisation and clinical diagnosis of depression in PD. Moreover, alleged differences in symptomatology for PD have been used to argue in favour of a "reactive" position regarding the origin of depressive symptoms (Farabaugh et al. 2009), whilst the lack of any differences is seen as endorsing a common neurobiological explanation for the symptoms of depression along with the classic motor symptoms of PD (Merschdorf et al. 2003).

Before turning to these specific questions however, it is worth considering the overall picture of depressive symptoms in PD. It is now generally accepted that PD is frequently associated with depression, and from a clinical point of view, the similarities with the symptoms of MDD are so strong, that it is frequently difficult to distinguish the two conditions, especially if the depressive morbidity precedes the onset of the motor symptoms (Merschdorf et al. 2003).

The preceding analyses have shown that in terms of its psychometric properties, the ADQ is a suitable instrument for the measurement of depression in both PD and MDD samples. The results of the principal component factor analysis of the ADQ for PD1 and PD2, with a total of 157 patients, representing a heterogeneous group of patients with PD, unselected for severity of depression, produced three components, suggesting a specific symptom structure for the depression of PD.

The three components were interpreted as (i) the "core symptoms" of depression in PD, (ii) "distinguishing symptoms" and (iii) "sleep disturbance". The core symptoms contained the key features of depressed mood and loss of interest or pleasure (anhedonia) required for a DSM-IV-TR diagnosis of depressive disorder. They also included: pessimism regarding the future, weepiness, worried pre-occupation, suicidal ideation, problems with concentration, health concerns and loss of appetite, that are typically characteristic of depressive symptomatology. The "distinguishing" symptoms, which included loss of feelings for other people, diurnal variation and self-blame and guilt, were so called, because they did not group together with the core symptoms and hence raised the possibility that they might be indicative of areas in which patients with PD showed a different pattern of symptoms, compared to patients with MDD. The third component represented problems with sleep, in the form of both initial and late insomnia. As these symptom groupings (i–iii) were aligned along different components of the principal components analysis, which are orthogonal to each other, it would appear that they represent distinct clusters of symptoms, unrelated to each other. Thus sleep disturbance does not appear to be associated with the core depressive symptoms of PD and the so-called "distinguishing" symptoms, also seem to be unrelated to either the sleep disturbance or the core symptoms of depression in PD.

One explanation for these findings is that components two and three of the analysis contain symptoms that are specifically associated with disturbances seen as part of PD rather than depression. Over the last 25 years, disorders of sleep and wakefulness have emerged as among the most common non-motor complications of PD, with as many as 90% of patients reporting difficulties with insomnia, hypersomnia, nightmares, nocturnal movements and other sleep complications (Stacy 2002; Janocha and Zawilska 2007). Complicating clinical factors that can additionally disrupt sleep in PD are parkinsonism, autonomic symptoms, and psychiatric and cognitive disorders (Weintraub and Burn 2011). Excessive daytime sleepiness and tiredness (both physical and mental) are also common (Tandberg, Larsen and Karlsen 1998). Sleep disturbances in PD are still not well understood, but it is possible that their loading on a separate component of the principal component analysis may reflect that they have more to do with the illness process, rather than being an expression of depressive symptoms. Indeed, Starkstein, Preziosi, Forrester et al. (1990) have previously suggested that sleep disturbances are not specific to depression in PD.

Similarly, it is possible that the allegedly "distinguishing" symptoms are reflective of dopaminergic dysfunction in PD, thus standing apart from the remaining depressive symptoms. There is evidence to suggest that dopaminergic dysfunction is responsible for the emotional blunting that may present as loss of feeling for other people (Halbig et al. 2011). Furthermore, feelings of guilt and self-blame have also been related to a putative dopaminergic disorder (Berrios et al. 1992). Diurnal variation too, may be related in this sample of patients to medication induced fluctuations in dopamine levels. This is likely, as the wording of this item on the ADQ did not specify a particular time of day when the patient might be expected to feel worse, leaving the possibility open. Patients may indeed feel much worse in the morning, before their medication has taken effect, or at other times of the day, in so-called "off" periods (Davies et al.

1999). All of these interpretations are speculative and require further investigation. It is also the case that the analysis under discussion was performed in a heterogeneous sample of patients with PD without making an appropriate comparison with depressed control patients. In order to examine the possibility that depression in PD is subtly different from idiopathic mood disorders, it is essential to include these control measures. The necessary comparison of symptom profiles for patients with PD and those with MDD and milder forms of depression is described next, after a brief consideration of the origins of depression in PD.

(iii) The origins of depression in PD

The nature and origins of depression in PD remain unclear. As understanding of the neurobiological substrates for depression in general, and the neuropsychological symptoms of PD in particular, has advanced, many of the old arguments regarding the aetiology of depression in terms of its "reactive" or "disease-related" properties have been abandoned in favour of the more sophisticated revelation of brain-behaviour relationships. Specifically, dopaminergic, noradrenergic and serotonergic neurotransmitter systems have been implicated in the depression arising in PD (Cummings and Masterman 1999; Remy et al. 2005; Tan et al. (2011). Nevertheless, even the more recent literature occasionally raises the question of distinguishing "reactive" from other forms of depression in PD (Farabaugh et al. 2009). However, the observation that depression often precedes the onset of motor symptoms in PD, together with the fact that people suffering from depressive disorders are more likely to go on to develop PD than other diseases, is one that is difficult to accommodate within the "reactive" model for PD depression (Nilsson et al. 2001; 2002; Schuurman et al. 2002; Todes and Lees 1985). Arguments regarding the aetiology of depression in PD have turned on an examination of the relationship between neuropsychological, neuropsychiatric and motor symptoms, with a view to identifying potential subgroups in the symptom presentation of PD which may be associated with particular neural substrates and represent variants of the disease (see chapter 3). However, these have been based almost exclusively on zero-order correlation statistics and so have been unable to account for multi-collinearity within the data, undermining the credibility of the findings. In order to overcome these problems, the relationship between symptoms representative of the three main symptom domains of PD, motor, affective and cognitive, was examined with the aid of multivariate statistical techniques, which are discussed below in relation to the results of stage II of the present study.

11.1.2 Symptom profiles for depression in PD and other forms of depressive disorder

A number of studies have claimed that there are notable differences in the symptom profile for PD as compared to MDD. These are presented in Chapter 3, table 3-5. An attempt was made to verify these findings in the present study, by identifying those items of the ADQ items which contributed most to the overall score for depression. Item analysis revealed that these included: low mood, pessimism regarding the future, lack of interest and enjoyment in activities, feeling weepy, concern about health, worried pre-occupation and poor concentration (see table 10-5). On the other hand, suicidal ideation, reduced feelings for others, diurnal variation, loss of appetite, sleep disturbance and guilt or self-blame contributed least to the total score for depression in the PD patients. It seems therefore, that the depression in PD, is characterised by the two symptoms which are crucial to a DSM-IV-TR diagnosis of depressive disorder, namely low mood and anhedonia. It is important to note, that previous studies (e.g. Ehrt et al. 2006), whilst arguing that the depression in PD is characterised by less severe sadness, have not challenged the notion that it remains a key characteristic in the depressive symptomatology of PD. With the exception of suicidal ideation, which in contrast to previous studies (e.g. Leentjens 2004), was not found to be prominent among the patients studied, the present findings appear to confirm the results of earlier research. The importance of symptoms such as concerns about health (also found by Gotham et al. 1986) pessimism (noted by Leentjens 2004) and worried preoccupation more generally, to the clinical picture in the depression of PD, is in keeping with reports that the clinical features of depression in PD have a high frequency of anxiety symptoms (Schiffer et al. 1988; Menza et al. 1993). Increased problems with concentration have also been found in previous studies (e.g. Ehrt et al. 2006; Farabaugh et al. 2009; Koerts et al. 2008). Moreover, the finding that patients with PD tend to be more tearful is in keeping with an early observation by Lewy (1923) who described them as "moody, irritable and weepy". Some authors have suggested that certain somatic symptoms such as sleep disturbances are increased (e.g. Koerts et al. 2008); this was not found in the present study, although many patients were taking medication to help them sleep at night and this may have confused the clinical picture. The relatively lower contribution of feelings of guilt and self-blame to the overall score for depression on the ADQ is in keeping with previous reports in the literature (Ehrt et al. 2006; Gotham et al. 1986; Farabaugh et al. 2009), as is the finding that diurnal variation (Merschdorf et al. 2003) and appetite loss (Brown and MacCarthy

1990) are less prominent. There are also relatively few reports of psychotic symptoms associated with depression (Brown and MacCarthy 1990) and although not assessed by the ADQ, a similar impression was gained in the present study.

However, whilst this way of evaluating symptom frequency may provide a broad impression of the clinical picture of depression in PD, and produces results that are in keeping with previous reports in the literature which argue for a differential pattern of symptoms in PD compared to non-PD depressive disorders, it is limited by at least two serious constraints. The first is that no comparison is made with an appropriate control group and this has equally been a difficulty for the majority of previous studies (e.g. Farabaugh et al. 2009). The second is that no attempt has been made to take account of the severity of the depressive symptoms, a factor which is likely to affect the profile of clinical symptoms of depression that is obtained.

To date, few studies have made the crucial direct clinical comparisons of depressive symptoms between groups of PD and MDD patients, the exceptions being the studies by Ehrt et al. (2006) and Merschdorf et al. (2003). These however, came to opposite conclusions, the former arguing in favour of differences in the symptom profile for depression in PD and DSM-defined depressive disorders, whilst the latter concluded that there was no evidence for a distinction. An attempt was made in the present study to clarify the position using data from the ADQ obtained in a sample of PD and MDD patients and using a different methodology, that it is contended, has several advantages over that used in previous studies. An important consideration in carrying out the required comparison between PD and MDD groups was that patients from both samples should be equated in terms of severity of depressive symptoms and that the range of severity should be clinically significant, i.e. above a cut-off point for at least moderate to severe levels of depression. Failure to control for levels of symptom severity may result in quantitative differences in symptomatology being incorrectly interpreted as qualitative differences. For example, there is evidence that suicidal ideation, psychotic features and vegetative symptoms are more prominent in severe forms of depression (Schrag et al. 2007) and may therefore not feature in the symptom profile at milder levels, hence giving rise to a misleading picture of qualitative differences. In so far as groups of equivalent severity are compared, this may not be a problem, but whilst the Ehrt et al. (2006) samples appear to have been within the mild range for symptom severity (the mean score on the MADRS for the PD group was 13.8 and for the MDD group was 14.8), they are likely to have been considerably heterogeneous, as only 26.2% of the PD patients satisfied the criteria for major depression at the time of the assessment compared to 100% of the MDD sample. Equally, although the Merschdorf et al. (2003) samples were at the upper end of the range for symptom severity (mean HAM-D scores of 17.7 and 18.3 for the PD and MDD groups respectively), the authors themselves draw attention to the fact that their results may be constrained by the fact that there was a wide range of depression severity in their samples and suggested that further studies need to be performed with more homogenous samples.

Achieving homogeneity in the samples is difficult to accomplish because, as has been demonstrated in (i) above, relatively few patients with PD score within the upper ranges for symptom severity on measures of depression, which are typical for MDD. In order to allow a comparison of this sort, it was necessary, in the present study, to use data from a larger sample of PD patients (PD1) who had participated in a postal questionnaire version of the study. This yielded the matched comparison sample of 30 patients in both PD and MDD groups, who were then examined in relation to their symptom profile for depressive symptoms. Patients from both of the clinical groups were matched individually for severity of symptoms, in order to achieve equivalently matched samples not only in terms of group mean scores, but also to ensure that the range of scores did not vary between the groups, in an attempt to achieve the homogeneity desired.

11.1.3 Comparison of patients with PD and MDD matched for severity of depression

With the aforementioned principles in mind, a comparison was made between depressed PD patients and patients with a DSM-IV-TR diagnosis of MDD at the upper range of symptom severity, with a mean ADQ score of 31.9 (± 7.2) and 31.8 (± 7.5) respectively, which is above the diagnostic cut-off for clinically significant depression. These samples would appear to represent a more homogeneous range of depression severity than has hitherto been studied.

A comparison between the mean scores on individual items of the ADQ for patients with PD and MDD revealed significant differences only in relation to three items: feeling weepy, health concerns and loss of appetite. On the first two, the PD patients had reliably higher scores, on the third, their scores were lower than those of the MDD patients, indicating that appetite was not affected to the same extent. These results provide little support for the proposition that PD patients differ in a significant way in their profile of depressive symptoms from patients with MDD. The increased tearfulness of the PD patients may reflect autonomic dysfunction, rather than being specific to a depressive disorder (Berrios et al. 1995). Equally, the greater health concerns of the PD patients may not be surprising in view of the fact that they are suffering from a progressive neurodegenerative disorder. Although the item on health concerns attempted to measure hypochondriasis, and was carefully worded so as to avoid the possibility that people would refer it to the condition of PD, this may have been only partially successful, hence patients' endorsement of this item on the ADQ. Appetite in PD does not appear to be affected, as has been noted in previous studies (Brown and MacCarthy 1990) and only this seems to be a discriminating feature of PD depression. No differences of the kind referred to above in relation to increased anxiety, concentration difficulties and suicidal ideation versus diminished cognitive symptoms of depression, such as guilt and self-blame, were identified between the two groups.

In view of these considerations, it would appear reasonable to conclude from this analysis, that the differences in depressive symptomatology between patients with PD and MDD are not significant. Such findings endorse the position held by Merschdorf et al. (2003), that differences in the symptom profile between patients with PD depression and MDD are negligible.

11.1.4 Comparison of patients with PD and controls matched for mild depression

A similar comparison between PD patients matched for milder depressive symptoms with control subjects revealed differences in mean scores only for the items concerning problems with concentration and diurnal variation. In both cases the PD patients endorsed the symptoms more strongly than the control subjects. As regards concentration problems, these results seem to add support to the findings reported in the literature (e.g. Koerts et al. 2008; Farabaugh et al. 2009). Stronger endorsement of diurnal variation however, may reflect fluctuations in mobility that are illness related; for example rigidity and bradykinesia may be more apparent in the morning before medication has taken effect (Davies et al. 1999).

It is also possible, however that these differences may not be reliable, as they were not sustained with application of the Bonferroni procedure for multiple comparisons. Even assuming that this correction procedure may be too conservative, and in view of the differences reported previously, the results of the present study suggest that when PD patients are compared to control groups in which the homogeneity of depression severity has been strictly controlled, any alleged differences between them become less apparent.

11.1.5 Comparison of symptom profiles for depression

Nevertheless, the way of arriving at this conclusion might be challenged on methodological grounds. Comparing the frequency with which symptoms are endorsed, or the consequent mean scores for individual scale items, overlooks the important fact that in order to establish differences in the profile of symptoms between groups, the comparison has to take into account not just differences that may appear for one scale item, but also the probability that the scale items are inter-correlated with each other. A particular item, for example, may have the highest mean score for all of the items, but does not have to make the highest contribution to the overall score on the scale, because of its correlation with other items. In the present study, item analysis was therefore used in order to establish a symptom profile for PD and MDD groups with severe symptoms of depression and PD and control groups with milder depression. Items on the ADQ were then compared in terms of their contribution to the overall score. This methodology allows items to be evaluated in relation to all of the other items on the scale, and overcomes the problems associated with making a simple comparison of individual means. It is thus contended, that this is a more appropriate method for establishing potential differences in symptom profiles, but it does not appear to have been used in previous research.

A comparison of the PD group matched for severity of depression with the MDD group, revealed significant differences between the groups in relation to only three symptoms. Two of these were the same as those reported above, namely loss of appetite and health concerns. The third however, was in relation to a change in feelings for other people. These symptoms differentiated between the two groups, in the extent to which they contributed to the overall score for depression. These findings should be interpreted with reference to the mean scores for the symptoms concerned and their variation between groups. Thus, as has already been mentioned, loss of appetite is not as marked in the PD patients, and contributes less to their overall score for depression, than is the case for the MDD patients. Health concerns on the other hand, are higher among the PD patients, and make a greater contribution to their overall depression score than in the MDD group. Finally, there are no differences between the two groups in their endorsement of the item relating to a change in feelings for other people, but this item is more significant in shaping the overall score for the PD patients in comparison to those with MDD.

Despite attempts to eliminate symptoms that overlap with the features of PD in the construction of the ADQ, it is evident that the three symptom areas in which PD patients appear to be differentiated as regards symptom profile from the MDD patients may in fact, reflect specific conditions prevailing in PD. It is perhaps not surprising that this group of patients should report greater preoccupation with health, given the nature of their illness and the consequent disability that it causes. On the other hand, the fact that they report fewer problems with appetite, despite being depressed, is perhaps surprising. PD itself, is frequently associated with appetite loss and dopaminergic medication is further known to exacerbate the problem (The Columbia Encyclopedia 2011). Patients' failure to endorse this symptom may reflect the fact that they have adjusted to having a diminished appetite as part of their illness and therefore do not report it as a change in their normal pattern. Finally, emotional blunting expressed in the form of changes in feelings towards others has been linked to dopaminergic dysfunction (Halbig et al. 2011) and may thus also be a feature PD rather than depression *per se*.

As regards the comparison of PD patients matched for milder symptoms of depression with control subjects, differences in profile were established as relating to only two symptoms: problems with concentration and guilt and self blame (the latter difference was almost significant at the p=0.07 level). Concentration difficulties appeared to be making a greater contribution, and guilt a smaller contribution to the overall depression score for the PD patients, in keeping with previous reports in the literature (Ehrt et al. 2006).

The replication of these findings for the symptoms of concentration and guilt feelings, together with a tendency, albeit insignificant, for low mood to be less important in the overall depression score for the PD patients with milder depression, is in contrast to the results obtained for patients with severe depression. It would appear to suggest, that the symptoms that are allegedly different in the profile for depression in PD may be characteristic of milder types of depression. The profile for severe depression in PD, on the other hand, is not different from that of MDD along the dimensions that have been proposed in the literature. It seems likely therefore, that any apparent differences in symptom profile may be related to the severity of depression, rather than specifically being characteristic of depression in PD.

11.1.6 Power considerations

One possibility for the failure to show differences between groups on the symptom profile for depression is that the evaluation did not have sufficient statistical power to demonstrate differences. In order to address this issue, *q,* an index of the effect size (Cohen 1992, 157) for the evaluation of the significance of the differences between the correlation coefficients for the ADQ items between the groups was calculated for both severe and mild depression. Values for the effect size *q* are presented in table 10.1.15. For the correlations obtained for the groups with severe depression, small effect sizes (defined in the region of q=0.1; Cohen 1992, 158) were obtained for the following items: worried preoccupation, pessimism regarding the future, loss of interest and enjoyment, suicidal ideation, early morning waking, self blame and guilt, and diurnal variation. With such small effect sizes, the sample size required to obtain a significant result (p=.05) and undisputed levels of power (.80) would be in excess of N=1,500. Sample sizes of this order of magnitude are clearly impractical in clinical studies of the kind described here. Instead, the inference from the power analysis is that it would be extremely unlikely that significant differences between the severely depressed samples could be established for these items of the ADQ. It is thus unlikely that type II errors are responsible for the failure to demonstrate differences between the groups on these items and that it is reasonable to accept that they do not differ in this respect. A similar conclusion might also be drawn for the remaining items (low mood, concentration difficulties, feeling weepy and difficulty in falling asleep), which fell within the medium range (q=0.3) for effect size, although here, there is the possibility that with sample sizes in excess of N=177 (Cohen 1992, 158), significance might be reached. Nevertheless, even such sample sizes are unlikely to be within the scope of most clinical studies, bearing in mind the difficulty in matching patients with PD for severity of depression with MDD patients.

As regards a power analysis of the comparisons between the mildly depressed groups, it can be seen from table 10-15 that only for the items of low mood, guilt and concentration difficulties is the effect size above the medium range (q=0.3). All the comparisons for the remaining ADQ items demonstrate a small effect size, which would require unrealistically high sample sizes in order to reach significance. As above, the parsimonious conclusion must be, that with respect to these symptoms, the differences between the groups are insignificant and unlikely to be the result of type II errors.

Taken together, these analyses suggest that under strictly controlled conditions, where both the severity of depression and the homogeneity of samples is accounted for, there do not appear to be differences in the profile of depressive symptoms between PD patients with severe levels of depression and MDD patients with equally severe symptoms. The differences that do occur (in appetite, health concerns and emotional blunting in the form of changes in feelings for other people) may be explained in terms of illness factors related to PD. Equally, few differences were found between the PD and control samples with milder depression. Those that were established for decreased feelings of guilt and increased problems with concentration are in keeping with previous reports in the literature (Ehrt et al. 2006), but there is some doubt as to their validity, as they did not withstand the Bonferroni correction procedure. Neither do they represent a comprehensive replication of the symptoms that allegedly differ in PD. For example, no differences were found with respect to anxiety (worry), suicidal ideation, loss of interest and enjoyment of previous activities, and pessimism regarding the future, which are representative of the cognitive symptoms for which differences are most commonly reported. The only difference that was established between the groups, matched for severe depression, related to consistency in responding to individual items on the ADQ. The patients with PD were significantly more systematic in their responses than patients with MDD. However this finding is inconsistent with the alleged cognitive differences for PD, in which concentration difficulties are paramount (Koerts et al. 2008). In view of the patterns found in this study, it seems that the previously reported differences in symptom profile for PD patients are dependent on: (1) the severity of depression – alleged differences are more likely to reflect quantitative rather than qualitative differences in symptomatology, and (2) when the range of symptom severity is not appropriately controlled, i.e. samples lack homogeneity.

In conclusion it is unlikely that any of the differences found, represent significant differences in the phenomenology of depression seen in PD. This is indirectly supported by the fact that mildly depressed patients with PD appeared to differ from the MDD patients according to the dimensions previously discussed in the literature, particularly with respect to the more cognitive features of depression. However, since these differences were not sustained in the more severely depressed PD group, a parsimonious conclusion would be to assume that they are more likely to be reflective of differences in depression severity and not in the phenomenology of the depression in PD. The failure to find differences in symptom profiles for the severely depressed patients with PD and those with MDD is in keeping with the suggestion that the neuropathological basis for the affective disorder in both conditions is the same (see chapter 3, section 3.6.2).

11.2 Stage II

Stage II of the study focused on attempting to establish relationships among the main symptom domains of PD using exploratory factor analytic techniques to identify patterns in the data. Surprisingly few previous studies have taken this approach: an early study by Reynolds and Montgomery (1987) and more recently van Rooden et al. (2009a) both used a factor analytic procedure, but only to explore the relationships among motor symptoms. A study using factor analysis to explore groupings among non-motor symptoms found a separate factor accounting for scores on the MADRS depression scale and other neuropsychiatric symptoms, but it did not include cognitive and motor symptoms (Lloret et al. 2011). There appears to have been only one previous study that also took account of the three main symptom domains of PD (van Rooden et al. 2009b).

An attempt was also made to differentiate potential subgroups in the sample, which might be characterised by a predominance of psychological symptoms, using cluster analysis. Two independent samples of patients were studied: PD2 (N=60) and PD3 (N=75). Exploratory factor analysis was performed on the motor and non-motor symptoms of PD in the first sample (PD2). The findings were confirmed in the second, independent sample of patients with PD (PD3).

11.2.1 Stage II: discussion of results

In a study of this kind, it is necessary, as indicated in chapter 9, to meet certain criteria. Firstly, care should be taken to ensure that the measures chosen to reflect the domains of interest (motor, affective and cognitive) should be as representative as possible. To this end, at least two measures relating to each of the symptom domains were included in the analysis pertaining to stage II of the study. Secondly, it is important to select measures that have adequate sensitivity in the samples studied, avoiding possible floor and ceiling effects. The measures entered in the principal component analysis showed appreciable variation across the sample, thereby supporting the idea that they were of adequate sensitivity, thus giving the opportunity for correlations between variables to arise. However, no significant correlations were consistently obtained between any of the three types of variables representing the main symptom domains of PD, thus suggesting that the motor, affective and cognitive manifestations of the illness are independent of each other. Given the limitations of zero-order correlations for exploring patterns of symptom alignment among the data, factor analysis was used to help determine the structure of the underlying constructs. Four factors were identified in the spectrum of motor and non-motor symptoms and from among the background variables for the PD2 sample. These corresponded to the somatic or illness features of PD, depression, chronicity and cognitive dysfunction. This factor structure was replicated almost exactly by the replication factor analysis in the PD3 sample thereby giving additional strength to the results (see section 10.3.8.). The first and strongest factor, in both of the analyses, was a somatic factor comprising the measures of motor performance and duration of illness. A second factor was characterised by cognitive performance and included medication, especially benzhexol, which is an anticholinergic agent especially useful in the treatment of tremor in PD. In the exploratory factor analysis, the cognitive factor also included a measure of physical functional disability (NUDS), and this could be taken as suggesting a possible, albeit weak, association between cognitive and motor variables. Such an interpretation seems unlikely however, because the NUDS is a measure of general competence in everyday life activities (for example, dressing and other self-care skills), and thus is likely to include a cognitive component in addition to motor ability. It is most likely that the cognitive content of this scale causes it to feature in this factor. This explanation is reinforced by the fact that the Hoehn and Yahr scale, which is a pure motor measure does not appear in the cognitive factor. The depression factor comprised purely the depression measures used in the two analyses. The exploratory factor analysis also yielded a chronicity factor which included age at onset and examination, the number of admissions to the hospital neurology department and duration of medication for benzhexol. A similar factor was evident in the replication factor analysis, but had an eigenvalue below the stricter value of 1.5 adopted for these studies and so was not reported. The replication factor analysis explained 64.7% of the variance in the data with the inclusion of all four factors (eigenvalue>1).

As the individual factors are orthogonal to each other, this suggests that the motor, affective and cognitive aspects of PD appear to be independent of one another. Results broadly in keeping with those of the present study were reported by van Rooden et al. (2009b), which is the only other factor analytic study that it has been possible to identify from the literature, that also took account of the three main symptom domains of PD. These authors also found that the motor symptoms were not associated with either neuropsychological deficits or neuropsychiatric disorders, such as depression. The non-motor features of PD, in the form of cognitive impairment, psychotic symptoms and depression were found to be associated with autonomic dysfunction, daytime sleepiness and axial symptoms such as freezing, swallowing and speech difficulties, but not with the motor impairment *per se*. These, rather than pure motor deficits, were considered to reflect disease severity. This was the strongest factor in the study, consisting predominantly of non-motor symptoms and axial features. The findings of the present study differ in this respect, in that they additionally differentiate between the affective and cognitive symptoms of PD, providing evidence for their independence. In view of the neuropsychological nature of the present study, less emphasis was placed on the other non-motor symptoms of PD and this is almost certainly reflected in the results. A second factor identified in the van Rooden et al. (2009b) study, reflected the motor complications of therapy and was related to dopaminergic medication. The third factor reflected an association between sleep and depression and the fourth was a somatic factor containing the key motor features of PD, in the form of tremor, bradykinesia and rigidity. The association between sleep and depression was not replicated in the present study, as shown in the preceding analysis of the ADQ. This may be related to differences in sampling and in the assessment procedures used.

Establishing independence among the symptom domains of PD has both practical and theoretical implications. From a practical point of view, focusing management exclusively on the motor symptoms of the illness, which is still commonly the case, may not be sufficient: depression, which appears to be a separate component of the illness in its own right, may need separate treatment. Indeed there is evidence in support of this view, as L-dopa does not appear to alleviate the affective symptoms in PD (Eskow et al. 2011). Moreover, this has clinical significance, as depression in PD is under-treated. It is estimated that the affective disorder is recognised in only about half of the patients with PD who have significant clinical symptoms of depression (Shulman et al. 2002) and that only about 20-25% of depressed PD patients receive treatment for the disorder (Mayeux et al. 1986; Weintraub et al. 2003). In the present study about one-third of the depressed PD patients were receiving anti-depressant medication, which still represents a significant shortfall in treatment, especially as depression has a crucial impact on the quality of life of both the patient (Schrag 2006) and his/her carer (Schrag, Hovris et al. 2006).

The theoretical implications are more complex, as there are a number of ways to account for the relationship between motor, affective and cognitive symptoms in PD. As described in chapter 3 (section 3.6.1), depression may be regarded as "reactive" to the chronic and progressive motor disorder and the cognitive impairment may be consequent upon depression, i.e. a form of pseudodementia (Berrios and Quemada 1990; Bulbena and Berrios 1986; Klepac et al. 2008; Taylor, Saint-Cyr, Lang and Kenny 1986). Indeed, some authors (Jellinger 2013; Marder et al. 1995) have suggested that depression may be a risk factor for cognitive impairment in PD. This cascade effect would predict a linear correlation between the three symptom domains. In a factor analysis, the reactive position would imply that a common illness factor, containing the features of all three types of symptom should be obtained. This was not found in the present analyses.

Two other models are possible, both of which would be compatible with the independent factors found. The simplest position would be based upon the assumption that the three symptom domains have independent causation. Although the present findings do not offer evidence against this model, it seems implausible, because of all the evidence linking PD to increased rates of depression and cognitive dysfunction (see chapters 3 and 4). The alternative model is that the three types of symptom share the same underlying causal mechanism. At first sight, this latter position might seem to indicate that motor and psychological variables should intercorrelate in PD. In practice, this is not necessarily the case, as the expression of the separate symptom domains may be subject to the influence of intervening variables which could enhance or attenuate their manifestation. Assuming, on the grounds of parsimony, that the notion of several independent causal mechanisms can be discounted, the lack of correlations leading to a common illness factor is thus more likely to be consistent with the common cause hypothesis, which regards motor, affective and cognitive changes in PD as all being fundamental to the underlying disease process. Indeed, it is now accepted that differential degeneration of individual frontostriatal circuits or pathways linking the frontal cortex with the basal ganglia and subserving motor and non-motor functions are distinctively associated with the deficits seen in PD (see chapter 3, section 3.6.2 and chapter 4, section 4.9).

A logical extension of the common cause hypothesis, would therefore predict considerable heterogeneity in the clinical picture for PD and this is precisely what is observed (Foltynie, Brayne and Barker 2002; van Rooden et al. 2010; 2011). Consequently, it might be reasonable to expect the existence of clinical subtypes of the disorder. Indeed, three motor subtypes have been proposed in which different patterns of motor symptoms predominate and these have been described as: a hypokinetic-rigid form, a tremor-dominant form and a postural instability-gait disorder form (Zetusky, Jankovic and Pirozzolo 1985; Jankovic et al. 1990). Although these alleged subtypes appear to have validity in terms of clinical presentation, few studies have addressed the question in any systematic way. Even fewer studies have examined the possibility that non-motor symptoms might be associated with particular motor subtypes of PD. PD with depression has been regarded as a distinct subtype in some investigations (e.g. Mayeux et al. 1984; Santamaria et al. 1986) and it has been suggested that depression may be associated with the hypokinetic-rigid form of PD (Starkstein et al. 1998). Graham and Sagar (1999) have differentiated three distinct subtypes of PD characterised by cognitive impairment. The first is a "pure" form of the motor disorder unaccompanied by intellectual decline, in the second type, motor symptom progression is accompanied by deficits in executive functions which eventually proceed to a global cognitive impairment, and the third is a "rapid progression" subtype, characterised by an older age at onset, rapid progression of motor symptoms and cognitive decline. Faster rates of cognitive decline have also been associated with the postural instability-gait disorder subtype (Alves et al. 2006; Burn et al. 2006). However, Factor et al. (2011) have distinguished between postural instability with falling and freezing of gait in the postural instability-gait disorder form and suggest that the former type is associated with depression. The possibility that affective or cognitive variables might be associated with a clinical subtype of PD was explored in the present study by means of cluster analysis, which is an objective method for classifying patients into subtypes.

11.2.2 Identification of possible subgroups within the sample

The cluster analysis revealed two clusters characterised on clinical and demographic variables. One was characterised by late onset, shorter illness duration, taking less medication (especially benzhexol), with good control of motor symptoms, normal free recall and Schonell (IQ) performance and with only a slight decline on the Benton visuospatial test. A second cluster was characterised by early onset, long duration of illness, taking higher doses of benzhexol, poorer motor control and impaired free recall and Schonell scores. However, depression did not appear to discriminate any subgroups in this sample. Previous work has produced inconclusive results. Some studies suggest that depression is associated with a younger age at onset of PD (Ehrt et al. 2007) and that patients with early onset PD are more depressed than those with late onset, even when disease duration is controlled (Starkstein et al. 1989). However, controlling for disease duration eradicated the difference between early and late onset groups in at least one study (Kostic et al. 1994) and another did not find that depression differentiated between groups, in common with the present findings (Filho, Teive and Werneck 2007). Nevertheless, the pattern characterised by a distinction between early versus late onset of PD is one that is beginning to achieve recognition in the literature, although associations with affective changes do not appear to have been sustained (e.g. van Rooden et al. 2010). The results of the present study are in keeping with this trend.

However, the association of early disease onset with marked cognitive impairment in this sample is different from the pattern commonly reported in the literature (Garron, Klawans and Narin 1972; Hietanen and Teravainen 1988; Lieberman 1974; Martilla and Rinne 1976; van Rooden et al. 2010*)*, where late onset is alleged to be associated with faster disease progression and cognitive decline. This discrepancy may simply reflect differences in sampling and use of different criteria for defining early and late onset categories. The selection criteria for patients included in this study were strict in order to obtain a representative sample of patients with idiopathic PD and in an effort to limit age-related comorbidities. The cut-off age of 70 was intended to protect against the confounding effects of other age related diseases, in particular, cognitive dysfunctions associated with ageing *per se,* but some studies have defined their older onset groups with an age above 70 (Friedman 1994; Reid et al. 1989). Early onset is usually defined as presenting with the symptoms of PD before the age of 40, but some authors include up to age 50 in this category (Samii, Nutt and Ransom 2004; Schrag and Schott 2006). The distinction in the present study was derived on the basis of the clusters identified, the mean age at illness onset for patients in one cluster being 50 years, leading to the definition of "early onset" in comparison to those in the other cluster whose mean age at onset was 61 years and who were defined as "late onset" cases. Nonetheless, clear differences between these subtypes were evident. Age cut-off criteria defined by researchers may differ from those that are data driven and this may have consequences for the subtypes identified (van Rooden et al. 2010).

Entry criteria to the study also imposed a minimal illness duration of 3 years, intended to avoid diagnostic uncertainties and to allow symptoms to develop and stabilise (Mathews and Haaland 1979). This and the upper age limit for the study means that only a proportion of late-onset cases may have been captured for this analysis, and these selection criteria may have produced a bias against cases in which cognitive decline was associated with late onset. Nevertheless, the advantages of this "purer" sample were that it has been possible to demonstrate that cognitive deficits are not simply associated with ageing in PD. Indeed, the findings from the present study would support evidence suggesting that cognitive deficits in PD are evident even in patients with an early disease onset and may be associated with a variety of causal factors.

One possibility accounting for the higher rates of cognitive decline in the early onset group, may be the difference in disease duration between the two groups. For the early onset group, disease duration is over three times that for the older onset group. Thus the patients who were affected by the disorder at a younger age may simply have been exposed to the degenerative process for longer and in that time, the cognitive dysfunctions had developed. Implicit in this, is the assumption that cognitive deficits take longer to develop, or emerge later in the disease process, a possibility that is supported by clinical impressions as far as PD-related dementia is concerned (Hely et al. 2008). However mild cognitive impairments are frequently present in PD from early in the disease process (e.g. Foltynie et al. 2004; Hietanen and Teravainen 1988; Jellinger 2013; Tsai et al. 1994) and may increase the risk of developing dementia (Janvin et al. 2006). There is also some indication that cognitive functions demonstrate differential rates of impairment in PD, visuospatial abilities being among the most sensitive in this respect (Johnson and Galvin 2011). This is in keeping with the observation in the present study showing that in the late onset group which was cognitively intact, only performance on the Benton spatial relations test was slightly impaired. The only way to test these hypotheses would be to compare groups of patients with early versus late disease onset, controlling for disease duration.

It may also be the case that some deficits, especially those related to memory, are iatrogenic, at least in part, and related to anticholinergic medication (e.g. benzhexol) (Miller et al. 1987; Campbell et al. 2009). Clearly these are also likely to be exacerbated by the length of time that such medication has been taken and thus related to longer disease duration. For example, it is possible that the deficit in verbal memory found in the long duration-early onset group may simply reflect its greater exposure to treatment with benzhexol. More will be said about the effects of anticholinergic medication in the discussion of stage III. Suffice it to say at this point, that these findings illustrate the general point that passage of time alone (as in duration of illness) cannot be used as an explanatory variable. Time can only provide the opportunity for other events to take place (e.g. treatment, further degeneration of brain systems). Finally, because of the multiplicity of potentially relevant variables and the fact that in practice investigators cannot control them all (e.g. treatment history), statements about various aspects of the illness, such as the characteristics of early versus late onset should not be made in an absolute way, as if they applied to all samples of people with PD.

11.2.2.1 Variables which characterise sub-groups in the sample

One further finding is worthy of note. Of the grouping variables examined by discriminant function analysis (gender, age at onset, L-dopa dose and benzhexol dose) gender emerged as a useful indicator. Being male was associated with early disease onset, poor motor control, and high doses of medication. Over 71% of patients were correctly classified according to gender by these variables. This result was further reinforced by groupings according to age at onset and L-dopa dosage where gender also appeared as the major discriminator. Gender has previously been associated with the differential progression of PD (Hely et al. 1999), women being found to have poorer motor control with the earlier development of dyskinesias; although these differences had disappeared after 10 years, the gender difference remained, with women having poorer Hoehn and Yahr scores. These diverse findings may again be due to differences in sampling. Gender differences may either not have emerged as a significant variable in previous studies, or may show variations, because these have generally included older subjects, where any effects may have been swamped by age related factors. The previously noted association between memory impairment and benzhexol dosage is also confirmed by the discriminant analysis.

The results of stage II of the study, as demonstrated by the cluster analysis, emphasise the importance of the particular characteristics of the sample that is under investigation. The significance of the age range of subjects used has already been mentioned. In the U.K. at least, not all cases of PD are referred to neurologists and, not all so referred are admitted to hospital. The source from which subjects are obtained and whether outpatients are included together with hospital in-patients could therefore affect the results. The indication for studies of this kind, is that it is important to use samples that are truly representative of cases of PD in the community. In practice, this means that studies may need to be based on an adequate case register covering a defined geographical area as in the Norwegian ParkWest study (Alves et al. 2009).

In conclusion, two clusters with clinical meaning (early versus late onset of PD) were identified, which could be distinguished by neuropsychological test performance. No subtypes of PD appeared to be differentiated on the basis of depression. Evaluating these results in the context of previously published studies, highlights the need to draw comparisons between samples of patients that are equivalent with respect to key features of interest, such as age at onset of PD, in order to defend the generalizability of findings. However, it also points to the importance of using data-driven approaches, such as cluster analysis, in order that variables which differentiate between clinical subtypes of PD might be revealed. A case in point is the differentiation of the two clusters in the present study, showing a pattern of cognitive impairment that might otherwise not have come to light. PD subtypes are likely to be characterised by complex interactions arising among disease mechanisms, treatment, age and chronicity variables, and gender, which may not be readily identified, unless critical variables are controlled.

CHAPTER TWELVE

THE RESEARCH STUDY: DISCUSSION – STAGE III

12.1 Introduction

The main purpose of the research reported in the preceding pages was to gain a better understanding of how the neuropsychological features of a neurodegenerative disorder such as Parkinson's disease may affect the lives of people suffering from the condition. Hence, the discussion so far has sought to clarify a number of unresolved issues concerning, in particular, the affective disturbances concomitant upon Parkinson's disease. The third and final stage of the research undertook an investigation of the task of caring for a spouse with Parkinson's disease, the foundations for which were laid on important conclusions drawn from the first two stages of the study discussed in chapter 11.

The work undertaken in stages I-II of the research was concerned with establishing any relationships between the main symptom domains of PD and was considered to be an important prerequisite to testing the effects of these independent variables on the outcome or dependent variables for the carer, pursuant to testing the main hypothesis in stage III of the study. If the variables representing the different symptom domains were to show high levels of association, not only would this have implications for their origin in PD, as discussed in relation to stage II, but it would have important indications for the design of the third stage of the study, concerned with care-giving. Demonstrating that the motor, affective and cognitive manifestations of the disorder were independent of one another was thus an important precursor to stage III of the present study. Specifically, it provided a rationale for assuming that the three symptom domains had an independent influence on the care-giving situation. Other studies have sometimes made this assumption, without first verifying it.

The model which provided a background to stage III of the study was the stress process model of caring (Pearlin et al. 1990), which is widely used in studies of care-giving. Within the context of this model, it was assumed that the fundamental hardships of caring for a person with PD arise from the three main symptom domains of the condition. Motor symptoms affecting functional performance bring about a situation in which patients increasingly require help with the basic activities of daily living. Affective symptoms, in the form of anxiety and depression, and less frequently psychotic symptoms, may also influence the patient's functional performance, particularly if s/he is withdrawn and depressed. Equally, cognitive dysfunction is likely to affect the patient's self-care abilities and reduce independence. Thus, the disease symptoms may be viewed as specific domains from which stressors originate for both the carer and the person with PD, who is increasingly unable to function without assistance. In addition, the limitations imposed by the disease related symptoms lead to a proliferation of stressors. For example, the care recipient's restricted mobility may mean that the couple are no longer able to maintain social activities or to take holidays to the same extent as prior to the illness. Depressive symptoms may result in withdrawal on the part of the care recipient, and an unwillingness to receive visitors, even family members, at home. This has a rebound effect on carers, restricting their former life-style and access to different forms of support. Many of the changes wrought by the illness in the form of psychological symptoms (both cognitive and affective) may be particularly distressing for carers, as they are sometimes perceived as changes in the personality of the care recipient, as discussed in chapter 8. These in turn are likely to affect the carer's satisfaction with the marital relationship, which may be perceived as having deteriorated along with the evolution of the illness, thereby diminishing another significant area of support for the carer. Alternatively, a satisfactory marital relationship may help to buffer the ill-effects of having to provide care for a spouse with whom marital and affectional ties remain strong.

The purpose of the third part of the study was to evaluate a model of the care-giving process in PD, taking into account the characteristic aspects of disease presentation, but attempting to include variables reflecting the dyadic and transactional nature of the care-giving process. It would be impossible for any study to include all aspects of care-giving but these were considered to reflect some of the more important aspects, which have so far received relatively little attention. Care-giving outcomes were measured in terms of the strain resulting from the task of providing care to a spouse with PD and psychological morbidity in the form of depression. It was hypothesised that care-giving strain might act as a mediating variable between PD-related illness variables and carer outcomes in the form of depression, as well as an outcome variable in its own right. Measurement variables were selected in order to reflect important dimensions within the care-giving process and at least two measures relating to each of the symptom domains were included in the analysis. In order to obtain as full a description of these symptoms as possible, and in keeping with the dyadic approach to the care-giving situation that was adopted for this research, the perspectives of both the care recipient and the carer were taken into account in the assessment. Thus both patient-rated and carer-rated accounts of neuropsychological and neuropsychiatric symptoms (using the Cognitive Failures Questionnaire – Other) were obtained, and these were supplemented with observer ratings gathered during a standardised clinical interview with the couple.

The fact that the neuropsychological and neuropsychiatric symptoms are generally not as severe in PD as in patients with either a DSM diagnosis of major depression or dementia, provided a model of a clinical disorder that was not dominated by one or other of the symptom domains, thus making it possible to examine the relationships between them and carer outcomes avoiding possible floor or ceiling effects in the data. The measures used had adequate sensitivity in the samples studied. This was confirmed by the principal component factor analysis, which showed appreciable variation across the sample, thus giving the opportunity for correlations between variables to arise.

The study exclusion criteria were designed to impose some control over the complexities of the situation studied. Age criteria were used, as in stage II of the study, to reduce the risk of comorbidities especially in the area of possible neuropsychological impairments and the study was restricted to couples in which one person suffered from PD and was living with a spouse, who was defined as the main carer. Because this part of the study was an exploration of factors affecting the well-being of family carers, it was also restricted to those living in their own homes in the community. Sampling methods were designed to ensure that the patients recruited to the study were representative of patients with PD and their carers living in the community.

12.1.1 Limitations of the study

No study is without limitations and several weaknesses of the present study need to be pointed out. Perhaps the most significant one is that this was a cross-sectional rather than a longitudinal study. The latter, by providing information on the trajectories with which variables of interest change over time, would allow causal relationships between variables to be established. Nevertheless, the causal steps analysis (Baron and Kenny

1986) used in the present study permitted some insight into the questions of major interest in this respect.

A further possible limitation is that whilst it is recognised that a range of potential mediators may act to modify the effects of the primary, disease related stressors upon the outcomes for carers, not all of these could be accommodated in the model tested. In particular, those traditionally associated with theories of stress (Lazarus and Folkman 1984) and adapted to take account of the care-giving process (Pearlin et al. 1990) including the remedial effects of social support and carer coping strategies were not evaluated. Previous studies in PD have addressed these issues with varying results, e.g. Miller et al. (1996) did not find any effects of social support with regard to care-giving outcomes, possibly because levels of support were comparatively low. However, even where these factors have been shown to mediate care-giving outcomes, their effects are relatively small. Nevertheless, had they been included in the present analysis, they may have helped to account for some of the hardship of care-giving. In addition, because of the geographical area on which the study was based, it was not possible to include culture-specific aspects of care-giving among the variables examined.

Finally, whilst not considered a limitation of the present study, the lack of control groups deserves some explanation. In view of existing findings which demonstrate that the impact of caring for a spouse with PD has negative implications for the carer in terms of raised levels of strain and depression, it was deemed unnecessary to examine a control group of elderly carers of people without neurodegenerative disorders for the purposes of comparison. Indeed, control groups appear to have limited utility in a study of the kind reported here, for a number of reasons. Firstly, as with dementia carers, spouse carers of people with PD report greater levels of distress than adult children and other family carers, so mixed groups of carers lack homogeneity, which is likely to influence findings (Aarsland, Larsen, Karlsen et al. 1999). As a result, only spouse carers were included in the study. In order to match controls to the index sample it would be necessary to ask one member of a healthy, age-matched control couple to identify with being the "carer" and the other, the "patient". Presenting such couples with many of the items in the protocol used to examine care-giving lacks validity, quite simply because they do not perceive themselves in these categories. Measures of care-giving strain or burden are thus inappropriate with control groups and the use of depression scales, somewhat redundant, as established norms for the instruments exist. Secondly, control groups may be useful for testing specific hypotheses related to the nature of the disorder in PD, for example, in attempting to separate physical components of the disorder, such as restricted mobility, and making comparisons with patients with functionally equivalent limitations arising from different aetiologies, such as arthritis. However, the criteria for determining the choice of conditions for comparison are not at all clear and may result in groups that are too heterogeneous for useful comparisons to be made. In terms of determining which aspects of the care-giving situation are most distressing for carers, the unique feature of PD is that patients may act as their own controls as the characteristic presentation of the illness is in the three main symptom domains of interest, namely motor, affective and cognitive disturbances. The purpose of the present study was to go beyond a purely descriptive account of carer distress and attempt to suggest explanatory mechanisms to account for the way in which the care-giving situation is shaped in PD. This required a different approach, with a focus on the symptoms of PD and examination of the extent to which they actually account for variation in carer strain and depression. In addition, the role of potential mediators in the care-giving process was evaluated.

12.1.2 Strengths of the study

One of the most important attributes of the stress process model has been to draw attention to the fact that it is not the strength and quality of the stressor *per se*, that determines strain-related outcomes, but the transactional nature of the process, involving various mediators of care-giving such as the social support and coping strategies mentioned. Their ability to either attenuate or exacerbate the effect of the primary stressors helps to explain the observation that given apparently similar care-giving situations, no two carers cope in the same way. It can only be logical to assume that a multitude of factors affecting the care-giving situation, which may be subsumed, one way or another under the general headings of social support and coping strategies used by the carer, are the mediating factors which modify care-giving outcomes. No study is capable of identifying and then examining in detail, all of the potential modifying variables in relation to care-giving. Those selected for special attention in the present analysis included an evaluation of the quality of the relationship between the carer and the care-recipient and the carers' perceptions of the psychological symptoms in the care recipient; the former have so far been given relatively little attention in relation to care-giving in PD, whilst the latter do not appear to have come under empirical scrutiny at all.

An important feature of the study is that it attempted to examine the relationships between different aspects of the care-giving situation and the outcome for carers through the use of multivariate statistics. In a study of this complexity, where multiple correlations are likely to occur within the data, and covariance patterns emerge, it is important to examine patterns in the database as a whole and not to focus on selected comparisons. Thus, factor analysis was used to identify systematic patterns of alignment among the variables and causal steps analysis (Baron and Kenny 1986), which is based on multiple regression analyses, to establish potential mediation effects. In so doing the study sought to clarify the distinction between the concepts of strain or burden and outcome for the carer, as well as elucidating the role of selected variables as mediators in the relationship between patient and carer variables.

12.1.3 Recruitment of subjects to stage III of the study

The age constraints imposed meant that the sample of patients selected for the study included mainly younger representatives of the population of people with PD living in the community, which served to increase the homogeneity of the sample. However, this made recruitment to stage III of the study, where a spouse carer was also required to be living in the same household as the patient, particularly difficult, as more than half of the patients identified did not meet the age or carer criteria for inclusion in the study. The difficulties encountered reflect the general demographic characteristics of people with PD and similar findings have been reported in other community studies of this population (e.g. Jones et al. 1999; Mutch et al. 1986). Table 12-1 shows the age distribution of the study participants in comparison to previously published studies carried out in the U.K.

It can be seen from table 12-1 that at least 40% of patients with PD participating in the studies reported were over the age of 70. This helps to explain why recruitment to the present study proved difficult, with the restrictive age criteria originally imposed and thus for practical reasons, in stage III, it was necessary to raise the upper limit for patient age to 80 years.

A further bias is evident in the data obtained in the present study relating to the gender distribution of the patients recruited to the study. This bias is particularly evident in samples PD1 and PD3 where the entry criteria to the study included having a spouse-carer; no such gender bias was evident in sample PD2, where the presence of a carer was not required.

PD is known to be more common in men than in women (Ben-Shlomo 1997; Van Den Eeden et al. 2003; Wooten et al. 2004) so the gender bias in the samples included in the present study is representative of the gender distributions of patients with PD more generally. This gender bias is reflected in the literature on care-giving in PD, in that there appear to be more men than women with PD living in a marital or other close partnership in the community (e.g. Aarsland, Bronnick et al. 2007; Aarsland, Larsen, Karlsen et al. 1999; Carter et al. 2008; Hooker et al. 2000; Leiknes et al. 2010). In so far as carers in general tend to be women, this is in keeping with trends reported in the literature, but it is somewhat surprising in relation to spouse carers who might be expected to be more evenly distributed. However data from two of the surveys referred to in table 12-1 (Jones et al. 1999; Oxtoby 1982) revealed that significantly more women with PD were single or had been widowed or divorced than men with the disorder. The process of recruitment to the present study elicited more records for women with PD living alone without a carer than for men, possibly reflecting the differential death rates for older men and women, but it also appears to be the case, that more female PD sufferers are accommodated in residential care (Calder et al. 1991; Jones et al. 1999).

Table 12-1. Age distributions of patients with Parkinson's disease by gender in selected UK studies in comparison to the present study.

	Study			
Patient's age	**Oxtoby (1982)**	**Mutch et al. (1986)**	**Jones et al. (1999)**	**Present study**
Men	%	%	%	%
< 55 years	11	12	5	10
55-69 years	52	27	37	82
70+ years	37	61	58	8
Totals (N)	N=129	N=109	N=278	N=141
Women	%	%	%	%
< 55 years	12	2	2	7
55-69 years	62	14	21	81
70+ years	45	83	77	12
Totals	N=123	N=140	N=243	N=91

These complex considerations highlight the importance of having an awareness of the factors which may influence the selection of patients with PD for research purposes. It is clear, that unless very large numbers of patients are used in research studies it is not possible to control for the different biases introduced by patient selection. It is therefore important to have a precise formulation of the way in which patients should be selected in order to meet the aims and requirements for the optimal examination of a specified research question. In practice this means that different selection criteria are required, matched to the specific research question under consideration. Hence in the present study, age and other exclusion criteria referred to above were used to minimise the risk of including patients with additional complications that might detract from the clinical picture of PD and the requirement for having a spouse carer was specifically related to the main question of interest for the research. The justification for this lay in the main purpose of the study, which was to gain a better understanding of the mechanisms involved in bringing about different care-giving outcomes (better adjusted versus highly strained) and thus examination of the issues in as closely a homogeneous group as possible was considered desirable. Thus, whilst the patients and carers recruited to stage III of the study were not fully representative of the entire population of people with PD, they formed a representative sample of patients with PD living with spouse carers in their own homes in the community. These selection criteria were considered justifiable as the aim of the research was not epidemiological and the purpose was not to gain information on the extent of the care-giving problem in general, as studies of this kind are widely available.

12.1.4 Clinical characteristics of the patients with PD

The patients with PD participating in stage III of the study had well established symptoms of the disease, at moderate levels of severity (Hoehn and Yahr grades 3/4). Assessment revealed also that they were suffering significant levels of affective disorder, with 57.2% of the sample above the cut-off ($\geq$ 11) for depression (both mild and severe) on the GDS and 20.0% using the stricter criterion score of $>$ 17 on the HAM-D. These results are in keeping with the levels of depression found for patients in stage II of the present study and previous reports in the literature (Reijnders et al. 2008). Symptoms of anxiety were also prominent among the sample with over 33% of the patients demonstrating at least mild levels of anxiety on the Hamilton Anxiety Scale.

The age selection criteria imposed on the study were designed to exclude, as far as possible, patients who might be suffering from concomitant age related illnesses, and probably also served to exclude patients with PD-dementia. Nevertheless, cognitive deficits were evident in a significant proportion (over 30%) of the sample, and this figure is in keeping with previous reports for patients with PD (Buntington and Fitzsimmons 1991). These findings lend support to the emerging view of PD as a condition in which non-motor symptoms contribute significantly to the overall morbidity of the condition, thus making it a "quintessential neuropsychiatric disorder" (Weintraub and Burn 2011).

12.2 The relationship between symptom domains in PD

12.2.1 A replication study

Extending the range of instruments to measure physical functioning in PD and including different scales for the measurement of depression and anxiety, which are among the most common of the non-motor symptoms in PD (Aarsland, Bronnick et al. 2007), did not alter the nature of the relationships revealed in the factor analysis among the motor, affective and cognitive manifestations of the disease in PD3, which remained independent of each other. Neither depressive symptoms nor cognitive abilities were related to disease severity (Hoehn and Yahr scale) or to motor and autonomic symptoms as measured on the Webster scale. In addition, functional impairment (NUDS) was unrelated to depression and cognition. Cognitive performance was associated with medication taken for PD in a common factor. These findings endorse similar conclusions drawn from stage II of the study and previous reports in the literature (e.g. Carter et al. 2008), although the latter did not take account of the multicollinearity in their data, using only simple correlations to establish relationships. This replication in an independent sample of patients with PD, using a wider range of instruments to measure the symptoms of interest, and multivariate statistics to take account of multiple correlations in the data, means that it appears reasonable to conclude that the three symptom domains are independent of one another, as argued in the discussion of the results for stage II of the study. As previously suggested, the independence of the symptom domains in PD is seen as supporting the idea that all three physical, affective and cognitive domains represent symptomatology intrinsic to the disease itself.

12.3 The effects of care-giving in Parkinson's disease

The principal aim of stage III of the study was to provide an analysis of the conditions influencing care-giving in PD. In keeping with previous studies which are summarised in chapter 7, the consequences of providing help and support to a spouse with PD were found to be significant in terms of the care-giving strain and psychological morbidity reported by carers. In addition, carers' levels of marital satisfaction were evaluated. Both carer depression and marital satisfaction represented more generic measures, it being recognised that factors other than care-giving might also shape the underlying constructs determining carer outcomes.

12.3.1 Levels of care-giving strain among carers

The levels of strain established for carers were considerable and in keeping with reports from previous studies using the Machin Strain Scale (or an adaptation of it in the form of the Relatives' Strain Scale) with PD spouse carers, when differences in scoring are taken into account (e.g. Miller et al. 1996; Aarsland, Larsen, Karlsen et al. 1999; Thommessen et al. 2002). Although the Cognitive Failures Questionnaire (CFQ-carer) might also be regarded as a measure of strain, though not specifically related to care-giving, carers in the present study did not achieve high scores on this instrument. Their scores were significantly lower than those obtained with a sample of PD carers studied by Poliakoff and Smith-Spark, (2008) and did not differ from scores obtained in a group of healthy, older adults (Hohman et al. 2011). Nonetheless about 20% of carers had scores representing significant levels of both care-giving and more general strain. This figure, however, should not be treated as differentiating a group of carers who may have reached some critical level of care-giving strain, as cut-off values are generally not available for scales measuring the strain or burden of care-giving.

The levels of care-giving strain found in the present study contribute to the growing body of literature demonstrating that elevated strain levels are characteristic of care-giving in PD (e.g. Calder et al. 1991; Lyons et al. 2009; Miller et al. 1996; Thommessen et al. 2002). It remains uncertain whether the strain of care-giving may be affected by the nature of the neurodegenerative condition and the consequent care needs of the care recipient, although intuitively, this might appear to be the case. There are very few comparative studies which include PD. Two studies comparing carers of people with PD and those with DAT did not find differences between carers in terms of depression or care-giving strain (Dura, Haywood-Niler and Kiecolt-Glaser 1990; Thommessen et al. 2002); however, a third found that caring for someone with DAT led to greater psychiatric morbidity, but only for women carers (Hooker et al. 2000). These findings suggest that factors other than those implicated in meeting specific care needs may be of primary importance in shaping carers' responses to the care-giving task (e.g. carer gender).

Care-giving research in PD has more frequently used measures of strain or burden specifically related to care-giving, rather than psychological morbidity more generally, in order to evaluate the hardships experienced by carers. Whilst it is important to sample a representative range of care-giving-specific variables in order to gain an understanding of the care-giving experience, it should be remembered that the construct of care-giving strain or burden is multidimensional and remains poorly understood. For example, the relationship between care-giving strain and psychological morbidity in carers is somewhat inscrutable: not all carers who admit to being under considerable levels of strain, concurrently report more serious forms of psychological morbidity in the form of depression. It is not known what levels of care-giving strain, and under what conditions, may be predictive of damaging effects on the carer's physical and psychological health or of the decision to terminate the provision of home care. Indeed, as was hypothesised in this and other studies (e.g. Shim, Landerman and Davis 2011), absolute levels of strain may not be the crucial factor, because their effects may be modified by a variety of intervening variables, such as social support or the quality of the relationship between the carer and the care recipient. These intervening or mediating variables are in themselves of considerable interest, as they can help to identify critical factors affecting the care-giving process, which serve to ameliorate (or worsen) the outcome for carers. Thus, for the purposes of the research described here, it was considered important to choose a less equivocal and more robust outcome measure for determining the well-being of carers, preferably one with established clinical properties. A measure meeting these requirements is that of disturbed affect in the form of depression.

12.3.2 Levels of depression among carers

It is now well-documented that some carers of people with PD demonstrate levels of psychological morbidity in excess of the norms established for the general population, matched for age (e.g. Dura, Haywood-Niler and Kiecolt-Glaser 1990; O'Reilly et al. 1996; Martinez-Martin et al. 2008). Spouse carers appear to be particularly at risk (Aarsland, Larsen, Karlsen et al. 1999; O'Reilly et al. 1996). 32% of carers participating in the current research qualified as probable "cases" on the GHQ and the proportion found to be at least mildly depressed (25-30%, depending on the measure used) was compatible with the figure of 35% reported by Meara et al. (1999) and of 30% found by Happe, Berger and the FAQT study (2002), although a study by Schrag, Hovris et al.

(2006) reported a higher rate of 54%. Moderately severe depression was found in 5% of carers in the present study and in 7% of those reported by Schrag, Hovris et al. (2006), though in the Aarsland, Larsen, Karlsen et al. (1999) study this rate was doubled at 13%. These differences are most likely to result from the use of a variety of different measurement instruments among the studies and the relatively small samples studied; the proportions serve only to indicate that substantial numbers of carers fall within the mild to moderate range for depressive symptomatology and therefore suffer from considerable levels of psychological morbidity. Comparison with the age-matched, healthy control group reported in stage I of this study, confirmed that the carers of people with PD reported higher levels of depressive symptoms on all of the measures used.

Previous studies viewing depression as a carer outcome have used widely differing methods of assessment, making comparisons difficult. Using the GDS, D'Amelio et al. (2009) reported a mean score for carers of 9.3 in comparison to the score of 7.8±6.3 found in the present study. Two other studies using the BDI with spouse carers have reported similar mean scores: 8.3±6.6 (Aarsland, Larsen, Karlsen et al. 1999) and 8.5±6.5 (Schrag, Hovris et al. 2006) in comparison to the slightly lower mean score of 7.2±6.1 for the present study. The carers in the present study demonstrated mean depression scores that are slightly lower than in previous studies, and this may be a result of the entry criteria used, which may have eliminated cases at the more severe end of the spectrum of PD requiring greater carer involvement over longer periods of time.

12.3.3 Levels of marital satisfaction among carers

Nearly one-third of carers also reported diminished levels of marital satisfaction; this would appear to be relatively high compared to people in this age range in the general population (Bookwala and Jacobs 2004), suggesting that care-giving may be compromising the quality of the perceived carer-care recipient relationship. The majority of carers reporting dissatisfaction with their marital relationship were female, but it should be remembered that the majority of carers in this study were women, and that men, in general, report being more satisfied with their marriages than women (Levenson et al. 1993; Franco, Franco and Alishahie 2008).

Few studies have addressed the way in which care-giving relationships may affect carer well-being, but a recent study of the carers of people with DAT and PD (Shim et al. 2011) found that poorer relationship quality (described as low mutuality) was associated with caring for care recipients with lower functional ability, having had less care-giving experience and depressive symptoms in carers. However this study did not take account of the non-motor symptoms of the two conditions, and there is evidence that cognitive impairment may have a negative impact on carer mutuality in care-giving more generally (Lawrence et al. 1998; Williamson, Schaffer and The Family Relationships in Late Life Project 2001). Perhaps somewhat counter-intuitively, because previous reports in the literature have suggested that care recipient affective changes such as depression and apathy, affect carer well-being in a specifically detrimental way, leading to depression (e.g. Miller et al. 1996; Aarsland, Larsen, Karlsen et al. 1999), a study by Lyons et al. (2002) did not reveal any association between depression in the care recipient and carer perceptions of strain in their relationship. This suggests that the marital relationship is unlikely to mediate the relationship between patient and carer depression.

12.3.4 Carers' perceptions of psychological symptoms in the care recipient

Previous work on care-giving has raised the suggestion that carer outcomes may have more to do with features that are characteristic of the carer, than stressors deriving from the primary symptoms of the care recipient. In particular, attention has been focused on carer personality variables and other individual characteristics that might influence carer attitudes to care-giving, such as the quality of their relationship with the care recipient, as discussed in the previous section. Furthermore, the dyadic perspective adopted in the present study, would predict that not only the patient's representation of his/her situation in the context of the illness, but equally the carer's view and consequent actions taken, determine the way in which the care-giving process unfolds and the consequences that it has for the protagonists involved. From the neuropsychological perspective taken in this study, of particular interest were the carer's perceptions of the psychological symptoms in the care recipient. It would seem logical to expect that the care needs of the patient would be determined by the carer, not just from the point of view of the physical disability, but also from his/her appraisal of the patient's psychological functioning.

The results showed that carers viewed their spouses with PD as demonstrating relatively high levels of psychological morbidity, especially in the area of cognitive impairment; these were in excess of the levels reported in a study using the same instrument (CFQ-other) by Poliakoff and Smith-Spark (2008), but comparisons are difficult to make, because of the dearth of studies in this area.

Examination of the zero order correlations between the variables in question (see table 10-29) revealed some interesting dependencies. Whilst carer perceptions of depression in the patient were correlated with both patient self reported symptoms and clinician assessments, carers' perceptions of their spouses' levels of cognitive dysfunction failed to demonstrate any correlation with "objective", i.e. clinician rated assessments. On the other hand, perceptions of cognitive dysfunction were correlated with patients' self-rated symptoms of depression (GDS), but not with clinician rated symptoms using the HAM-D. The implication of this may be that while carers are reasonably accurate in their judgements of depression concerning their spouse, their assessment of cognitive function appears to be wide off the mark in relation to "objective" assessments. This was confirmed by statistical analyses which showed that carers' appraisals of depression in their spouses were congruent with both patient and clinician ratings, but that their evaluation of the care recipients' cognitive functioning showed no relationship to the results of neuropsychological test performance. The carers' evaluation of the patients' physical disability was also divergent with that of the clinician.

The data also showed that there exists a positive correlation between carers' perceptions of cognitive dysfunction in their spouse and their own outcomes in terms of depression, and this relationship was supported by the regression analyses in relation to carer outcomes in the form of depression on the BDI. It is logical to assume that carers' negative affective state may be related to their tendency to overestimate levels of cognitive dysfunction in their spouses, but also that they may be unable to distinguish between their spouses' affective and cognitive symptoms.

12.4 Pathways in care-giving

The main objective of stage III of the study was to provide an analysis of the conditions influencing care-giving in PD. Having established the independence of the symptom domains characteristic of the illness, the next step in the analytical procedure was to examine patterns in the data reflecting both patient and carer variables, in order to establish linkages between them. This might suggest how the constructs of interest, namely carer outcomes in the form of strain and depression, are shaped and influenced by a variety of factors in the care-giving situation. The aim of the analyses was to elicit the pathways of association among the variables using the general framework of the stress process model of care-giving.

12.4.1 Relationships between patient and carer-related measures in the data: a factor analytic approach

The four factors identified within the spectrum of variables reflecting the characteristics of the PD3 sample and their carers corresponded to the somatic/illness, cognitive and affective features of PD together with a carer "well-being" factor. The strongest of these was the somatic factor which included measures of symptom severity and functional performance, together with illness duration and a measure of anxiety derived from the HAM-A. The association of anxiety with the somatic features of PD is not surprising, particularly in view of the strong focus on somatic anxiety within the Hamilton Scale. In addition, there is considerable overlap between the somatic symptoms of anxiety and the physical symptoms of PD (Berrios et al. 1995). Adoption of an "inclusive" method of scoring symptoms on the HAM-A is likely to have potentiated this effect (Schrag et al. 2007). Of particular interest to the present study, is the fact that carer strain was also represented in this factor, suggesting that the physical symptoms of PD in particular, appear to be associated with the strain of care-giving. The somatic factor accounted for the largest proportion (33.1%) of the variance in the data. The relationships among variables established in the factor analysis are illustrated in figure 12-1.

Figure 12-1. Associations among selected variables in the care-giving situation revealed through factor analysis.

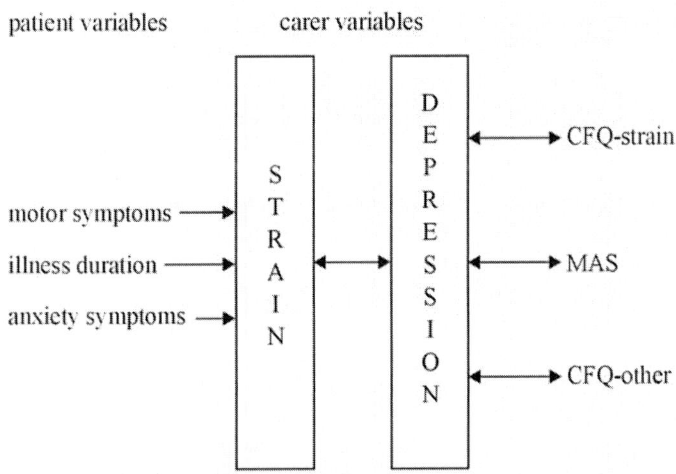

CFQ-strain: general strain reported by carer
MAS: Marital satisfaction reported by carer
CFQ-other: perceptions of psychological symptoms in patient reported by carer

A straightforward and plausible explanation of the relationships revealed in the first factor, is that more advanced disease, characterised by longer illness duration and leading to increased levels of disease severity and greater functional impairments is associated with higher degrees of strain in carers. This is a common finding in PD care-giving studies as discussed in section 12.4.2 below.

However, the relationship between carer strain and the somatic features of PD was the only instance in which carer-related variables showed an association with any of the patient-related variables in the factor analysis. Measures of patient affective and cognitive symptoms loaded on separate factors, the latter being associated, as in previous analyses, with the medication prescribed for PD. Some of the reasons for the interaction between PD medication and cognitive function have been discussed in stage II of the study. To reiterate, it has been shown that benzhexol, an anticholinergic drug used in PD for the control of motor symptoms, in particular tremor, has detrimental effects on cognitive functioning, especially memory (Miller et al. 1987; Campbell et al. 2009). The association with L-dopa may reflect the potentially beneficial effects of this drug on cognitive performance, especially aspects of executive functions which tap into fronto-striatal dopamine pathways (Cools et al. 2003; Lewis, Slabosz et al. 2005). Verbal free recall tasks of the kind used in the study are known to be dependent on executive functions (e.g. Baldo et al. 2002) and so may be sensitive to the effects of medication. Alternatively dopamine overdose to the ventral striatal areas of the brain may have detrimental effects on cognitive functioning (Kehagia, Barker and Robbins 2010). It can be seen from the factor loadings that there appear to be differential effects associated with cognitive performance on the different tasks used, but in view of the complex relationship between L-dopa and cognitive function it would be an over-interpretation of the data from this analysis to attempt to draw any further conclusions.

From the factor analysis it was apparent that neither the neuropsychiatric symptoms, nor the cognitive performance of the care recipient appeared to be associated with any of the carer variables. These results contrast with previous studies, which have shown an association between carer depression and neuropsychiatric symptoms (in particular depression) in the care recipient (e.g. Miller et al. 1996; Aarsland, Larsen, Karlsen et al. 1999). One reason for this may lie in the fact that variables with greater explanatory potential were included in this study, compared to previous ones. In particular, the present study included the carers' appraisal of psychological functioning in the care recipient, and this may have affected the pattern of results.

The carer's perception of cognitive dysfunction and depression in the care recipient were associated with other carer variables in the factor described as "carer well-being". Carer depression was most strongly represented in this dimension along with satisfaction with the marital relationship and the CFQ for the carer. In so far as the CFQ, which is a self-assessment of meta-memory, is indicative of perceived strain on the part of carers (Wagle et al. 1999), it is in keeping with the interpretation of this factor as a dimension reflecting "carer well-being". The indicator of care-giving strain (scores on the Machin Strain scale) also appeared in this factor, with virtually the same loading as on the somatic factor. This makes strain a so-called "multivocal" item in the analysis and confirms the difficulties previously discussed with the concept of care-giving strain. The cross-loading suggests that the scale is measuring two separate constructs, neither of which have been defined, or possibly that it is reflecting a third, that is different from, but related to, the factors that it is loading on. Thus care-giving strain requires further investigation. One possibility is that strain should be measured separately in relation to different types of impairment (physical, affective and cognitive) because these may impact differently on care-giving outcomes.

None of the self-reported or clinician rated measures for care-recipient symptoms loaded on this factor, suggesting that they are not directly associated with carer outcomes. Rather, it appears that what seems to be of primary importance in carer outcome, is the carers' ***perception*** of the neuropsychological and neuropsychiatric symptoms in the care recipient. This result is of considerable significance as it appears to indicate that the changes which are perceived to be occurring in the patient, particularly in the cognitive domain, may be potentially the strongest predictors of depression in the carer. This possibility is addressed with further statistical analyses that are discussed later.

The significance of the fact that the current daily dose of L-dopa also loads on the carer well-being factor, albeit weakly, is more difficult to interpret; it is unlikely to be a reflection of disease severity *per se*, because medication used in PD does not appear in the somatic factor, which contains illness related symptoms. Furthermore, there is some evidence to show that the relationship between disease severity and medication in PD is not a straightforward one, and dosage levels may not reflect severity (Van Rooden et al. 2009b). As the dose of L-dopa is also contained in the cognitive factor, it may reflect an association between cognitive deficits in the care recipient and carer distress. There is evidence to link L-dopa (especially in doses that ameliorate the motor symptoms) with inappropriate cognitive responses associated with excessive dose side effects in the ventral striatal areas of the brain, leading to impulsive responding and a failure to switch stimuli when reward patterns change (Kehagia et al. 2010). The consequences of such behaviour in daily life may have distressing effects for carers. Alternatively, it may mean that carer strain plays some role in determining the treatment regime for patients, perhaps reflecting a mechanism by which carers reporting higher levels of psychological strain may intervene more strongly on behalf of their spouses with clinicians, who may respond (without necessarily being aware of this) by raising levels of medication for the patient. Although these interpretations are somewhat speculative, it seems less likely that the result simply reflects an association between poorer psychological outcomes for carers and disease variables, as measures of motor and functional disability for the care recipient are not associated with carer variables in any of the factors. The possibility that carer strain and depression is associated with levels of medication for the care recipient requires further investigation, but it is an interesting observation which may describe a potentially unwarranted consequence of carer strain for the treatment of patients with PD. This also serves to emphasize the need to improve our understanding of mechanisms affecting the outcomes for carers and the complex way in which they may affect care-giving situations for both carers and carer recipients.

As the individual factors identified are orthogonal to each other, one conclusion from the factor analysis is that not only the motor, affective and cognitive aspects of PD are independent of each other, but also that carer outcomes do not appear to be specifically affected by the separate symptom domains of PD. The exception to this is the relationship between illness related variables and care-giving strain, which is not surprising in view of the emphasis of the strain scale on measuring the need for care and ways in which the couples' lifestyle has been affected by the illness.

Patterns in the data revealed by the factor analysis point to two important features that appear to characterise care-giving. Firstly, strain and depression outcomes for carers are associated in the same factor, implying that they share common variance. The second point however, is that they do not appear to be measuring exactly the same properties of the care-giving situation. In particular, carer depression, unlike care-giving strain, is not associated with the somatic features of PD. Both therefore appear to have explanatory power and it would be premature to retain one, at the cost of the other, in a theoretical model. However the relationship between them remains imperfectly understood and deserves further investigation. This was attempted through additional analyses of the data.

Before turning to these, the dynamics of strain across the course of care-giving will be examined briefly.

12.4.2 The dynamics of carer strain

The results obtained in stage III of the study showed a progressive increase in carer strain (Machin Strain Scale) with stage of illness as measured on the Hoehn and Yahr, presumably reflecting an increase in the number of care-giving tasks required and negative changes in lifestyle for the couple. Although carer strain was manifest at all stages of the disease, the increase in levels appeared to accelerate from Hoehn and Yahr stage 2 onwards, a finding that is in keeping with results from previous studies (Carter et al. 1998; D'Amelio, et al. 2009). As this was not a longitudinal study, these interpretations need to be treated with caution, as they refer to different groups of patients and carers in the stages of the disease process.

12.4.3 Factors associated with strain in carers: motor symptoms

One of the main conclusions to be drawn from the factor analysis was that carer strain was associated with the somatic symptoms of PD. An association of this kind has been described in virtually all previous reports in the literature using measures of strain or burden to evaluate the effects of care-giving for carers of people with PD (e.g. Aarsland, Larsen, Karlsen et al. 1999; Caap-Ahlgren and Dehlin 2002; Calder et al. 1991; Carter et al. 1998; 2008; Cifu et al. 2006; D'Amelio et al. 2009; Edwards and Scheetz 2002; Kim et al. 2007; Leiknes et al. 2010; Lökk 2008; Martinez-Martin et al. 2007; 2008; Razali et al. 2011; Roland, Jenkins and Johnson 2010). The majority of these studies have focused on the demands resulting from the physical impairment in the care recipient (e.g. Roland et al. 2010) without taking other, non-motor symptoms into consideration. In so doing, they have followed the path taken by the abundant literature on studies of carers of people with DAT and other forms of dementia.

Care-giving strain has thus largely been perceived in terms of the carer's feelings of being able to cope with the level of care required to assist with the activities of daily living for the patient, quality of symptom management, perceived ability to control the disease and its progression, knowledge of the disease, financial resources, and levels of perceived support in the form of social, professional, healthcare, publications and technological resources (Edwards and Ruettiger 2002; McRae et al. 1999). Scales designed to measure carer strain (or burden) reflect these concerns, but no instruments have been developed specifically for use in PD. This means that many of the characteristic features of the illness, such as difficulties arising from "on/off phenomena", motor fluctuations and dyskinesias which are the cause of considerable unpredictability in terms of functioning in PD (Carter et al. 1998), as well as the fact that PD is still perceived by many patients, carers and neurologists alike, as mainly a motor disorder, may not be adequately reflected in existing scales for carer strain, despite being particularly problematic in PD.

However, whilst the alleged association between motor impairments and carer strain appears to be robust, it is an association that is only one of many that may potentially have an impact on carer strain. Most previous studies have based their findings on univariate analyses (zero order correlations), which fail to take into account that the association between carer strain and PD motor impairments, for example, may be weaker than those between carer strain and patient depression. Thus carer strain is unlikely to be influenced by motor symptoms independently of mental symptoms, such as patient depression and cognitive disturbances. Indeed, in spite of the overwhelming focus of care-giving strain scales on the physical aspects of the disease and its management, as described above, in measuring the carer's perceptions of his/her ability to cope with the delivery of care that is required, they frequently also refer to aspects of the care-giving situation that may be much broader than those mentioned. Examples of such items from strain scales include questions such as: "Do you ever get depressed (or frustrated) about the situation?" (Machin 1980) or "Do you feel angry (or strained) when you are around your relative?" (Zarit et al. 1980), without giving a more specific referent. It is therefore unclear which aspects of care-giving, carer responses may be referring to. It is equally plausible that both physical and behavioural changes in the care recipient may generate such feelings. Thus strain scales are clearly multidimensional measures involving carer reactions to a variety of care-giving stressors, but also registering their impact in a variety of different ways, from feelings of burden in having to provide additional assistance to the care recipient to emotional responses in the carer. Both would appear to be valid measures, but an important aim of research on care-giving should be to differentiate factors that influence these outcomes, separately and in common.

Although the factor analysis did not demonstrate any association between the strain reported by the carer and patient affective and/or cognitive symptoms in the present study, this is likely to be because these effects were masked by the much stronger association that was revealed between carer perceptions of the psychological symptoms in the care recipient and carer outcomes in the form of strain and depression.

Another important consideration in evaluating the relationship between carer strain and disease related variables in PD is in relation to the instruments used to measure the motor impairment. These vary in the extent to which they can be considered to provide "pure" measures of motor symptoms, as discussed in stage II. Instruments designed to measure functional performance, such as the NUDS or the Karnofsky and WHO scales, are likely to reflect both states of depression and cognitive impairment in the patients, in addition to their physical abilities. Indeed, they may also partially reflect carer variables; for example, clinical observations show that some carers demonstrate their devotion to their spouses with PD by intervening with help more than is actually needed (Davies et al. 1999). Thus, reported levels of patients' functional disability, even when elicited from the patients themselves, may represent an outcome constructed in terms of a complexity of both patient and carer influences. There is some empirical evidence to support this: a study by Lyons et al. (2002) found that although carer and care recipients were broadly in agreement in their perceptions of the care recipient's IADL needs, there was a tendency for carers to rate the care recipients as being more dependent than they themselves did. Moreover, it is not inconceivable that even the Webster scale, which is regarded as a virtually "pure" measure of motor and autonomic impairment in PD, might also be affected by the patient's neuropsychiatric symptoms, because of the problem of "symptom overlap" discussed in chapter 3.

12.4.4 Understanding the notion of strain: the association with neuropsychological symptoms in PD

Guided by the results of the factor analysis and a modified version of the stress process model for care-giving (Pearlin et al. 1990), the correlates of carer strain were further examined in order to determine which aspects of the care-giving situation appear to be making the greatest contribution to strain in carers. A significant contribution in the form of PD-related illness variables was identified as shaping the construct of strain: these included patient depression, disease stage and duration. In addition, the carer's appraisal of marital satisfaction and affective symptoms in the care recipient also formed part of the model for carer strain obtained with linear regression. The fact that disease severity is associated with strain is consistent with previous studies as described in section 12.4.2 above and is not surprising, as many of the items on the Machin Strain Scale reflect concern with advancing motor and/or other somatic symptomatology. For example, subjective feelings of worry, frustration or embarrassment in relation to the spouse may well be connected with advances in physical disability and dopamine related symptoms such as sexual disinhibition and other impulsive behaviours. However, the strongest predictor of carer strain was not the motor or physical dysfunction associated with PD, which accounted for 18% of the variance in the measure, but rather the care recipient's affective symptomatology in the form of depression, primarily as perceived by the carer, with the patients' self-reported symptoms having a smaller effect (accounting for only 5% of the variance in the strain measure). Carers' perceptions of depression in their spouses accounted for 36% of the variance in their reported feelings of strain and showed a good correlation with the clinician rated assessment of depression in the patient (r=0.49), though it was higher with the patients' self-rated reports (r=0.61), indicating that carers are good judges of affective changes in their spouses. Thus when other, more important factors are taken into account simultaneously in multivariate analyses of the kind described here, the apparent effects of somatic symptoms on carer strain are shown to diminish considerably, and in some studies have been found to disappear entirely (e.g. Aarsland, Larsen, Karlsen et al. 1999). Thus, patient-depression was found to be making a major contribution to the strain of care-giving, irrespective of whether it was rated by the patient him/herself, the clinician or the carer; ratings by the carer had the greatest influence on his/her levels of reported strain.

Carer strain also appeared to be affected by carers' reported satisfaction with their marital relationship with the care recipient. Whilst it may seem understandable that someone who is unhappy with their marital relationship may be resentful of having to care for their partner and thus reports higher levels of strain, such a conclusion would be unjustified from the present study. Despite the independent variables in multiple regression being referred to as "predictor" variables, it should be remembered that the relationship between them and the dependent variable, in this case strain, is only correlational and does not specify the direction of the relationship. Thus it is equally likely that high levels of carer strain might be the cause of diminished levels of marital satisfaction. Nevertheless, studies of this kind have some justification in assuming that because the strain measure chosen is specifically focused on the care-giving situation, it is providing a valid criterion variable for which predictive variables may be sought through the experimental procedure used. In summary, the variables contributing to the regression model for strain accounted for some two-thirds of the variance in this measure.

One way of confirming whether these variables have a significant influence on the construct of strain is the extent to which they help to distinguish between groups of carers with reported high and low levels of strain. The results of the discriminant function analysis showed that a high proportion of carers (83.1%) were correctly classified according to their scores on the Machin Strain Scale. Classification of those with high levels of strain was 85.7% with duration of illness, patient depression and marital satisfaction as significant predictor variables. For those with low strain, the classification was correct for 80.6% of carers, indicating that additional factors not accounted for in the analysis must be contributing to the lower levels of care-giving strain reported by these carers. Since duration of illness and not disease severity, appears to be the important discriminating variable, it may represent a chronicity factor, rather than more advanced disease. Thus it is possible to conclude that high levels of carer strain are mainly associated with long-lasting disturbances in mood in the care recipient, together with the carer's dissatisfaction with the marital relationship, possibly over longer periods of time.

It is somewhat remarkable that there continues to be a lack of consensus regarding the conceptualization of care-giving strain or burden, given that it has been at the centre of studies of care-giving for almost 30 years. Scales such as the one used in this study to measure care-giving strain are typically composed of items designed to reflect problems for the carer considered to be emanating from the care recipient's illness (e.g. Savundranayagam et al. 2011; Zarit et al. 1980) and this distinctive feature is seen as being their uniquely positive attribute. All other measures of carer outcome in terms of physical health, psychological morbidity, emotional distress and various other factors reflecting their life situation are more general and not specific to care-giving. This distinction is theoretically important and means that strain should not be used interchangeably with these terms (Maurin and Boyd 1990), a consideration that is not always observed in care-giving studies of PD (e.g. D'Amelio et al. 2009; Miller et al. 1996).

Moreover, research into care-giving in PD has viewed carer strain both as a predictor and as an outcome variable. Of particular interest are those studies which included both measures of care-giving strain and of psychological morbidity in carers, usually in the form of depression. In cases where strain is seen as a risk factor for psychological morbidity in carers, it is effectively acting as an additional stressor contributing to depression (e.g. Lyons et al. 2002). Alternatively, in some studies, strain has been viewed as an outcome variable with carer depression contributing to it, presumably on the basis that depressed carers are likely to report greater levels of care-giving strain (e.g. Caap-Ahlgren et al. 2002; Martinez-Martin et al. 2007; Deuel et al. 2010). These theoretical positions are rarely made explicit or justified by researchers. However, the raised prevalence of clinically significant symptoms of depression in carers of people with PD demonstrated in this and other studies, requires not only description, but explanation if the care-giving process, in all of its complexities, is to be understood. The position adopted in the present study was that carer depression should be treated as a dependent or outcome variable, and strain was conceptualised either as a secondary stressor or as a mediating variable, as described later in the discussion. It was deemed reasonable to assume that the alternative view, in which carer depression is primarily a contributor to care-giving strain, required justification of the position that carers may be depressed for reasons other than finding themselves in the situation of care-giving. Whilst this may also be true, the raised prevalence rates for depression found in carers would have to be accounted for by some other systematic explanation. The parsimonious view would seem to be that rates of depression are raised among carers because of the difficult situation in which they find themselves, namely that of care-giving. Hence the theoretical position adopted for the present study, viewed carer depression as primarily an outcome measure.

12.4.5 Factors associated with depression in carers: PD motor symptoms

The extent to which depression in carers may be associated with the various symptom domains of PD has been unclear, as previous studies have given contradicting results. As regards the present research, no relationship of any kind was found with disease stage, severity of the motor impairment or degree of functional ability and carer depression in either zero order correlational or multivariate statistical analyses. The only disease related variable to be associated with carer affect was the duration of illness, and this occurred only with one of the carer outcome measures for depression (the GDS). It is a finding that is difficult to interpret for a number of reasons. Firstly, disease duration may be a reflection of other factors in the care-giving situation, such as the length of time for which the carer has provided care. The results of the study also show that carer depression is mainly affected by the strain of care-giving and it would be reasonable to assume that strain accumulates over time, eventually leading to depression. Secondly, it is equally likely that illness duration may be a reflection of the length of time for which the care recipient has been depressed, as this is the main primary symptom domain to be associated with carer depression. Finally, illness duration may be reflecting a range of other influences on the care-giving situation that are difficult to determine; as argued in stage II, not time itself, but the opportunity that arises for other events to take place over a certain period, such as the evolution of depression, for example, may be the main effects that are reflected in the illness duration variable.

Few previous studies appear to have used standardised depression scales as a measure of carer outcome in PD; only six were identified from the relevant literature. In these studies, the contribution of motor impairment to carer depression is somewhat controversial. For example, in keeping with the results of the present study, no association has been reported between carer depression and severity of motor symptoms (Meara et al. 1999) or disease stage (Fernandez et al. 2001), except at the most severe, end-stage of the illness (Carter et al. 1998). However, other studies have found significant correlations between carer depression and disease stage (Aarsland, Larsen, Karlsen et al. 1999; Schrag, Hovris et al. 2006), duration of illness (Fernandez et al. 2001; Martinez-Martin et al. 2008), severity of the motor impairment and functional ability (Aarsland, Larsen, Karlsen et al. 1999; Carter et al. 2008; Schrag, Hovris et al. 2006). The reasons for the discrepant findings between the two groups of studies remain unclear.

12.4.6 Factors associated with depression in carers: PD neuropsychological symptoms

However, as argued above, drawing conclusions about complex, multi-factorial situations such as care-giving on the basis of simple, zero-order correlations is inappropriate and can be misleading, especially in situations where variables are highly inter-correlated. Hence, regression analyses were used to control for the shared variance among variables in determining the predictors of carer depression. Of the main PD symptom domains examined, only depression was found to be associated with carer affective status, irrespective of the way in which it was measured. Between 14-22% of the variance in carer depression was explained by care recipient depression, in a model which did not include carer variables. The importance of patient-related depression in determining carer depression in PD was originally described by Miller et al. (1996) and together with other non-motor symptoms, including cognitive deficits, has more recently been confirmed in a number of other studies (e.g. Aarsland, Larsen, Karlsen et al. 1999; Schrag, Hovris et al. 2006; Carter et al. 2008). The proportion of the variance explained by the non-motor symptoms of PD varies among studies, for example care recipient depression was responsible for just 1%

in the study by Carter et al. (2008), but they also reported a significant influence of cognitive symptoms, which together with depression, were more important than motor symptoms in explaining the variance in carer depression. The relatively high contribution of care recipient depressive symptoms in the present study is probably due to the absence of any effects of the other patient variables. The patients in this study were also in a more advanced stage of PD than in the study by Carter et al. (2008) and this too may have affected the extent to which their affective symptoms might have influenced carer depression, bearing in mind the importance of illness duration revealed in these analyses.

The failure to find any effects of cognitive symptoms on carer outcomes in the current research may be a result of the strict entry criteria used, which were designed to eliminate patients with other concomitant age-related conditions. This may have resulted in a sample of patients, in whom cognitive impairment was relatively mild or in whom it had not yet developed, as the selection bias may have inadvertently also excluded a possible subgroup of PD patients in whom PD is characterised by cognitive failure. The additional difficulties of coping with cognitively impaired spouses with PD on the carers may have therefore been reduced. The significance of this should not be underestimated, as there is evidence that cognitive changes following either stroke or PD have an adverse impact on carers and the strength of this association is significantly greater than in the case of carers of people with DAT (Thommessen et al. 2002; Shin, Youn et al. 2012).

However, when carer variables were added to the model tested as an explanation of carer depression, the regression model derived changed substantially. Carer depression was in all cases, irrespective of the instruments used for its measurement, primarily affected by care-giving strain, which accounted for around 30% of the variance in each of the indices used. Each measure of depression was further associated with a different predictive variable, but in no case did any of these variables contribute more than an additional 10% to the variance in outcome. The quality of the marital relationship (MAS) further contributed to the GDS, the carer's perceptions of cognitive dysfunction in the patient (CFQ-other-cognitive) to the BDI and the age of the carer to the GHQ. This suggests that apart from the main association with strain, carers may be more depressed when the marital relationship is poor and/or when they perceive their spouse as suffering from cognitive decline. Furthermore, there was a tendency for younger carers to be more depressed, a finding that is in keeping with previous work which has found younger spouse carers to be at higher risk for depression (Schneider et al. 1999) and strain (Carter et al.

2010). However, at best, these variables accounted for just under half of the overall variance in carer depression. This means that other factors, unconnected with those studied, must also be determining depression for the carer.

High levels of classification, discriminating depressed from non-depressed carers were achieved using discriminant function analysis for all three depression instruments: the GHQ (86.2%), the GDS (83.9%) and the BDI (77.8%). The discriminant functions were more accurate in predicting the grouping variables for the non-depressed carers, once more suggesting that additional factors, not taken into account in the model were responsible for depression in carers. Classifications based on carer age and gender could be not be achieved according to the variables used for the discriminant analysis procedure. The variables contributing to the classifications are broadly in keeping with those shown by the regression analysis to be contributing to depression in the carer. Indices of depression based on the GHQ and the GDS were associated with carer strain and in the case of the former with duration of illness, and in that of the latter with marital satisfaction. Depression on the BDI however, appeared to be determined by the carer's perceptions of cognitive dysfunction in the care recipient and the carer's age. As these relationships are partly dependent on different measures of depression for the carer, the need to take a multi-dimensional approach to the assessment of carer outcomes is emphasized.

12.4.7 The course of depression in carers

Carer depression appears to follow a different pattern from carer strain in relation to disease progression. A sharp rise in depression was observed for those carers looking after patients in Hoehn and Yahr stage 2 as compared to stage 1, but in contrast to strain, levels of depression were lower for those carers with care recipients in stage 3 and remained at a similar level for those in stage 4. Little can be reliably said about stage 5, as there were only two patients in this category (probably as a result of the entry criteria to the study), but at least one previous study has reported that carer depression was found to increase towards the end-stage of the disease process (Carter et al. 1998). These results suggest not only that the dynamics of carer strain and depression follow a different path over the course of PD, but that they may be affected by different processes over the course of disease progression. The interpretation of these results is somewhat limited by the cross-sectional nature of the data and therefore firm conclusions cannot be drawn about the longitudinal course of carer strain and depression in caring for someone with PD. The pattern of carer depression in relation to disease stage seen in this study is interesting, but needs to be replicated in further research. A preliminary conclusion would seem to suggest that depression affects carers in the relatively early stages of care-giving and this would be in keeping with the finding that neither motor or functional impairment associated with PD appear to be its main determinants.

Nevertheless, it does appear that a clear distinction should be made between the concepts of strain and depression as outcome measures for carers. The present findings would seem to indicate that although carers may report greater levels of strain (or burden) with disease progression, this does not necessarily automatically translate into higher levels of psychopathology in the form of depression. Other factors appear to be implicated in determining carer depression in PD and these were explored through analyses of the data which focused on attempting to understand the role of potential mediating variables in the chain of relationships which constitute care-giving, from the primary disease related stressors, through carer strain to the final outcome measured in terms of the affective status of the carer.

12.4.8 Factors associated with the marital satisfaction

Poor marital satisfaction reported by carers was associated with care recipient depression, but not with any of the other illness-related factors, in a model which took account only of the PD-related illness variables. However, when carer variables were added to the model, marital satisfaction was most closely associated with care-giving strain. Carers were classified into two groups – those satisfied with their marital relationship and those not – with an accuracy of about 78%, male carers suffering high levels of care-giving strain reporting the highest levels of marital dissatisfaction.

12.4.9 Factors associated with the CFQ-carer

The more generic measure of strain employed in the study in the form of the CFQ for the carer was not found to be associated with any of the independent variables used in the regression analyses. This is perhaps not surprising, as carers' scores on the CFQ did not differ from those of a group of healthy, older adults reported by Hohman et al. (2011). As no relationship was found between the CFQ-carer and care-giving strain, it would appear that the two measures are sampling distinctly separate types of strain among the carers. This is confirmed by the results of the discriminant analysis, with carers grouped according to their levels of strain on the CFQ-carer. Correct classification was achieved for almost 70% of carers with low marital satisfaction and high levels of carer depression found to be the strongest determinants of high levels of more general feelings of strain among carers. Hence the CFQ cannot be considered to be a sensitive measure of strain in the care-giving process, although it is shaped by more generic factors, which themselves are partially shaped by the effects of care-giving.

The findings of the present study emphasize that as indicators of the effects of care-giving, strain and depression are strongly related to each other (see figure 12-2). Both care recipient and carer-related variables are associated with care-giving strain in the form of the primary disease-related stressors (including motor and affective, but not cognitive variables) and carer appraisals of depression in the care recipient and marital satisfaction. Carer depression on the other hand, is determined solely by carer-related variables in the form of care-giving strain, carer age and carer appraisal of cognitive dysfunction in the care recipient.

Figure 12-2. Associations among selected variables in the care-giving situation revealed through multiple regression and discriminant function analyses.

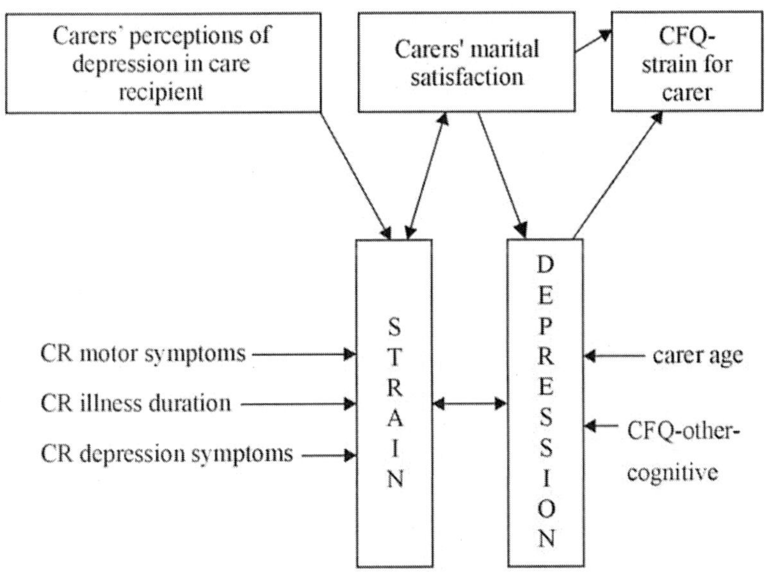

Note: CR – care recipient

12.5 Models of care-giving: the relationship between carer strain and depression in PD care-giving

In addition to the difficulties associated with the conceptualisation of the construct of care-giving strain, research in this area also lacks the guidance of a clear theoretical framework. That is not to say that such frameworks do not exist. The main theoretical approaches in care-giving research have evolved from stress theory (Lazarus and Folkman 1984) and have been elaborated in a number of forms as described in chapter 6. Confusion arises, however, as few of the studies on care-giving in PD have made their theoretical underpinnings explicit, and as a result, the relationship between care-giving strain and psychological morbidity is variously interpreted. This is not unimportant as the relationship between the two has implications for theoretical models of care-giving, yet has received very little attention in the care-giving literature on PD.

Previous studies have generally viewed both strain and depression as measures reflecting different aspects of carer outcomes (e.g. Aarsland, Larsen, Karlsen et al. 1999; Carter et al. 2008; D'Amelio et al. 2009; Miller et al. 1996; Schrag, Hovris et al. 2006), or as mentioned above, have treated carer depression as an additional contributor to strain (e.g. Caap-Ahlgren et al. 2002; Martinez-Martin et al. 2007; Deuel et al. 2010). Decisions regarding the nature of outcome indicators are theoretically important; although treating both strain and depression as different forms of outcome for carers appears relatively neutral in theoretical terms, this position often ignores the fact that whilst they are related, each is associated with different sets of variables, as demonstrated in the present study. Equally, the assumption that carer depression is a determinant of carer strain represents a definite theoretical stance. This assumption cannot be justified without empirical investigation as correlation statistics are unable to demonstrate causality. No studies of this kind appear to have been conducted in PD.

Another problem in interpreting studies is that they frequently report their findings in relation to undefined concepts such as carer distress; this appears to be an amalgamation of both strain and depression measures, although how the notion of distress is reached, is not fully explicated (e.g. D'Amelio et al. 2009).

According to the stress process model of care-giving (Pearlin et al. 1990), primary stressors consist of objective indicators such as illness-related symptoms, problematic behaviour and ADL and IADL dependencies of the care recipient. They also include two subjective indicators of the hardships experienced by carers as a result of the objective indicators. The first of these relates to the overload or burnout experienced by carers and involves their feelings of fatigue, but also the extent to which they perceive their task as unremitting and overwhelming in its demands. The second aspect is referred to as relational deprivation, which reflects changes in the carer-care recipient relationship, and losses in reciprocity between the couple. These primary stressors are seen as giving rise to secondary role strains in the form of family conflict, job-care-giving conflict, financial problems and restrictions on social life. A major premise of the model is that one set of stressors may lead to another, a process that has been described as stress proliferation (Aneshensel et al. 1995). It is not surprising that carers exposed to both the primary stressors and secondary role strains should react with diminished psychological well-being, referred to as intrapsychic strains. These are conceived as primarily involving dimensions of self-concept: one, a more global type, reflecting changes in the carer's self-esteem and feelings of mastery, the other situational, associated with loss of self, role captivity, feelings of competence and possible gains. Primary stressors, secondary role strains and secondary intrapsychic strains are seen as being the antecedents of carer outcomes and therefore are conceptualised as stressors. The model acknowledges the importance of mediators in accounting for the observation common to stress research, that individuals exposed to apparently similar stressors may respond to them in strikingly dissimilar ways. Mediation is recognised as having occurred if the relationship between a stressor and an outcome is attenuated or reinforced under different mediating conditions. Pearlin et al. (1990) assume that the same kinds of mediators are relevant to care-giving research as to stress research more generally. Thus, in the main, carers' coping strategies and levels of social support have been investigated as potential mediators of care-giving. Finally, the crucial choice of outcome indicators is guided, in this model, by reference to how an understanding of stress processes may help "to highlight the structural arrangements of the society and its institutional forces that affect peoples' lives (Pearlin et al. 1990, 590). These indicators have generally been construed in terms that reflect the well-being of people, their physical and mental health and their ability to sustain social roles. Similarly, in the Pearlin et al. (1990) model of care-giving, carers' physical and mental health, including depression, anxiety and cognitive difficulties are evaluated as well as limitations imposed on usual activities and the decision to place the care recipient in institutional care.

Certain modifications to the theoretical model proposed by Pearlin et al. (1990) are suggested as a result of the data-driven approach using multivariate analyses in the present study are shown in figure 12.2. It can be seen that PD-illness-related symptoms were similarly conceptualised as the primary stressors in care-giving. Essentially, without them, the care-giving situation would not arise. However, Pearlin et al.'s (1990) subjective indicators are seen as representing separate dimensions of care-giving and within the dyadic view of caring adopted for the study, are not viewed as primary stressors, as they represent a reaction of the carer to the demands elicited by the PD-illness related symptoms. Thus carer appraisals are involved in their feelings of overload, consequent upon their care-giving duties. These subjective feelings are thus a consequence of the primary stressors and in this sense, a step further along in the stress process. It is acknowledged however, that this is not a major departure from the original model, as carers' subjective reactions can be held to be "primary" stressors in the sense that they are elicited by the primary illness symptoms. The distinction is seen to be useful in terms of discerning which of the stressors, i.e. those directly related to PD-illness symptoms or those modified by carer appraisals in the form of care-giving strain, contribute most to outcomes. Furthermore, changes in the relationship between the carer and the care recipient were not conceptualised as primary stressors, but as potential mediators of the association between care-giving strain and carer outcome, again more appropriately reflecting the carer's perceptions within a dyadic process and taking into account the fact that negative changes were not inevitable. Equally, the carers' perceptions of psychological symptoms in the care recipient are evaluated in terms of their potential mediating properties in relation to care-giving strain and carer depression. These modifications to the Pearlin et al. (1990) model of the care-giving process were considered justified on the basis of the empirical results of the multivariate analyses which revealed patterns in the data compatible with a theoretical understanding of this kind. Perhaps most importantly however, in keeping with the stress process theory, care-giving strain was regarded as contributing to carer outcomes in the form of depression and cognitive failures. Hence the relationship between care-giving strain and carer depression was explicitly defined as the former being antecedent to the latter.

The theoretical model thus formulated was used to guide further analyses of the data in an effort to arrive at a better understanding of the care-giving process. Although it is useful to know that the greatest contribution to carer depression is made by care-giving strain, as shown in the previous analyses, this result is difficult to interpret for a number of reasons. Firstly, the levels of strain at which carers might be at risk of developing psychiatric morbidity is unknown. Secondly, it is difficult to make comparisons between studies because of the use different scales, in which strain or burden is conceptualised in various ways (Hunt 2003). Nevertheless the ability to identify individuals who may be at risk is crucial to the clinical utility of these scales. A third complication lies in determining which aspects of care-giving are especially problematic for carers. Ideally, a measure of care-giving strain or burden ought to capture the different aspects of care-giving which give rise to difficulties for carers and identify individuals at risk of developing mental health problems as a result of their care duties. Unfortunately, despite growing understanding that care-giving strain is a multidimensional construct, this is rarely recognised in the continued use of global summary scores to reflect levels of strain, especially in the care-giving literature on PD. At least two studies have demonstrated that the items in the Relatives' Strain Scale (which is a close derivation of the Machin Strain Scale) may be grouped according to separate categories which are differentially related to each other (Greene et al. 1982; Ulstein et al. 2007) and a two factor structure has been reported for the Zarit Burden Interview (Hérbert, Bravo and Préville 2000). For the purposes of constructing appropriate interventions with carers it is also essential to know if any of the underlying constructs of care-giving strain have particular saliency in contributing to psychiatric morbidity. In addition, Ulstein et al. (2007) point out that in clinical settings it may be easier and more acceptable to use a strain scale, than to carry out a full psychiatric interview with the carer. Hence the properties of such scales need to be understood.

A fourth problem lies in identifying different conditions which may modify levels of care-giving strain. From a theoretical perspective, factors which help to explain the occurrence of care-giving strain, may act either to reinforce or to attenuate its ill-effects for the carer. For example, based on evidence from the literature (see chapter 7) increased levels of marital satisfaction, carer age and longer experience of the task should diminish the risk of care-giving strain, whilst increased carer perceptions of psychological dysfunction in the patient might be expected to increase it. Thus differential effects of variables reflecting properties of the care-giving situation may have a simultaneous effect on carer outcomes, possibly cancelling each other out. Such effects are considered to reflect mediational properties in the variables. Those evaluated in the present study included the quality of the marital relationship and the carer's perceptions of psychological symptoms in the patient and it was hypothesised that these would exert their effects at different junctures in the care-giving process, as illustrated in figure 12.2.

Finally, despite a wealth of literature on carer burden, especially in relation to dementia care, the relationship between carer strain and psychiatric morbidity remains poorly understood. Somewhat surprisingly, it has rarely been the subject of investigation in care-giving studies (Bedard et al. 2000). Nor is it understood how the transition from suffering high levels of strain to developing clinically significant levels of depression may occur. This too, is a question involving the buffering effects of potential mediators. Although the relationship between care-giving strain and carer depression is a positive one, it is by no means perfect, indicating that carer strain does not always raise the risk of depression for the carer, even above certain critical values. The majority of carers in the present study appear to experience manageable levels of strain and respond adaptively to the situation of care-giving. This does not mean however, that their scores on the Machin Strain Scale are uniformly low, but that despite considerable levels of strain they are able to deal successfully with the difficulties engendered by the care-giving situation. Equally, all of the carers who reported raised levels of depressive symptoms did not necessarily report greater levels of strain. Similar sub-groupings of carers have been reported by Ulstein et al. (2007) and they reflect the fact that the more serious psychopathology affecting carers is not attributable in this and other studies to the primary disease related stressors (e.g. Bedard et al. 2000). It therefore seems likely that other factors intervene in the process of care-giving either to ameliorate or to intensify the strain experienced by the carer and thus determine the final outcome. It is also important to remember that although cross-sectional studies such as the one reported here, appear to give a somewhat static picture of the care-giving situation and carer outcomes in particular, the processes involved are ongoing and cyclical.

In view of these considerations, although care-giving strain was viewed in the present study as both a stressor contributing to, and as an outcome of care-giving, it was also investigated as a potential mediating variable between the disease-related stressors and carer outcomes in the form of depression. The main symptom domains of PD were hypothesized as resulting in differing levels of care-giving strain, which in turn was posited to be an antecedent of carer depression.

12.5.1 Possibilities for mediation in the care-giving pathway

The mediation hypothesis for care-giving strain in the proposed model of care-giving illustrated in figure 12.2. was tested using the causal steps analysis of Baron and Kenny (1986) for determining direct and indirect effects of chosen variables on specified outcome variables. Carer depression as measured on the GDS was chosen as the outcome measure in view of the results of the regression analysis which demonstrated that the greatest amount of variance could be accounted for by this variable. Care-giving strain was viewed as an intervening or mediating variable, in seeking to provide a more accurate account of the effect of the independent variables (disease-related stressors) on carer outcome. The proposed mechanism is one of mediation and it implies a causal hypothesis whereby patient-related symptoms are considered to cause the mediator, in this case care-giving strain, which in turn is the cause of carer depression (Holland 1988; Sobel 1990). The approach assumes that the mediator provides a better explanation of the relationship between the disease-related stressors and carer depression than the direct route from the stressors to depression; it represents an attempt to establish causal links among the three variables. Nevertheless, it should be remembered that causation cannot be inferred from any statistical procedure that is based on correlations, as is the case with the multiple regression analyses used to compute the estimates of these relationships. Frazier et al. (2004) suggest that three primary criteria are necessary in order to conclude that one variable is caused by another. These are that: (a) an association exists between the two variables, (b) the association is not spurious, and (c) the cause precedes the effect in time.

Finally, mediation analyses can be performed with either multiple regression or structural equation modelling (SEM). The logic of the analyses is the same in both cases, but SEM is considered the preferred method because of its heightened possibilities in controlling for measurement error and providing information on the degree of fit of the entire model. It is also much more flexible than regression, allowing the inclusion of multiple predictor variables, multiple outcome variables and multiple mediators in the model, as well as other potential causes of the mediator and outcome (Frazier et al. 2004). Nonetheless, in clinical research of the kind described here, where it is difficult to recruit sufficiently large numbers to perform SEM analyses (e.g. at least 200; see Quintana and Maxwell 1999), the use of multiple regression is to be preferred (Holmbeck 1997).

12.5.2 Carer strain as a mediator of the relationship between PD-related symptoms and carer depression

A question of central interest to this study was the relationship between care-giving strain and depression. Analysis of the data revealed that the main contribution to carer depression was made by care-giving strain, a finding that has been frequently reported in the literature on dementia care-giving (e.g. Chapell and Reid 2002; Pearlin et al. 1990). This raises the possibility that strain might act as an important juncture along the care-giving path to carer depression. Of the other independent variables, only patient depression was associated with carer depression (in the absence of carer predictive variables) suggesting that its effects were mediated in the full model by the more powerful strain variable. In addition, as neither the motor or cognitive symptoms of PD appeared to have a direct effect on carer outcomes, it is proposed that their effects might be exerted indirectly through the mediating effects of care-giving strain. Although the lack of a direct effect of an independent variable on the dependent variable (carer depression) breaches the conditions of step 1 in the causal steps procedure, it does not preclude the occurrence of mediation (Kenny 2012). For the model under consideration this would imply that, as a potential mediator, strain acts as a buffer with regard to the direct effects of disease-related symptoms, and in turn, diminishes their effects on carer depression. Whilst at first sight, this might appear counter-intuitive, what it means is that although motor symptoms are contributing to care-giving strain, a simultaneous process is occurring by which strain appears to be suppressing these effects on carer depression. A similar process may be occurring in the case of cognitive symptoms, although the case for this is less strong, as cognitive symptoms are associated with strain only on univariate, not multivariate analyses. The potential attenuating, or indeed amplifying, effects of strain might be exerted through additional characteristics of the care-giving situation, acting upon this variable, and these will be examined later.

The results of the causal steps procedure to establish mediation indicated that care-giving strain partially mediated the relationship between patient-depression and carer-depression, accounting for 76% of the effect. Since strain is a carer variable, this suggests that a large proportion of the effect of PD illness related depressive symptoms on carer depression is modulated through the prism of carer perceptions. In other words, the effects of patient depression for the carer are magnified through the carer's appraisals in terms of care-giving strain, leading to negative affect. Care-giving burden has also been found to mediate the path from care recipient symptoms to depression for spouse carers in the dementia care literature (e.g. Lawton et al. 1991).

Strain was also found to mediate the relationship between motor and cognitive symptoms and carer depression, but here mediation was inconsistent. This implies that strain was acting as a suppressor variable in this case, attenuating the effects of the motor and possibly cognitive symptoms on carer depression. A strong case can be made for causation in the chain of events from patient symptoms to carer depression, as there can be (virtually) no doubt that the symptoms of PD preceded both care-giving strain and carer depression. There may always be some possibility that certain carers would have been depressed independently of their care-giving role, but this is unlikely to apply to the group as a whole.

These analyses provide interesting insights into the data. Carer strain appears to act differentially with respect to the main symptom domains of PD, amplifying the effects of patient depression, but suppressing any potentially negative impact of the motor and cognitive symptoms on carer depression. This suggests that something important is occurring at this stage in the care-giving process, which may ameliorate the effects of some illness symptoms (motor and cognitive) but not others (depression). All of the symptom domains have a positive association with care-giving strain[2] indicating that strain increases in line with care-giving duties that are consequent upon the manifestations of PD. It is not unreasonable to conclude that apart from the direct effect of patient depression on carer psycho-morbidity, it also has indirect effects, which are magnified by the subjective feelings of strain in the carer. As motor (and to a lesser extent cognitive) symptoms also result in care-giving strain, it is more difficult to interpret the suppressive effect that occurs for these symptoms along the indirect pathway (via the strain mediator) to carer depression. It is only possible to assume that the effects of strain must have been differentially reduced in relation to these symptoms. It would seem logical that other factors are acting on the strain variable to produce these effects.

One such possibility is the carer's level of marital satisfaction with the care recipient, which may act upon the relationship between care-giving strain and carer depression, by "cushioning the blow", either as a means of providing valued support to the carer or because s/he may feel that caring for his/her spouse is a means of reciprocating the rewards of a previously positive relationship. Equally, an unsatisfactory relationship may generate resentment in relation to the care-giving role and increase levels of strain. These possibilities were examined by testing the potential mediating effects of marital satisfaction on the relationship between carer strain and depression.

---

[2] A significant relationship is found when patient cognitive symptoms alone are regressed on care-giving strain, but not with multiple regression analyses.

12.5.3 The role of marital satisfaction in care-giving in PD

In the context of care-giving, it is possible to conceptualise the quality of the relationship between the carer and the care recipient in a number of ways, all of which may be elements of the stress process model of care-giving as described by Pearlin et al. (1990). It is evident from the study that the relationship between care-giving strain and marital satisfaction is reciprocal: in addition, both increases in carer strain and lower marital satisfaction are associated with a greater likelihood of depression in carers (see figure 12-3).

Figure 12-3. Revised model of care-giving in PD based on causal steps analyses.

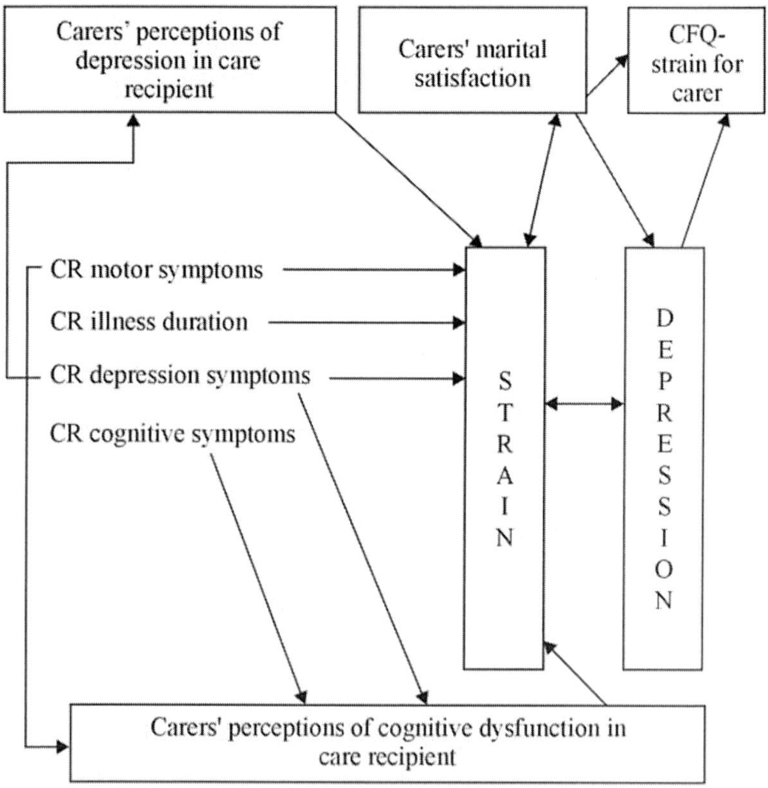

Note: CR – care recipient

One way of viewing the quality of the marital relationship is as a personal resource of the carer in the form of coping with the care-giving situation. This approach has been explicated by Kramer (1993a) to extend the notion of coping beyond the traditional problem and emotion focused strategies, to include ones that are focused on maintaining social relationships. There has long been evidence from the care-giving literature generally, that worse outcomes for carers are associated with disrupted relationships with the care recipient (Cantor 1983; Poulshock and Deimling 1984), but where affectional bonds are strong, carers perceive lower levels of stress (Cantor 1983; Horowitz and Shindleman 1983). It is not unreasonable to expect that relationships may become disrupted during the care-giving process, as the emergence of psychological symptoms in particular, cause behavioural changes in the care recipient. It has been shown in this and previous studies, that those changes associated with depression are especially difficult for carers to come to terms with, but bizarre and problematic behaviours, are also among the most disruptive (Pinquart and Sörensen 2003; Savundranaygam et al. 2005). In PD these may include the impulse control disorders that have been associated with dopamine agonists (see chapter 3). Hence even formerly valued and satisfying relationships may be shaken, as the disease or iatrogenic processes transform previously kind, stable and reliable partners into unpredictable or emotionally labile individuals, who may become withdrawn, suspicious, fearful or unusually impulsive and induce behaviours, such as gambling or sexual demands that were inconceivable before the onset of the illness. This is seen most dramatically in the descriptions of carers, when they speak of the person they used to know, as no longer being there, by which they are reflecting their experiences in terms of a complete severance of the previous relationship (Kramer 1993a).

These considerations lead to the conclusion that if relationship quality is to be characterised as a form of coping resource for carers, it is the quality of the current relationship (rather than any pre-existing one) that is of primary importance in determining carer outcomes. It is not entirely obvious however, that relationship quality is best conceptualised as one of coping or whether it would not be more appropriately seen as a form of social support. A fairly consistent finding in the literature is that greater perceived satisfaction with support by the carer is linked to lower levels of care-giving strain, depression and health problems in general (Edwards and Scheetz 2002). However, not all studies have been in agreement on this. For example, Lawton et al. (1991) did not find any effects of instrumental social support for carers of people with dementia and social support was not found to influence care-giving strain or depression in PD (Miller et al. 1996), although the size of the social network was found to be significantly reduced in comparison to an age-matched control group, possibly preventing opportunities for social support to arise. However, the quality of the marital relationship with the care recipient may represent a special form of social support, which is particularly important for spouses caring for partners with PD, as other relationships and contacts, even with family members gradually diminish with disease progression (Miller et al. 1996). Hence the role of the marital relationship, which represents a specific and uniquely intimate relationship in the lives of most people, may be particularly significant to the well-being of both the carer and the care recipient. Notwithstanding this, it would still seem that present rather than past marital satisfaction may be more relevant to either coping or social support for the carer.

The scale used to measure relationship quality in the present study was the Marital Adjustment Test designed by Locke and Wallace (1959). It is probably the best established measure of marital satisfaction (or distress) and has been the most comprehensively researched of all the measures available, in terms of its psychometric features (Cohen 1985), so that it may be regarded as a "gold standard" in this respect (Whiting and Crane 2003). Locke and Wallace (1959, 251) defined marital adjustment as the "accommodation of a husband and wife to each other at a given time". This suggests that the measure is attempting to tap a dyadic process rather than an attitudinal variable, and that it is focused on the present not the past, making it an appropriate tool for evaluating carers' marital satisfaction in the context of either a coping or social support resource, as described above. Seen in this way, marital satisfaction becomes a potential mediating variable in the care-giving process. Because of the evidence from previous research cited above, that carers who assess their marital relationship with the care recipient as being strong in affectional ties, perceive the task of care-giving as less onerous, marital satisfaction may be hypothesised as a mediating variable between carer strain and outcome in the form of depression. A supportive relationship might be helpful in defraying the strain of care-giving and protecting carers from going on to develop depression. Alternatively, those carers whose relationships are unsatisfactory, might be at greater risk of depression.

Evaluation of the mediating effect of marital satisfaction gave support to this hypothesis. Although the effect was relatively small, it was reliable: approximately 24% of the effect of strain on depression appears to be mediated by the marital relationship. This suggests that higher levels of care-giving strain result in carer depression, partly because they have a negative impact on the marital relationship, which in turn leads to higher levels of depression for the carer. In other words, higher levels of strain may cause resentment in carers, thereby negatively affecting the marital relationship, with the consequent loss of mutuality leading to depression.

Satisfaction with the marital relationship is likely to reflect various aspects of the couple's life together, including affectional ties, mutual concern for each other, intimacy and degree of caring. These have been conceptualised as reflecting the mutuality of the relationship (Steadman et al. 2007). Previous studies have shown an association between mutuality and carer burden and depression in PD, although being based on correlational statistics, they have been unable to establish the direction of these effects (Carter et al. 1998; Edwards and Scheetz 2002; Schrag, Hovris et al. 2006).

An equally plausible position to that described above, is that marital satisfaction may affect the carer's appraisal of the care-giving situation, in effect diminishing (or exacerbating) perceptions of stressors. This is thought to be an important factor in ameliorating the negative effects of care-giving (Archbold et al. 1990), one which may have diminished the impact of the motor and cognitive symptoms on carer outcomes in the present study. This theoretical position does not view marital satisfaction as a mediator in the care-giving pathway, but as causal in determining both carer strain and depression and opens possibilities for treating carer strain and depression as potential mediators. Supplementary analyses revealed that care-giving strain mediated approximately 50% of the relationship between marital satisfaction and carer depression, (Sobel Z=-3.182, S.E.=0.02, p=0.001). The importance of marital satisfaction in determining both strain and depression outcomes for the carer appears stronger than the possibility examined earlier, in which relationship satisfaction was viewed as mediating the carer strain-depression pathway. Nevertheless, this does not preclude the possibility, that given the appropriate circumstances, both pathways may have explanatory value.

Positive appraisals of care-giving, which allow the carer to take the hardships of the caring task in his/her stride, are likely to be qualities of the couple's previous marital history in which they built up reserves of loyalty and trust towards each other as the result of mutual experiences. They are frequently expressed in carers' convictions that "he (or she) would do the same for me, if the situation were reversed". Thus although the task of care-giving is hard, carers are not resentful. Negative appraisals, on the other hand, magnify stressful events, increasing the likelihood of poorer outcomes for carers. Marital history, and in particular the quality of the relationship prior to the onset of PD, has also been conceptualised as a vulnerability factor in care-giving (Kramer 1993b), in so far as it may predispose the carer to making negative appraisals of the situation. For example, a previously abusive relationship is unlikely to engender a caring attitude towards the care recipient on the part of the aggrieved husband or wife, even when ill-health makes them no longer capable of causing distress, as in the past. Such extreme examples are probably rare, but perhaps even lesser misdemeanours in earlier stages of the relationship, such as occasional indifference or preoccupation with oneself may build up resentments as opposed to the benefits or more positive relationships.

One further possibility might account for the relationship between care-giving strain and the marital relationship established in the study; this encompasses a view of carer depression as having mediational properties for the relationship. There is considerable evidence in the general population to link depression and marital discord (e.g. Du Rocher Schudlich, Papp and Cummings 2011) and some to suggest that depression may precede marital disharmony (Johnson and Jacob 2000; Benazon and Coyne 2000). Although it is most likely that there is a cyclical relationship between the two, the possibility that carer depression might act as a mediator for the pathway between care-giving strain and marital satisfaction was also considered for the sake of completion. Testing this alternative model revealed that carer depression could be regarded as a significant mediator, accounting for approximately 39% of the relationship between strain and marital satisfaction (Sobel Z=-2.18, S.E.=0.49, p=0.03). Thus there are alternative models that are consistent with these data and should be investigated in further studies. However, it is at least plausible, that all of these mechanisms may be present under different circumstances, and so awareness of these interdependencies is crucial to an understanding of care-giving.

The present study provides empirical support for the view that marital satisfaction in the carers of people suffering from PD may protect against the strain experienced in the wake of the hardships of care-giving, but that low marital satisfaction contributes to depression in carers, both directly and indirectly by mediating the impact of care-giving strain on carer depression. It is presumably the effects of marital satisfaction on care-giving strain that allow the latter to suppress the potentially harmful effects of motor and cognitive symptoms on carer outcomes in terms of depression. This is not evident in the case of patient depressive symptoms, as these have both a direct and an indirect effect on carer depression.

Caring for someone with a neurodegenerative condition such as PD involves high levels of interpersonal contact between the carer and the care recipient, not only in the area of meeting physical care needs, but also in terms of negotiating agreement with regard to virtually all aspects of everyday life, such as taking medication, maintaining a social life and the more intimate aspects of the couple's relationship. All of these areas may potentially be the source of considerable interpersonal strain, if one partner appears to have changed as a result of the disease process or the other is seen as lacking in empathy in regard to the changes by remaining inflexible, demonstrating irritation and lacking acceptance or even becoming unduly overprotective. Above all, these strains may impact on the manner of interaction between the couple and alter the use of interpersonal strategies, affecting core aspects of their relationship such as their sense of mutuality and coherence as a couple. De Longis and O'Brien (1990) have defined positive carer strategies aimed at nurturing the relationship with the care recipient in terms of negotiation, compromise, consideration of the other person's limitations, compassion and empathy. Negative strategies are damaging and disruptive to the relationship and consist of critical, hostile or confrontational attitudes and behaviours, minimizing communication and ignoring the care recipient. These strategies may help to maintain or destroy relationship mutuality and are thus considered to be important mechanisms in determining the outcomes of care-giving.

Yet it seems inconceivable that the mechanism of negative interaction strategies outlined above, could have universal explanatory power for the deterioration of marital relations in care-giving. If these strategies are trait dependent features of carers, such individuals would also be expected to have poor pre-existing relationships with their spouses. Although a few couples where this might have been the case were identified among the sample, it was without doubt only a tiny minority. This is not surprising, as the majority of couples had been together for the greater part of their lives and the survival of marriage into later life is associated with greater stability and satisfaction (Franco et al. 2008). Indeed, whilst speculative, an impression gained from interviewing the couples was that those who were in relationships of shorter duration (second marriages) were ones in which the carer was prone to express greater frustration with his/her situation.

The alternative is that negative interaction strategies may be state dependent and come to the fore in stressful situations such as care-giving, especially when the care recipient's behaviour is difficult to understand. An example of this is that when carers do not feel appreciated, they experience care-giving as a burden and conflicts arise, which result in reduced marital satisfaction (Franco et al. 2008). Other challenges to carers may come in the form of having to cope with changes to the marital relationship, ranging from adjustments that have to be made in taking on responsibilities that were formerly those of the care recipient, to more intimate aspects of the relationship including expressions of affection and sexual relations (see chapter 5). Depressed patients with PD are characteristically withdrawn and have difficulty in demonstrating interest in others and their surroundings; it may be partly for these reasons that PD related depression is acutely distressing to carers, who are not fully aware that the care recipient's behaviour is an expression of the affective disorder and not a rejection of the carer's concern. Other behavioural disorders, including the manifestations of cognitive impairments or impulse control disorders may be equally disturbing to carers. In the case of the former, ironically it may be the relatively mild initial presentation of the cognitive deficits of PD that causes most problems, in not being recognised as such. The person suffering from PD may thus be perceived by those most closely involved in his/her care as having changed in "personality" as a result of the illness, or as just being "plain difficult". Neither of these perceptions is likely to generate empathy on the part of the carer, the former perhaps introducing a fearful strangeness to the relationship, the latter a form of distancing, as the result of a perceived lack of willingness to co-operate on the part of the care recipient in the face of all the difficulties facing the couple. Negotiation and compromise which lie at the heart of empathic understanding are thus made exceedingly difficult for the carer. Identification with the spouse suffering from PD in order to understand his/her perspective, is blocked not only by difficulties in understanding that the psychological changes are a manifestation of the illness, but by the almost insurmountable problem of understanding these changes in the same way as the patient. Yet at the same time, an empathic understanding of the patient also requires the carer to maintain his/her own separateness in order to be able to continue to provide care appropriately. Carers who merge inappropriately with the care recipient are those who become over-protective and in effect cause harm, by depriving the person of independence and autonomy.

Carers who are able to manage the fine line that requires maintaining a dynamic balance between proximity and distance in their relationship with the care recipient represent individuals with secure adult attachment relationships. They are able to regulate optimal levels of proximity with their partner, thereby ensuring that the equilibrium between anxiety and security in the relationship is maintained. Illness factors, especially those affecting the psychological well-being of the care recipient, deregulate these mechanisms and when this happens, there is a tendency to respond with anxious (e.g. clinging) or avoidant behaviours (e.g. withdrawing), which may be a further threat to the relationship with the carer. But it would be unreasonable to expect patients with significant levels of psychological morbidity to be the main force in maintaining adult attachment relationships, as they are unlikely to have the resources to do so. This does not mean that they are totally incapable of responding in ways that facilitate rapport: in a study by Gallagher-Thompson et al. (2001) moderately impaired husbands with probable dementia were found to smile more than either their care-giving wives or a control group of non-care-giving couples in the context of a task to plan a future event. Nevertheless, the primary responsibility for the relationship rests with the carer. Those with secure attachments would be expected to find ways of dealing with disruptions to the relationship brought about by uncharacteristic or inappropriate behaviours of the care recipient, by making the necessary adaptations to allow for his/her incapacity. Insecure attachments on the part of the carer are unlikely to engender an empathic response, because the carer's own needs for reducing the anxiety emanating from the disruption to the marital relationship, are paramount. In these circumstances, carers may respond with the avoidant negative strategies outlined by DeLongis and O'Brien (1990), namely by assuming a hostile, deprecating stance, dismissing the relationship and escaping into self-sufficiency or adopting the over-protective attitudes already mentioned. The result, inevitably, is a reduction in satisfaction with the marital relationship.

A factor then, that may lie at the root of these relationship difficulties is not so much the attachment style of carers, nor their coping resources in terms of relationship focused strategies, although these are undoubtedly engaged in shaping outcomes, but the way in which carers perceive and interpret care recipient behaviours, and this may ultimately contribute to their distress. To the best of the author's knowledge, these relationships do not appear to have been considered previously in the literature on care-giving.

12.6 The role of carer appraisals of psychological symptoms in the care recipient

Stress process models in general, and of care-giving in particular, emphasise the importance of carers' appraisals of stressors as having a critical role in determining outcomes (e.g. Lazarus and Folkman 1984; Pearlin et al. 1990; Lawton et al. 1991). In accordance with these views, two types of appraisal are distinguished. Primary appraisal refers to carers' assessment of disease-related aspects in the care-giving situation which are potentially harmful or threatening; for example these might include having to undertake additional physical tasks, such as helping their spouse to turn over in bed at night or dealing with incontinence, as well as taking over responsibility for household administration, because of their spouse's mental incapacity. If judged to be unduly onerous, a process of secondary appraisal is initiated in which carers assess whether their resources for dealing with the situation are adequate (i.e. coping mechanisms).

Secondary appraisal has been conceptualised as the subjective response to care-giving (Lawton et al. 1991) and is therefore the equivalent of care-giving strain or burden (Montgomery et al. 1985; Poulshock and Deimling 1984).

Previous work has measured primary appraisals in terms of the amount of time spent on care-giving activities (e.g. Chappell and Reid 2002; Lawton et al. 1991; Yates et al. 1999). Not surprisingly, there is usually a strong positive relationship between primary and secondary appraisals (Chappell and Reid 2002). However, primary appraisals that are focused on informal hours of care provision, in PD are perhaps more likely to reflect the physical disabilities of the care recipient, or cognitive dysfunction in demented patients. In view of the emerging consensus in the literature, supported by the results of this study, that it is the non-motor symptoms of PD that have the greatest impact on carer outcomes (e.g. Aarsland, Larsen, Karlsen et al. 1999; Carter et al. 2008; Happe and Berger 2002; Leiknes et al. 2010; Meara et al. 1999; Miller et al. 1996), the logical corollary was to investigate the explanatory potential of carers' primary appraisals of psychological functioning in the care recipient. Hence, the mediational role of carer appraisals was examined in relation to the affective and cognitive symptoms of PD. The results of the causal steps analysis confirmed the prediction that carers' perceptions of depressive symptoms in the care recipient appeared to partially mediate the relationship between patient-depression and care-giving strain, accounting for approximately 44% of the effect on strain; their effect was to strengthen the impact of affective disturbances in the patient on carers' subjective feelings of the strain. Despite the fact that patient depressive symptoms, when seen through the eyes of carers, are intensified in terms of their impact on care-giving strain, there is a congruity between patient reported symptoms of depression and the carers' perceptions. Carers are thus sensitive to affective changes in their spouses and their perceptions were specific to the depressive symptoms demonstrated by patients.

As regards a similar evaluation of carers' ratings of their spouses' propensity for making cognitive errors, the implications for care-giving strain were unexpected and therefore revealing. Here it seems, carers' perceptions of cognitive failures in their spouses partially mediated the relationship between all three symptom domains (motor, affective and cognitive) and care-giving strain (see figure 12-3). Approximately 29% of the effect of patient motor symptoms, 37% of patient depression and 63% of cognitive dysfunction on care-giving strain seem to be mediated by the carer's perception of cognitive failure in the care recipient. The effect is to increase the impact of symptoms on care-giving strain, but clearly it is not specific to cognitive symptoms. Thus carers' appraisal of cognitive failure in their spouses serves to intensify the effects of both motor and affective symptoms on their subjective feelings of strain, in addition to those of cognitive dysfunction. It seems therefore, that it is not the affective or cognitive, or indeed motor status of the care recipient ***per se,*** that determines the associated strain experienced by the carer, but the carers' ***perceptions*** of the decline in the psychological functioning of the care recipient. This result adds to the body of research suggesting that care-giving outcomes may be more strongly influenced by the characteristics of the carer, than those associated with the care recipient (Hooker et al. 1998; Lyons et al. 2009).

A surprising feature of these findings was that they were unspecific, carers' appraisals of their spouses' cognitive failures mediating the effects of both motor and affective symptoms. Moreover, the indirect effect of cognitive symptoms, via carers' appraisals, made a significant contribution to care-giving strain, whereas the direct effect of more "objective" neuropsychological measures was more controversial, appearing only in univariate, but not multivariate statistical analyses. This implies that carers perceptions of cognitive decline in their spouses generalises to their physical disability and to their affective state, having a cumulative impact on care-giving strain. Interestingly, carers' perceptions of the cognitive dysfunction in PD correlate with functional disability in their spouses, but not with motor symptoms. Thus it would seem that characteristic features of the illness, presenting as functional difficulties in the form of slowness and increased clumsiness affecting the activities of daily living, may be mistaken for cognitive deficits. This, in another form, is essentially the problem of symptom overlap, discussed in relation to depressive symptoms in chapter 3. A similar process may occur with affective symptoms being taken for cognitive failure. The difficulty in recognising symptoms and understanding the underlying processes that they represent is not surprising, as it frequently presents a problem even for clinicians. Hence the diagnostic challenge of pseudodementia, for example (Bulbena and Berrios 1986). There is even an aspect in which carers' perceptions may be entirely accurate, for example, as when apraxia may interfere with dressing and low mood with a loss of interest in current events, which may suggest memory problems, signalling diminishing cognitive capacity. Nevertheless, the findings serve as a reminder of the fact, that carers are not passive bystanders in the care-giving process, whose task is merely reactive to the care recipient's needs. For married couples who had lived together for many years, it would be most unlikely that carers should be unaware of changes in their spouse's behaviour and this sensitivity would undoubtedly lead them to draw interpretations as to their origin. Although it may at first be surprising that carers appear to over-generalise as to the cognitive nature of the symptoms they observe, similar difficulties might well affect routine clinical judgements, unsupported by specialist assessments in neurodegenerative disorders and neuropsychology.

A striking aspect of these findings is that it is the carers' perceptions of cognitive dysfunction that are of greatest importance to shaping the construct of strain, rather than neuropsychological test performance, which had no direct impact when multiple correlations in the data were accounted for using multivariate statistical analyses. The lack of association between patients' cognitive functioning and care-giving strain or burden is not in itself surprising as it is a common finding in the dementia care literature (Mahoney et al. 2005), although evidence is emerging that it has more significance to care-giving in PD (Thommessen et al. 2002; Shin, Youn et al. 2012). It is interesting to speculate that carers' strain levels may be affected by being present during the neuropsychological evaluation of the care recipient, as this may increase their fears regarding his/her cognitive functioning.

These findings suggest the potential for helping carers to recognise the symptoms of PD (especially non-motor ones) and to differentiate among them. This might have several advantages, such as helping to identify those patients with significant depressive symptomatology and directing them towards treatment. Equally having a better understanding of certain behaviours would help carers to have clearer strategies for how to deal with specific problems that arise in the course of care-giving. For example, these might include knowing when requesting help from formal services might be useful as opposed to seeking other forms of possible support. An example here might be illustrative of the point. Behavioural changes characterised by withdrawal and apparent loss of interest in activities that were previously enjoyed, might be interpreted in a variety of ways by a carer. They might be attributed to the physical difficulties imposed by PD or to lowered mood. They might equally be seen as a sign of diminishing cognitive capacity. Each of these interpretations is likely to hold different meanings for the carer. It might be easiest to empathise with physical disability, whereas lowered mood might be understood, but some of its consequences may leave the carer feeling isolated and rejected. Cognitive loss may be especially feared because of the changes that it wreaks in personal identity and relationships. In addition, carers are likely to have views regarding the efficacy of possible treatment, which too may affect their outlook. These aspects of carers' appraisals have not been investigated, but are likely to influence their secondary appraisals or the way in which they arrive at their construction of care-giving strain. It would be helpful for further work to address the concepts underlying carers' perceptions of non-motor symptoms in PD in order to ascertain why they appear particularly damaging to their welfare. It cannot be precluded however, that carers suffering from strain and depression might be more inclined to interpret their spouses' functioning in a negative light and this possibility should therefore be explored in future studies. In either case, there would be obvious implications for intervention to ease the hardship of care-giving.

12.7 Carers as proxy informants

The pattern that emerged for carers' perceptions of psychological symptoms in the care recipient deserves closer scrutiny from the point of view of their reliability as proxy informants on behalf of the care recipient. Carers' ratings of mood disturbances in their spouses correlated with both clinician and patients' reports of depressive symptoms, but not with their neuropsychological test performance. This was confirmed by statistical analyses comparing carer evaluations with those of patients and the research clinician. Hence their judgements regarding affect appear both sensitive and specific. However, carers' assessment of the patient's cognitive performance did not correlate with neuropsychological test measurements, although it was associated with functional (though not motor) disability and affective status. There may be a number of reasons for this. One is that the neuropsychological tests used, may lack sensitivity in a group of patients who, because of the age selection criteria for the study, might be expected to show only relatively mild cognitive impairment, but do not meet the diagnostic criteria for dementia. However, this is unlikely to be the case, as about one-third of the patients were identified as having deficits in memory and visuospatial function on formal testing. Nevertheless, it may be that such tests lack ecological validity, as test performance may not correlate well with the problems of everyday life (Hickox & Sunderland 1992). Thus, a second reason may be that carer judgements concerning cognitive impairment in their spouses are more sensitive than neuropsychological tests, because carers have good long-term knowledge of their spouses and are able to detect subtle changes in cognitive performance, which the tests are not. This point has been made by Naismith et al. (2011) who suggest that carers' capacity to rate mild cognitive changes in PD might act as an early warning sign for cognitive decline, indicating the need for screening and intervention. In their study, carers reported more changes affecting memory and behaviour for PD patients with mild cognitive impairment than for those without, compared to other areas of functioning such as self-care activities, mood, eating and sleep. Here however, carer ratings of change in memory, but not behaviour, were related to neuropsychological test performance. Carers in the present study also identified cognitive changes in their care recipients, but these failed to correlate with test performance, suggesting that carers tended to over-estimate, or at least over-generalised the effects of these changes. As proposed in the foregoing discussion, carers may therefore interpret alterations in mood and the functional ability of the patient, together with the concomitant behavioural changes (e.g. withdrawal or decreased levels of communication), as indicators of cognitive impairment. Thus carers' apparent sensitivity to subtle changes in cognitive performance may reflect a tendency to over-generalise, in applying explanations of cognitive failure to account for other difficulties experienced by the care recipient, a fact that does not seem to have been considered by Naismith et al. (2011). Indeed there is evidence to show that whilst carers may provide descriptions of their care recipients' cognitive status which are predictive of a clinical diagnosis of dementia, this is dependent on information being gathered from a wide variety of cognitive domains (Monnot, Brosey and Ross 2005; Isella et al. 2006). When restricted to an enquiry about memory performance, the predictive power of such reports is low (Watson, Lewis and Fillenbaum 2005). Further work is required to acquire a better understanding of the relationships among the inter-related factors governing carer perceptions of the psychological presentation of PD.

Nevertheless, carer reports of patient functioning in PD are important in a variety of clinical situations, especially when the patient is suffering from significant levels of cognitive impairment. Studies show that spouses provide the most reliable reports (Ready, Ott and Grace 2004), although a tendency has been recognised for proxy informants to exaggerate the intensity of symptoms in comparison to the patient's own account (Fleming et al. 2005). Other studies have shown that carers' assessments of motor (Hoehn and Yahr 1967) and functional performance (Schwab and

England 1969) show concordance with clinicians' and patients' ratings, but only when both patient and carer attend the clinic together (McRae et al. 2002). Carers are best able to replicate patients' responses in relation to concrete variables, although Fleming et al. (2005) did not find this to be true in relation to the amount of physical activity undertaken by patients with PD. More subjective questions related to quality of life issues, focusing on anxiety, depression and concentration show greater disparities (Martinez-Martin et al. 2004). Certain features associated with the groups examined also appear to determine the concordance of patient and carer reports: agreement is higher for patients with better functional abilities and those who are more severely depressed; it is lower for those with more advanced disease (Fleming et al. 2005). This is of particular concern, because it is precisely in situations of severe disability that proxy evaluations may be most needed.

These indications from the literature regarding the extent to which carer judgements concur with those of patients and clinicians, form an important background to the present study. They provide support for the notion that carers are competent in recognising depression and functional disabilities, especially in less advanced disease, despite their tendency to rate these difficulties higher than patients themselves. In the same way, carers also evaluate cognitive dysfunctions as being more problematic (Fleming et al. 2005), though it would probably be inappropriate to expect patients to be accurate in this regard, except perhaps in the early stages of cognitive impairment (Hickox and Sunderland 1992). Only one previous study has made the appropriate comparison with the results of psychometric testing, finding good correlations with carers' reports of more change in memory and behaviour for patients with mild cognitive impairment, than those without (Naismith et al. 2011). The authors interpreted these findings as evidence of carers' ability to pick up subtle cognitive changes, that could not be detected on routine clinical assessment. However, it would appear that many of the instruments designed for making proxy measurements of the kind described, such as the Cambridge Behavioural Inventory-Revised used by Naismith et al. (2011; Wear et al. 2008) and the CFQ-other-cognitive scale (Broadbent et al. 1982) used in the present study, may lack specificity with regard to cognitive performance. For example, many of the questions (in both) which enquire about everyday problems such as being more forgetful, having difficulty with concentration and making decisions, being easily distracted and irritable, are questions equally relevant to the assessment of the cognitive symptoms of depression. It is therefore not surprising that in the present study, the results for the CFQ-other-cognition correlated with the patients' self-rated depression scores on the GDS. Similarly, in the Naismith et al. (2011) study, carers' apparently greater sensitivity to subtle signs of cognitive decline in the care recipients, may have reflected the affective rather than cognitive symptoms of PD. The relationship to functional performance, in areas such as bathing and dressing etc. is also in keeping with this notion, as self-care activities are likely to be affected not only by cognitive impairments but also by depression. The questionable specificity of the CFQ-other-cognition, means that it is probably best to treat it as a more general measure of the carer's ability to detect psychological symptoms in the care recipient.

Several points emerge from the preceding analysis. Firstly, carers appear to make reasonably accurate judgements about the depressive symptomatology of the care recipient. This is in keeping with previous reports that there is higher concordance between both parties when the patient is suffering from higher levels of depression (Martinez-Martin et al. 2004). Secondly, carers' perceptions of cognitive dysfunction are unrelated to findings on neuropsychological testing and are negatively skewed, indicating a greater tendency for some carers to view their spouses as suffering impairments in this area. Carers showed a greater propensity for judging their spouses to be cognitively impaired than in a previous study using the same instrument (Poliakoff and Smith-Spark 2008), but this may have reflected differences in the samples. Thirdly, although it might be argued that these results reflect carers' greater sensitivity to cognitive changes in the patient than that revealed by formal testing, this is an assumption that cannot be justified on the grounds that carers do not show specificity with regard to cognitive deficits, broadening their judgements to include both motor and affective symptoms. This is in keeping with the literature which shows that carers have a tendency to produce inflated assessments of the care recipient's disability (e.g. Fleming et al. 2005). Fourthly, it is important to be aware that in making judgements concerning the depressive and cognitive symptoms, carers need not be aware of the underlying domains that these symptoms represent i.e. they are making a phenomenological judgement not a classificatory one. Finally, the instrument used in the present study to measure carer perceptions of cognitive dysfunctions in the patient may not have discriminated sufficiently between the cognitive symptoms of an affective disorder and cognitive dysfunction more generally. This would explain carers' apparent tendency to overestimate levels of cognitive difficulties in the sample and the correlation of their judgements with other measures of affective symptoms. A similar argument might be made with respect to motor symptoms. These difficulties need to be addressed in future studies and they should be borne in mind when proxy judgements from carers are used in aiding clinical decisions.

Although the stress process model adopted for the present study conceptualises carer depression as an outcome of care-giving, it is important to remember that the process is a dynamic and recurrent one, where outcomes may feedback into the system, affecting carer appraisals and acting as mediators. For example, it is well established that there is considerable concordance for depressive illness among spouses (Meyler, Stimpson and Peek 2007) and this is equally true for older married couples (Druley et al. 2003; Eagles, Walker, et al. 1987) although it does not appear to be related to the duration of the relationship (McLeod 1993). Thus, although carer depression may be the result of care-giving for some individuals, once established, it may become an additional stressor, affecting carer perceptions at both the primary and secondary appraisal level, and driving the care-giving process in a relentless spiral towards further depression for the carer. Cross sectional studies are almost certainly observing care-giving relationships characterised by these dyadic forms of interaction between carer and care recipient. However, it is important to remember, that only a proportion of carers are depressed, and that other factors, such as marital satisfaction, offer some protection against the negative consequences of care-giving, especially in situations where the care recipient is not depressed.

12.8 Applications for clinical practice

One important aspect of the findings from the study lies in their potential for guiding practical interventions with carers and their spouses. A key finding in this respect is that carer outcomes in the form of depression are most closely associated with care-giving situations in which the care recipient is also depressed. Depression appears to be specifically destructive, because of its effects on care-giving strain and carer depression, but also because it reverses the protective effects of marital satisfaction for the carer. This points to the need to identify and treat depressive illness in patients with PD, in order to alleviate their own suffering and to prevent depression in their carers. Although it was estimated that around half of the patients in the present study were suffering from clinically significant levels of depression, fewer than 20% were receiving treatment for their depressive disorder.

Treatment of depression in carers is also indicated in view of the substantial proportions of carers (25-30%) in the study, in whom clinically significant depressive symptoms were identified. From a clinical neuropsychological point of view this requires that a formal evaluation of both the care recipient and the carer should form part of a regular, standardised assessment procedure for couples in whom one person has PD. In the U.K. this is a measure to be implemented in legislation that is currently under review in the form of the "Care and Support" Bill, which is to be enacted in 2013. The present research adds to the already existing empirical support for ensuring that carers are included, alongside the care recipient in an assessment, as this makes it more likely that their needs may be recognised and addressed. In view of the heightened risk for neuropsychiatric and neuropsychological complications associated with PD, the assessment should clearly include an evaluation of the patient from this perspective. Carers should be offered an assessment, which among other concerns, should screen for depression. Moreover, clinicians should be alerted to the fact, that carers who report high levels of psychological morbidity in their spouses, may themselves be at increased risk of depression.

Given the importance of carer perceptions of psychological symptoms in the care recipient to shaping the construct of care-giving strain, and ultimately depression, two approaches might be useful. The first, essentially of an educational nature, might be targeted at helping carers to recognise the non-motor symptoms of PD and to place them within the context of the disease process. The second approach might focus on helping carers to identify the meaning attributed to the non-motor symptoms and provide opportunities for modifying any dysfunctional thoughts associated with their perceptions of the psychological symptoms. Cognitive-behavioural therapy (CBT) might thus prove useful in providing a promising way of helping to modify the negative consequences of primary appraisals of symptoms made in the context of care-giving in PD. There is some preliminary evidence to suggest that CBT may be useful in reducing depression in the carers of people with PD (Secker and Brown 2005), and the results of the present study provide a rationale for targeting areas of dysfunctional thinking for modification.

The study also provides potentially useful information for developing guidelines for interventions with carers of people with PD. The overriding importance of carers' perceptions of psychological symptoms in the care recipients to determining care-giving strain indicates a useful starting point for planning interventions, which might focus on the apparent tendency of carers to over-generalise and thereby overestimate the occurrence of cognitive dysfunction in their spouses. The question of over-generalisation in this respect is of course somewhat controversial, as there is a sense in which carers' perceptions are, for those carers involved, the only "real" perceptions in the care-giving situation. However, it is always at the extremes of any distribution, in this case, in the way in which these perceptions serve to form care-giving attitudes, that problems arise. And so a failure to understand the needs of the patient (low levels of perception of psychological symptoms on the part of carers) may result in neglect, whilst an over-sensitivity (exacerbated perceptions) might generate an over-protective attitude, an unwillingness to share aspects of care with other family members or institutions, and over engagement to the point where the strain of caring becomes intolerable.

Alternatively, incorrect perceptions or their inappropriate interpretation may give rise to personalisation of the meaning attributed to specific behaviours, and generate feelings of heightened anxiety, anger or rejection. Thus, as already suggested, carers might benefit from educational interventions to help them recognise and understand the symptoms of PD, with particular focus on the non-motor manifestations of the disorder. It might be particularly useful to explore the meanings that they attribute to certain symptoms, in order to comprehend why these attributions have such weighty consequences for care-giving strain. This understanding should then generate possibilities for helping carers to modify the distortions in their perception of psychological symptoms.

In conclusion, the study provided important findings to inform the design of intervention strategies to reduce carer strain and influence the provision of better support services. In particular it highlighted the need to focus more on understanding the way in which carers may perceive the care recipient's symptoms and disabilities, so that appropriately focused educational and therapeutic strategies may be developed to minimise the strain of caring. This would appear to be particularly important as the results of the study suggest, that carer perceptions are more important than patient or clinician ratings of potential care-giving stressors, in contributing to both the strain and consequent depression with which they have to contend.

12.9 Final conclusions

The aim of the research described in this book was to adopt a clinical neuropsychological approach to examining (primarily) the non-motor symptoms of PD and their effects for care-giving. This presented a task of considerable complexity, requiring an analysis of the neuropsychiatric and neuropsychological presentation of the condition, in order to identify areas of controversy or issues that have been relatively unexplored, and yet have potentially significant implications for care-giving. From the start, it was apparent that the affective disorder in PD was one of the most important considerations in this respect.

Previous research co-authored by the investigator was among the first studies to demonstrate that depression in PD was paramount in determining poor mental health outcomes for carers (Miller et al. 1996). This provided the inspiration for the present study, but before undertaking a more comprehensive analysis of how the psychological symptoms of PD, and in particular depression, influence care-giving, it was deemed necessary to clarify several questions concerning the presentation of depression in PD. These were addressed in stage I of the study.

In the first instance, a new research instrument, the ADQ, for the measurement of affective symptoms in PD was designed, which accounted for overlap between motor and depressive symptoms and allowed specific hypotheses about the nature of the depressive disorder in PD to be tested. Its psychometric properties were established as being satisfactory. The ADQ was then used, together with other standardised instruments recommended for use in PD, to examine various questions regarding the depression of PD. Although it was not a primary aim of the study, confirmation was obtained for the picture that has emerged from the literature in recent years, suggesting that around 50% of patients with PD are affected by depression, but that in the main, the depression is of a type characterised by milder symptoms than in MDD (Reijnders et al. 2008; Starkstein et al. 2011). This figure is considerably higher than for age-matched, healthy, older people and represents a distinctly increased risk for depression in people with PD.

Although several studies have claimed that the profile of depressive symptoms in PD differs from that in depressed patients without PD (see chapter 3, section 3.5.4), the conclusion from the present study was that this is due to the confounding effects of depression severity. When depressed patients with PD were matched for severity of symptoms with patients diagnosed as having MDD, no significant differences in symptom profile could be identified. A similar result was obtained when equivalent matching was achieved for milder levels of depression between PD and non-PD groups. It was concluded that the alleged differences in symptom profile cannot be attributed to qualitative differences, and merely reflect quantitative differences in depression. The only exception to this appears to be that patients with PD are more consistent in their responses, than those with MDD, possibly reflecting fewer problems with decision-making.

The question of the relationship between the main symptom domains of PD, physical, neuropsychiatric and neurocognitive, is one that has been insufficiently explored and yet is vital to a better understanding of PD as a neuropsychiatric (or neuropsychological) disorder. It also has implications for determining the origins of these symptoms in PD. This question was addressed in stage II of the study. It was concluded that the symptoms are independent of one another, and it is argued that this position is reinforced by the fact that it was reached on the basis of multivariate statistical methods, which can account for collinearity in the data. This formed the basis of an argument in favour of a theoretical position which views the affective and cognitive symptoms of PD primarily as an inherent part of the disorder and contends that they are likely to share a common underlying biological substrate as part of the disease process. This is not to say that motor, affective and cognitive dysfunctions are the result of disturbances to the same brain regions (which clearly they are not), but to endorse the view that they are likely to arise from a common underlying pathology. A critical feature of this theoretical position is that it rejects the reactive view of depression in PD, along with the possibility that cognitive deficits may be consequent upon the affective disorder, as a form of "pseudo-dementia". Equally, it is not keeping with the notion of concurrent co-morbidities in the form of "endogenous" depression or DAT. Nevertheless, it is recognised that depression is a risk factor for cognitive impairment in PD, although the neurobiological basis for each may be different (Marder et al. 1995; Poletti et al. 2012), but still the result of a common pathological process.

An attempt to identify sub-groups of patients characterised by constellations of affective and motor symptoms proved unsuccessful, but a distinction between patients with younger versus older onset of symptoms and impaired cognition was found, in keeping with previous reports in the literature (van Rooden et al. 2010). However, these groups did not follow the pattern previously reported: younger patients were shown to be more cognitively impaired, but this may have been an iatrogenic effect associated with anticholinergic medication.

Finally, in stage III the effects of the three main symptom domains of PD for care-giving were investigated, in a study design that also included an analysis of carer-related variables. The aim was to determine how different aspects of the care-giving process might influence the strain and psychological well-being of spouse carers of people with PD. A variety of instruments were used in order to provide a comprehensive range of measures reflecting aspects of care-giving, identified from the literature as being central elements of the process. A path model of care-giving was derived, which attempted to capture the complexities of the process and took into account factors that appeared to mediate relationships between key variables. Among those of particular interest were carer perceptions of the psychological functioning of the care recipient and the extent to which these may have mediated the relationship between primary stressors in the form of illness variables and care-giving strain. Additionally, the carer's satisfaction with the marital relationship with the care recipient was evaluated as a mediator of the relationship between strain and psychological morbidity in the carer. Finally, the mediating properties of strain itself were considered, as a means of helping to clarify the concept of care-giving strain in relation to measures of psychological morbidity for the carer.

Carer outcomes were measured in terms of the physical and mental health of the carer. It was found that about one-third of carers were suffering from clinically significant levels of depressive symptoms. Only 5% had a previous psychiatric history and so on the grounds of parsimony, it was concluded that the most likely cause lay in their current life situation, reflected in the sustained hardship of providing care for their spouse with PD. Carers in the present study were not found to have higher rates of physical ill-health, despite evidence from previous studies of both dementia and PD care-giving that carers are more prone to poorer health and even mortality (Hooker et al. 1998; Schulz and Beach 1999).

The results of the study add to the emerging consensus, that the risk of developing symptoms of depression, which in some cases reach clinical significance, as a consequence of caring for a spouse with PD, appears to be primarily related to the non-motor symptoms of the condition, in particular, to the depression of PD. Carer depression was related to care recipient depression both directly and indirectly, through care-giving strain and marital satisfaction. Carers whose spouses were depressed, reported higher levels of care-giving strain and lower levels of marital satisfaction, which in turn had repercussions for the carer in terms of increased psychological morbidity. However, there seem to be junctures in the process of care-giving, where carer appraisals of the situation appear to have a deciding role for the way in which the process may evolve, affecting their psychological well-being.

Before turning to these appraisals however, a critical juncture – indeed one which appears to represent a pivotal point in the care-giving process – will be considered. This is the stage at which the carer's subjective feelings of strain or burden in relation to carrying out care-giving tasks and meeting other demands of the care-giving situation are conceptualised as accumulating. An unresolved question in care-giving research relates to why carers, experiencing apparently similar levels of strain or burden, show such wide variations in their psychological reactions. As is evident from this and other studies, the majority, in fact, cope well and do not seem to experience exceptional difficulties. However, not so much in spite of this, but rather because of it, it seemed particularly important to reach an understanding of the circumstances under which a significant proportion of carers (about one-third) had reached a stage, where their mental health had been seriously compromised. Hence a major focus of the present study was directed towards gaining a better understanding of care-giving strain and its relationship to carer outcomes.

The final path diagram for the care-giving process in PD, showing the relationships between patient and carer variables is presented in figure 12-4. The findings make it possible to attempt to answer the questions raised in stage III of the study.

As can be seen from figure 12-4, care-giving strain itself is determined by both patient and carer-related variables. The former, primary stressors include motor and affective symptoms, as well as illness duration, and the latter involve marital satisfaction and the carer's perceptions of depression and cognitive dysfunction in the care recipient. A large proportion (65%) of the variance in carer strain is explained by these variables. The study failed to demonstrate any consequences of cognitive dysfunction for care-giving and although this is a common finding in the dementia care literature (e.g. Mahoney et al. 2005), it is at variance with two previous studies in PD that have investigated this question (Thommessen et al. 2002; Shin, Youn et al. 2012). This may reflect differences in the measures used or more likely, the selection criteria for the present study, which were intended to screen out patients with PD dementia. Therefore, it should not be concluded that cognitive decline in the care recipient does not have significant effects for caring for someone with PD.

PD is still diagnosed on the basis of the presentation of the motor symptoms and estimates of illness duration are most likely to reflect this. However, patients often remain independent for some considerable time following initial diagnosis, so the duration of illness may not be an indicator of the length of time for which the carer has been involved in physical care-giving duties, but may reflect the duration of non-motor symptoms (especially depression), which may even precede the diagnosis, and it is contended, are particularly harmful to carer well-being. Thus motor and affective symptoms, together with illness duration appear to have a direct effect in shaping care-giving strain. This is not surprising, in view of the focus of strain measures on the specific conditions of care-giving. Apart from these primary, illness-related stressors (Pearlin et al 1990), it was also evident that carer variables may influence strain. One of these was the appraisal of the illness-related symptoms by the carer, as mentioned above. The influence of subjective judgements on the evolution of strain has been recognised in the theoretical model underpinning the majority of research in this area, which was derived from the stress and coping framework originally formulated by Lazarus and Folkman (1984) and adapted for care-giving by Pearlin et al. (1990). In accordance with these conceptualisations, the key to understanding the effects of stressors (illness variables) on the carer's well-being, together with the individual differences that are observed in carer outcomes, is the notion of cognitive appraisal. This refers to the carer's perceptions of various aspects of the care-giving situation. Adaptations to the stress process model of care-giving have taken account of this subjectivity, treating care-giving strain or burden as a secondary appraisal variable (Lawton et al. 1991; Chappell and Reid 2002). Primary appraisal refers to the carer's response to the demands of the care-giving situation, in terms of the kind of tasks that are undertaken as part of caring and the time devoted to them, whilst secondary appraisal relates to the carer's consequent experience of hardship and psychological strain.

The majority of previous studies, most of them in dementia-care, have investigated the carer's perceptions of care-giving with respect to secondary appraisals (i.e. care-giving strain). They have also improved the sophistication of the analysis by including factors considered to affect appraisal, such as the personality characteristics of the carer (Hooker et al. 1998) and the resources and vulnerabilities of the carer in the form of gender, education, individual coping strategies, attitudinal style, social support and the relationship with the carer recipient (e.g. Aneshensel et al. 1995; Lyons et al. 2009; see chapter 7). The present study provided empirical support for the equal importance of secondary appraisals in care-giving in PD, highlighting care-giving strain and its potential for modification, as representing a critical factor in determining outcomes.

Far less attention has been focused on primary appraisals, except in the context of allegedly more "objective" measures, such as time spent on caring tasks. These of course, are not really objective, as they are not determined by care recipient needs *per se,* but by the carer's perception of them. They therefore show large individual differences and are not well correlated with direct measures of illness-related symptoms. It is likely that primary appraisals mainly reflect aspects of physical care, because it is difficult to quantify caring activities related to more psychological symptoms, such as engagement with the care recipient in order to reduce his/her anxiety or encouraging him/her to become involved in activities. In the context of spousal care-giving this is even more difficult to disentangle from "non-caring" activities. Thus, even if a measure of this sort were to be used for assessing carer's appraisals of psychological symptoms, it would, most likely be a poor and non-specific indicator.

Figure 12-4. Path diagram based on regression analyses to predict carer depression in the stress process model of care-giving in PD.

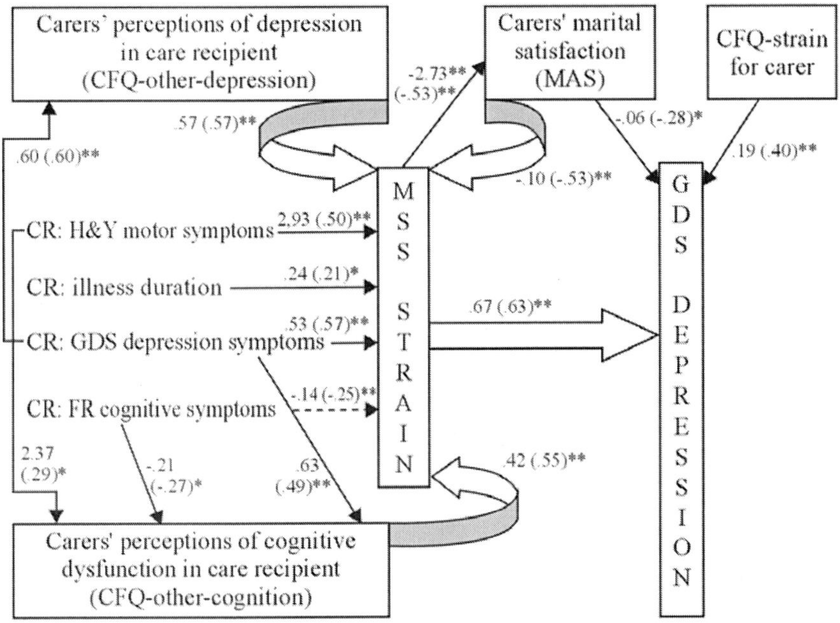

Unstandardised coefficients (B) and standardised betas (in parentheses) are shown. Thick arrows show the relationships that are demonstrated as being most important, when the effects of mediation are taken into account. The broken line indicates that the relationship between CR cognitive symptoms is present in univariate analysis, but not for multiple regression.

Perhaps because of these difficulties, as far as could be ascertained, the investigation of carer appraisals has not hitherto specifically focused on the effects of primary appraisals of non-motor or non-physical symptoms for care-giving. In view of the importance of non-motor symptoms, in particular depression, to shaping carer outcomes, this is an oversight long in need of rectification. An instrument designed to obtain carers' proxy ratings of patients' psychological symptoms was used in this study to gain a measure of their primary appraisal of these symptoms. These appraisals were seen as potentially mediating the effects of the illness-related symptoms on care-giving strain.

Carer perceptions of the psychological symptoms in the patient were found to have substantial consequences for care-giving strain, increasing the impact of the illness-related symptoms in comparison to both patient and clinician rated assessments. The carer's perceptions of depressive symptoms were better predictors of care-giving strain than the direct influence of patient depression, the effect of their recognising these symptoms being, as might be expected, to increase care-giving strain. The carer's perceptions of cognitive dysfunction in the patient had even wider implications. Difficulties arising in all three domains of PD symptomatology, motor, affective and cognitive were affected by the carer's appraisals in this regard. These indirect effects served to increase the subjective feelings of care-giving strain. Thus it seems, that it is not the symptoms themselves or the functional impairments to which they lead, that give rise to greater engagement in care-giving tasks, and the consequent subjective overload for the carer, but the carer's *interpretation* of these symptoms and disabilities.

This is a significant finding that does not appear to have been reported previously. It helps to provide an explanation for the long-established findings in the literature which have frequently been unable to demonstrate associations between various forms of carer outcomes and direct measures of physical deterioration in care recipients (see chapter 7). Previous studies have also shown that the non-motor symptoms in PD are more important in contributing to the mental ill-health of carers (e.g. Aarsland, Larsen, Karlsen et al. 1999; Carter et al. 2008; Happe and Berger 2002; Leiknes et al. 2010; Meara et al. 1999; Miller et al. 1996). The present study takes this research one step further, by demonstrating that it is the carer's awareness of the deterioration of his/her spouse in the area of psychological functioning that proves to be particularly damaging in terms of the strain and subsequent psychological morbidity that s/he suffers.

Without further research, explanations for the singular impact of psychological symptoms on carer outcomes can only be speculative. It seems likely that psychological changes have the greatest impact in causing carers to despair that their spouse is no longer "the person that s/he used to be". This means that the losses incurred in the wake of neurodegenerative illnesses such as PD are exceptionally heavy, because of their toll on intimate relationships. But a more fundamental question is: what causes carers' judgements of the psychological changes in their spouses to be excessively negatively biased, especially with regard to poorer cognitive function, as found in this study? One reason may be poor specificity on the part of carers in recognising symptoms, causing them to overestimate levels of cognitive dysfunction. This tendency may be exacerbated as a result of their close emotional ties with the care recipient and empathy for his/her condition, which cause them to fear the worst. An explanation of this kind would be in keeping with carers' observed tendency to underestimate the quality of life of those they care for, in relation to the care recipient's own evaluations (Martinez-Martin et al. 2004), especially in areas of psychological functioning. Another reason may be heightened apprehension, resulting from greater awareness of dementia and its consequences, which in recent years has been highlighted by the media and systematic campaigns by patients' and carers' organisations. These intensified efforts to draw attention to the needs of people with neurodegenerative illnesses and their carers are of unquestionable importance in providing education, support and stimulating the provision of improved services. However, it may be that campaigns designed to inform, while alerting carers' sensitivity to the possibility of cognitive impairment in PD, also engender excessive or unrealistic fears, driven by their perceptions of the intractable and relentless progression of such disorders. In addition, carers who are depressed themselves, may have an increased tendency to focus on the threat of negative outcomes for the care recipient. These possibilities provide directions for further studies. They also suggest that interventions might usefully be targeted at identifying carers who may be unduly concerned about the psychological changes affecting their spouses, in particular with regard to their cognitive limitations. There might also be benefit in designing educational programmes and therapeutic interventions to modify the unfavourable biases in carers' perceptions, giving rise to dysfunctional thinking concerning their spouse's cognitive abilities and the inevitability of decline in this area.

In view of these findings, carers' limitations in providing proxy judgements of cognitive impairment in the care recipient should be recognised. However, their sensitivity in this area should alert clinicians to the possibility that they may be suffering levels of care-giving strain that may be detrimental to their mental health and possibly signal the need for formal neuropsychological assessment of the care recipient. On the other hand, carers should be recognised as providing more accurate judgements of depression in their spouses and because of the importance of affective disorders to the quality of life of both parties (Miller et al. 1996; Schrag 2006; Schrag, Hovris et al. 2006), this emphasises the need for their being involved in consultations concerning the assessment of the person for whom they provide care (clause 9 of the draft Care and Support Bill 2012).

Care-giving strain was found to be the single most important indicator of carer outcomes in the form of depression, replicating a finding that is well established in the dementia care literature (Chappell and Reid 2002). Additional factors contributing to depression in carers included, carer age, younger carers experiencing more severe symptoms, lower levels of marital satisfaction and carer appraisals of cognitive dysfunction in the care recipient. These additional factors were differentially associated with the various instruments used to measure depression and indicate the utility of this approach to ensuring that as much variance as possible is captured in the data. In this model of care-giving, accommodating both care recipient and carer variables, primary stressors in the form of motor, affective and cognitive symptoms, are seen as leading indirectly to carer depression through care-giving strain. This characterisation of strain as a mediating variable between PD-illness-related variables and carer depressive outcomes, means that as a result of its subjective qualities arising out of carer appraisals, strain has the ability to modify the effects of the primary stressors. A mechanism by which this occurs is through the carer's perceptions of the psychological symptoms of PD, as described.

The analyses revealed that care-giving strain does indeed have the properties of a mediating variable. In the case of patient depressive symptoms, strain is a strong mediator, enhancing their effects on carer depression. For motor and cognitive symptoms it appears to act as a suppressor, eliminating the direct effect of these variables on carer depression. This confirms the impression, that although carers may report considerable strain as a result of their care-giving obligations, this does not necessarily translate into a direct risk for depression. It also provides an explanation for the individual differences observed in carer responses to ostensibly similar situations. For example, whilst PD mobility problems may restrict the couples' lifestyle and cause additional burdens in the form of providing assistance with the activities of daily living for the carer, which are reported in studies of this kind as contributing to the strain of care-giving, carers appear to be able to take these in their stride (at least up to a certain point). A similar suppressive pattern is seen with the cognitive deficits associated with PD, even though their direct effect on care-giving strain was questionable, but evident via carer perceptions. Care-giving strain therefore seems to exacerbate the symptoms of patient-depression, making it more likely that the carer will become depressed. On the other hand, it ameliorates the effects of motor and cognitive symptoms on carer depression.

At first sight, these findings may appear somewhat discrepant. Although there is no difficulty with the notion that feelings of strain in the carer may act as a prism or lens, intensifying the negative effects of care recipient depression, and leading to a deterioration in their own mental health, it is more difficult to envisage how they may act as a filter with regard to motor and cognitive symptoms. The problem arises because of the common conceptualisation of strain as an entirely negative entity, and so it is likely to be, when its intensity exceeds a critical threshold. This appears to be the situation as regards care recipient depression. With regard to motor and cognitive symptoms however, the critical threshold for strain to become unduly burdensome is presumably not reached and although the symptoms may still contribute to strain, these effects are suppressed. Care-giving strain then, appears to act as a relay station, to use a common metaphor, boosting the effect of some signals, whilst attenuating others. The effects are likely to partially cancel each other out, and thus to mask global scores on strain measures. However, attempting to disaggregate them in this way reveals the complex processes underlying care-giving. An interpretation of this kind is in keeping with the findings of the factor analysis, demonstrating that strain is likely to be a multidimensional concept.

The question then arises as to how care-giving strain is exerting its mediating role. It may do so, simply in accordance with the putative filtering mechanism with respect to certain symptoms, whilst others are magnified, as outlined above. However it is still necessary to explain how these mechanisms come about. An obvious possibility is that additional factors are acting on the relationship between strain and carer depression, mediating the outcome. Marital satisfaction for the carer appeared partially to fulfil the role of a mediator, but other models of the relationship among these variables were equally plausible; although care-giving strain did have negative effects for marital satisfaction, the reverse effect was considerably stronger. Thus whilst in a small number of cases, the effects of care-giving may have caused resentment in carers, diminishing their levels of relationship satisfaction, in the main, the opposite of this was evident, marital satisfaction having a strong buffering effect on care-giving strain. The mediating qualities of marital satisfaction also help to explain why care-giving strain does not inevitably lead to poor carer outcomes. The carer's positive feelings for the patient may help to "neutralise" feelings of subjective strain in relation to care-giving duties resulting from motor and cognitive disabilities. This may not be as readily achieved with regard to the patient's depressive symptoms. A high proportion of the effect of patient depressive symptoms on carer depression was mediated by care-giving strain, suggesting that carers found affective changes in the care recipient particularly difficult to cope with, and were more likely to become depressed themselves as a result. Affective changes are more likely to have damaging effects for the quality of the present relationship with the carer and to reinforce his/her feelings of isolation and alienation. As a result of being depressed the patient may withdraw from family and friends and previous activities, which in turn may diminish sources of social support for the carer. It is acknowledged that similar changes may occur with severe cognitive decline, but these are unlikely to have been evident in the present study because of the selection criteria for patients, which most likely served to eliminate those with severe forms of cognitive impairment. Thus rather than the buffering effect seen in the case of motor and cognitive symptoms, depressive symptoms, either directly, or by increasing care-giving strain, which in turn decreased marital satisfaction, elicited a mediation effect that amplified the effect of care-giving strain on carer depression. This explanation is reinforced by the observation that neither motor, nor cognitive symptoms, had any effect on marital satisfaction.

None of the care recipient variables representing the domains of motor, affective and cognitive functioning were found to have a direct effect on carer outcome in the form of depression, confirming the impression from previous research, that the ill-effects of care-giving may have more to do with the characteristics of carers, than those they help to look after (Hooker et al. 1998; Lyons et al. 2009). Choosing to use clinician assessments of depression in the patient as opposed to patient self-reported measures did not significantly alter the results in this respect. The main predictor of carer depression is care-giving strain, a subjective measure, which showed a positive relationship with carer depression such that higher levels of strain were associated with greater depression in the carer.

In this and other research (e.g. Chwalisz 1996) carers adjustment to their role has been shown to be influenced by their subjective (secondary) appraisal of the task as onerous and personally distressing. Indeed the greater susceptibility of some carers to suffer higher levels of emotional strain appears to be unconnected to any objective definition of caring commitments (Hooker et al. 1992). Rather, personality characteristics of the carer (Hooker et al. 1998), attitudinal variables, such as an optimistic as opposed to pessimistic outlook (Lyons et al. 2009) and coping strategies (Chwalisz 1996) have been found to differentiate among those carers who fare well and those who do not. These individual and personal qualities are seen as providing a protective effect in a situation that is inherently stressful.

What then of those carers who are more vulnerable to the stressors of care-giving? Are they to be regarded as lacking the qualities mentioned, which allegedly provide a buffer against the hardships of care-giving? It is important to guard against overly simplistic interpretations, and this one carries the additional danger of adding to the difficulties already faced by carers, by suggesting that they are not doing enough to cope. On the contrary, the results of the present study suggest that carers may be worn down partly because of their greater sensitivity to the psychological symptoms they recognise in their spouses. These perceptions then drive a sequence of further appraisals, which determine the outcome of the care-giving process. But it is carers' awareness of the changes in their spouses affective and cognitive mental state, and their consequent concern, that may provide an important starting-point in the cascade of subsequent events that constitute the process of care-giving.

One final point needs to be made regarding the choice of outcome measures in care-giving research. The results of the present study add further support to the theoretical distinction between care-giving strain or burden and more general outcomes for carers, as for example, in the form of depression. Although related, these are nonetheless separate concepts, as evidenced by the fact that they are affected by different factors in the course of care-giving. Specifically, carer appraisals of psychological symptoms in the care recipient are strongly associated with care-giving strain, but not with carer depression. On the other hand, the carer's perception of the quality of the relationship with the care recipient is related to both strain and depression. Previous studies of care-giving in dementia have found that other mediators show the reverse pattern; social support, for example, seems to be related to carers' quality of life, but not to burden (Chappell and Reid 2002; Yates et al. 1999). Moreover, because care-giving strain is a broader concept than depression, but as has been shown, is strongly related to it, it is important to further understanding of how this secondary appraisal mechanism is contributing to carer depression. The present study has provided some clarification, in highlighting the importance of carer perceptions, especially of the psychological symptoms of PD, to this construct, but it has also emphasised it multidimensional nature. The term therefore needs to be used carefully and not interchangeably with other, more generic concepts, to describe care-giving outcomes. Indeed, the definition of strain should move towards differentiating its different aspects in relation to specific care-giving domains. This was recommended by Poulshock and Deimling in 1984, but has not found reflection in the literature, especially that of care-giving in PD. Thus while care-giving strain remains a useful construct in the evaluation of the care-giving process, it continues to require greater clarification. For so long as the meaning of this measure remains relatively obscure and it is not possible to use to identify carers at risk of psychological ill-health, its utility as an outcome measure is limited. It is recommended that it is more appropriately viewed as a mediator in the care-giving process.

Carer depression has distinct advantages over the notion of care-giving strain as a measure of carer outcome, because of its established clinical validity. However, no more than 50% of the variance in this measure could be explained in the present study. This is perhaps not surprising in a more generic measure of outcome, but emphasises the need for greater precision in accounting for carer depression. Two points are of relevance here. The first is, that ideally, for the purposes of clinical intervention in care-giving situations, it would be helpful to have reliable risk indicators for depression, so that preventative action could be taken to help carers, rather than only being able to identify them, once they had crossed a clinical threshold for depressive illness. The second point is a more general one, namely that outcome indicators, should be tailored to the purposes for which they are to be used. Hence for more general purposes, it would be helpful to know what is meant by "high" levels of strain, but in clinical situations greater specificity is required.

Finally, it is worth addressing the usefulness of other more generic measures, sometimes used for the purposes of assessing outcomes in care-giving research, two of which were used in the present study. Although marital satisfaction for the carer, has sometimes been treated as an outcome variable (see chapter 7), only a small proportion (7%) of the variance in this measure was accounted for in the study by patient depression and just 25%, by the effects of care-giving strain. Neither patient nor carer variables, on the other hand, were adequate predictors of the more generalised measure of carer strain in the form of the CFQ. It is concluded therefore that neither of these measures are satisfactory indices of care-giving outcomes.

It is in the nature of a study of the kind described in this book that it should build on previous research in related areas and aim to further understanding in the designated field. It is hoped that the work reported here realizes these principles of scientific enquiry at least to a modest degree. If the results were to contribute even in a small way to advancing knowledge upon which future policies for care-giving might be structured, this would constitute a tribute to those patients and their carers who, despite the demands of PD, were willing to participate in the study and share their experiences, demonstrating a generosity and fortitude that will remain with the author, as a reminder of the very human face of living with a long-term neurodegenerative condition.

APPENDIX A

Legislation Affecting Carers in the UK

The first legislation in the UK to recognize carers was enacted in 1986 and since then, there have been successive moves to take account of the needs (and rights) of carers through the introduction of legally recognized measures, which are summarized below.

Disabled Persons (Services, Consultation & Representation) Act 1986

Section 8 of this Act (Department of Health (DOH) 1986) required that during an assessment of a disabled person the ability of carers who 'provide a substantial amount of care on a regular basis' should be taken into account. However, this was more a reflection of the provisions of the Act to check that the disabled person had appropriate care, than concern with meeting the needs of carers themselves. Nevertheless, the term "carer" to describe people providing informal care for family members had entered the statute books.

The Carers (Recognition and Services) Act 1995

The recognition of carers was strengthened further in legislation under the terms of the Carers (Recognition and Services) Act (DOH 1995) which gave carers important new rights and a clear legal status. It was "the first piece of legislation to recognize fully the role of carers within community care law" (Tinker et al. 1999); the Act made provision for carers involved in substantial levels of care on a regular basis to receive an assessment of their ability to care and to continue caring, independently of the needs of the care recipient. Local authorities who are responsible for the provision of care services in the U.K., were required to take into account the results of this assessment in the process of making decisions about the type and level of community care services to be provided to the older or disabled care recipient. However a drawback of this legislation was that it placed no obligations on the local authorities, to provide services to carers following an assessment of their needs.

The Carers and Disabled Children Act 2000

The Carers and Disabled Children Act (DOH 2000) corrected the deficiencies in previous legislation by giving local authorities mandatory duties to supply services directly to carers. Carers were eligible to request an assessment and to receive services, regardless of whether the care recipient was willing to be assessed or not. The delivery of services could be focused on meeting the needs of the carer or the older/disabled person and the Act empowered local authorities to make direct payments to carers. The Act also delivered greater flexibility in service provisions by addressing one of the central needs of carers – that of having access to respite care. A short break voucher scheme was introduced in order to facilitate carers in taking a brief respite from caring.

The National Strategy for Carers 1999

A further initiative came in the form of the National Strategy for Carers (DOH 1999) which outlined three key approaches for interventions to assist carers: provision of information, support and care. One of the most important unmet needs of carers addressed in the strategy under the section on "care for carers" was recognized as being the need for breaks from caring duties. This initiative was supported by a new Carers Special Grant with funding of £140 million for England initially over a three-year period reserved for the specific purpose of providing breaks and direct services to carers to support them in their caring role. In 2008 the carer's strategy was revised and included an additional £150 million, specifically for the purpose of accommodating breaks for carers. The grant was subsequently renewed on a regular basis and by 2010/11 the funding had been increased to £256 million. Following a general election in the UK in 2010, the coalition government pledged a further £400 million over four years in support of respite for carers as part of its "Vision for adult social care" (Arksey and Glendinning 2012).

The Carers (Equal Opportunities) Act 2004

This Act introduced three modifications to the existing law concerning the availability of services for carers. Firstly, it strengthened the initiative to make carer assessments available by requiring local authorities to inform carers of their right to a needs assessment. Secondly, it required local authorities to take into account carers' commitments and wishes regarding work, education, training and leisure activities. Thirdly, its aim was to assist co-operation between different authorities providing services to carers (DOH 2004b).

The Work and Families Act 2006

Although mainly concerned with childcare arrangements, this Act extended the right to request flexible working hours to employees who care for adults (Department of Trade and Industry 2006).

Carers at the Heart of 21st Century Families and Communities 2008

This was intended to be a ten year vision for carers and became known as the "Carers' Strategy". It set out a wide range of commitments including: the provision of information and advice; a provision for facilitating breaks for carers; improved support from the NHS; and support to help carers in managing their work and care duties. The strategy also pledged that: "Carers will be supported so that they are not forced into financial hardship by their caring role" (H.M. Government 2008:83). However the funding of benefits for carers was not addressed and only identified as a long-term priority from 2011 onwards.

The legislation described in the next section evolved out of the Carers' Strategy, although it was never enacted. The strategy was not entirely abandoned however, although wider consultations were sought regarding the enactment of proposals to support carers.

The Personal Care at Home Act 2010

This Act (DOH 2010) was introduced to Parliament on November 25th 2009 and received Royal Assent on April 8th 2010 but its implementation was never commenced owing to a general election in the U.K. which brought about a change of government and new policy directions. It was to be the first stage in a three-step process towards establishing a national care service which, broadly speaking, had received cross-party support and was considered likely to be enacted, if in a modified way, after the election. A controversial feature of the Act's provisions was the intention to introduce free personal care for people with high levels of need. It was estimated that the legislation would initially have benefitted an estimated 280,000 people who either paid for care privately or were charged by councils for the care provided. The intention was to improve the equity of access to free care across England and Wales. Each stage of the legislation steering the process of creating a national care service was to widen the provision of care, the second stage providing for free personal care to those living in residential homes after two years and in the third stage free personal care for all was to be available by 2015 with the introduction of a compulsory comprehensive insurance scheme. Under the legislation, people entering the care system were to be given access to a "re-ablement" programme for a period of six weeks in order that their need for care might be reduced or obviated and that they might remain independent. A further 130,000 people, it was estimated might benefit from these plans. Part of the funding (approximately two-thirds £420m) for the implementation of these initiatives was to come from the National Health Service and the remainder (£250m) was to be provided by local authorities through efficiency savings. Opponents of the Act argued that the proposals were not affordable and would place too heavy a burden on local authorities and working-age people (The Guardian 2010).

Recognised, valued and supported: next steps for the Carers' Strategy 2010

The new Coalition Government published this policy document in which the actions that it intended to take over the next four years to support its priorities in ensuring the best possible outcomes for carers and those they support were identified. These included:

- supporting those with caring responsibilities to identify themselves as carers at an early stage, recognising the value of their contribution and involving them from the outset both in designing local care provision and in planning individual care packages
- enabling those with caring responsibilities to fulfil their educational and employment potential
- personalised support both for carers and those they support, enabling them to have a family and community life
- supporting carers to remain mentally and physically well
- enabling carers to have a life outside of caring (H.M. Government 2010)

Vision for adult social care 2010

The proposed legislation for a creating a national care service was ultimately abandoned and superseded by new plans for care reforms presented by the government in November 2010 under the title of "A vision for adult social care" (DOH 2010b).

The new proposals were guided by a number of principles which included the greater personalization of services to older and disabled people and their carers. This was to be achieved, in part, through the introduction of "personal budgets" for all those in need of care by 2013. Personal budgets were introduced in 1996, but only 13% of those estimated as needing one, were in fact receiving one. The aim of the government was to accelerate the pace with which personal budgets were allocated, preferably as direct payments to those in need. Personal budgets were intended to be a way of making better use of resources by giving people more flexibility in terms of choice and control over the social services they received. Where appropriate, carers were to have the management of these budgets so that they were no longer in the position of having to accept (or reject) the standardised services offered to them by the local authority, but would be able to select services tailored to meet their assessed eligible care needs and agreed outcomes, in line with a personalized support plan. This presented somewhat of a challenge to the existing day care services offered by local authorities as the funding could be used to design and purchase support from a range of service providers, including public, private and other sectors, increasing peoples' autonomy over decisions regarding their care and support. The intention was to stimulate a greater diversity of service provisions with a broad market of high-quality service providers and thus to address the plurality of peoples' needs. Services were required to provide safeguards against the risk of abuse and neglect of vulnerable people in the community.

The long evident demand for respite from caring responsibilities was recognized in these proposals in so far as the intention was that personal budgets should enable carers to take regular breaks in order to rest or pursue their own activities, whilst at the same time ensuring that the care-recipient was guaranteed continuity of care in his/her own home. As mentioned above, a further £400 million was made available through the NHS over the following four years to support carers' breaks. There was some concern from carers' support groups that this funding had not been ring-fenced and thus might not, as in the past, actually reach carers and would be used for purposes other than those for which it is intended (eg. Princess Royal Trust for Carers). Indeed, there are claims that this is the case (Neary 2012).

The principle of personalisation, through giving individuals control of their care and autonomy in decision-making, brought about an important change in the philosophy guiding the delivery of care to people in need. It heralded a shift in emphasis from the state to the individual, both in terms of the responsibility for care and with regard to the provision of essential services:

> The vision sets out a new direction for adult social care, putting people, personalised services and outcomes centre stage and returning social care to its foundations of reciprocity and constructive action by individuals on behalf of the whole community.
> (Burstow 2010).

This new agenda for adult social care places the responsibility for care squarely on the shoulders of the family, friends and neighbours and the local community, in keeping with the flagship policy idea of the 2010 UK Conservative Party general election manifesto referred to as the "Big Society" and forms part of the legislative programme of the Conservative – Liberal Democrat Coalition Agreement (H.M. Government 2010a). It greatly diminishes the role of the state in the provision of care and support services, which are to be delivered in partnership between individuals, communities, the voluntary sector, the NHS and local authorities. A further aim of the plans is one of prevention, namely taking action in local communities to keep people independent and helping to build the "Big Society". It is also intended that the greater local accountability implicit in these plans will drive improvements and innovations to intensify the production and availability of high-quality care and support services. Quality outcomes are to be monitored and the information published in order to ensure full accountability and transparency of the services offered.

The plans published as "A vision for social care" were the first stage of a consultation process which included a report from the Law Commission (2010) and the independent Commission on the Funding of Care and Support (2011) chaired by Andrew Dilnot which presented its recommendations to the government in the report, "Fairer Care Funding", and were intended to guide the development of the White Paper that would give rise to future legislation in 2012. A clear message emerging from the consultation procedure was that the existing legislation for residential and community care, adult protection and support for carers was "inadequate, often incomprehensible and outdated" (Law Commission 2012). There was widespread agreement that the present law, based on an accumulation of statutes enacted over a period of 60 years was both confusing and led to conflicting interpretations. Furthermore, Dilnot (2011) described the funding of the care system as ".... confusing, unfair and unsustainable .... [it] is not fit for purpose and needs urgent and lasting reform".

This indictment of the present system of care appears to be consensual with the government declaring its support, in principle, for the proposed reforms. The real issue however, is one of political priorities, as Henwood (2012) has pointed out. Without dedicating funding to a new model of social care there can be no progress, but the scale of the problem is so vast, that successive governments have failed to deal effectively with the problem of long-term care. Care provision is an issue that is likely to affect every citizen living in the U.K.: nearly 90% of women and 70% of men are currently estimated to need care in retirement and the number of older people needing support services is expected to continue rising (H.M. Government 2010b). It is thus likely that most people will have family members or friends in need of care and support. Sustaining services at adequate levels to meet the anticipated needs requires a fundamental review of the ways in which they are to be delivered. This message is carried in the government's proposals:

> We can draw on a work force who can provide care and support with skill, compassion and imagination, and who are given the freedom and support to do so. We need the whole work force, including care workers, nurses, occupational therapists, physiotherapists and social workers, alongside carers and the people who use services, to lead the changes set out in the vision.
> (Burstow 2010)

Caring for our future: progress report on funding reform 2012

Following the publication of the report by the Commission on the Funding of Care and Support (2011) the government held consultations with service users, family carers, formal care organizations and local authorities in order to ascertain their views on the Commission's recommendations. The main findings were published in the form of a progress report (DOH 2012a) which concurred with the recommendations of the Commission that:

- an upper limit should be fixed for the amount that individuals would be expected to pay for their care
- people should not have to sell their homes at the time they enter formal residential care (allowing a system of deferred payments),
- the same rules governing eligibility for care and support should apply equally across the country in order to create a fairer and more coherent system of care
- there was a need for clear information to be made available to allow people to plan and prepare for their care needs

- continuity of care would be strengthened by affirming the portability of care assessments, allowing people to move more easily between local authorities
- a commitment would be made to improving the integration of adult care with other services in the wider care and support system by placing clear duties on the NHS and local authorities to co-operate in providing integrated services.
(DOH 2012a).

A number of these commitments were to be guaranteed by the Health and Social Act (2012) and the draft Care and Support Bill (2012), but the report emphasised, that whilst agreeing with the principles of the recommendations made by the Commission on the Funding of Care and Support (2011) and confirming the government's intention to base a new funding model for social care and support on them, it was unable to guarantee that changes would be made in the direction indicated given the current economic climate. Indeed, the likelihood that the proposed reforms will be shelved for some considerable time was made evident by Jeremy Hunt, the U.K. Health Secretary, who described the estimate of £1.7bn for a cap on individual liability for care costs as being "unaffordable" (Hunt 2012).

The progress report (DOH 2012a) laid out a timetable for the proposed enactment of the measures contained in the draft Care and Support Bill (2012b), which includes pre-legislative scrutiny of the proposed Bill and further consultations on the financial arrangements, establishing a working group to provide the public with adequate information to help them plan for their care needs and publication of an integration framework providing guidance on how modernisation of the NHS (through the measures taken in the Health and Social Act 2012) might improve older peoples' experience of moving between health and social care agencies. These actions were to be completed in the second half of 2012. The Care and Support Bill is to be introduced in 2013 while consultations continue on the deferred payments scheme for residential care, and is to be followed by a spending review in order to make decisions on the capped cost model and extended means test threshold against other priorities for government spending. 2015 is seen as the year in which the deferred payments scheme might be introduced along with national eligibility criteria for care and support. However there is considerable disappointment among the charitable support organisations such as Parkinson's U.K. (2012) which have emphasised that whilst they welcome the proposed changes, reforms to the care system are urgently needed and service users and their carers are unable to wait for their implementation. The concern is that there are no provisions in the draft Bill for the funding reforms and that as these are only to be considered in 2013 as part of a comprehensive spending review, there can be no guarantee that they will be delivered.

Draft Care and Support Bill 2012

One of the main aims of the draft Care and Support Bill (DOH 2012b) is to introduce modern legislation on adult care by consolidating the existing provisions and proposing a new structure for regulations and guidance issued under the new act. This guidance will form a single code of practice to replace the confusing and sometimes contradictory mass of guidelines currently in effect, which are drawn on statutes enacted over the last 60 years. The Bill accommodates most of the recommendations of the Law Commission (2010), including a commitment to extend and increase the rights of carers along with proposals for how this should be implemented. The following provisions are proposed:

- A general duty to promote the wellbeing of service users (including carers) will become the underlying principle used as a basis for interpreting the rest of the legislation (clause 1);
- Local authorities will have a duty to "establish and maintain a service for providing people with information and advice relating to care and support for adults and carers" (clause 2);
- A new duty to promote diversity and quality in the provision of services (clause 3);
- A duty to promote co-operation between partners in the provision of care arrangements (clause 4-6);
- A duty on local authorities to provide services that help prevent or delay the needs for care and support (clause 7);
- There will be a new national framework for eligibility for care and support - the White Paper accompanying the draft Bill (DOH 2012c) also promises a new (extended) minimum threshold for eligibility by 2015 although this is not in the draft Bill (clause 13);People who do not meet eligibility criteria will still have rights to advice and information;
- The entitlement will be portable if users and carers move to another area, with local authorities required to maintain services at the pre-existing level (clause 31);
- A new right for carers to be consulted on the assessment of the adult in need of care (clause 9);

- The right to an assessment will be extended to all carers (currently only those with "substantial caring responsibilities" have this entitlement) and give carers a clear entitlement to support for their own wellbeing (clause 10);
- The needs assessment should include an assessment of the whole family (clause 12);
- Charging for carers' services is optional but local authorities have the power to impose charges for meeting carers' needs for support (clause 14 and 15);
- A new duty to meet carers' needs for support (clause 19)
- A duty to consult and involve carers in care and support plans: they are entitled to be involved in their preparation and to receive a copy of the plan (clause 24)
- A new entitlement to a personal budget and the right to request direct payments which can be paid to the carer or the adult needing care (clause 25 and 28);
- Legislation to safeguard adults at risk of abuse, giving local Adult Safeguarding Boards statutory authority (clauses 34-38).
- Additional resources will be transferred from the NHS to local government: £100 million in 2013/14 and £200 million in 2014/15 to help better integrate care and support. 10 per cent of this will be used to meet reform implementation costs.
  (Local Government Association 2012; Age UK 2012; Carers Trust 2012).

A Care and Support Transformation Board and Care and Support Implementation Board will oversee the reforms.

Benefits currently available to people with Parkinson's disease and their carers.

Invalid Care Allowance was introduced in 1975 and was the first benefit specifically for carers and has remained so to the present day. In its original form it was extremely restrictive, being available only to those of working age, caring for older or disabled people. Married women caring for close relatives were excluded until a judgement of the European Court of Justice in 1986, as were people of pensionable age (Thane 2009). It was the precursor of the present-day Carers' Allowance, which is a taxable benefit intended to help those who look after a disabled person, receiving either disability living allowance or attendance allowance. Eligibility criteria involve a minimum age of 16, do not allow the carer to be in full-time education and require that s/he is available to the person receiving care for at least 35 hours a week, which excludes a great number of people who do not live in the same household as the care recipient. The allowance is means tested: carers may not earn more than £100 per week after deduction of tax, and the flat rate of £53.90 per week is reduced by the amount of other benefits, including the State pension (The National Archives 2012).

Until quite recently, people below the statutory retirement age in the UK were entitled to receive Incapacity Benefit (IB), if they could not work because of illness or disability and had made National Insurance contributions. Incapacity Benefit was originally introduced to replace Invalidity Benefit and Sickness Benefit in 1995 and was in its turn, replaced by Employment and Support Allowance (ESA) in 2008. The two benefits continue to co-exist alongside each other, to the extent that some individuals who qualified for Incapacity Benefit before the introduction of ESA have, on the basis of periodic assessments, remained eligible to receive it. At the time of writing, all Incapacity Benefit claimants are to undergo a "Work Capability Assessment" started in April 2011 and to be completed by March 2014, to establish if they continue to have a limited capacity to work. Assuming they remain incapacitated, they are to be transferred to the new benefit (Disability Alliance 2012). These benefits would only apply to younger people with PD, who may still be able to maintain restricted levels of employment.

At the time of writing there are two social security benefits available to older people with disabilities who have a need for care: these are Disability Living Allowance (DLA) and Attendance Allowance. The first of these is a non-means-tested, non-contributory benefit which can be claimed by a UK resident aged under 65 years who has care and/or mobility needs as a result of a mental or physical disability. It is not subject to taxation. The benefit is made up of two components each of which correspond to different classes of need: help with personal care and help with mobility. There are detailed rules regarding eligibility, which make its implementation extremely complex and it has recently come under review by the government in connection with the new social care proposals. The intention is to replace DLA with a new form of care provision, known as the personal independence payment (PIP). Under the new proposals, those receiving PIP will be more rigorously assessed in order to continue receiving benefits. It is estimated that the new scheme will generate savings for the government of around 20% or £2bn, from the current £12.6bn spent on provisions of this kind. Although the new assessments are intended to reduce abuses of the benefit scheme for disabled people, a great deal of controversy surrounding these measures has been generated and arguments to this effect presented to Parliament (Hames 2011). For example, there is genuine concern on the part of disabled peoples' support organizations, such as Parkinson's UK, that in view of the fluctuating nature of PD, there is the danger that the intended assessments will be prone to error unless conducted by specialists. There is also the question of whether they need to be repeated at regular intervals in the case of a degenerative condition such as PD, bearing in mind the inconvenience, anxiety and disruption they are likely to generate for predominantly older patients, who have problems with mobility.

Disabled people over the age of 65 are eligible for attendance allowance, which was introduced in 1971, with intention of providing help with the care needs of older and disabled people needing frequent attention and constant supervision at home. In 1976, it was supplemented by mobility allowance to help those with severe mobility problems.

AFTERWORD

It is a pleasure to write an afterword to Barbara Politynska's magnificent volume on Parkinson's disease (PD), in which she offers a comprehensive conceptual framework for the study of neurodegenerative disorders from a neuropsychological perspective, drawing on this knowledge to inform understanding of the care-giving process. This book is the culmination of the author's long-term interest in Parkinson's disease as a prototypical neuropsychological disorder and represents a blending of expertise in neuropsychology with clinical experience in the psychological assessment and management of neurodegenerative diseases. It is also a timely publication, helping to consolidate research in this area by recognizing that the management of Parkinson's disease requires a delicate dovetailing of knowledge of this terrible disease with an understanding of the difficulties faced by carers of people with the disorder. This process of integration could only start when PD was redefined as a condition in which the mental and neuropsychological complaints were recognized as playing a central role in both the diagnosis and management of the condition. The fact that it took many years before this was achieved can only be understood by delving into the history of PD.

James Parkinson (after whom PD was named by Charcot in 1862) defined the 'Shaking palsy' (*paralysis agitans*) as: "Involuntary tremulous motion, with lessened muscular power, in parts not in action and even when supported; with a propensity to bend the trunk forwards, and to pass from a walking to a running pace: the senses and intellects being uninjured". Coached in early 19th century medical concepts, his definition is often anachronistically understood as claiming that the shaking palsy was a pure 'neurological disease' free from mental and cognitive symptoms.

By 1800, the medical meaning of 'paralysis' was still very broad. For example, both Sauvages and Vogel defined it as a loss of both motion and sensation. Likewise, 'senses' meant 'sensory modalities' (e.g. vision or touch) and not 'reason' (as it came to mean later on). Parkinson wanted to differentiate his shaking palsy from the common garden paralysis of stroke where the 'senses' might be involved. By 'intellects', Parkinson meant cognition. His wanting to deny the presence of cognitive symptoms makes sense for at the time 'intellectual impairment' was also considered to be part and parcel of the definition of 'paralysis'. Indeed, none of the nine patients reported by Parkinson seems to have shown 'dementia'. This syndrome only began to be reported in the context of PD after the 1850s, when anti-muscarinic agents became popular in the treatment of the disease.

Until the time of Charcot, PD had been classified as a 'Neurosis' (in Cullen's sense): "*Paralysis agitans* is considered at the moment a *Névrose* in the sense that we cannot identify any characteristic lesion"; Axenfeld concurred: "PD must provisionally remain in the class of the neuroses given that it is not characterised by an identical and constant lesion". However, during this period advances in Neuropathology had started to challenge the Cullean definition of 'Neuroses'. Indeed, after the 1860s the new medical specialism of Neurology was constructed out of the accumulation of 'Neuroses' in which focal lesions had been found.

In this regard, Meynert suggested that PD might be associated with a disorder of the basal ganglia and Blocq and Marinesco reported a case of unilateral Parkinsonism caused by a tuberculous destruction of the Substantia Nigra. Based on these findings, Brissaud favoured the *Locus Niger* and Lewy went on to report 60 cases showing lesions in Striatum and Globus Pallidus and identifying the inclusion bodies that since have carried his name.

It was only towards the very end of the 19th century that personality changes, insanity, depression, and cognitive impairment began to be reported in relation to PD. The tide started in 1881, when Benjamin Ball reported three cases: one with hallucinations and two with irritability and depression. He concluded: "… a large number of Parkinsonian patients present psychological disorders extending from simple irritability to psychosis; far from being an exception I would say that a slight degree of cognitive disorganization (*perturbation intellectuelle*) is the rule." As against Ball, Bucknill (an English alienist) argued that only "statistical evidence" could substantiate his claim. Tuke dismissed Ball's cases as Kahlbaumian Catatonias exhibiting severe motor disturbance.

Reports supporting Ball's claim continued. Parant described a case with nocturnal delusions and another who complained that his extremities were much larger than normal. In a later paper, the same author suggested that a causal link (mediated by the cortex) existed between the neurological and psychological manifestations of PD. By then alienists had moved away from the conventional 'spinal theory' of PD so that they could accommodate the 'psychiatric' complaints. In regards to the status of the latter, some (e.g. Charcot, Brissaud and others) believed that the association between psychiatric symptoms and PD was artifactual; others (e.g. Ball, Parant, Régis, Luys, Roger and Bechet) were convinced that mental symptoms were part of the disease. Régis went on to distinguish between 'Elementary psychological disturbances' (mood disorder, intellectual apathy, hypersensitivity, irritability, asthenia, torpidity, lethargy, nightmares and deterioration of mental functions) and 'delusional or psychotic states' (depression with delusions of ruin, guilt, hypochondria and suicidal ideation). To these he added a third group: Dementia, confusion, oneiric states and nocturnal hallucinosis.

The neurological view of PD was popular on this side of the Channel. Gowers believed that mental symptoms were reactive and not-specific: "The intellect may be unaffected throughout, except by the irritability which usually accompanies the physical restlessness, or by mental depression, which is chiefly the natural result of the physical ailment". Years later, Kinnier Wilson was to iterate the same view: "mental symptoms are mostly limited to depression and irritability, the natural outcome, perhaps, of an incurable disease, anything beyond these is to be ascribed to accompanying arteriosclerosis or some incidental condition ... on the intellectual side there may be noted some bradyphrenia or slowness of thought yet it is probably more apparent than real." Against this reactivity view, Mjönes in 1949 found that the severity of depression was out of proportion with the neurological deficit and was unlikely to be reactive. Warburton went on to explain that the severity of the depression bore no relation to illness severity for it only occurred in vulnerable personalities.

Concerning dementia, it was only during the early 1860s that Charcot reported 'blurring of intellect and loss of memory'. This point is of some interest as it historically coincides with the early usage of anti-muscarinic agents. For the rest of the century, most writers, including neurologists, refer to intellectual weakness during the terminal stage of the illness (and one wonders how often these patients were already in delirium). No psychometric studies seem to have been carried out until after the First World War. The reason for this is not necessarily a lack of instruments or psychometric methodology for both were available by the 1910s.

Under the supervision of Guillain and Piéron, Witold Aubrun wrote a doctoral thesis in 1937 on the cognitive state of patients with PD. This work is interesting on three accounts: it is one of the earliest experimental studies of cognitive functions in PD; it makes use of standardized psychometric instruments; and it excluded from the 20 subject sample, subjects who might be suffering from 'senile dementia'. The protocol evaluated perception, state of consciousness, cognitive function, attention, remote and recent memory, orientation, praxis, mood, personality, and sleep. On the basis of the wealth of data obtained, the author concluded that patients suffering from PD were more often than not cognitively impaired.

Why did it take so long for mental disorders and dementia to be accepted as an intrinsic expression of PD? Observational bias is an obvious explanation: patients did not live for long enough to show the symptoms. A more likely explanation is theoretical expectation: it was part of the clinical canon that in the context of general medicine mental symptoms had to be interpreted first as reactive.

Since those days adequate evidence has accumulated to support the view that depression, hallucinations, obsessions, paranoid beliefs, cognitive impairment and other behavioural disturbances are part and parcel of PD, making it a quintessentially neuropsychological disorder. Dr Politynska's book offers a masterly summary of this work, showing how central the mental symptoms of PD are to the understanding of the disease and to successful management of patient and carer alike. For regardless of how well the physical symptoms are controlled, the overall management of patients with PD is difficult if they remain depressed, akathisic, irritable, hallucinating, paranoid, sleepless or obsessional.

The author's starting point is the presentation of a cogent rationale for undertaking research of the kind that is described in later sections of the book. She justifies the case for studying PD and care-giving within the context of a neuropsychological paradigm, emphasizing the fact that the intractable and progressive nature of the disease draws both patient and carer into a specific inter-dependency that may last for many years. This demands an integrated approach to the care of both the patient and his/her carer, which needs to be informed by a better understanding of the dyadic nature of the relationship between them. An important aspect of this approach is to provide both clinicians and policy-makers with an empirical foundation for the organization of services for patients and their carers, and is particularly timely for countries such as the UK, currently on the verge of implementing a major overhaul in legislation concerning care and support services for people with long-term illnesses who are cared for by relatives at home. The introduction provides a clear formulation of the problem with which the book is concerned, outlining the main goals of the research and the way in which they are to be achieved.

The three chapters that follow provide a theoretical account of the main symptom domains of PD. The first of these deals with the epidemiology and clinical presentation of the physical symptoms of the disorder, the diagnostic criteria for the idiopathic form of the disease within the broader syndrome of parkinsonism, possible aetiological factors, neuropathological mechanisms and treatment, with a particular focus on the role of dopaminergic medication. It is a concise and focused account in which the author demonstrates a good grasp of PD from the broader perspective of its basic medical aspects and sets an example of the essential need in neuropsychology for an interdisciplinary understanding of the subject matter.

The chapter on the neuropsychiatric aspects of PD is an impressive review of the mental changes that are characteristic of PD. Its primary focus is on the affective disorder in PD, for this has been the subject of serious controversies in the scientific literature over the last twenty years and more. Considerable disagreement has prevailed in relation to the prevalence, nature and origins of depression in PD. The author offers an in-depth analysis of issues concerning disparities in definitions of depression and methodological deficiencies which undoubtedly lie at the heart of these controversies, but also addresses more complex questions such as the difficulties of assessing depressive disorders in neurological populations. These include the tricky problem of "symptom overlap" which refers to the fact that PD and depressive disorders have a number of symptoms in common, resulting in difficulties in accurately attributing them to the right cause. A further unresolved and contentious issue is the claim that a different profile of depressive symptoms is typically associated with PD, leading to speculations that the affective disorder has a phenomenologically distinct presentation or even that it is merely a phenocopy of depression. Dr Politynska deals with the challenges posed by the continuing debate in these areas skilfully and with considerable scientific acumen; her discussion of the issues at stake and critical evaluation of the literature is a model for research in this area.

She also achieves a complex integration of research in the neuropsychology of PD: starting with a brief description of the historical background to work in this area, the discussion guides the reader through the forest of diverse positions adopted in order to explain the considerable heterogeneity in clinical observations relating to the cognitive impairment in PD. Here the author distinguishes herself in providing a state of the art exposition of a highly complex body of knowledge, selecting, integrating and evaluating evidence from the most up to date studies in the field.

The chapter concerning the psychosocial aspects of PD once again demonstrates a more interdisciplinary approach, examining the subjective experience of PD as a chronic illness, together with the patient and carer's adaptation to living with the ensuing disability. Key concepts are illustrated with examples from the author's clinical experience, which add considerable value to the discussion. This is followed by two chapters which provide a critical analysis of issues in care-giving, addressing in particular, the question of why, despite considerable research experience in this area, so little has been achieved in terms of developing an informed approach for helping carers, either in terms of policy decisions or beneficial interventions. Methodological issues are dealt with first, raising fundamental concerns regarding the measurement of carer outcomes; the author argues convincingly for the use of more generic measures of psychopathology, which have recognised clinical significance, whilst retaining the notion of burden or strain (the latter being her preference) as an intermediary or mediating variable in the care-giving process. This leads to an explication of theoretical models of care-giving, and how they have evolved from the basic transactional stress model. There follows a comprehensive review of factors affecting the well-being of carers ranging from background socio-economic variables to those that are specific to PD, namely the physical, affective and cognitive changes that occur in the wake of the disease process. The particular strength of the discussion lies in the fact that because far less evidence is available for PD itself, the author draws upon the wider body of research on dementia, where appropriate, pointing to differences in the effects of the two conditions in terms of care-giving. Additionally factors with potential for ameliorating (or indeed exacerbating) the harmful effects of care-giving are explored, including family and marital relationships, attachment and cultural influences, and the predisposition of carers to the task. The broad conclusion is that psychological rather than physical changes affecting the patient have greatest impact on the carer. However, there is also the troubling suggestion that care-giving difficulties may have more to do with the carer's attitudes and personality, rather than characteristics of the person with PD. These indications from the literature formed the basis of the research enquiry that is presented in later sections of the book.

The theoretical part of the book (the first seven chapters) is in itself, sufficient evidence of the author's research skills in selecting and organizing appropriate materials for analysis and her capacity for critical evaluation, thus providing unquestionable evidence of her original contribution to research in this area. Each chapter, whether it be concerned with the symptoms of PD or caring for someone with the condition maintains a focus on care-giving and ends with a succinct summary, highlighting empirical questions which are addressed in the research that follows. This lends a useful organization to the text which serves to provide the reader with a coherent background to the later empirical study.

The study itself is described with meticulous attention to the rigours of research methodology. The author provides a reasoned justification for the research with a clear definition of her hypotheses and the research questions that emerge from them. She also addresses the contentious issue of control groups and how they should be used. Here she makes the important point, that the symptom complex of PD provides the researcher with a rare internal control, dispensing with the need for control groups for each of the symptom areas, which would in fact, merely add undesirable "noise" to the data. The description of research methods, which includes the detailed methodology required for selecting items and evaluating the psychometric properties of a new scale to measure depression in PD, designed for the purposes of the research, is worthy of attention for two reasons. The first is that it serves to reflect the author's skill and mature understanding of research methodology. The second is that it confirms her sensitivity to clinical issues in the context of research: indeed the value of the book as a whole is enhanced by the fact that throughout, the author does not lose sight of implications for clinical practice.

The study is carefully planned, following a logical sequence of enquiry in order to attain the specified goal of achieving a better understanding of the conditions influencing the welfare of both the person with PD and his/her carer. The first question to be addressed relates to the unresolved dispute concerning alleged differences in symptom profile for depression in PD. Here, in taking steps to correct methodological deficiencies in previous research, the author has ensured, first of all, that PD patients and those with major depressive disorder were precisely matched for severity of depression for the purposes of comparison. Furthermore her statistical analyses, take account of the fact that the sensitivity with which a particular symptom contributes to establishing the presence of depression (its contribution to the overall score on a depression scale) may vary between groups, and so a comparison of mean scores for individual scale items is insufficient to verify potential differences. Neither of these conditions have been adequately met to date. When properly satisfied, no differences were seen in symptom presentation, suggesting that there are no qualitative differences between patients with PD and those with major depression, when severity of symptoms is controlled. This is an important result, not only because it helps to resolve a long-standing dispute in the literature, but also because it elucidates the nature of the affective disorder in PD. Having thus demonstrated that the depression of PD is not atypical in any way, the author recognizes the need to establish the relationship between the main symptom domains in the disorder. This is not merely a theoretical exercise, used to clarify arguments regarding the origins of psychological symptoms (in particular depression) in PD, but an important foundation for further stages of the investigation, demonstrating the author's awareness of more complex methodological issues. Her application of multivariate statistics demonstrates appreciation of the fact that covariance patterns are likely to arise in data from a study of this kind, which cannot be dealt with by simple correlational approaches – a problem which she identifies as continuing to cause difficulties with the interpretation of published research in this area. Indeed, the study as a whole reflects the author's excellent grasp of more complex statistical methods, including causal steps (a form of structural equation modelling) and power analyses. It is also worth drawing attention to the fact that the use of multiple groups allows a replication of the study confirming that the symptom areas of PD are relatively independent of one another, in two independent groups of patients with PD. These findings provide justification for the model of care-giving tested in stage III of the study – one in which the nature of the variables is clearly specified and mediating variables accounted for. The results confirm that the perceived strain of care-giving is the best predictor of psychological morbidity in the form of depression for the carer. Strain is however, somewhat inconsistent in mediating the care-giving pathway between the symptoms of PD and carer depression, especially as far as motor and cognitive symptoms are concerned, and it seems likely that other mediation factors, such as marital satisfaction, may come into play. Hence carers whose relationship with their partners suffering from PD is satisfying and supportive may be "protected" to some extent, against the hardships of care-giving and vice versa, those with poor mutuality experiencing greater strain. As regards patient depression, however, no buffering effect appears to occur, indicating that it is more difficult for carers to be shielded against the symptoms of depression in their spouses, causing them to experience higher levels of strain and ultimately raising the risk of their becoming depressed.

Since strain is a subjective carer variable, these results might be interpreted as adding strength to previous observations that carer characteristics are the best indicators of care-giving outcomes. However, the author takes her investigation further, drawing attention to the dangers of making an over-simplified interpretation of these findings. She goes on to probe other potential mediating effects in the form of the carer's perception of psychological symptoms in his/her spouse, which it might be argued, are key constituents of a dyadic approach to the understanding of care-giving. Carers' appraisals appear to be a crucial factor in determining care-giving strain, a finding which in itself may not be surprising, but seen in the context of there being little common ground between carers' judgements and more objective, clinical measurements, creates a new and important perspective on care-giving. The significance of these findings is noteworthy, not only from a theoretical standpoint, but also because of their clear implications for clinical practice and policy decisions. They help to provide a meaningful interpretation of several still unresolved questions in the literature such as why it is, that in ostensibly similar situations, no two carers appear to cope in the same way and the fact that carer characteristics, rather than those relating to the disability of the patient, appear to be primarily associated with care-giving outcomes. Moreover, they signal the direction for intervention procedures to develop and provide a foundation for addressing certain aspects of policy decisions.

As members of PD clinics will know only too well, fine control of the psychiatry and neuropsychology of PD is central to an integrated approach to care. In this regard, it becomes an ethical imperative to extend the treatment to the carers themselves if patient-rejection is to be prevented. For, much as the neurobiological management of the patient with PD has progressed in the last decades, what it has to offer is neither sufficient nor apposite to deal with the psychological and social consequences of the disease. That is the message of this book and one which PD experts and therapists cannot afford to forget.

Dr Politynska's book represents a comprehensive study of the neuropsychology of PD and the effects of caring for someone with the condition. The presentation of research in book-form bestows a continuity which allows a systematic approach to be taken to a complex problem, such as that raised in the present text and enables the author to plan and execute a logical, step-wise approach to the task in hand, demonstrating the quality of her analytical research skills at every stage of the work. This is a well-written text, illustrated throughout with excellent graphics and demonstrating the author's scientific scholarship. I consider that it makes a significant contribution to advances in research in this area.

Professor G E Berrios
Chair of the Epistemology of Psychiatry
Consultant Neuropsychiatrist & Head of Neuropsychiatry Department
University of Cambridge, UK
Fellow & Honorary Fellow of the Royal College of Psychiatrists
Fellow of the Academy of Medical Sciences
Fellow of the British Psychological Society

January 2013

REFERENCES

Aarsland, D., Andersen, K., Larsen, J.P., Lolk, A. & Kragh-Sorensen, P. (2003). Prevalence and characteristics of dementia in Parkinson's disease: an 8 year prospective study. *Archives of Neurology*, *60,* 387-392.

Aarsland, D., Andersen, K., Larsen, J.P., Lolk, A., Nielsen, H. & Kragh-Sorensen, P. (2001). Risk of dementia in Parkinson's disease: A community-based, prospective study. *Neurology, 56*, 730-736.

Aarsland, D., Beyer, M.K. & Kurz, M.W. (2008). Dementia in Parkinson's disease. *Current Opinion in Neurology, 21(6),* 676-682.

Aarsland, D., Bronnick, K., Ehrt, U., De Deyn, P.P., Tekin, S., Emre, M. & Cummings, J.L. (2007). Neuropsychiatric symptoms in patients with Parkinson's disease and dementia: frequency, profile and associated care giver stress. *Journal of Neurology, Neurosurgery and Psychiatry, 78,* 36-42.

Aarsland, D., Bronnick, K., Williams-Gray, C., Weintraub, D., Marder, K., Kulisevsky, J., Burn, D., Barone, P., Pagonabarraga, J., Allcock, L., Santangelo, G., Foltynie, T., Janvin, C., Larsen, J.P., Barker, R.A. & Emre, M. (2010). Mild cognitive impairment in Parkinson disease: a multicenter pooled analysis. *Neurology, 75(12),*1062-1069.

Aarsland, D. & Karlsen, K. (1999). Neuropsychiatric aspects of Parkinson's disease. *Current Psychiatry Reports,1(1),* 61-68.

Aarsland, D. & Kurz, M.W. (2010). The epidemiology of dementia associated with Parkinson's disease. *Journal of the Neurological Sciences, 289,* 18-22.

Aarsland, D., Kvaloy, J.T., Andersen, K., Larsen, J.P., Tang, M.X., Lolk, A., Kragh-Sorensen, P. & Marder, K. (2007). The effect of age of onset of PD on risk of dementia. *Journal of Neurology, 254(1),* 38-45.

Aarsland, D., Larsen, J.P., Karlsen, K., Lim, N.G. & Tandberg, E. (1999). Mental symptoms in Parkinson's disease are important contributors to caregiver distress. *International Journal of Geriatric Psychiatry,14,* 866-874.

Aarsland, D., Larsen, J.P., Tandberg, E. & Laake, K. (2000). Predictors of nursing home placement in Parkinson's disease: a population-based, prospective study. *Journal of the American Geriatrics Society. 48(8)*, 938-942.

Aarsland, D., Litvan, I., Salmon, D., Galasko, D., Wentzel-Larsen, T. & Larsen, J.P. (2003). Performance on the dementia rating scale in Parkinson's disease with dementia and dementia with Lewy bodies: comparison with progressive supranuclear palsy and Alzheimer's disease. *Journal of Neurology, Neurosurgery and Psychiatry, 74(9),*1215-1220.

Aarsland, D., Marsh, L. & Schrag, A. (2009). Neuropsychiatric symptoms in Parkinson's disease. *Movement Disorders*, *24,* 2175-2186.

Aarsland, D., Påhlhagen, S., Ballard, C.G., Ehrt, U. & Svenningsson, P. (2012). Depression in Parkinson's disease – epidemiology, mechanisms and management. *Nature Reviews Neurology*, 8, 35-47.

Aarsland, D., Perry, R., Brown, A., Larsen, J.P. and Ballard C. (2005). Neuropathology of dementia in parkinson's disease: a prospective, community based study. *Annals of Neurology, 58,* 773-776.

Aarsland, D., Tandberg, E., Larsen, J.P. & Cummings, J.L. (1996). Frequency of dementia in Parkinson's disease. *Archives of Neurology, 53,* 538-542.

Aarsland, D., Zaccai, J. & Brayne, C.A. (2005). A systematic review of prevalence studies of dementia in Parkinson's disease. *Movement Disorders, 20(10),* 1255-63.

Acitelli, L.K. & Antonucci, T.C. (1994) Gender difference in the link between marital support and satisfaction in older couples, *Journal of Personality and Social Psychology, 67*, 688-698.

Adams, K.B. (2001). Depressive symptoms, depletion or developmental change? Withdrawal, apathy and lack of vigour in the Geriatric Depression Scale. *The Gerontologist, 41*(6), 768-777.

Adler, C.H. (2009). Mild cognitive impairment in Parkinson's disease. *Parkinsonism and Related Disorders, 15S3,* S81-S82.

Afifi, A.A. and Clark, V. (1984). *Computer-Aided Multivariate Analysis.* Van Nostrand Reinhold Company.

Age UK (2012). Worth waiting for? The Draft Care and Support Bill. Retrieved: http://ageukblog.org.uk/2012/08/07/worth-waiting-for-the-draft-care-and-support-bill/

Ahlskog, J.E. (2011). Pathological behaviours provoked by dopamine agonist therapy of Parkinson's disease. *Physiology and Behaviour, 104*(1), 168-172.

Ahlskog, J.E. & Muenter, J.D. (2001). Frequency of levodopa related dyskinesias and motor fluctuations as estimated from the cumulative literature. *Movement Disorders*, *16,* 448-458.

Ainsworth, M.D.S., Blehar, M.C., Waters, E. & Wall, S. (1978). *Patterns of attachment: A psychological study of the strange situation.* New Jersey: Lawrence Erlbaum.

Albert, M.S., Butters, N. & Levin, J. (1979). Temporal gradients in the retrograde amnesia of patients with alcoholic Korsakoff's disease. *Archives of Neurology, 36,* 211-216.

Albert, M.L., Feldman, R.G. & Willis, A.L. (1974). The 'subcortical dementia' of progressive supranuclear palsy. *Journal of Neurology, Neurosurgery and Psychiatry. 37(2),*121-130.

Alexander, G.E., DeLong, M.R. & Strick, P.L. (1986). Parallel organisation of functionally segregated circuits linking basal ganglia and cortex. *Annual Review of Neurosciences, 9,* 357-381.

All Party Parliamentary Group for Parkinson's Disease. (2009). Please mind the gap: Parkinson's disease services today. Retrieved from: http://www.parkinsons.org.uk/PDF/APPG_Report_Please_Mind_the_Gap.pdf

Almberg, B., Grafström, M., & Winblad, B. (1997a). Caring for a demented elderly person - burden and burnout among caregiving relatives. *Journal of Advanced Nursing, 25*(1), 109-116.

Almberg, B., Grafström, M., & Winblad, B. (1997b). Major strain and coping strategies as reported by family members who care for aged demented relatives. *Journal of Advanced Nursing, 26*(4), 683-691.

Almberg, B., Jansson, W., Grafstrom, M. & Winblad, B. (1998). Differences between and within genders in caregiving strain: A comparison between caregivers of demented and non-caregivers of non-demented elderly people. *Journal of Advanced Nursing, 28*, 840-858.

Alves, G., Larsen, J.P., Emre, M., Wentzel-Larsen, T. & Aarsland, D. (2006). Changes in motor subtype and risk for incident dementia in Parkinson's disease. *Movement Disorders, 21(8),* 1123-1130.

Alves, G., Müller, B., Herlofson, K., HogenEsch, I., Telstad, W., Aarsland, D., Tysnes, O.B., Larsen, J.P.; Norwegian ParkWest study group. (2009). Incidence of Parkinson's disease in Norway: the Norwegian ParkWest study. *Journal of Neurology, Neurosurgery and Psychiatry, 80(8),*851-857.

Alves, G., Wentzel-Larsen, T. & Larsen, J.P. (2004). Is fatigue an independent and persistent symptom in patients with Parkinson's disease? *Neurology*, 63, 1908-1911.

American Psychiatric Association. (2000). Diagnostic and Statistical Manual of Mental Disorders, 4th Edition, Text Revision. Washington, DC: American Psychiatric Association.

Anderson, R. & Bury, M. (Eds.)(1988). *Living with chronic illness. The experience of patients and their families.* London: Unwin Hyman.

Andersson, L. & Stevens, N. (1993). Associations between early experiences with parents and well-being in old age. *Journal of Gerontology, 48B*(3), 109-116.

Androutsellis-Theotokis, A., Rueger, M.A., Park, D.M., Mkhikian, H., Korb,E., Poser, S.W. Walbridge, S., Munasinghe, J., Koretsky, A.P., Lonser, R.R. & McKay, R.D. (2009). Targeting neural precursors in the adult brain rescues injured dopamine neurons. *Proceedings of the National Academy of Sciences of the United States of America (PNAS) 106(32),* 13570-13575.

Aneshensel, C.S., Pearlin, L.I. Mullan, J.T., Zarit, S.H. & Whitlach, C.J. (1995). *Profiles in caregiving. The unexpected career.* London: Academic Press.

Ankri, J., Andrieu, S., Beaufils, B., Grand, A., & Henrard, J.C. (2005). Beyond the global score of the Zarit Burden Interview: Useful dimensions for clinicians. *International Journal of Geriatric Psychiatry, 20*(3), 254-260.

Annerstedt, L., Elmståhl, S., Ingvad, B. & Samuelsson, S.M. (2000). Family caregiving in dementia - an analysis of the caregiver's burden and the "breaking-point" when home care becomes inadequate. *Scandinavian Journal of Public Health, 28*(1), 23-31.

Arabia, G., Grossardt, B.R., Geda, Y.E., Carlin, J.M., Bower, J.H., Ahlskog, E., Maraganore, D.M. & Rocca, W.A. (2007). Increased risk of depressive and anxiety disorders in relatives of patients with Parkinson's disease. *Archives of General Psychiatry*, *64(12),* 1385-1392.

Archbold, P.G., Stewart, B.J., Greenlick, M.R. & Harvath, T.A. (1990). Mutuality and preparedness as predictors of caregiver role strain. *Research in Nursing and Health, 13*, 375-384.

Arksey, H. & Glendinning, (2012). Informal welfare. In P. Alcock, M. May & S. Wright, (Eds.) *The student's companion to social policy (pp. 234-241)* 4th Edition, Chichester, U.K.: Wiley-Blackwell.

Asada, T., Kinoshita, T., & Kakuma, T. (2000). Analysis of behavioral disturbances among community-dwelling elderly with Alzheimer disease. *Alzheimer's Disease and Associated Disorders, 14(3),* 160-167.

Ascher, E.A., Sturm, V.E., Seider, B.H., Holley, S.R., Miller, B.L. & Levenson, R.W. (2010) Relationship satisfaction and emotional language in frontotemporal dementia and Alzheimer disease patients and spousal caregivers. *Alzheimer's Disease and Associated Disorders, 24*(1), 49-55.

Ascherio, A., Chen, H., Weisskopf, M.G., O'Reilly, E., McCullough, M.L., Calle, E.E., Schwarzschild, M.A. & Thun, M.J. (2006). Pesticide exposure and risk for Parkinson's disease. *Annals of Neurology, 60(2),* 197–203.

Athey, R.J., Porter, R.W. & Walker, R.W. (2005). Cognitive assessment of a representative community population with Parkinson's disease (PD) using the Cambridge Cognitive Assessment-Revised (CAMCOG-R). *Age and Ageing, 34(3),* 268-273.

Auriacombe, S., Grossman, M., Carvell, S., Gollomp, S., Stern, M.B. & Hurtig, H.I. (1993). Verbal fluency deficits in Parkinson's disease. *Neuropsychology, 7,* 182-192.

Avanzi, M., Baratti, M., Cabrini, S., Uber, E., Brighetti, G. & Bonfa, F. (2006). Prevalence of pathological gambling in patients with Parkinson's disease. *Movement Disorders, 21,* 2068-2072.

Baddeley, A.D. (1986). *Working Memory.* New York: Oxford University Press.

Badr, H., Acitelli, L.K. & Carmack Taylor, C.I. (2007) Does couple identity mediate the stress experienced by caregiving spouses? *Psychology and Health, 22*(2): 211-229.

Baird, J.C. & Noma, E. (1978). Fundamentals of scaling and psychophysics. New York: Wiley.

Baker, C. & Stern, P.N. (1993). Finding meaning in chronic illness as the key to self-care. *Canadian Journal of Nursing Research, 25*(2), 23-36.

Baker, K.L., Robertson, N., & Connelly, D. (2010). Men caring for wives or partners with dementia: masculinity, strain and gain. *Aging and Mental Health, 14*(3), 319-327.

Baldo, J.V., Delis, D., Kramer, J. & Shimamura, A.P. (2002). Memory performance on the California Verbal Learning Test-II: findings from patients with focal frontal lesions. *Journal of the International Neuropsychological Society, 8(4),* 539-546.

Baldwin, S. & Parker, G. (1989). The Griffiths Report on Community Care. In M.Brenton & C. Ungerson. *Social Policy Review 1988-89.* London: Longman.

Ballard, C.G., Aarsland, D., McKeith, I., O'Brien, J., Gray, A., Cormack, F., Burn, D., Cassidy, T., Starfeldt, R., Larsen, J.P., Brown, R. & Tovee, M. (2002). Fluctuations in attention: PD dementia vs DLB with parkinsonism. *Neurology, 59(11),* 1714-1720.

Baltes, M.M. & Baltes, P.B. (Eds.). (1986). The psychology of control and aging. Hillsdale, N.J.:Erlbaum.

Barbeau, A. (1971). Long-term side-effects of levodopa. *Lancet, 1(7695),* 395.

—. (1973). Aging and the extrapyramidal system. *Journal of the American Geriatric Society, 21,* 145-149.

Barbeau, A., Mars, H. & Gillo-Joffroy, L. (1971). Adverse clinical side effects of levodopa therapy. *Contemporary Neurology Series, 8,* 203-237.

Barnard, D. (1990). Healing the damaged self: identity, intimacy, and meaning in the lives of the chronically ill. *Perspectives in Biology and Medicine, 33*(4):535-546.

Baron, R.M., & Kenny, D.A. (1986). The moderator-mediator variable distinction in social psychological research: conceptual, strategic, and statistical considerations. *Journal of Personality and Social Psychology, 51*(6), 1173-1182.

Barone, P., Aarsland, D., Burn, D., Emre, M., Kulisevsky, J. & Weintraub, D. (2011). Cognitive impairment in nondemented Parkinson's disease. *Movement Disorders, 26(14),* 2483-2495.

Bartholomew, K. & Horowitz, L.M. (1991). Attachment styles among young adults: a test of a four-category model. *Journal of Personality and Social Psychology, 61*, 226-244.

Barusch, A.S. & Spaid, W.M. (1989). Gender differences in caregiving: Why do wives report greater burden? *The Gerontologist, 29*, 667-676.

Bass, D.M., Noelker, L.S. & Rechlin, L.R. (1996). The moderating influence of service use on negative caregiving consequences. *Journal of Gerontology, 51B(3),* S121-S131.

Bauer, M.J., Maddox, M.K., Kirk, L.N., Burns, T. and Kuskowski, M.A. (2001) Progressive dementia: personal and relational impact on caregiving wives. *American Journal of Alzheimer's Disease and Other Dementias, 16,* 329-334.

Bauld, L., Chesterman, J., Davies, B., Judge, K. & Mangalore, R. (2000). *Caring for Older People: An Assessment of Community Care in the 1990s.* Aldershot: Ashgate.

Baumgarten, M. (1989). The health of persons giving care to the demented elderly: a critical review of the literature. *Journal of Clinical Epidemiology, 42*(12), 1137-1148.

Bayles, K.A., Trosset, M.W., Tomoeda, C.K., Montgomery, E.B. & Wilson, J. (1993). Generative naming in Parkinson's disease patients. *Journal of Clinical and Experimental Neuropsychology, 15(4),* 547-562.

Beardsley, J.V. & Puletti, F. (1971). Personality (MMPI) and cognitive (WAIS) changes after levodopa treatment. *Archives of Neurology, 25(2),* 145-150.

Beato, R., Levy, R., Pillon, B., Vidal, C., Tezenas du Montcel, S., Deweer, B., Bonnet, A.M., Houeto, J.L., Dubois, B. & Cardoso. F. (2008). Working memory in Parkinson's disease patients. *Arquivos Neuropsiquiatria, 66(2-A),* 147-151.

Beatty, W.W. (1994). Remote memory in retrospect. In L.S. Cermak (Ed.) *Neuropsychological explorations of memory and cognition: Essays in honour of Nelson Butters* (pp.215-221). New York: Plenum Press.

Beatty, W.W. & Monson, N. (1989). Lexical processing in Parkinson's disease and multiple sclerosis. *Journal of Geriatric Psychiatry and Neurology, 2,* 145-152.

Beatty, W.W., Monson, N. & Goodkin, D.E. (1989). Access to semantic memory in Parkinson's disease and multiple sclerosis. *Journal of Geriatric Psychiatry and Neurology, 2,* 22-33.

Beatty, W.W., Staton, R.D., Weir, W.S., Monson, N. & Whitaker, H.A. (1989). Cognitive disturbances in Parkinson's disease. *Journal of Geriatric Psychiatry and Neurology, 2,* 22-33.

Beats, B.C., Sahakian, B.J. & Levy, R. (1996). Cognitive performance in tests sensitive to frontal lobe dysfunction in the elderly depressed. *Psychological Medicine, 26,* 591-603.

Bebb, G.L. (1925). A study of memory deterioration in encephalitis lethargica. *Journal of Nervous and Mental Disease, 61,* 356-365.

Bech, P. (1993). The Hamilton disorders. *Psychotherapy and Psychosomatics, 60,* 113-115.

Beck, A.T., Rush, A.J., Shaw, B.F. & Emery, G. (1979). *Cognitive therapy of depression.* New York: Guilford Press.

Beck, A.T., Ward, C.H., Mendelson, M., Mock, J. & Erbaugh, J. (1961). An inventory for measuring depression. *Archives of General Psychiatry, 4,* 561-71.

Becker, C., Brobert, G.P., Johansson, S., Jick, S.S. & Meier, C.R. (2011). Risk of incident depression in patients with Parkinson disease in the U.K. *European Journal of Neurology, 18,* 448-453.

Bedard, M., Pedlar, D., Martin, N., Malott, O. & Stones, M. (2000). Burden in caregivers of cognitively impaired older adults living in the community: methodological issues and determinants. *International Psychogeriatrics, 12(3),* 307-332.

Beekman, A.T., Copeland, J.R. & Prince, M.J. (1999). Review of community prevalence of depression in later life. *British Journal of Psychiatry, 174,* 307-311.

Beeri, M.S., Werner, P., Davidson, M. & Noy, S. (2002). The cost of behavioral and psychological symptoms of dementia (BPSD) in community dwelling Alzheimer's disease patients. *International Journal of Geriatric Psychiatry,17*(5):403-408.

Benazon, N. R., & Coyne, J. C. (2000). Living with a depressed spouse. *Journal of Family Psychology*, *14*, 71-79.

Benjamin, S., Decalmer, P. & Haran, D. (1982). Community screening for mental illness: a validity study of the General Health Questionnaire. *British Journal of Psychiatry, 140*, 174-180.

Ben-Shlomo, Y. (1997). The epidemiology of Parkinson's disease. In N.P. Quinn, (Ed.), *Parkinsonism*, (pp 55-68). London, Bailliere-Tindall.

Bentin, S., Silverberg, R. & Gordon, H.W. (1981). Asymmetrical cognitive deterioration in demented and Parkinson patients. *Cortex, 17,* 533-544.

Benton, A.L., Hannay, H.J. & Varney, N.R. (1975). Visual perception of line direction in patients with unilateral brain disease. *Neurology*, *25,* 907-910.

Ben-Zeev, D., & Young, M.A. (2010). Accuracy of hospitalized depressed patients' and healthy controls' retrospective symptom reports: an experience sampling study. *Journal of Nervous and Mental Disorders, 198*(4), 280-285.

Berardelli, A., Accornero, N., Argenta, M., Meco, G. & Manfredi, M. (1986). Fast complex arm movements in Parkinson's disease. *Journal of Neurology, Neurosurgery and Psychiatry, 49,* 1146-1149.

Berg, C.A. & Upchurch, R. (2007) A developmental-contextual model of couples coping with chronic illness across the adult life span. *Psychological Bulletin, 133*(6), 920-954.

Berg, D., Merz, B., Reiners, K., Naumann, M. & Becker, G. (2005). Five-year follow-up study of hyperechogenicity of the substantia nigra in Parkinson's disease. *Movement Disorders*, *20,* 383-385.

Berg, D., Supprian, T., Hofmann, E., Zeiler, B., Jäger, A., Lange, K.W., Reiners, K., Becker, T. & Becker, G. (1999). Depression in Parkinson's disease: brainstem midline alteration on transcranial sonography and magnetic resonance imaging. *Journal of Neurology, 246(12),* 1186-1193.

Bergmann, K., Foster, E.M., Justice, A.W. & Mathews, V. (1978). Management of the demented elderly in the community. *International Journal of Psychiatry, 132,* 441-449.

Bergmann, K. & Jacoby, R. (1983). The limitations and possibilities of community care for the elderly demented. In Department of Health and

Social Services (Ed.). *Elderly people in the community: Their service needs*. London: HMSO.

Bergvall, N., Brinck, P., Eek, D., Gustavsson, A., Wimo, A., Winblad, B. & Jönsson, L. (2011). Relative importance of patient disease indicators on informal care and caregiver burden in Alzheimer's disease. *International Psychogeriatriatrics, 23*(1), 73-85.

Berrios, G.E. (1995). Parkinson's Disease (Paralysis Agitans). In G.E. Berrios & R. Porter (Eds). *A History of Clinical Psychiatry: The Origin and History of Psychiatric Disorders*. London: The Athlone Press.

Berrios, G.E., Bulbena, A., Bakshi, N., Dening, T.R., Jenaway, A., Markar, H., Martin-Santos, R. & Mitchell, S.L. (1992). Feelings of guilt in major depression. Conceptual and psychometric aspects. *British Journal of Psychiatry, 160,* 781-787.

Berrios, G.E., Campbell, C. & Politynska B. (1995). Autonomic failure, depression and anxiety in Parkinson's Disease. *British Journal of Psychiatry*, *166,* 789-792.

Berrios, G.E. & Quemada, J.I. (1990). Depressive illness in multiple sclerosis: clinical and theoretical aspects of the association. *British Journal of Psychiatry*, *156,* 10-16.

Berrios, G.E. & Samuel, C. (1987). Affective disorder in the neurological patient. *Journal of Nervous and Mental Diseases*. *175(3),* 173-176.

Beyer, M.K., Janvin, C.C., Larsen, J.P. & Aarsland, D. (2007). A magnetic resonance imaging study of patients with Parkinson's disease with mild cognitive impairment and dementia using voxel-based morphometry. *Journal of Neurology, Neurosurgery and Psychiatry, 78(3),* 254-259.

Bhidayasiri, R. & Truong, D.D. (2012). Therapeutic strategies for nonmotor symptoms in early Parkinson's disease: the case for a higher priority and stronger evidence. *Parkinsonism and Related Disorders*, *18S1,* S110-S113.

Bieliauskas, L.A. & Glantz, R.H. (1989). Depression type in Parkinson's disease. *Journal of Clinical and Experimental Neuropsychology, 11(5),* 597-604.

Billenkamp, K. (1959). Untersuchungen zur psychologie des Parkinsonismus. *Archiv für Psychiatrie und Nervenkranz, 198,* 673-686.

Birchler, G.R. & Webb, L.T. (1977). Discriminating interaction behaviors in happy and unhappy marriages. *Journal of Consulting and Clinical Psychology*, *45,* 494-495.

Birn, R.M., Kenworthy, L., Case, L., Caravella, R., Jones, T.B., Bandettini, P.A. & Martin, A. (2010). Neural systems supporting lexical search guided by letter and semantic category cues: a self-paced overt response fMRI study of verbal fluency. *Neuroimage, 49(1),* 1099-107.

Bishop M. (2005). Quality of life and psychosocial adaptation to chronic illness and acquired disability: a conceptual and theoretical synthesis. *Journal of Rehabilitation, 71(2),* 5-14.

Bjelland, I., Dahl, A.A., Haug, T.T., Neckelmann, D. (2002). The validity of the Hospital Anxiety and Depression Scale. An updated literature review. *Journal of Psychosomatic Research, 52(2),* 69-77.

Blackwell, A.D., Sahakian, B.J., Vesey, R., Semple, J.M., Robbins, T.W. & Hodges, J.R. (2004). Detecting dementia: novel neuropsychological markers of preclinical Alzheimer's disease. *Dementia and Geriatric Cognitive Disorders, 17(1-2)*, 42-48.

Blazer, D. (1989). Major depression in later life. *Hospital Practice, (Off Ed), 24(9A),* 69-76.

Bohnen, N.I., Kaufer, D.I., Hendrickson, R., Constantine, G.M., Mathis, C.A., Moore, R.Y. (2007). Cortical cholinergic denervation is associated with depressive symptoms in Parkinson's disease and parkinsonian dementia. *Journal of Neurology, Neurosurgery and Psychiatry, 78(6),* 641-643.

Boller, F. (1980). Mental status of patients with Parkinson disease. *Journal of Clinical Neuropsychology, 2(3),* 157-172.

Boller, F., Mizutani, T., Roessmann, U. & Gambetti, P. (1980). Parkinson disease, dementia and Alzheimer disease: clinicopathological correlations. *Annals of Neurology, 7,* 329-335.

Bond, M.J. & Clark, M.S. (2002). Predictors of the decision to yield care of a person with dementia. *Australasian Journal on Ageing, 21*(2), 86-91.

Bondi, M.W. & Kaszniak, A.W. (1991). Implicit and explicit memory in Alzheimer's disease and Parkinson's disease. *Journal of Clinical and Experimental Neuropsychology, 13,* 339-358.

Bondi, M.W., Kaszniak, A.W., Bayles, K.A. & Vance, K.T. (1993). Contributions of frontal system dysfunction to memory and perceptual abilities in Parkinson's disease. *Neuropsychology, 7,* 89-102.

Bondi, M.W., Salmon, D.P. & Butters, N. (1994). Neuropsychological features of memory disorders in Alzheimer's disease. In R.D. Terry, R. Katzman & K.L. Bick (Eds.) *Alzheimer's Disease* (pp. 41-63). New York: Raven Press.

Bondi, M.W. & Troster, A.I. (1997). Parkinson's disease: Neurobehavioural consequences of basal ganglia dysfunction. In P.D. Nussbaum (Ed.) *Handbook of Neuropsychology and Aging* (pp. 216-245). New York and London: Plenum Press.

Bonifati, V. (2005). Genetics of Parkinson's disease. *Minerva Medicine, 96(3),* 175-186.

Bonifati, V., Rizzu, P., van Baren, M.J., Schaap, O., Breedveld, G.J., Krieger, E., Dekker, M.C., Squitieri, F., Ibanez, P., Joosse, M., van Dongen, J.W., Vanacore, N., van Swieten, J.C., Brice, A., Meco, G., van Duijn, C.M., Oostra, B.A., & Heutink, P. (2003). Mutations in the DJ-1 gene associated with autosomal recessive early-onset parkinsonism. *Science, 299(5604),* 256-259.

Bookwala, J. & Franks, M.M. (2005) Moderating role of marital quality in older adults' depressed affect: beyond the main-effects model. *Journal of Gerontology, 60B*(2), P338-P341.

Bookwala, J. & Jacobs, J. (2004). Age, marital processes and depressed affect. *The Gerontologist,* 44(3), 328-338.

Bookwala, J., & Schulz, R. (1996). Spousal similarity in well-being: The Cardiovascular Health Study. *Psychology & Aging, 11*, 582-590.

Borek, L.L. & Friedman, J.H. (2005). Levodopa addiction in idiopathic Parkinson disease. *Neurology*, *65,* 1508.

Bosboom, J.L.W., Stoffers, D. & Wolters E.Ch. (2004). Cognitive dysfunction and dementia in Parkinson's disease. *Journal of Neural Transmission, 111,* 1303-1315.

Boss, P., Caron, W. & Horbal, J. (1988). Alzheimer's disease and ambiguous loss. In C. Chilman, E. Nunnally & F. Cox (Eds.). *Chronic Illness and Disability* (pp. 123-140). Newbury Park, CA: Sage.

Boss, P., Caron, W., Horbal, J. & Mortimer, J. (1990) Predictors of depression in caregivers of dementia patients: boundary ambiguity and mastery. *Family Process, 29,* 245-254.

Botez, M.I. & Barbeau, A. (1973). Letter: Long term mental changes in levodopa-treated patients. *Lancet, 302(7836),* 1028-1029.

Bowen, F.P. (1976). Behavioural alternations in patients with basal ganglia disorders. In M.D. Yahr (Ed.), *The Basal Ganglia*, (pp.169-177). New York: Raven Press.

Bowen, F.P., Hoehn, M.M. & Yahr, M.D. (1972). Parkinsonism: Alterations in spatial orientation as determined by a route-walking test. *Neuropsychologia, 10,* 355-361.

Bower, J.H., Maraganore, D.M., Peterson, B.J., McDonnell, S.K., Ahlskog, J.E. & Rocca, W.A. (2003). Head trauma preceding Parkinson's disease. *Neurology*, *60(10),* 1610–1615.

Bowlby, J. (1973). *Attachment and loss: Separation, anxiety and anger.* New York: Basic Books.

—. (1969/1982). *Attachment and loss:* Attachment. New York: Basic Books.

—. (1988). A secure base. New York: Basic Books.

Bowling, A. (1997). *Measuring Disease. A review of disease-specific quality of life measurement scales.* Buckingham: Open University Press.

Boyd, J.H. & Weissman, M.M. (1982). Epidemiology. In E.S. Paykel (Ed.). *Handbook of Affective Disorders* (pp.110-125). New York: Guilford Press.

Braak, H., Bohl, J.R., Muller, C.M., Rub, U., de Vos, R.A.I. & Del Tredici, K. (2006). Stanley Fahn Lecture 2005: The staging procedure for the inclusion body pathology associated with sporadic Parkinson's disease reconsidered. *Movement Disorders*, *21(12),* 2042-2051.

Braak, H., Braak, E., Yilmazer, D., de Vos, R.A., Jansen, E.N. & Bohl, J. (1996). New aspects of pathology in Parkinson's disease with concomitant incipient Alzheimer's disease. *Journal of Neural Transmission, Supplement, 48,* 1-6.

Braak, H. & Del Tredici, K. (2008). Nervous system pathology in sporadic Parkinson disease. *Neurology*, *70,* 1916-1925.

Bradburn, N.M. (1969). *The structure of psychological well-being.* Cicago: Aldine.

Brain, Lord, (1962). *Diseases of the Nervous System* (6th ed.). London: Oxford University Press.

Braithwaite, V. (1996). Between stressors and outcomes: Can we simplify caregiving process variables? *The Gerontologist, 36,* 42-53.

Brandt-Christensen, M., Lopez, A.G., Nilsson, F.M., Andersen, P.K. & Kessing, L.V. (2007). Depressive disorders and anti-parkinson drug treatment: a case register study. *Acta Psychiatrica Scandinavica,115(6),* 466-472.

Brannan, A.M. & Heflinger, C.A. (2001). Distinguishing caregiver strain from psychological distress: Modelling the relationship between child, family and caregiver variables. *Journal of Child and Family Studies, 10*(4), 405-418.

Braun, M., Mikulincer, M., Rydall, A., Walsh, A. & Rodin, G. (2007). Hidden morbidity in cancer: spouse caregivers. *Journal of Clinical Oncology, 25*(30), 4829-4834.

Braun, M., Mura, K., Peter-Wright, M. Hornung, R. & Scholz, U. (2010) Toward a better understanding of psychological well-being in dementia caregivers: the link between marital communication and depression. *Family Process, 49*(2), 185-203.

Brearley, G. & Birchley, P. (1994). *Counselling in disability and illness.* London: Mosby.

Breen, E.K. (1993). Recall and recognition memory in Parkinson's disease. *Cortex, 29,* 91-102.

Bretherton, I. & Munholland, K.A. (1999). Internal working models in attachment relationships: A construct revisited. In J. Cassidy & P.R. Shaver (Eds.), *Handbook of attachment: Theory, research and clinical implications* (pp. 89-111). New York: Guilford.

Brink, S. (2004). *Elder Care: The nexus for family, work, and health policy.* Caledon Institute of Social Policy.

Broadbent, D.E., Cooper, P.F., Fitzgerald, P. & Parkes, K.R. (1982). The cognitive failures questionnaire (CFQ) and its correlates. *British Journal of Clinical Psychology, 21,* 1-16.

Bronner, G., Royter, V., Korczyn, A.D. and Giladi, N. (2004) Sexual dysfunction in Parkinson's disease. *Journal of Sex and Marital Therapy, 30*, 95-105.

Bronnick, K. Emre, M., Lane, R., Tekin, S. & Aarsland, D. (2007). Profile of cognitive impairment in dementia associated with Parkinson's disease compared with Alzheimer's disease. *Journal of Neurology, Neurosurgery and Psychiatry,78,* 1064-1068.

Brooks, D.J. (2012). Parkinson's disease: diagnosis. *Parkinsonism and Related Disorders, 18S1,* S31-S33.

Brown, A.S. & Gershon, S. (1993). Dopamine and depression. *Journal of Neural Transmission, General Section, 91(2-3),* 75-109.

Brown, G.W. & Harris, T. (1978). *Social origins of depression. A study of psychiatric disorder in women.* London, Great Britain: Tavistock Publications Limited.

Brown, R. & Jahanshahi, M. (1995). Depression in Parkinson's disease: a psychosocial viewpoint. *Advances in Neurology, 65,* 61-84.

Brown, R.G., Jahanshahi, M., Quinn, N. & Marsden, C.D. (1990) Sexual function in patients with Parkinson's disease and their partners. *Journal of Neurology, Neurosurgery and Psychiatry, 53,* 480-486.

Brown, R.G. & Marsden, C.D. (1984). How common is dementia in Parkinson's disease? *Lancet, 2,* 1262-1265.

Brown, R.G. & Marsden, C.D. (1986). Visuospatial function in Parkinson's disease. *Brain, 109,* 987-1002.

Brown, R.G. & MacCarthy, B. (1990). Psychiatric morbidity in patients with Parkinson's disease. *Psychological Medicine, 20,* 77-87.

Brown, R.G., MacCarthy, B., Gotham, A.M., Der, G.J. & Marsden, C.D. (1988). Depression and disability in Parkinson's disease: a follow-up of 132 cases. *Psychological Medicine, 18(1),* 49-55.

Brown, G.W., & Prudo, R. (1981) Psychiatric disorder in a rural and an urban population: Aetiology of depression. *Psychological Medicine, 11*(3), 581-599.

Browne, C.J. & Shlosberg, E. (2005). Attachment behaviours and parent fixation in people with dementia: the role of cognitive functioning and pre-morbid attachment style. *Aging and Mental Health, 9*(2), 1-9.

Browne, C.J. & Shlosberg, E. (2006). Attachment theory, ageing and dementia: a review of the literature. *Aging and Mental Health, 10*(2),134-142.

Brzeziński, J. (1996). *Metodologia badań psychologicznych*. Warszawa: Wydawnictwo Naukowe, PWN. (In Polish).

Bschor, T. (2002). Masked depression: the rise and fall of a diagnosis. *Psychiatrische Praxis*. 29(4), 207-210.

Buchner, L. & Yeandle, S. (2011). *Valuing carers 2011: Calculating the value of carers' support*. London: Carers UK. Retrieved: http://www.carersuk. org/media/k2/ attachments/Valuing_carers_2011___Carers_UK.pdf

Bulbena, A. & Berrios, G.E. (1986). Pseudodementia: facts and figures. The British Journal of Psychiatry, 148, 87-94.

Bulbena, A. & Berrios, G.E. (1993). Cognitive function in the affective disorders: a prospective study. *Psychopathology, 26(1),* 6-12.

Bullock, R. (2004). The needs of the caregiver in the long-term treatment of Alzheimer disease. *Alzheimer Disease and Associated Disorders, 18* (Supplement 1), S17-23.

Buntington, L.K. & Fitzsimmons, B. (1991). Depression in Parkinson's disease. *Journal of Neuroscience Nursing, 23,* 158-164.

Burgener, S.C. & Berger, B. (2008). Measuring perceived stigma in persons with progressive neurological disease: Alzheimer's dementia and Parkinson's disease. *Dementia, 7*, 31-53.

Burn, D.J., Rowan, E.N., Allan, L.M., Molloy, S., O'Brien, J.T. & McKeith, I.G. (2006). Motor subtype and cognitive decline in Parkinson's disease, Parkinson's disease with dementia, and dementia with Lewy bodies. *Journal of Neurology, Neurosurgery and Psychiatry. 77(5)*,585-589.

Burns, A., Lawlor, B. & Craig, S., (2002). Rating scales in old age psychiatry. *British Journal of Psychiatry, 180,* 161-167.

Burns, A., Lawlor, B. & Craig, S., Eds. (2004). *Assessment scales in old age psychiatry*. London & New York: Martin Dunitz.

Burstow, P. (2010). Adult Social Care. Written Ministerial statement retrieved:

http://www.publications.parliament.uk/pa/cm201011/cmhansrd/cm101116/wmstext/101116m0001.htm.

Burton, E.J., McKeith, I.G., Burn, D.J., Williams, E.D. & O'Brien, J.T. (2004). Cerebral atrophy in Parkinson's disease with and without dementia: a comparison with Alzheimer's disease, dementia with Lewy bodies and controls. *Brain, 127,* 791-800.

Bury, M. (1982). Chronic illness as biographical disruption. *Sociology of Health and Illness, 4(2),* 167-182.

—. (1991). The sociology of chronic illness: a review of research and prospects. *Sociology of Health and Illness,13*(4), 451-468.

—. (2000). On chronic illness and disability. In C.E. Bird, P. Conrad & A.M. Fremont (Eds.). *Handbook of Medical Sociology* (5th edition). New Jersey, P.A.: Prentice Hall.

Butcher, H.K., Holkup, P.A. & Buckwalter, K.C. (2001). The experience of caring for a family member with Alzheimer's disease. *Western Journal of Nursing Research, 23*(1): 33-55.

Buytenhuijs, E.L., Berger, H.J.C., Van Spaendonck, K.P.M., Horstink, W.I.M., Borm, G.F. & Cools, A.R. (1994). Memory and learning strategies in patients with Parkinson's disease. *Neuropsychologia, 32,* 335-342.

Caap-Ahlgren, M. & Dehlin, O. (2001). Insomnia and depressive symptoms in patients with Parkinson's disease: relationship to health-related quality of life. An interview study of patients living at home. *Archives of Gerontology and Geriatrics*, *32,* 23-33.

Caap-Ahlgren, M., & Dehlin, O. (2002). Factors of importance to the caregiver burden experienced by family caregivers of Parkinson's disease patients. *Aging Clinical and Experimental Research, 14*(5), 371-377.

Calder, S.A., Ebmeier, K.P., Stewart, L., Crawford, J.R. & Besson, J.A.O. (1991). The prediction of stress in carers – the role of behavior, reported self-care and dementia in patients with idiopathic Parkinson's disease. *International Journal of Geriatric Psychiatry*, *6*(10), 737-742.

Calderon, V., & Tennstedt, S. (1998). Ethnic differences in the expression of caregiver burden: Results of a qualitative study. *Journal of Gerontological Social Work, 30,* 159-178.

Callahan, J.J. (1989). Play it again Sam – There is no impact. *The Gerontologist, 29*, 5-6.

Caltagirone, C., Carlesimo, A., Nocentini, U. & Vicari, S. (1989). Defective concept formation in Parkinsonians is independent from mental deterioration. *Journal of Neurology, Neurosurgery and Psychiatry, 52,* 334-337.

Cameron, J.I., Franche, R.L., Cheung, A.M., Stewart, D.E. (2002). Lifestyle interference and emotional distress in family caregivers of advanced cancer patients. *Cancer, 94*(2), 521-527.

Campbell, N., Boustani, M., Limbil, T., Ott, C., Fox, C., Maidment, I., Schubert, C.C., Munger, S., Fick, D., Miller, D. & Gulati, R. (2009). The cognitive impact of anticholinergics: a clinical review. *Clinical Interventions in Aging, 4,* 225-233.

Campbell, P., Wright, J., Oyebode, J., Job, D., Crome, P., Bentham, P., Jones, L. & Lendon, C. (2008). Determinants of burden in those who care for someone with dementia. *International Journal of Geriatric Psychiatry, 23*(10):1078-1085.

Cantello, R., Gilli, M., Riccio, A. & Bergamasco, B. (1986). Mood changes associated with "end of dose deterioration" in Parkinson's disease: a controlled study. *Journal of Neurology, Neurosurgery and Psychiatry*, *49,* 1182-1190.

Canter, G.J., de la Torre, R., & Mier, M. (1961). A method for evaluating disability in patients with Parkinson's disease. *Journal of Nervous and Mental Diseases, 133*, 143-147.

Cantor, M. (1983). Strain among caregivers: A study of experience in the United States. *The Gerontologist, 26,*597-604.

Carers Trust (2012). *Draft Care and Support Bill, July 2012. Briefing 2: detailed briefing clause by clause*. Retrieved from: http://www.carers.org/sites/default/files/carers_trust_briefing_2_-__draft_care_and_support_bill_detailed_briefing_clause_by_clause_3.pdf

Carnelley, K.B., Pietromonaco, P.R., & Jaffe, K. (1996). Attachment, caregiving and relationship functioning in couples: Effects of self and partner. *Personal Relationships, 3,* 257-278.

Carrafa, G.P., Schultz, C.L. & Smyrnios, K.X. (1997). Differences between Anglo-Celtic and Italian Caregivers of Dependent Elderly Persons: a Pilot Study. *Ageing and Society, 17,* 699-712.

Carpenter, B.D. (2001) Attachment bonds between adult daughters and their older mothers: associations with contemporary caregiving. *Journal of Gerontology, 56B*(5), P257-P266.

Carter, J.H., Lyons, K.S., Stewart, B.J., Archbold, P.G., & Scobee, R. (2010), Does age make a difference in caregiver strain? Comparison of young versus older caregivers in early-stage Parkinson's disease. *Movement Disorders, 25*(6), 724-730.

Carter, J.H., Stewart, B.J., Archbold, P.G., Inoue, I., Jaglin, J., Lannon, M., Rost-Ruffner, E., Tennis, M., McDermott, M.P., Amyot, D., Barter, R., Cornelius, L., Demong, C., Dobson, J., Duff, J., Erickson,

J., Gardiner, N., Gauger, L., Gray, P., Kanigan, B., Kiryluk, B., Lewis, P., Mistura, K., Malapira, T., Zoog, K., et al. (1998). Living with a person who has Parkinson's disease: the spouse's perspective by stage of disease. Parkinson's Study Group. *Movement Disorders, 13*(1), 20-28.

Carter, J.H., Stewart, B.J,, Lyons, K.S., Archbold, P.G. (2008). Do motor and nonmotor symptoms in PD patients predict caregiver strain and depression? *Movement Disorders, 23*(9), 1211-1216.

Casado, B. & Sacco, P. (2012). Correlates of caregiver burden among family caregivers of older Korean Americans. *The Journal of Gerontology, 67B(3),* 331-336.

Caslake, R., Moore, J.N., Gordon, J.C., Harris, C.E. & Counsell, C. (2008). Changes in diagnosis with follow-up in an incident cohort of patients with parkinsonism. *Journal of Neurology, Neurosurgery and Psychiatry*, *79,* 1202-1207.

Cassidy, J. (1994). Emotion regulation: influences of attachment relationships. *Monographs of the Society for Research in Child Development, 59*(2-3), 228-249.

Cassidy, J., & Shaver, P. R. (Eds). (1999). *Handbook of attachment: Theory, research, and clinical applications.* New York: Guilford Press.

Celesia, G.G. & Wanamaker, W.M. (1972). Psychiatric disturbances in Parkinson's disease. *Diseases of the Nervous System*, *33(9),* 577-583.

Cepoiu, M., McCusker, J., Cole, M.G., Sewitch, M., Belzile, E. & Ciampi, A. (2008). Recognition of depression by non-psychiatric physicians - a systematic literature review and meta-analysis. *Journal of General Internal Medicine, 23(1),* 25-36.

Ceravolo, R., Frosini, D., Rossi, C. & Bonuccelli, U. (2009). Impulse control disorders in Parkinson's disease: definition, epidemiology, risk factors, neurobiology and management. *Parkinsonism and Related Disorders*, *155,* S111-S115.

Chan, A.C.N., Ng, C.K.M., Chan, L.C.K. & Phillips, D.R. (2003).The meaning of care for older Chinese caregivers: an exploratory model of positive caring. Working Paper Series, No. 10. Asia-Pacific Institute of Ageing Studies, Lingnan University, Hong Kong. Accessed on 24th June 2012 from:
http://www.library.ln.edu.hk/eresources/etext/apws/apws_010.pdf

Chappell, N.L. (2001). Caregiving in old age. In N.J. Smelsen & P.B. Baltes (Eds.) *International encyclopedia of social and behavioural sciences* (pp. 1479-1481). Oxford, England: Pergamon Press.

Chappell, N.L. & Penning, M. (1996). Behavioural Problems and distress among caregivers of people with dementia. *Ageing and Society, 16,* 57-73.

Chappell, N.L., & Reid, R.C. (2002). Burden and well-being among caregivers: examining the distinction. *The Gerontologist, 42*(6), 772-780.

Charmaz, K. (1983). Loss of self: a fundamental form of suffering in the chronically ill. *Sociology of Health and Illness, 5(2),* 168-195.

—. (1987). Struggling for a self: Identity levels of the chronically ill. In J.Roth & P. Conrad (Eds.). *Research in the sociology of health care.* Greemwich, CT: JAI Press.

—. (1995). The body, identity and self: adapting to impairment. *Sociological Quarterly, 36,* 656-680.

—. (2006). *Constructing grounded theory. A practical guide through qualitative analysis.* London: Sage.

Chartier-Harlin, M,C., Dachsel, J.C., Vilariño-Güell, C., Lincoln, S.J., Leprêtre, F., Hulihan, M.M., Kachergus, J., Milnerwood, A.J., Tapia, L., Song, M.S., Le Rhun, E., Mutez, E., Larvor, L., Duflot, A., Vanbesien-Mailliot, C., Kreisler, A., Ross, O.A., Nishioka, K., Soto-Ortolaza, A.I., Cobb, S.A., Melrose, H.L., Behrouz, B., Keeling, B.H., Bacon, J.A., Hentati, E., Williams, L., Yanagiya, A., Sonenberg, N., Lockhart, P.J., Zubair, A.C., Uitti, R.J., Aasly, J.O., Krygowska-Wajs, A., Opala, G., Wszolek, Z.K., Frigerio, R., Maraganore, D.M., Gosal, D., Lynch, T., Hutchinson, M., Bentivoglio, A.R., Valente, E.M., Nichols, W.C., Pankratz, N., Foroud ,T., Gibson, R.A., Hentati, F., Dickson, D.W., Destée, A. & Farrer, M.J. (2011). Translation initiator EIF4G1 mutations in familial Parkinson disease. *American Journal of Human Genetics, 89(3),* 398-406.

Chattat, R., Cortesi, V., Izzicupo, F., Del Re, M.L., Sgarbi, C., Fabbo, A., & Bergonzini, E. (2011). The Italian version of the Zarit Burden Interview: a validation study. *International Psychogeriatrics, 23*(5), 797-805.

Chaudhuri, K.R. (2011). Parkinson's disease and quality of life – A clinician's perspective. *European Neurological Review, 6*(Supplement 1), 9-12.

Chaudhuri, K.R., Healy, D.G. & Schapira, A.H. (2006). Non-motor symptoms of Parkinson's disease: diagnosis and management. *Lancet Neurology, 5,* 235-245.

Chaudhuri, K.R., Prieto-Jurcynska, C., Naidu, Y., Mitra, T., Frades-Payo, B., Tluk, S., Ruessmann, A., Odin, P., Macphee, G., Stocchi, F., Ondo, W., Sethi, K., Schapira, A.H., Martinez Castrillo, J.C. & Martinez-

Martin, P. (2010). The nondeclaration of nonmotor symptoms of Parkinson's disease to health care professionals: an international study using the nonmotor symptoms questionnaire. *Movement Disorders*, *25,* 697–701.

Chaudhuri, K.R. & Schapira, A.H. (2009). Non-motor symptoms of Parkinson's disease: dopaminergic pathophysiology and treatment. *Lancet Neurology, 8(5),* 464-474.

Chen, P., Kales, H.C., Weintraub, D., Blow, F.C., Jiang, L., Ignacio, R.V. & Mellow, A.M. (2007). Depression in veterans with Parkinson's disease: frequency, co-morbidity and healthcare utilization. *International Journal of Geriatric Psychiatry*, *22(6),* 543-548.

Cheng, E.M., Tonn, S., Swain-Eng, R., Factor, S.A., Weiner, W.J., Bever, C.T. Jr; American Academy of Neurology Parkinson Disease Measure Development Panel. (2010). Quality improvement in neurology: AAN Parkinson disease quality measures: report of the Quality Measurement and Reporting Subcommittee of the American Academy of Neurology. *Neurology, 75(22),* 2021-2027.

Chia, L.G., Cheng, L.J., Chuo, L.J., Cheng, F.C. & Cu, J.S. (1995). Studies of dementia, depression, electrophysiology and cerebrospinal fluid monoamine metabolites in patients with Parkinson's disease. *Journal of Neurological Sciences,133(1-2),* 73-78.

Choi, C., Sohn, Y.H., Lee, J.H. & Kim, J.S. (2000). The effect of long-term levodopa therapy on depression level in de novo patients with Parkinson's disease. *Journal of the Neurological Sciences, 172,* 12-16.

Choonara, Y.E., Pillay, V., du Toit, L.C., Modi, G., Naidoo, D., Ndesendo V.M.K. & Sibanbo, S.R. (2009). Trends in the molecular pathogenesis and clinical therapeutics of common neurodegenerative disorders. *International Journal of Moelcular Science*, *10,* 2510-2557.

Chou, K.R. (2000). Caregiver burden: a concept analysis. *Journal of Pediatric Nursing, 15*(6), 398-407.

Chumbler, N.R., Grimm, J.W., Cody, M., & Beck, C. (2003). Gender, kinship and caregiver burden: the case of community-dwelling memory impaired seniors. *International Journal of Geriatric Psychiatry, 18*(8), 722-732.

Chwalisz, K. (1996). The perceived stress model of caregiver burden: Evidence from the spouses of persons with brain injuries. *Rehabilitation Psychology, 41,* 91-114.

Cicirelli, V.G. (1981). *Helping elderly parents: The role of adult children.* Boston: Auburn House.

Cicirelli, V. (1983). Adult children's attachment and helping behaviour to elderly parents: a path model. *Journal of Marriage and the Family, 45*, 815-822.

—. (1986) Family relationships and care/management of the dementing elderly. Chapter 5. In M.L.M. Gilhooly, S.H. Zarit & J.E. Birren (Eds.), *The Dementias: Policy Management* (pp. 93-109). Englewood Cliffs, N.J.: Prentice-Hall.

—. (1991). Attachment theory in old age: Protection of the attached figure. In K. Pillemer & K. McCartney (Eds.), *Parent-child relations throughout life* (pp. 25-42). New Jersey: Erlbaum.

—. (1993) Attachment and obligation as daughters' motives for caregiving behaviour and subsequent effect on subjective burden. *Psychology and Aging, 8*(2), 144-155.

Cifu, D.X., Carne, W., Brown, R., Pegg, P., Ong, J., Qutubuddin, A. & Baron, M.S. (2006). Caregiver distress in parkinsonism. *Journal of Rehabilitation Research and Development, 43*(4), 499-508.

Clark, L.A. & Watson, D. (1995). Constructing validity: Basic issues in objective scale development. *Psychological Assessment, 7,* 309-319.

Coen, R.F., O'Boyle, C.A., Coakley, D., & Lawlor, B.A. (2002). Individual quality of life factors distinguishing low-burden and high-burden caregivers of dementia patients. *Dementia and Geriatric Cognitive Disorders, 13*(3), 164-170.

Cohen C.A., Colantonio A. & Vernich L. (2002). Positive aspects of caregiving: rounding out the caregiver experience. *International Journal of Geriatric Psychiatry, 17,* 184-188.

Cohen, H., Bouchard, S., Scherzer, P. & Whitaker, H. (1994). Language and verbal reasoning in Parkinson's disease. *Neuropsychiatry, Neuropsychology and Behavioural Neurology, 7,* 166-175.

Cohen, J. (1992). A power primer. *Psychological Bulletin, 112(1),* 155-159.

Cohen, P.M. (1985). Family measurement techniques: Locke marital adjustment scale and the dyadic adjustment scale. *American Journal of Family Therapy, 13*(2), 66-71.

Cole, S.A., Woodard, J.L., Juncos, J.L., Kogos, J.L., Youngstrom, E.A. & Watts, R.L. (1996) Depression and disability in Parkinson's disease. *Journal of Neuropsychiatry and Clinical Neuroscience,* 8, 20-25.

Colerick, E.J. & George, L.K. (1986). Predictors of institutionalization among caregivers of patients with Alzheimer's disease. *Journal of the American Geriatrics Society, 34*, 493-498.

Collin, C., Wade, D.T., Davies, S. & Horne, V. (1988). The Barthel ADL Index: a reliability study. *International Disability Studies, (2),*61-63.

Collins Dictionary (1992). *Collins Softback English Dictionary*. Glasgow: Harper Collins Publishers.

Collins, N.L. & Feeney, B.C. (2000) A safe haven: an attachment theory perspective on support seeking and caregiving in intimate relationships. *Journal of Personality and Social Psychology, 78*(6), 1053-1073.

Collins, N.L. & Read, S.J. (1990). Adult attachment, working models and relationship quality in dating couples. *Journal of Personality and Social Psychology, 58*, 644-663.

Commission on Funding of Care and Support (2011). Fairer Care Funding: The Report of the Commission on Funding of Care and Support. Retrieved from: https://www.wp.dh.gov.uk/carecommission/files/2011/07/Fairer-Care-Funding-Report.pdf

Compta, Y., Parkkinen, L., O'Sullivan, S.S., Vandrovcova, J., Holton, J.L., Collins, C., Lashley, T., Kallis, C., Williams, D.R., de Silva, R., Lees, A.J. and Revesz, T. (2011). Lewy- and Alzheimer-type pathologies in Parkinson's disease dementia: which is more important? *Brain, 134(Pt 5),* 1493-1505.

Consedine, N.S., Magai, C., Cohen, C., & Gillespie, M. (2002). Ethnic variation in the impactof negative emotion and emotion inhibition on the health of older adults. *Journal of Gerontology, 57B,* P396-P408.

Cools, R., Barker, R.A., Sahakian, B.J. & Robbins, T.W. (2001). Enhanced or impaired cognitive function in Parkinson's disease as a function of dopaminergic medication and task demands. *Cerebral Cortex, 11,* 1136-1143.

Cools, R., Barker, R.A., Sahakian, B.J. & Robbins, T.W. (2003). L-dopa medication remediates cognitive inflexibility, but increases impulsivity in patients with Parkinson's disease. *Neuropsychologia, 41,* 1431-1441.

Cools, R. & Robbins, T.W. (2004). Chemistry of the adaptive mind. *Philosophical Transactions of the Royal Society, A, 362,* 2871-2888.

Cools, A.R., Van den Bercken, J.H.L., Horstink, M.W.I., Van Spaendonck, K.P.M. & Berger, H.J.C. (1984). Cognitive and motor shifting aptitude disorder in Parkinson's disease. *Journal of Neurology, Neurosurgery and Psychiatry, 47,* 443-453.

Cooper, C.L. (Ed.) 2005. *Handbook of stress medicine and health.* 2nd ed. London: CRC Press.

Cooper, C.L. & Dewe, P. (2004). *Stress. A brief history.*Oxford: Blackwell Publishing Ltd.

Cooper, C., Selwood, A., Blanchard, M., Walker, Z., Blizard, R., & Livingston, G. (2010). The determinants of family carers' abusive behaviour to people with dementia: results of the CARD study. *Journal of Affective Disorders, 121*(1-2), 136-142.

Cooper, J.A., Sagar, H.J., Jordan, N., Harvey, N.S. & Sullivan, E.V. (1991). Cognitive impairment in early untreated Parkinson' disease and its relationship to motor disability. *Brain, 114,* 2095-2122.

Cooper, J.A., Sagar, H.J., Tidswell, P. & Jordan, N. (1994). Slowed central processing in simple and go/no-go reaction time tasks in Parkinson's disease. *Brain, 117(3),* 517-529.

Copeland, J.R., Davidson, I.A., Dewey, M.E., Gilmore, C., Larkin, B.A., McWilliam, C., Saunders, P.A., Scott, A., Sharma, V. & Sullivan, C. (1992). Alzheimer's disease, other dementias, depression and pseudodementia: prevalence, incidence and three-year outcome in Liverpool. *British Journal of Psychiatry*, *161,* 230-239.

Cousins, R., Davies, A.D.M., Turnbull, C.J. & Playfer J.R. (2002). Assessing caregiving distress: A conceptual analysis and a brief scale. *British Journal of Clinical Psychology*, *41,* 387-403.

Crane, D.R., Allgood, S.M., Larson, J.H. & Griffin, W. (1990). Assessing marital quality with distressed and nondistressed couples: a comparison and equivalency table for three frequently used measures. *Journal of Marriage and the Family*, *52(1),* 87-93.

Crispi, E.L., Schiaffino, K. & Berman, W.H. (1997) The contribution of attachment to burden in adult children of institutionalised parents with dementia. *The Gerontologist, 37*(1), 52-60.

Critchley, M. (1929). Arteriosclerotic Parkinsonism. *Brain*, *52,* 23-83.

Cubo, E., Bernard, B., Leurgans, S. & Raman, R. (2000). Cognitive and motor function in patients with Parkinson's disease with and without depression. *Clinical Neuropharmacology*, *23(6),* 331-334.

Cummings, J.L. (1988). The dementias of Parkinson's disease: Prevalence, characteristics, neurobiology and comparison with dementia of the Alzheimer type. *European Neurology, 28(Suppl.1),* 15-23.

—. (1992). Depression and Parkinson's disease: a review. *The American Journal of Psychiatry*, 149(4), 443-454.

—. (2003). *The Neuropsychiatry of Alzheimer's Disease and Related Dementias*. London, Martin Dunitz.

Cummings, J.L. & Benson, D.F. (1984). Subcortical dementia: Review of an emerging concept. *Archives of Neurology*, 41, 874-879.

Cummings, J.L. & Benson, D.F. (1988). Psychological dysfunction accompanying subcortical dementia. *Annual Review of Medicine, 39,* 53-61.

Cummings, J.L. & Benson, D.F. (1992). *Dementia. A clinical approach* (2nd ed.) Boston: Butterworth-Heinemann.

Cummings, J.L., Darkins, A., Mendez, M., Hill, M.A. & Benson, D.F. (1988). Alzheimer's disease and Parkinson's disease: comparison of speech and language alterations. *Neurology, 38,* 680-684.

Cummings, J.L. & Masterman, D.L. (1999). Depression in patients with Parkinson's disease. *International Journal of Geriatric Psychiatry*, *14,* 711-718.

Curtin, M. & Lubkin, I. (1995). What is chronicity? In I. Lubkin (Ed). *Chronic Illness: Impact and interventions* (3rd edition). (pp. 3-25). Sudbury, M.A.: Jones and Bartlett.

Dagher, A., Owen, A.M., Boecker, H. & Brooks, D.J. (1999). Mapping the network for planning: a correlational PET activation study with the Tower of London task. *Brain, 122(10),* 1973-1987.

Dagher, A., Owen, A.M., Boecker, H. & Brooks, D.J. (2001). The role of the striatum and hippocampus in planning: a PET activation study in Parkinson's disease. *Brain, 124,* 1020-1032.

Daire, A.P. (2002) The influence of parental bonding on emotional distress in caregiving sons for a parent with dementia. *The Gerontologist, 42*(6), 766-771.

Damasio A.R. (1996). *Descartes' Error*. London: Papermac, Macmillan Publishers Ltd.

D'Amelio, M., Terruso, V., Palmeri, B., Di Benedetto, N., Famoso, G., Cottone, P., Aridon P., Ragonese, P. & Savettieri, G. (2009). Predictors of caregiver burden in partners of patients with Parkinson's disease. *Neurological Science, 30*(2), 171-174.

Davidson, P.S.R., Anaki, D., Saint-Cyr, J.A., Chow, T.W. & Moscovitch, M. (2006). Exploring the recognition memory deficit in Parkinson's disease: estimates of recollection versus familiarity. *Brain, 129,* 1768-1779.

Davie, C.A. (2008). A review of Parkinson's disease. *British Medical Bulletin*, *86,* 109-127.

Davies, A.D.M.**,** Cousins, R., Turnbull, C.J., Playfer, J.R. & Bromley, D.B. (1999). The experience of caregiving in Parkinson's disease. In R. Percival & P. Hobson, (Eds.) *Parkinson's Disease: Studies in Psychological and Social Care.* (pp. 154-198). Leicester: BPS Books.

Davila, J., Burge, D., & Hammen, C. (1997). Why does attachment style change? *Journal of Personality and Social Psychology, 73*, 826-838.

Davila, J., & Cobb, R. (2003). Predicting change in self-reported and interviewer-assessed adult attachment: Tests of the individual difference and life stress models of attachment change. *Personality and Social Psychology Bulletin, 29*, 859-870.

Davila, J., & Sargent, E. (2003). The meaning of life (events) predicts change in attachment security. *Personality and Social Psychology Bulletin, 29*, 1383-1395.

Deeken, J.F., Taylor, K.L., Mangan, P., Yabroff, K.R., & Ingham, J.M. (2003). Care for the caregivers: A review of self-report instruments developed to measure the burden, needs and quality of life of informal caregivers. *Journal of Pain and Symptom Management, 26*(4), 922-953.

De Groot, M., Anderson, R., Freedland, K.E., Clouse, R.E. & Lustman, P.J. (2001). Association of Depression and Diabetes Complications: A Meta-Analysis. *Psychosomatic Medicine*, *63,* 619-630.

Deimling, G.T. & Poulshock, S.W. (1985). The transition from family in-home care to institutional care. Focus on health and attitudinal issues as predisposing factors. *Research on Aging, 7*(4), 563-576.

Deimling, G.T., Smerglia, V.L. & Schaefer, M.L. (2001) The impact of family environment and decision-making satisfaction and caregiver depression: a path analytic model. *Journal of Aging and Health,13,* 47-71.

De Lau, L.M.L. & Breteler M.M.B. (2006). Epidemiology of Parkinson's disease. *Lancet Neurology, 5,* 525-535.

De Lau, L.M., Schipper, C.M., Hofman, A., Koudstaal, P.J. & Breteler, M.M. (2005). Prognosis of Parkinson's disease: risk of dementia and mortality: the Rotterdam Study. *Archives of Neurology, 62(8),* 1265-1269.

Della Salla, S., Di Lorenzo, G., Giordana, A. & Spinnler, H. (1986). Is there a specific visuo-spatial impairment in parkinsonians? *Journal of Neurology, Neurosurgery and Psychiatry, 49,* 1258-1265.

De Long, M.R., Georgeopoulos, A.P. & Crutcher, M.D. (1983). Cortico-basal ganglia relations and coding of motor performance. *Experimental Brain Research, 49(suppl. 7),* 30-40.

De Long, M. & Wichmann, T. (2007). Circuits and circuit disorders of the basal ganglia. *Archives of Neurology*, *64,* 20-24.

De Longis, A. & O'Brien, T. (1990). An interpersonal framework for stress and coping: An application to the family of Alzheimer's patients. In M.A.P. Stephens, J.H. Crowther, S.E. Hobfoll, & D.L. Tennenbaum (Eds.), *Stress and coping in later life families* (pp.221-240). New York: Hemisphere.

Department of Health (1986). *Disabled Persons (Services, Consultation & Representation)* ***Act.*** London: HMSO.

—. (1986). *The Carers (Recognition and Services) Act.* London: HMSO.

—. (1999). *Caring about carers: a national strategy for carers.* London: HMSO.

—. (2000). *Carers and Disabled Children Act.* London: HMSO.

—. (2004a). *Chronic disease management: A compendium of information.* London: Department of Health.

—. (2004b). *The Carers (Equal Opportunities) Act.* London: HMSO.

—. (2008). *Carers at the heart of 21st century families and communities: a caring system on your side, a life of your own.* London: Department of Health.

—. (2010a). *Recognised, valued and supported: next steps for the Carers Strategy.* London: Department of Health.

—. (2010b). *A vision for adult social care: Capable communities and active citizens.* London: Department of Health.

—. (2010c). *The Personal Care at Home Act.* London: HMSO.

—. (2012a). Caring for our future: progress report on funding reform. London: HMSO.

—. (2012b). *Draft Care and Support Bill.* London: HMSO.

—. (2012c). *Caring for our future: reforming care and support.* White Paper, London: HMSO.

Department of Trade and Industry (2006). *The Work and Families Act 2006.* London: HMSO.

De Smet, Y., Ruberg, M., Serdaru, M., Dubois, B., Lhermitte, F. & Agid, Y. (1982). Confusion, dementia and anticholinergics in Parkinson's disease. *Journal of Neurology, Neurosurgery and Psychiatry, 45,* 1161-1164.

Detweiler-Bedell, J.B., Friedman, M.A., Leventhal, H., Miller, I.W. & Leventhal, E.A. (2008). Integrating co-morbid depression and chronic physical disease management: identifying and resolving failures in self-regulation. *Clinical Psychology Review, 28(8),* 1426-1446.

Deuel, L.M., Chesire, A.M., Eason, S., Como, P.G., & Biglan, K.M. (2010). Reply: An exploration of the burden experienced by spousal caregivers of individuals with Parkinson's disease. *Movement Disorders, 25(13),* 2254-2255.

De Vugt, M.E., Riedijk, S.R., Aalten, P., Tibben, A., van Swieten, J.C., Verhey, F.R. (2006). Impact of behavioural problems on spousal caregivers: a comparison between Alzheimer's disease and frontotemporal dementia. *Dementia and Geriatric Cognitive Disorders, 22(1),* 35-41.

De Vugt, M.E., Stevens, F., Aalten, P., Lousberg, R., Jaspers, N., Winkens, I., Jolles, J., &Verhey, F.R. (2003). Behavioural disturbances in dementia patients and quality of the marital relationship. *International Journal of Geriatric Psychiatry, 18(2),* 149-154.

Dickson, D.W. & Orr, C.F. (2011). Neuropathology of dementia in Parkinson's disease. In C.W. Olanow, F. Stocchi & A. Lang (Eds.). *Parkinson's disease. Non-motor and non-dopaminergic features.* Wiley.

Diehl, M., Elnick, A.B., Bourbeau, L.S. & Labouvie-Vief, G. (1998) Adult attachment styles: their relations to family context and personality. *Journal of Personality and Social Psychology, 74*, 1656-1669.

Diener, E. & Suh, E. (1997). Measuring quality of life: economic, social and subjective indicators. *Social Indicators Research, 40,* 189-216.

Dijkers, M. (2007). "What's in a name?" The indiscriminate use of the "Quality of life" label, and the need to bring about clarity in conceptualizations. *International Journal of Nursing Studies, 44,* 153-155.

Diller, L. & Riklan, M. (1956). Psychosocial factors in Parkinson's disease. *Journal of the American Geriatrics Society, 4,* 1291-1300.

Dilnot, A. (2011). Commission on funding of care and support: Our report. Retrieved from: http://www.dilnotcommission.dh.gov.uk/our-report/.

Dilworth-Anderson, P., Williams, I.C., & Gibson, B.E. (2002). Issues of race, ethnicity, and culture in caregiving research: a 20-year review (1980-2000). *The Gerontologist, 42(2),* 237-272.

Disability Alliance (2012). Disability Alliance factsheet: incapacity benefit. www.disabilityalliance.org/fact.htm.

Dobkin, R.D., Menza, M., Allen, L.A., Gara, M.A., Mark, M.H., Tiu, J., Bienfait, K.L. & Friedman, J. (2011). Cognitive behavior therapy for depression in Parkinson's disease: a randomized controlled trial. *American Journal of Psychiatry, 168(10),* 1066-1074.

Dodd, M.L., Klos, K.J., Bower, J.H., Geda, Y.E., Josephs, K.A., Ahlskog, J.E. (2005). Pathological gambling caused by drugs used to treat Parkinson disease. *Archives of Neurology, 62(9),* 1377-1381.

Dooneief, G., Mirabello, E., Bell, K., Marder, K., Stern, Y. & Mayeux, R. (1992). An estimate of the incidence of depression in idiopathic Parkinson's disease. *Archives of Neurology*, *49,* 305-307.

Dorfman, L.T., Holmes, C.A. & Berlin, K.L. (1996). Wife caregivers of frail elderly veterans: Correlates of caregiver satisfaction and caregiver strain. *Family Relations, 45*, 46-55.

Doty, P., Jackson, M.E. & Crown, W. (1998). The impact of female caregivers' employment status on patterns of formal and informal eldercare. *The Gerontologist, 38(3),* 331-341.

Downes, J.J., Roberts, A.C., Sahakian, B.J., Evenden, J.L., Morris, R.G. &

Robbins, T.W. (1989). Impaired extra-dimensional shift performance in medicated and unmedicated Parkinson's disease: evidence for a specific attentional dysfunction. *Neuropsychologia, 27(11-12),* 1329-1343.

Downes, J.J. Sharp, H.M., Costall, B.M., Sagar, H.J. & Howe, J. (1993). Alternating fluency in Parkinson's disease: An evaluation of the attentional control theory of cognitive impairment. *Brain, 116,* 887-902.

Drachman, D.A. & Stahl, S. (1975). Letter: Extrapyramidal dementia and levodopa. *Lancet, 1(7910),* 809.

Druley, J.A., Stephens, M.A.P. & Coyne, J.C. (1997). Emotional and physical intimacy in coping with Lupus: women's dilemmas of disclosure and approach. *Health Psychology, 16*, 506-514.

Druley, J.A., Stephens, M.A.P., Martire, L.M., Ennis, N. & Wojno, W.C. (2003). Emotional congruence in older couples coping with wives' osteoarthritis: exacerbating effects of pain behaviour. *Psychology and Aging, 18*, 406-414.

Dubois, B., Danzé, F., Pillon, B., Cusimano, G., Lhermitte, F. & Agid, Y. (1987). Cholinergic-dependent cognitive deficits in Parkinson's disease. *Annals of Neurology, 22(1),* 26-30.

Dubois, B. & Pillon, B. (1997). Cognitive deficits in Parkinson's disease. *Journal of Neurology, 244,* 2-8.

Dubois, B., Pillon, B., Lhermitte, F. & Agid, Y. (1990). Cholinergic deficiency and frontal dysfunction in Parkinson's disease. *Annals of Neurology, 28,* 117-121.

Dubois, B., Ruberg, M., Javoy-Agid, F., Ploska, A. & Agid, Y. (1983). A subcortico-cortical cholinergic system is affected in Parkinson's disease. *Brain Research, 288(1-2)*, 213-218.

Dunkin, J.J., & Anderson-Hanley, C. (1998). Dementia caregiver burden: a review of the literature and guidelines for assessment and intervention. *Neurology, 51(1 Supplement 1),* S53-S60.

Dunne, F.J. (1993). Subcortical dementia. *British Medical Journal, 307,* 1-2.

Dupart, T. (2005). Attachment styles in caregivers of loved ones with Alzheimer's disease. http://proquest.umi.com/pqdlink?did=1313901771&Fmt=7&clientId=79356 &RQT=309&VName=PQD

Dura, J.A. & Haywood-Niler, E. (1990). Husbands caring for demented wives: sequelae of loss of wife as a support. *The American Journal of Alzheimer's Care and Related Disorders and Research,* 11-16.

Dura, J.R., Haywood-Niler, E. & Kiecolt-Glaser, J.K. (1990). Spousal caregivers of persons with Alzheimer's and Parkinson's disease dementia: a preliminary comparison. *The Gerontologist, 30(3),* 332-336.

Du Rocher Schudlich, T. D., Papp, L. M. & Cummings, E. M. (2011). Relations between spouses' depressive symptoms and marital conflict: a longitudinal investigation of the role of conflict resolution styles. *Journal of Family Psychology, 25*(4), 531-540.

Duxbury, L., Higgins, C. & Schroeder, B. (2009). Balancing paid work and caregiving responsibilities: a closer look at family caregivers in Canada. Retrieved from: http://www.cprn.org/documents/51061_EN.pdf

Eagles J.M., Beattie J.A.G., Blackwood G.W., Restall D.B. & Ashcroft G.W. (1987a). The mental health of elderly couples. I. The effects of a cognitively impaired spouse. *British Journal of Psychiatry, 150,* 299-303.

Eagles J.M., Walker L.G., Blackwood G.W., Beattie J.A.G. & Restall D.B. (1987b). The mental health of elderly couples. II. Concordance for psychiatric morbidity in spouses. *British Journal of Psychiatry, 150*, 303-308.

Eatough, V.M., Kempster, P.A., Stern, G.M. & Lees, A.J. (1990). Premorbid personality and idiopathic Parkinson's disease. *Advances in Neurology, 53*, 335-337.

Ebmeier, K.P., Calder, S.A., Crawford, J.R., Stewart, L., Besson, J.A.O. & Mutch, W.J. (1990). Clinical features predicting dementia in idiopathic Parkinson's disease: a follow-up study. *Neurology, 40,* 1222-1224.

Edwards, N.E., & Ruettiger, K.M. (2002). The influence of caregiver burden on patients' management of Parkinson's disease: implications for rehabilitation nursing. *Rehabilitation Nursing, 27*(5), 182-186.

Edwards, N.E. & Scheetz, P.S. (2002). Predictors of burden for caregivers of patients with Parkinson's disease. *Journal of Neuroscience Nursing, 34(4),*184-190.

Ehmann, T.S., Beninger, R.J., Gawel, M.J. & Riopelle, R.J. (1990). Depressive symptoms in Parkinson's disease: a comparison with disabled control subjects. *Journal of Geriatric Psychiatry and Neurology, 3,* 3-9.

Ehrt, U. (2009). Depression in Parkinson's Disease. Unpublished doctoral thesis, University of Bergen, Norway. https://bora.uib.no/bitstream/handle/1956/4068/Dr.thesis_Uwe%20Ehrt.pdf;jsessionid=CCD465CC527475FA5DE769936609E4D0.bora-uib_worker?sequence=1

Ehrt, U., Bronnick, K., De Deyn, P.P., Emre, M., Tekin, S., Lane, R. &

Aarsland, D. (2007). Subthreshold depression in patients with Parkinson's disease and dementia – clinical and demographic correlates. *International Journal of Geriatric Psychiatry, 22,* 980-985.

Ehrt, U., Bronnick, K., Leentjens, A.F.G., Larsen, J.P. & Aarsland, D. (2006). Depressive symptom profile in Parkinson's disease: a comparison with depression in elderly patients without Parkinson's disease. *International Journal of Geriatric Psychiatry, 21,* 252-258.

Ehrt, U., Pedersen, K.F. & Aarsland, D. (2011). Lesions associated with depression and apathy. In G.M. Halliday, R.A. Barker & D.B. Rowe (Eds.) *Non-dopamine lesions in Parkinson's disease* (pp.187-214). Oxford: Oxford University Press.

Elbaz, A., Grigoletto, F., Baldereschi, M., Breteler, M.M., Manubens-Bertran, J.M., Lopez-Pousa, S., Dartigues, J.F., Alperovitch, A., Tzourio, C. & Rocca, W.A. (1999). Familial aggregation of Parkinson's disease a population-based case control study in Europe. Europarkinson Study Group. *Neurology, 52,*1876 -1882.

Elliott, T.R. (1994). A place for theory in the study of psychological adjustment among persons with neuromuscular disorders: A reply to Livneh and Antonak. *Journal of Social Behaviour and Personality, 9,* 231-236.

Emre, M. (2003). Dementia associated with Parkinson's disease. *The Lancet Neurology, 2,* 229-237.

—. (2004). Dementia in Parkinson's disease: cause and treatment. *Current Opinion in Neurology, 17(4),* 399-404.

Emre, M., Aarsland, D., Brown, R., Burn, D.J., Duyckaerts, C., Mizuno, Y., Broe, G.A., Cummings, J., Dickson, D.W., Gauthier, S., Goldman, J., Goetz, C., Korczyn, A., Lees, A., Levy, R., Litvan, I., McKeith, I., Olanow, W., Poewe, W., Quinn, N., Sampaio, C., Tolosa, E. & Dubois, B. (2007). Clinical diagnostic criteria for dementia associated with Parkinson's disease. *Movement Disorders, 22,* 1689-1707.

Erdal, K.J. (2001). Depressive symptom patterns in patients with Parkinson's disease and other older adults. *Journal of Clinical Psychology, 57(12),*1559-1569.

Erlanger, D.M., Kutner, K.C., Barth, J.T. and Barnes, R. (1999). Neuropsychology of sports-related head injury: Dementia pugilistica to post concussion syndrome. *The Clinical Neuropsychologist, 13(2),* 193–209.

Erro, R., Picillo, M., Vitale, C., Amboni, M., Moccia, M., Longo, K., Cozzolino, A., Giordano, F., DeRosa, A., DeMichele, G., Pellecchia, M.T. and Barone, P. (2013). Non-motor symptoms in early Parkinson's disease: a 2-year follow-up study on previously untreated patients.

Journal of Neurology, Neurosurgery and Psychiatry, 84(1), 14-17.

Ertran, F.S., Ertran, T., Kizilta, G. & Uygucgil, H. (2005). Reliability and validity of the Geriatric Depression Scale in depression in Parkinson's disease. *Journal of Neurology, Neurosurgery and Psychiatry*, 76, 1445-1447.

Eskow Jaunarajs, K.L., Angoa-Perez, M., Kuhn, D.M. & Bishop, C. (2011). Potential mechanisms underlying anxiety and depression in Parkinson's disease: consequences of l-DOPA treatment. *Neuroscience and Biobehavioral Reviews, 35(3),* 556-564.

Essen-Möller, E. & Hagnell, O. (1961). The frequency and risk of depression within a rural population group in Scania. *Acta Psychiatrica Scandinavica, 162,* 28-32.

Evandrou, M. (1995). Employment and care, paid and unpaid work: the socio-economic position of informal carers in Britain. In J. Phillips (Ed.). *Working Carers*. Aldershot: Avebury.

Factor, S.A., Steenland, N.K., Higgins, D.S., Molho, E.S., Kay, D.M., Montimurro, J., Rosen, A.R., Zabetian, C.P. & Payami, H.(2011). Postural instability/gait disturbance in Parkinson's disease has distinct subtypes: an exploratory analysis. *Journal of Neurology, Neurosurgery and Psychiatry, 82(5),* 564-568.

Fahn, S. (2003). Description of Parkinson's disease as a clinical syndrome. *Annals of the New York Academy of Sciences*, *991*, 1-14.

Fahn, S. & Elton, R.L. Members of the UPDRS Development Committee. (1987). Unified Parkinson's Disease Rating Scale. In S. Fahn, C.D. Marsden & M. Goldstein (Eds.), *Recent Developments in Parkinson's Disease II,* (pp.153-163). Florham Park, N.J., Macmillan Healthcare Information.

Fahn, S. & Przedborski, S. (2005). Parkinsonism. In: L.P. Rowland (ed.), *Merritt's Neurology*, 11th edition, (pp.828-845). Philadelphia, Lippincott Williams & Wilkins.

Faircloth, C.A., Boylstein, C., Rittman, M., Young, M.E. & Gubrium, J. (2004). Sudden illness and biographical flow in narratives of stroke recovery. *Sociology of Health and Illness, 26(2),* 242-261.

Farabaugh, A.H., Locascio, J.J., Yap, L., Fava, M., Bitran, S., Sousa, J.L. & Growdon, J.H. (2011). Assessing depression and factors possibly associated with depression during the course of Parkinson's disease. *Annals of Clinical Psychiatry, 23(3),*171-177.

Farabaugh, A.H., Locascio, J.L., Yap, L., Weintraub, D., McDonald, W.M., Agoston, M., Alpert, J.E., Growdon, J. & Fava, M. (2009). Pattern of depressive symptoms in Parkinson's disease. *Psychosomatics, 50(5),* 448-454.

Farran, C.J., Keane-Hagerty, E., Salloway, S., Kupferer, S., & Wilken, C.S. (1991). Finding meaning: an alternative paradigm for Alzheimer's disease family caregivers. *The Gerontologist, 31(4),* 483-489.

Farran, C.J. & Kuhn, D.R. (1998). Finding meaning through caring for an elderly person with Alzheimer's disease: Assessment and Intervention. In P.T.P. Wong & P.S. Fry (Eds.) *Handbook of personal meaning: Theory, research and applications* (pp.335-358). Hillsdale, N.J.: Lawrence Erlbaum Associates.

Farran, C.J., Miller, B.H., Kaufman, J.E., & Davis, L. (1997). Race, finding meaning, and caregiver distress. *Journal of Aging and Health, 9(3),* 316-333.

Farran, C.J., Miller, B.H., Kaufman, J.E., Donner, E., & Fogg, L. (1999). Finding meaning through caregiving: development of an instrument for family caregivers of persons with Alzheimer's disease. *Journal of Clinical Psychology, 55(9),* 1107-1125.

Fearon, M., Donaldson, C., Burns, A. & Tarrier, N. (1998) Intimacy as a determinant of expressed emotion in caregivers of people with Alzheimer's disease. *Psychological Medicine, 28(5),* 1085–1090.

Feeney, J.A. (1996). Attachment, caregiving and marital satisfaction. *Personal Relationships, 3,* 401-416.

Feeney, B.C. & Collins, N.L. (2001) Predictors of caregiving in adult intimate relationships: an attachment theoretical perspective. *Journal of Personality and Social Psychology, 80(6),* 972-994.

Feeney, J.A., & Noller, P. (1996). *Adult Attachment.* London: Sage.

Fengler A.P. & Goodrich N. (1979). Wives of elderly disabled men: the hidden patient. *The Gerontologist, 18,* 175-183.

Fernandez, H.H. & Chen, J.J. (2007). Monoamine oxidase inhibitors: current and emerging agents for Parkinson disease. *Clinical Neuropharmacology, 30,* 150-168.

Fernandez, H.H. & Durso, R. (1998). Clozapine for dopaminergic-induced paraphilias in Parkinson's disease. *Movement Disorders,13(3),* 597-598.

Fernandez, H.H., Tabamo, R.E., David, R.R. & Friedman, J.H. (2001). Predictors of depressive symptoms among spouse caregivers in Parkinson's disease. *Movement Disorders, 16(6),* 1123-1125.

Filho, D.B., Teive, H.A.G. & Werneck, L.C. (2007). Early-onset Parkinson's disease and depression. *Arquivos Neuropsiquiatria,*65(1), 5-10.

Findley, L., Aujla, M., Bain, P.G., Baker, M., Beech, C., Bowman, C., Holmes, J., Kingdom, W.K., MacMahon, D.G., Peto, V. & Playfer, J.R. (2003). Direct economic impact of Parkinson's disease: a research survey in the United Kingdom. *Movement Disorders, 18(10),*1139-1145.

Finley, N., Roberts, M., & Banahan, B. (1988). Motivators and inhibitors of attitudes of filial obligation toward aging parents. *The Gerontologist, 28*, 73-78.

Fiori, K.L., Consedine, N.S. & Magai, C. (2009). Late life attachment in context: patterns of relating among men and women from seven ethnic groups. *Journal Cross Cultural Gerontology, 24,*121-141.

First, M.B., Spitzer, R.L., Gibbon, M., & Williams, J. B.W. (2002). *Structured Clinical Interview for DSM-IV-TR Axis I Disorders, Research Version, Patient Edition.* (SCID-I/P) New York: Biometrics Research, New York State Psychiatric Institute.

Fisher, L. & Lieberman, M.A. (1994) Alzheimer disease: the impact of the family on spouses, offspring and in-laws. *Family Process, 33*, 305-325.

Fiske, S.T., Kenny, D.A. & Taylor, S.E. (1982). Structural models for the mediation of salience effects on attribution. *Journal of Experimental Social Psychology, 18,* 105-127.

Fitting, M., Rabins, P., Lucas, J.M. & Eastham, J. (1986). Caregivers for dementia patients: a comparison of husbands and wives. *The Gerontologist, 26,* 248-252.

Flannery, R.B. (2002). Disrupted caring attachments: implications for long-term care. *American Journal of Alzheimer's Disease and Other Dementias, 17(4),* 227-231.

Fleming, A., Cook, K.F., Nelson, N.D. & Lai, E.C. (2005). Proxy reports in Parkinson's disease: caregiver and patient self-reports of quality of life and physical activity. *Movement Disorders, 20(11),* 1462-1468.

Fleming, V., Tolson, D. & Schartau, E. (2004). Changing perceptions of womanhood: living with Parkinson's disease. *International Journal of Nursing Studies, 41*, 515-524.

Flowers, K.A., Pearce, I. & Pearce, J.M.S. (1984). Recognition memory in Parkinson's disease. *Journal of Neurology, Neurosurgery and Psychiatry, 47,* 1174-1181.

Flowers, K.A. & Robertson, C. (1985). The effect of Parkinson's disease on the ability to maintain a mental set. *Journal of Neurology, Neurosurgery and Psychiatry, 48,* 517-529.

Flowers, K.A., Robertson, C. & Sheridan, M.R. (1995). Some characteristics of word fluency in Parkinson's disease. *Journal of Neurolinguistics, 9(1),* 33-46.

Folkman, S. (1997). Positive psychological states and coping with severe stress. *Social Science and Medicine, 45(8),* 1207-1221.

Folkman, S. & Lazarus, R.S. (1985). If it changes it must be a process:

Study of emotion and coping during three stages of a college examination. *Journal of Personality and Social Psychology, 48,* 150-170.

Folstein, M.S., Folstein, S.E. & McHugh, P.R. (1975). Mini-mental state. A practical method for grading the mental state of patients for the clinician. *Journal of Psychiatric Research, 12,* 189-198.

Foltynie, T., Brayne, C.E.G. & Barker, R.A. (2002). The heterogeneity of idiopathic Parkinson's disease. *Journal of Neurology, 249,* 138-145.

Foltynie, T., Brayne, C.E.G., Robbins, T.W. & Barker, R.A. (2004). The cognitive ability of an incident cohort of Parkinson's patients in the U.K. The CamPaIGN study. *Brain, 127,* 550-560.

Forno, L.S. (1996). Neuropathology of Parkinson's disease. *Journal of Neuropathology and Experimental Neurology*, *55,* 259-272.

Forrest, G. & Berg, I. (1982). Correspondence: Leeds scales and the GHQ in women who had recently lost a baby. *British Journal of Psychiatry, 141*, 429-430.

Forsaa, E.B., Larsen, J.P. Wentzel-Larsen, T. Goetz, C.G., Stebbins, G.T., Aarsland, D. & Alves, G. (2010). A 12-Year Population-Based Study of Psychosis in Parkinson Disease. *Archives of Neurology, 67(8),* 996-1001.

Forsell, Y., Jorm, A.F., Fratiglioni, L., Grut, M. & Winblad, B. (1993). Application of DSM-III-R criteria for major depressive episode to elderly subjects with and without dementia. *American Journal of Psychiatry*, *150(8),* 1199-1202.

Förstl, H. (1999). The Lewy body variant of Alzheimer's disease: clinical, pathophysiological and conceptual issues. *European Archives of Psychiatry and Clinical Neuroscience, 249, Supplement 3,* III/64-III/67.

Förstl, H. & Levy, R. (1991). F.H. Lewy on Lewy bodies, parkinsonism and dementia. *International Journal of Geriatric Psychiatry, 6,* 757-766.

Fox, M.J. (2002). *Lucky Man.* New York: Hyperion Books.

Fraley, R. C. (2002). Attachment stability from infancy to adulthood: Meta-analysis and dynamic modeling of developmental mechanisms. *Personality and Social Psychology Review*, *6*, 123-151.

Fraley, R. C., & Brumbaugh, C. C. (2004). A dynamical systems approach to understanding stability and change in attachment security. In W. S. Rholes & J. A. Simpson (Eds.), *Adult attachment : Theory, research, and clinical implications* (pp. 86-132). New York: Guilford Press.

Franco, K., Franco, J., & Alishahie, M. (2008). Marital Status. In S. Loue & M. Sajatovic (Eds.), *Encyclopedia of Aging and Public Health*, (pp.

526-528). New York: Springer Science.

Frank, R.G. & Elliott, T. (2000). Rehabilitation psychology: Hope for a psychology of chronic conditions. In R.G. Frank & T. Elliott (Eds.). *Handbook of rehabilitation psychology* (pp.3-8). Washington, D.C.: American psychological Association Press.

Frazier, L.D., Cotrell, V. & Hooker, K. (2003). Possible selves and illness: A comparison of individuals with Parkinson's disease, early-stage Alzheimer's disease, and healthy older adults. *International Journal of Behavioural Development, 27*(1), 1-11.

Frazier, P.A., Tix, A.P. & Barron, K.E. (2004). Testing moderator and mediator effects in counseling psychology research. *Journal of Counseling Psychology, 51(1)*, 115-134.

Freedman, M., Rivoira, P., Butters, N., Sax, D.S. & Feldman, R.S. (1984). Retrograde amnesia in Parkinson's disease. *Canadian Journal of Neurological Sciences, 11,* 297-301.

Freidson, E. (1970). *Profession of medicine: A study of the sociology of applied knowledge.* New York: Harper and Row.

Friedman, A. (1994). Old-onset Parkinson's disease compared with young-onset disease: clinical differences and similarities. *Acta Neurologica Scandinavica*, 89, 258-261.

—. (1999). Epidemiologa, etiopatogeneza, rozpoznawanie i leczenie choroby Parkinsona. In A. Friedman (Ed.), *Choroba Parkinsona* (pp.30-55). α-medica press, Bielsko-Biała. (In Polish).

—. (2006). Epidemiologia, rozpoznawanie i leczenie choroby Parkinsona. In T. Sobowa and J. Sławek (Eds.), *Zaburzenia poznawcze i psychiczne w chorobie Parkinsona i w innych zespołach parkinsonowskich* (pp.11-23). Wydawnictwo Continuo, Wrocław. (In Polish).

Frisina, P.G., Haroutunian, V. & Libow, L.S. (2009). The neuropathological basis for depression in Parkinson's disease. *Parkinsonism and Related Disorders, 15(2),* 144-148.

Fritz, M.S., & Mackinnon, D.P. (2007). Required sample size to detect the mediated effect. *Psychological Science, 18*(3), 233-239.

Fujisawa, R. & Colombo, F. (2009). The long-term care workforce: Overview and strategies to adapt supply to a growing demand. OECD Health Working Papers, No.44., France: OECD Publishing.

Gabriel, B., Beach, S.R. & Bodenmann, G. (2010). Depression, marital satisfaction and communication in couples: investigating gender differences. *Behaviour Therapy, 41(3)*, 306-316.

Gabrylewicz, T., Styczynska, M., Pfeffer, A., Wasiak, B., Barczak, A., Luczywek, E., Androsiuk, W. & Barcikowska, M. (2004). Prevalence of major and minor depression in elderly persons with mild cognitive impairment—MADRS factor analysis. *International Journal of Geriatric Psychiatry*, 19(12), 1168–1172.

Gagnon, M.D., Hersen, M., Kabacoff, R.I., Van Hasselt, V.B. (1999). Interpersonal and psychological correlates of marital dissatisfaction in late life: a review. *Clinical Psychology Review, 19*(3), 359-78.

Gallagher-Thompson, D. & Powers, D.V. (1997). Primary stressors and depressive symptoms in caregivers of dementia patients. *Aging and Mental Health, 2*(3), 248-255.

Gallagher-Thompson, D., Dal Canto, P.G., Jacob, T. & Thompson, L.W. (2001). A comparison of marital interaction patterns between couples in which the husband does or does not have Alzheimer's disease. *The Journals of Gerontology, 56B*(3), S140-S150.

Gallant, M.P. & Connell, C.M. (1997). Predictors of decreased self-care among spouse caregivers of older adults with dementing illnesses. *Journal of Aging and Health, 9,* 373-395.

Gallicchio, L., Siddiqi, N., Langenberg, P., & Baumgarten, M. (2002). Gender differences in burden and depression among informal caregivers of demented elders in the community. *International Journal of Geriatric Psychiatry, 17*(2), 154-63.

Gallo, J.J., Anthony, J.C. & Muthén, B.O. (1994). Age differences in the symptoms of depression: a latent trait analysis. *Journal of Gerontology, 49(6)*, P251-264.

Galvin, J.E., Pollack, J. & Morris, J.C. (2006). Clinical phenotype of Parkinson disease dementia. *Neurology, 67(9),* 1605-1611.

Garand, L., Dew, M.A., Urda, B., Hagerty Lingler, J., DeKosky, S.T. & Reynolds, C.F. (2007) Marital quality in the context of mild cognitive impairment. *Western Journal of Nursing Research, 29*(8), 976-992.

García-Alberca, J.M., Cruz, B., Lara, J.P., Garrido, V., Gris, E., Lara, A., & Castilla, C. (2012). Disengagement coping partially mediates the relationship between caregiver burden and anxiety and depression in caregivers of people with Alzheimer's disease. Results from the MÁLAGA-AD study. *Journal of Affective Disorders, 136*(3), 848-56.

Gardiner, J.M. & Richardson-Klavehn, A. (2000). Remembering and knowing. In E.Tulving & F.I.M. Craik (Eds.). *The Oxford Handbook of Memory* (pp. 229-244.). Oxford: Oxford University Press.

Garret, J.F. & Levine, E.S. (1962). *Psychological practices with the physically disabled.* New York, Columbia University Press.

Garron, D.C., Klawans, H.L. & Narin, F. (1972). Intellectual functioning of persons with idiopathic Parkinsonism. *The Journal of Nervous and Mental Disease, 154(6),* 445-452.

Gaudiano, B.A., Young, D., Chelminski, I. & Zimmerman, M. (2008).

Depressive symptom profiles and severity patterns in outpatients with psychotic vs nonpsychotic major depression. *Comprehensive Psychiatry, 49(5),* 421-429.

Gaugler, J.E., Kane, R.L., Kane, R.A., Clay, T., & Newcomer, R.C. (2005). The effects of duration of caregiving on institutionalization. *The Gerontologist. 45*(1), 78-89.

Gaugler, J.E., Kane, R.L., Kane, R.A. & Newcomer, R. (2005). Unmet care needs and key outcomes in dementia. *Journal of the American Geriatrics Society,53,* 2098-2105.

Geminiani, G., Cesana, B.M., Tamma, F., Contri, P., Pacchetti, C., Carella, F., Piolti, R., Martignoni, E., Giovannini, P., Girotti, F. & Caraceni, T. (1991). Interobserver reliability between neurologists in training of Parkinson's disease rating scales. *Movement Disorders*, *6,* 330-335.

George, D. & Mallery, P. (2003). SPSS for Windows step by step: A simple guide and reference. 11.0 update (4th ed.) Boston: Allyn & Bacon.

George, L. (1990). Caregiver stress studies – There really is more to learn. *The Gerontologist, 30*(5), 580-581.

George, L.K. & Gwyther, L.P. (1986). Caregiver wellbeing: a multidimensional examination of family caregivers of demented adults. *The Gerontologist*, *26*(3), 253-259.

Gerhardt, U. (1989). The sociological image of medicine and the patient. *Social Science and Medicine, 29*(6), 721-728.

Ghazi-Noori, S., Chung, T.H., Deane, K.H.O., Rickards, H. & Clarke, C.E. (2003). Systematic review of antidepressant therapies in Parkinson's disease. *Parkinsonism and Related Disorders*, *10*(2), 59-65.

Ghazi-Noori, S., Chung, T.H., Deane, K.H.O., Rickards, H. & Clarke, C.E. (2009). Therapies for depression in Parkinson's disease. *Cochrane Database of Systematic Reviews*, *4*, 1-19.

Gibb, W.R.G. (1988). Accuracy in the clinical diagnosis of parkinsonian syndromes. *Postgraduate Medical Journal*, *64*, 345-351.

Giladi, N., Treves, T.A., Paleacu, D., Shabtai, H., Orlov, T., Kandinov, B., Simon, E.S. & Korczyn, A.D. (2000). Risk factors for dementia, depression and psychosis in long-standing Parkinson's disease. *Journal of Neural Transmission*, *107*, 59-71.

Gilhooly, M.L.M. (1984). The impact of care-giving on care-givers: factors associated with the psychological well-being of people supporting a dementing relative in the community. *British Journal of Medical Psychology, 57*(1), 35-44.

—. (1986). Senile dementia: factors associated with caregiver's preference for institutional care. *British Journal Medical Psychology, 59,* 165-171.

Gilhooly, M.L.M. & Whittick, J.E. (1989) Expressed emotion in caregivers of the dementing elderly. *British Journal of Medical Psychology, 62*, 265-272.

Gilleard C.J. (1984a). *Living with dementia*. London & Sydney: Croom Helm.

—. (1984b). Problems posed for supporting relatives of geriatric and psychogeriatric day patients. *Acta Psychiatrica Scandinavica*, *70*, 198-208.

—. (1987). Influence of emotional distress among supporters on the outcome of psychogeriatric day care. *British Journal of Psychiatry*, 150, 219-223.

Gilleard C.J., Belford H., Gilleard E., Whittick J.E. & Gledhill K. (1984). Emotional distress amongst the supporters of the elderly mentally infirm. *British Journal of Psychiatry*, *145*, 172-177.

Gilleard, C.J., Boyd, W.D. & Watt, G. (1982). Problems in caring for the elderly mentally infirm at home. *Archives of Gerontology and Geriatrics, 1*, 151-158.

Ginanneschi, A. Degl'Innocenti, F., Magnolfi, S., Maurello, M.T., Catarzi, P., Marini, P. & Amaducci, L. (1988). Evaluation of Parkinson's disease: reliability of three rating scales. *Neuroepidemiology*, 7, 38-41.

Giovannoni, G., O'Sullivan, J.D., Turner, K., Manson, A.J. & Lees, A.J. (2000). Hedonistic homeostatic dysregulation in patients with Parkinson's disease on dopamine replacement therapies. *Journal of Neurology, Neurosurgery and Psychiatry*, 68, 423-428.

Gisquet, E. (2008). Cerebral implants and Parkinson's disease: a unique form of biographical disruption? *Social Science and Medicine, 67*(11), 1847-1851.

Glatt, S.L., Hubble, J.P., Lyons, K., Paolo, A., Tröster, A.I., Hassanein, R.E.S. & Koller, W.C. (1996). Risk factors for dementia in Parkinson's disease: Effect of education. *Neuroepidemiology, 15,* 20-25.

Global Parkinson's Disease Survey Steering Committee (2002). Factors impacting on quality of life in Parkinson's disease: results from an international survey. *Movement Disorders, 17*, 60-67.

Globus, M., Mildworf, B. & Melamed, E. (1985). Cerebral blood flow and cognitive impairment in Parkinson's disease. *Neurology, 35,* 1135-1139.

Glozman, J.M. (2004). Quality of life of caregivers. *Neuropsychology Review, 14*(4), 183-196.

Goetz, C.G., Poewe, W., Rascol, O., Sampaio, C., Stebbins, G.T., Counsell, C., Giladi, N., Holloway, R.G., Moore, C.G., Wenning, G.K., Yahr, M.D. & Seidl L. (2004). Movement Disorder Society Task Force report on the Hoehn and Yahr Staging Scale: Status and recommendations. *Movement Disorders*, *19,* 1020-1028.

Goffman E. (1963) *Stigma: Notes on the Management of Spoiled Identity*. New Jersey: Prentice Hall.

Golbe, L.I. (1991). Young-onset Parkinson's disease: a clinical review. *Neurology, 41*(2), 168-173.

Gold, D.P., Franz, E., Reis, M. & Senneville, C. (1994). The influence of emotional awareness and expressiveness on caregiving burden and health complaints in women and men. *Sex Roles, 31,* 205-224.

Gold, D.P., Reis, M., Markiewicz, D. & Andres, D. (1995). When home caregiving ends: A longitudinal study of outcomes for caregivers of relatives with dementia. *Journal of the American Geriatrics Society, 43*(1)*,* 10-16.

Gold, S.M., Zakowski, S.G., Valdimarsdottir, H.B.& Bovbjerg, D.H. (2004). Higher Beck depression scores predict delayed epinephrine recovery after acute psychological stress independent of baseline levels of stress and mood. *Biological Psychology, 67(3),* 261-273.

Goldberg, D. (1978). *Manual of the General Health Questionnaire*. NFER Nelson Publishing Company.

Goldberg, D.P. & Hillier, V.F. (1979). A scaled version of the General Health Questionnaire. *Psychological Medicine*, *9,* 139-145.

Goldberg, D. & Williams, P. (1988). *A user's guide to the General Health Questionnaire.* Windsor, UK: NFER Nelson Publishing Company Ltd.

Goldenberg, G., Wimmer, A., Auff, E. & Schnaberth, G. (1986). Impairment of motor planning in patients with Parkinson's disease: Evidence from ideomotor apraxia. *Journal of Neurology, Neurosurgery and Psychiatry, 49,* 1266-1272.

Goldman, S.M., Quinlan, P.J., Ross, G.W., Marras, C., Meng, C., Bhudhikanok, G.S., Comyns, K., Korell, M., Chade, A.R., Kasten, M., Priestley, B., Chou, K.L., Fernandez, H.H., Cambi, F., Langston, J.W. & Tanner, C.M. (2011). Solvent exposures and Parkinson disease risk in twins. *Annals of Neurology, 71(6),* 776-784.

Goldman, S.M., Tanner, C.M., Oakes, D., Bhudhikanok, G.S., Gupta, A. & Langston, J.W. (2006). Head injury and Parkinson's disease risk in twins. *Annals of Neurology*, *60* (1), 65–72.

Goldsworthy, B. & Knowles, S. (2008). Caregiving for Parkinson's disease patients: an exploration of a stress-appraisal model for quality of life and burden. *Journal of Gerontology, 63B*(6), P372-P376.

Gómez-Esteban, J.C., Tijero, B., Somme, J., Bilbao, I., Fernández, J., Boyero, S., Velasco, F., Lezcano, E. & Zarranz, J.J. (2009). Application of depression criteria (DSM-IV) in patients with Parkinson's disease. *Clinical Neurology and Neurosurgery, 111(8),* 665-669.

Gonçalves-Pereira, M., Carmo, I., da Silva, J.A., Papoila, A.L., Mateos, R., & Zarit, S.H. (2010). Caregiving experiences and knowledge about dementia in Portuguese clinical outpatient settings. *International Psychogeriatrics, 22*(2), 270-280.

Gonyea, J.G., O'Connor, M., Carruthm, A. & Boyle, P.A. (2005). Subjective appraisal of Alzheimer's disease caregiving: the role of self-efficacy and depressive symptoms in the experience of burden. *American Journal of Alzheimer's Disease and Other Dementias, 20*(5), 273-280.

Górska, T. & Majczyński, H. (1997). Mechanizmy sterowania ruchami dowolnymi. In T. Górska, A. Grabowska and J. Zagrodzka, (Eds.), *Mózg a zachowanie* (pp. 214-23). Warszawa, Wydawnictwo Naukowe PWN. (In Polish).

Gort, A.M., Mingot, M. Gomez, X., Soler, T., Torres, G., Sacristan, O., Miguelsanz, S., Nicolas, F., Perez, A., de Miguel, M. & Cabau, J. (2007). Use of Zarit Scale for assessing caregiver burden and collapse in caregiving at home in dementias. *International Journal of Geriatric Psychiatry, 22,* 957-962.

Gotham, A.M., Brown, R.G. & Marsden, C.D. (1986). Depression in Parkinson's disease: a quantitative and qualitative analysis. *Journal of Neurology, Neurosurgery and Psychiatry*, *49,* 381-389.

Gotham, A.M., Brown, R.G. & Marsden, C.D. (1988). 'Frontal' cognitive function in patients with Parkinson's disease 'on' and 'off' levodopa. *Brain, 111,* 299-321.

Gottman, J.M. (1979). *Marital interaction: experimental investigations.* San Diego, California: Academic Press.

Grabowska, A. (1999). Lateralizacja emocji w mózgu-dane eksperymentalne i kliniczne. (Lateralization of emotion in the brain – experimental and clinical evidence). In A. Herzyk & A. Borkowska (Eds.). *Neuropsychologia emocji. Poglądy, badania, klinika (pp. 59-79).* Lublin: Wydawnictwo Uniwersytetu Marii Curie-Skłodowskiej. (In Polish).

Grad, J. & Sainsbury, P. (1963). Mental illness and the family. *Lancet, 1*(7280), 544-547.

Grad, J. & Sainsbury, P. (1966). Problems of caring for the mentally ill at home. *Proceedings of the Royal Society of Medicine, 59*(1), 20-23.

Graham, J.M. & Sagar, H.J. (1999). A data-driven approach to the study of heterogeneity in idiopathic Parkinson's disease: identification of three distinct subtypes. *Movement Disorders, 14(1)*,10-20.

Grahn, J.A., Parkinson, J.A. & Owen, A.M. (2008). The cognitive functions of the caudate nucleus. *Progress in Neurobiology, 86,* 141-155.

Greene J.G., Smith R., Gardiner M. & Timbury G.C. (1982). Measuring behavioural disturbance of elderly demented patients in the community and its effects on relatives: a factor analytic study. *Age and Ageing, 11*(2), 121-126.

Greene, J.G. & Timbury, G.C. (1979). A geriatric psychiatry day hospital service: a five-year review. *Age and Ageing, 8*(1), 49-53.

Greene ,V.L., & Ondrich, J.I. (1990). Risk factors for nursing home admissions and exits: a discrete-time hazard function approach. *Journal of Gerontology, 45B*(6), S250-S258.

Greenwald, B.S., Kramer-Ginsberg, E., Marin, D.B., Laitman, L.B., Hermann, C.K., Mohs, R.C. & Davis, K.L. (1989). Dementia with coexistent major depression. *American Journal Psychiatry, 146(11),* 1472-1478.

Grossman, M., Carvell, S., Gollomp, S., Stern, M.B., Vernon, G. & Hurtig, H.I. (1991). Sentence comprehension and praxis deficits in Parkinson's disease. *Neurology, 41,* 1620-1628.

Grujic, Z. (2007). Cognitive disturbances in Parkinson's disease. *Disorders a Month, 53,* 302-308.

Guiliano, A.I., Mitchell, R.E., Clark, P.G., Harlow, L.L. & Rosenbloom, D. (1990). The meaning in caregiving scale: Factorial and conceptual dimensions. *Poster session presented at the second annual convention of the American Psychological Society*, Dallas, Texas.

Gupta, A. & Bhatia, S. (2000a). Psychological functioning in patients with Parkinson's disease. *Parkinsonism and Related Disorders*, 6, 185-190.

Gupta, A. & Bhatia, S. (2000b). Depression in Parkinson's disease. *Clinical Gerontologist, 22(2),* 59-70.

Gurd, J.M. & Ward, C.D. (1989). Retrieval from semantic and letter-initial categories in patients with Parkinson's disease. *Neuropsychologia, 27(5),* 743-746.

Gurland, B., Copeland, J., Kuriansky, J., Kelleher, M., Sharpe, L. & Dean, L.L. (1983). *The Mind and Mood of Aging: Mental Health Problems of the Community Elderly in New York and London.* London: Croom Helm.

Guttman, M., Boileau, I., Warsh, J., Saint-Cyr, J.A., Ginovart, N., McCluskey, T., Houle, S., Wilson, A., Mundo, E., Rusjan, P., Meyer, J. & Kish, S.J. (2007). Brain serotonin transporter binding in non-depressed patients with Parkinson's disease. *European Journal of Neurology,* 14(5), 523-528.

Haahr, A., Kirkevold, M., Hall, E.O. & Ostergaard, K. (2011). Living with advanced Parkinson's disease: a constant struggle with unpredictability. *Journal of Advanced Nursing, 67*(2):408-417.

Haehner, A., Hummel, T. & Reichmann, H. (2011). Olfactory loss in Parkinson's disease. Parkinson's disease, Article ID 450939, doi: 10.4061/2011/450939.

Halbig, T.D., Assuras, S., Creighton, J., Borod, J.C., Tse, W., Frisina, P.G., Voustianiouk, A., Gracies, J.M. & Olanow, C.W. (2011). Differential role of dopamine in emotional attention and memory: evidence from Parkinson's disease. *Movement Disorders*, *26(9),* 1677-1683.

Haley, W.E., Gitlin, L.N. Wisniewski, S.R. Mahoney, D.F. Cood, D.W. Winter, L. Corcoran, M. Schinfeld, S., & Ory, M. (2004). Well-being, Appraisal, and Coping in African-American and Caucasian Dementia Caregivers: Findings from the REACH Study. *Aging and Mental Health*, *8,* 316-329.

Haley, W.E., Levine, E.G., Brown, S.L. & Bartolucci, A.A. (1987). Stress, appraisal, coping and social support as predictors of adaptational outcome among dementia caregivers. *Psychology and Aging, 2*, 323-330.

Haley, W.E., Roth, D.L., Coleton, M.I., Ford, G.R,, West, C.A., Collins, R.P., & Isobe, T.L. (1996). Appraisal, coping, and social support as mediators of well-being in black and white family caregivers of patients with Alzheimer's disease. *Journal of Consulting and Clinical Psychology, 64*(1), 121-129.

Halkias, I.C., Haq, I., Huang, Z. & Fernandez, H.H. (2007). When should levodopa therapy be initiated in patients with Parkinson's disease? *Drugs and Aging*, *24,* 261-273.

Halliday, G.M., Li, Y.W., Blumbergs, P.C., Joh, T.H., Cotton, R.G., Howe, P.R., Blessing, W.W. & Geffen, L.B. (1990). Neuropathology of immunohistochemically identified brainstem neurons in Parkinson's disease. *Annals of Neurology*, *27,* 373-385.

Halliday, G.M., Hely, M., Reid, W. & Morris, J. (2008). The progression of pathology in longitudinally followed patients with Parkinson's disease. *Acta Neuropathologica, 115(4),* 409-415.

Hames, D. (2011). Column 228WH. Daily Hansard, Westmister Hall (9.3. 2011).

Hamilton, M., (1959). The assessment of anxiety states by rating. *British Journal of Medical Psychology*, *32*, 50-55.

—. (1960). A rating scale for depression. *Journal of Neurology, Neurosurgery and Psychiatry*, *23*, 56-62.

Hamilton, R.L. (2000). Lewy bodies in Alzheimer's disease: a neuropathological review of 145 cases using alpha-synuclein immunohistochemistry. *Brain Pathology, 10(3),* 378-384.

Hanley, J.R., Dewick, H.C., Davies, A.D.M., Playfer, J. & Turnbull, C. (1990). Verbal fluency in Parkinson's disease. *Neuropsychologia, 28(7),* 737-741.

Hantz, P., Caradoc-Davies, G., Caradoc-Davies, T., Weatherall, M. & Dixon, G. (1994). Depression in Parkinson's disease. *American Journal of Psychiatry*, 151 (7), 1010-1014.

Happe, S., Berger, K. & the FAQT Study Investigators. (2002). The association between caregiver burden and sleep disturbances in partners of patients with Parkinson's disease. *Age and Ageing, 31*(5), 349-354.

Harkin, M. (2011). National Carers Strategy needed NOW. Retrieved: http://www.marianharkin.com/index.php?id=20&tx_ttnews[tt_news]=618&tx_ttnews[backPid]=4&cHash=0c9de69cd79e0c3e7fd7cfa399cbf526

Harrington, D.L., Haaland, K.Y., Yeo, R.A. & Marder, E. (1990). Procedural memory in Parkinson's disease: Impaired motor but not visuoperceptual learning. *Journal of Clinical and Experimental Neuropsychology, 12,* 323-339.

Harrison, J.E., Stow, I. & Owen, A.M. (2002). Parkinson's disease. In J.E. Harrison & A.M. Owen (Eds). *Cognitive Deficits in Brain Disorders.* London: Martin Dunitz Ltd.

Hart, R.P., Kwentus, J.A., Wade, J.B. & Taylor, J.R. (1988). Modified Wisconsin Card Sorting Test in elderly normal, depressed and demented patients. *Clinical Neuropsychologist, 2,* 49-56.

Hatano, T., Kubo, S.I., Shimo,Y., Nishioka, K. & Hattori, N. (2009). Unmet needs of patients with Parkinson's disease: Interview survey of patients and caregivers. *The Journal of International Medical Research, 37,* 717-726.

Haupt, M. & Kurz, A. (1993). Predictors of nursing home placement in patients with Alzheimer's disease. *International Journal of Geriatric Psychiatry, 8*, 741-746.

Hayes, L. (1994). Early onset Parkinson's disease. Part 1: The patient's story. *Canadian Family Physician, 40,* 506-508.

Hazan, C. & Shaver, P.R. (1987). Romantic love conceptualized as an attachment process. *Journal of Personality and Social Psychology, 52*(3), 511–24.

Hazan, C. & Shaver, P.R. (1990). Love and work: An attachment theoretical perspective. *Journal of Personality and Social Psychology,59,* 270-280.

Headey, B., Holmstrom, E. & Wearing, A. (1985). Models of well-being and ill-being. *Social Indicators Research, 17,* 211-234.

Health and Social Care Information Centre (2012). *Survey of Carers in Households - 2009/10 England.* Retrieved: http://www.ic.nhs.uk/pubs/carersurvey0910.

Heindel, W.C., Salmon, D.P., Shults, C.W., Walicke, P.A. & Butters, N. (1989). Neuropsychological evidence for multiple implicit memory systems: A comparison of Alzheimer's, Huntington's and Parkinson's disease patients. *Journal of Neuroscience, 9,* 582-587.

Heitanen, M. & Teravainen, H. (1988). The effect of age of disease onset on neuropsychological performance in Parkinson's disease. *Journal of Neurology, Neurosurgery and Psychiatry, 51,* 244-249.

Helkala, E.L., Laulumaa, V. Soininen, H. & Reikkinen, P.J. (1988). Recall and recognition memory in patients with Alzheimer's and Parkinson's diseases. *Annals of Neurology, 24,* 214-217.

Helman, C.G. (1994). *Culture, Health and Illness* (3rd edition). Oxford: Butterworth-Heinemann.

Hely, M.A., Morris, J.G., Reid, W.G. & Trafficante, R. (2005). Sydney Multicenter Study of Parkinson's disease: non-L-dopa-responsive problems dominate at 15 years. *Movement Disorders, 20(2),* 190-199.

Hely, M.A., Morris, J.G., Traficante, R., Reid, W.G., O'Sullivan, D.J. & Williamson, P.M. (1999). The Sydney multicentre study of Parkinson's disease: progression and mortality at 10 years. *Journal of Neurology, Neurosurgery and Psychiatry*, 67(3), 300-307.

Hely, M.A., Reid, W.G., Aldena, M.A., Halliday, G.M. & Morris, J.G. (2008). The Sydney multicenter study of Parkinson's disease: the inevitability of dementia at 20 years. *Movement Disorders, 23(6),* 837-844.

Henderson, L., Kennard, C., Crawford, T.J., Day, S., Everitt, B.S., Goodrich, S. Jones, F. & Park, D.M. (1991). Scales for rating motor impairment in Parkinson's disease: studies of reliability and convergent validity. *Journal of Neurology, Neurosurgery and Psychiatry*, *54,*18-24.

Henry, J.D. & Crawford, J.R. (2004). Verbal fluency deficits in Parkinson's disease: a meta-analysis. *Journal of the International Neuropsychological Society, 10(4)*, 608-622.

Hérbert, R., Bravo, G., & Préville, M. (2000). Reliability, validity, and reference values of the Zarit Burden Interview for assessing informal caregivers of community-dwelling older persons with dementia. *Canadian Journal on Aging*, 19, 494-507.

Heru, A.M., Ryan, C.E. & Iqbal, A. (2004) Family functioning in the caregivers of patients with dementia. *International Journal of Geriatric Psychiatry, 19*, 533-537.

Herz, M.I., Endicott, J. & Spitzer, R.L. (1976). Brief versus standard hospitalization: the families. *American Journal of Psychiatry, 133*(7), 795-801.

Herzyk, A. (1999). Neuropsychologiczne modele emocji. (Neuropsychological models of emotion). In A. Herzyk & A. Borkowska (Eds). *Neuropsychologia emocji: poglady, badania, klinika (pp. 13-40).* Lublin, Wydawnictwo Uniwersytetu Marii Curie-Skłodowskiej. Chapter in Polish.

—. (2000a). *Mózg, emocje, uczucia. Analiza neuropsychologiczna.* Lublin: Wydawnictwo Uniwersytetu Marii-Curie-Skłodowskiej.

—. (2000b). Diagnoza neuropsychologiczna – dokąd zmierza? Pytania, polemiki, propozycje rozwiązań. In A. Borkowska, E.M. Szepietowska (Eds.). *Diagnoza neuropsychologiczna – metodologia i metodyka* (pp.23-50). Lublin: Wydawnictwo UMCS.

Hickox, A. & Sunderland, A. (1992). Questionnaire and checklist approaches to assessment of everyday memory problems. In J.R. Crawford, D.M. Parker & W.W. McKinlay (Eds.), *A handbook of neuropsychological assessment* (pp. 103-113). Hillsdale, N.J.: Lawrence Erlbaum Associates Inc.

Hinkle, L.E. (1973). The concept of stress in the biological and social sciences. *Science, Medicine and Man, 1,* 31-48.

Hirschfield, M.J. (1981). Families living and coping with the cognitively impaired. In L.A. Copp (Ed.) *Care of the Ageing: Recent Advances in Nursing* (pp. 159-167). Edinburgh: Churchill-Livingstone.

H.M. Government (2008). *Carers at the heart of 21st-century families and communities: A caring system on your side. A life of your own.* Department of Health Policy Document, (p.83). Retrieved: http://www.dh.gov.uk/prod_consum_dh/groups/dh_digitalassets/@dh/@en/documents/digitalasset/dh_085338.pdf.

—. (2010a). The coalition: our programme for government. Retrieved: http://www.cabinetoffice.gov.uk/sites/default/files/resources/coalition_programme_for_government.pdf

—. (2010b). *Building the National Care Service*. London: The Stationery Office.

—. (2010c). *Recognised, valued and supported: next steps for the Carers' Strategy.* Retrieved: http://www.dh.gov.uk/prod_consum_dh/groups/

dh_digitalassets/@dh/@en/documents/digitalasset/dh_122393. pdf.
Hobson, P. & Meara, J. (1999). The detection of dementia and cognitive impairment in a community population of elderly people with Parkinson's disease by use of the CAMCOG neuropsychological test. *Age and Ageing, 28,* 39-43.
Hobson, P. & Meara, J. (2004). Risk and incidence of dementia in a cohort of older subjects with Parkinson's disease in the United Kingdom. *Movement Disorders, 19(9),* 1043-1049.
Hodgins, M.J., Wuest, J. & Malcolm, J. (2011). Modeling the effects of past relationship and obligation on changes in the health and health promotion of women caregivers of family members with dementia. *Research in Nursing and Health, 34(6)*, 440-456.
Hodgson, T.L., Tiesman, B., Owen, A.M. & Kennard, C. (2002). Abnormal gaze strategies during problem solving in Parkinson's disease. *Neuropsychologia, 40,* 411-422.
Hoehn M. & Yahr, M., (1967). Parkinsonism: onset, progression and mortality. *Neurology*, *17*(5), 427–442.
Hoenig, J. & Hamilton, M.W. (1966). The schizophrenic patient in the community and his effect on the household. *International Journal of Social Psychiatry, 12*(3), 165-176.
Hoenig, J. & Hamilton, M.W. (1967). Extramural psychiatric care and the elderly. *British Journal of Psychiatry, 113*(497), 435-443.
Hoenig, J. & Hamilton, M.W. (1969). *The desegregation of the mentally ill.* London: Routledge and Keegan Paul.
Hohman, T.J., Beason-Held, L.L., Lamar, M., & Resnick, S.M. (2011). Subjective cognitive complaints and longitudinal changes in memory and brain function. *Neuropsychology, 25*(1), 125-30.
Holland, P.W. (1988). Causal inference, path analysis, and recursive structural equation models. *Sociological Methodology, 18*, 449-484.
Holmbeck, G.N. (1997). Toward terminological, conceptual, and statistical clarity in the study of mediators and moderators: examples from the child-clinical and pediatric psychology literatures. *Journal of Consulting and Clinical Psychology, 65,* 599-610.
Holmes, T.H. & Rahe, R.H. (1967). The Social Readjustment Rating Scale. *Journal of Psychosomatic Research, 11 (2),* 213–218.
Holroyd, S., Currie, L.J. & Wooten, G.F. (2005). Depression is associated with impairment of ADL, not motor function in Parkinson's disease. *Neurology*, *64,* 2134-2135.
Hoogendijk, W.J.G., Sommer, I.E.C., Tissingh, G., Deeg, D.J.H. & Wolters, E.Ch. (1998). Depression in Parkinson's disease: the impact of symptom overlap on prevalence. *Psychosomatics*, *39(5),* 416-421.

Hooker, K., Frazier, L.D. & Monahan, D.J. (1994). Personality and coping among caregivers of spouses with dementia. *The Gerontologist, 34(3),* 386-392.

Hooker, K., Manoogian-O'Dell, M., Monahan, D.J., Frazier, L.D. & Shifren, K. (2000). Does type of disease matter? Gender differences among Alzheimer's and Parkinson's disease spouse caregivers. *The Gerontologist*, *40 (5),* 568-573.

Hooker, K., Monahan, D.J., Bowman, S.R., Frazier, L.D. & Shifren, K. (1998). Personality counts for a lot: Predictors of mental and physical health of spouse caregivers in two disease groups. *Journal of Gerontology*. *53B*(2), P73-P85.

Hooker, K., Monahan, D., Shifren, K. & Hutchinson, C. (1992). Mental and physical health of spouse caregivers: the role of personality. *Psychology and Aging. 7(3),* 367-375.

Hooyman, N., Gonyea, J. & Montgomery, R. (1985). The impact of in-home services termination on family caregivers. *The Gerontologist, 25,* 141-145.

Hope, T., Keene, J., Gedling, K., Fairburn, C.G. and Jacoby, R. (1998). Predictors of institutionalisation for people living at home with a carer. *International Journal of Geriatric Psychiatry, 13*, 682-690.

Horn, S. (1974). Some psychological factors in parkinsonism. *Journal of Neurology, Neurosurgery and Psychiatry*, *37,* 27-31.

Hornykiewicz, O. (2006). The discovery of dopamine deficiency in the parkinsonian brain. *Journal of Neural Transmission [Suppl] 70*, 9–15.

Hornykiewicz, O., Pifl, Ch., Kish, S.J. Shannak, K. & Schingnitz, **G.** (1989). Biochemical changes in idiopathic Parkinson's disease, aging and MPTP parkinsonism: similarities and differences. In: D.B. Calne, G. Comi, D. Crippa, R. Horowski, M. Trabucchi (Eds.), *Parkinsonism and Aging* (pp. 57-67). New York: Raven Press.

Horowitz, A. (1985a). Family caregiving to the frail elderly. *Annual Review of Gerontology and Geriatrics, 5,* 199-246.

—. (1985b). Sons and daughters as caregivers to older parents: Differences in role performance and consequences. *The Gerontologist, 25*, 612-617.

Horowitz, A. & Shindelman, L. (1983). Reciprocity and affection: Past influences on current caregiving. *Journal of Gerontological Social Work, 5*, 5-21.

House of Commons (1990). *The NHS and Community Care Act.* London: HMSO.

Hovestadt, A., De Jong, G.J. & Meerwaldt, J.D. (1987). Spatial disorientation as an early symptom of Parkinson's disease. *Neurology,*

37(3), 485-487.

Howell, D.C. (2002). *Statistical Methods for Psychology* (Fifth edition). Duxbury, Thomson Learning, U.K.

Huber, S.J., Freidenberg, D.L., Paulson, G.W., Shuttleworth, E.C. & Christy, J.A. (1990). The pattern of depressive symptoms varies with progression of Parkinson's disease. *Journal of Neurology, Neurosurgery and Psychiatry*, *53*, 275-278.

Huber, S.J., Freidenberg, D.L., Shuttleworth, E.C., Paulson, G.W. & Christy, L.E. (1989). Neuropsychological impairments associated with severity of Parkinson's disease. *Journal of Neuropsychiatry and Clinical Neurosciences, 1,* 155-159.

Huber, S.J. & Paulson, G.W. (1985). The concept of subcortical dementia. *American Journal of Psychiatry, 142(11),* 1312-1317.

Huber, S.J., Paulson, G.W. & Shuttleworth, E.C. (1988). Relationship of motor symptoms, intellectual impairment and depression in Parkinson's disease. *Journal of Neurology, Neurosurgery and Psychiatry*, *51(6),* 855-858.

Huber, S.J., Shuttleworth, E.C. & Freidenberg, D.L. (1989). Neuropsychological differences between the dementias of Alzheimer's and Parkinson's diseases. *Archives of Neurology*, 46, 1287-1291.

Huber, S.J., Shuttleworth, E.C. & Paulson, G.W. (1986). Dementia in Parkinson's disease. *Archives of Neurology, 43,* 987-990.

Huber, S.J., Shuttleworth, E.C., Paulson, G.W., Bellchambers, M.J.G. & Clapp, L.E. (1986). Cortical vs. subcortical dementia: Neuropsychological differences. *Archives of Neurology, 43,* 392-394.

Hughes, A.J., Daniel, S.E., Ben-Shlomo, Y. & Lees, A. (2002). The accuracy of diagnosis of parkinsonian syndromes in a specialist movement disorder service. *Brain*, 125, 861-870.

Hughes, A.J., Daniel, S.E., Blankson, S. & Lees, A.J. (1993). A clinicopathologic study of 100 cases of Parkinson's disease. *Archives of Neurology, 50(2),* 140-148.

Hughes, A.J., Daniel, S.E., Kilford, L. & Lees, A.J. (1992). Accuracy of clinical diagnosis of idiopathic Parkinson's disease: a clinic-pathological study of 100 cases. *Journal of Neurology, Neurosurgery and Psychiatry, 55,* 181-184.

Hughes, A.J., Daniel, S.E. & Lees, A. (2001). Improved accuracy of clinical diagnosis of Lewy body Parkinson's disease. *Neurology*, 57 (8), 1497-1499.

Hughes, T.A., Ross, H.F., Mindham, R.H.S. & Spokes, E.G.S. (2004). Mortality in Parkinson's disease and its association with dementia and depression. *Acta Neurologica Scandinavica*, *110,* 118-123.

Hunt, C.K. (2003). Concepts in caregiver research. *Journal Nursing Scholarship, 35(1),* 27-32.

Hunt, J. (2012). Jeremy Hunt dashes hopes of early reform of social care funding system. *The Guardian*. Retrieved: http://www.guardian.co.uk/politics/2012/ oct/10/ jeremy-hunt-social-care-funding.

Huse, D.M., Schulman, K., Orsini, L., Castelli-Haley, J., Kennedy, S. & Lenhart, G. (2005). Burden of illness in Parkinson's disease. *Movement Disorders, 20(11),* 1449-1454.

Hutchinson, S.A.& Wilson, H.S. (1998). The theory of unpleasant symptoms and Alzheimer's disease. *Scholarly Inquiry in Nursing Practice,12*(2),143-158.

Imamura, A., Uitti, R.J. & Wszolek, Z.K. (2006). Dopamine agonist therapy for Parkinson's disease and pathological gambling. *Parkinsonism and Related Disorders*, *12,* 506-508.

Ingebretsen, R. & Solem, P.E. (1997). Attachment, loss and coping in caring for a dementing spouse. In B.M.L. Miesen & Jones, G.M.M. (Eds.), *Care-Giving in Dementia: Research and Applications.* Vol. 2., London: Routledge.

Ingersoll-Dayton, B. & Raschick, M.R. (2004). The relationship between care-recipient behaviours and spousal caregiving stress. *The Gerontologist, 44*(3): 318-327.

Inoue ,T., Kitagawa, M., Tanaka, T., Nakagawa, S. & Koyama, T. (2010). Depression and major depressive disorder in patients with Parkinson's disease. *Movement Disorders, 25(1),* 44-49.

International Parkinson Disease Genomics Consortium (2011). Imputation of sequence variants for identification of genetic risks for Parkinson's disease: a meta-analysis of genome-wide association studies. *The Lancet*, *377,* 641-649.

Ironside, P.M., Scheckel, M., Wessels, C., Bailey, M.E., Powers, S. & Seeley, D.K. (2003). Experiencing chronic illness: cocreating new understandings. *Qualitative Health Research, 13(2),* 171-183.

Ishihara, L. & Brayne, C. (2006). A systematic review of depression and mental illness preceding Parkinson's disease. *Acta Neurologica Scandinavica*, *113,* 211-220.

Ishihara, L.S., Cheesbrough, A., Brayne, C. & Schrag, A. (2007). Estimated life expectancy of Parkinson's patients compared with the UK population. *Journal of Neurology, Neurosurgery and Psychiatry. 78(12),* 1304-1309.

Isaacs, B. (1992). *Challenge of geriatric medicine*. Oxford: Oxford University Press.

Isella,V., Villa, L., Russo, A., Regazzoni, R., Ferrarese, C. & Appollonio, I. (2006). Discriminative and predictive power of an informant report in mild cognitive impairment. *Journal of Neurology, Neurosurgery and Psychiatry*, *77,* 166-171.

Ito, K., Nagano-Saito, A., Kato, T., Arahata, Y., Nakamura, A., Kawasumi, Y., Hatano, K., Abe, Y., Yamada, T., Kachi, T. & Brooks, D.J. (2002). Striatal and extrastriatal dysfunction in Parkinson's disease with dementia: a 6-[18F]fluoro-L-dopa PET study. *Brain, 125,* 1358-1365.

Ivanco, L.S. & Bohnen, N.I. (2005). Effects of donepezil on compulsive hypersexual behavior in Parkinson disease: a single case study. *American Journal of Therapy, 12*(5), 467-468.

Jackson, H. (1884). Evolution and dissolution of the nervous system. Croonian lectures delivered at the Royal college of Physicians. *Lancet, 123(Issue 3163),* 555-558, 649-652, 739-744.

Jacobs, D.M., Marder, K., Côté, L.J., Sano, M., Stern, Y. & Mayeux, R. (1995). Neuropsychological characteristics of preclinical dementia in Parkinson's disease. *Neurology, 45(9),* 1691-1696.

Janevic, M.R., & Connell, C. (2001). Racial, ethnic and cultural differences in the dementia caregiving experience: Recent findings. *The Gerontologist, 4*, 334-347.

Jankovic J. (2008). Parkinson's disease: clinical features and diagnosis. *Journal of Neurology, Neurosurgery and Psychiatry*, 79(4), 368-376.

Jankovic, J., McDermott, M., Carter, J., Gauthier, S., Goetz, C., Golbe, L., Huber, S., Koller, W., Olanow, C., Shoulson, I., et al. (1990). Variable expression of Parkinson's disease: a base-line analysis of the DATATOP cohort. The Parkinson Study Group. *Neurology, 40(10),*1529-1534.

Jankovic, J., Rajput, A.H., McDermott, M.P. & Perl, D.P. for the Parkinson study group, (2000). The evolution of diagnosis in early Parkinson's disease. *Archives of Neurology*, 57(3), 369-372.

Janocha, A. & Zawilska, J.B. (2007). Zaburzenia snu w chorobie Parkinsona: charakterystyka i leczenie. *Via Medica, 7(1),* 14-24. In Polish.

Janvin, C. (2006). Cognitive impairment in patients with Parkinson's disease: profiles and implications for prognosis. Doctoral dissertation from the Norwegian Centre for Movement Disorders, Stavanger University Hospital and Institute for Biological and Medical Psychology, University of Bergen. Rerieved: https://bora.uib.no/bitstream/1956/2242/18/Main_Thesis_Carmen_ Janvin.pdf on 21/04/2010.

Janvin, C., Aarsland, D. & Larsen, J.P. (2005). Cognitive predictors of dementia in Parkinson's disease: a community-based, 4-year longitudinal study. *Journal of Geriatric Psychiatry and Neurology, 18,* 149-154.

Janvin, C., Aarsland, D., Larsen, J.P. & Hugdahl, K. (2003). Neuropsychological profile of patients with Parkinson's disease without dementia. *Dementia and Geriatric Cognitive Disorders, 15,* 126-131.

Janvin, C., Larsen, J.P., Aarsland, D. & Hugdahl, K. (2006). Subtypes of mild cognitive impairment in Parkinson's disease: progression to dementia. *Movement Disorders, 21(9),* 1343-1349.

Jarrott, S.E., Zarit, S.H., Stephens, M.A.P., Townsend, A.L. & Greene, R. (2000) Effects of adult day service programs on time usage by employed and non-employed caregivers. *Journal of Applied Gerontology, 19,* 371-388.

Jellinger, K.A. (2010). The neuropathologic substrate of Parkinson's disease dementia. *Acta Neuropathologica, 119,* 151-153.

—. (2013). Mild cognitive impairment in Parkinson's disease: heterogenous mechanisms. *Journal of Neural Transmission, 120,* 157-167.

Jenkinson, C., Fitzpatrick, R., Peto, V., Greenhall, R. & Hyman, N. (1997). The Parkinson's Disease Questionnaire (PDQ-39): development and validation of a Parkinson's disease summary index score. *Age and Ageing, 26*, 353-357.

Jerrom, B., Mian, I., Rukanyake, N.G., & Prothero, D. (1993). Stress on relative caregivers of dementia sufferers, and predictors of the breakdown of community care. *International Journal of Geriatric Psychiatry, 8*(4), 331–337.

Jiménez-Jiménez, F.J., Sayed, Y., García-Soldevilla, M.A. & Barcenilla, B. (2002). Possible zoophilia associated with dopaminergic therapy in Parkinson disease. *Annals of Pharmacotherapy, 36*(7-8), 1178-1179.

Johnson, C.L. and Catalona, D.J. (1982). A longitudinal study of family supports to impaired elderly. Paper presented at the 35th Annual Scientific Meeting of the Geontological Society of America, Boston, USA, November 1982.

Johnson, D.K. & Galvin, J.E. (2011). Longitudinal changes in cognition in Parkinson's disease with and without dementia. *Dementia and Geriatric Cognitive Disorders*, *31(2),* 98-108.

Johnson, S. L. & Jacob, T. (2000). Sequential interactions in the marital communication of depressed men and women. *Journal of Consulting and Clinical Psychology, 68***,** 4-12.

Jones, F. & Bright, J. (2001). *Stress: Myth, theory and research.* Harlow,

England: Prentice-Hall.

Jones, R.J., D'eath, C., Harnsford, J., Hutchinson, H., Hyde, L., Thurlow, L. & Spanton, L. (1999). The needs of people with Parkinson's disease and their families: The Parkinson's disease study, Devon and Cornwall, 1989-92. In R. Percival & P. Hobson (Eds.), *Parkinson's disease: Studies in psychological and social care*. Leicester: The British Psychological Society.

Joshi, H. (1995). The labour market and unpaid caring: conflict and compromise. In I. Allen & E. Perkins (Eds.). *The Future of Family Care for Older People*. London: HMSO.

Judd, C.M. & Kenny, D.A. (1981). Process analysis: Estimating mediation in evaluation research. *Evaluation Research, 5,* 602-619.

Junqué, C., Ramírez-Ruiz, B., Tolosa, E., Summerfield, C., Martí, M.J., Pastor, P., Gómez-Ansón, B. & Mercader, J.M. (2005). Amygdalar and hippocampal MRI volumetric reductions in Parkinson's disease with dementia. *Movement Disorders, 20(5),* 540-544.

Kaasinen, V. & Rinne, J.O. (2002). Functional imaging studies of dopamine system and cognition in normal aging and Parkinson's disease. *Neuroscience and Behavioural Reviews*, *26,* 785-793.

Kądzielawa, D. (1986). Asymetria półkul mózgowych w zakresie emocji. (Cerebral asymmetry with regard to emotions). *Studia Psychologiczne, 24*, 87-102. Article in Polish.

Kafetsios, K., & Sideridis, G. (2006). Attachment, social support, and well being in younger and older adults. *Journal of Health Psychology, 11*(6), 867-879.

Kahana, E., King, C., Kahana, K., Menne, H., Webster, N.J., Dan, A., Kercher, K., Bohne, A. & Lechner, C. (2005) Successful ageing in the face of chronic disease. In M.L.Wykle, P.J. Whitehouse & D.L. Morris (Eds.). *Successful ageing through the life span. Intergenerational issues in health* (pp.101-126). New York, Springer Publishing Company.

Kahana, E. & Young, R. (1990). Clarifying the caregiving paradigm: challenges for the future. In D.E. Biegel & Blum, A. (Eds.). *Ageing and Caregiving: Theory, research and policy.* Newbury Park, CA: Sage Publications.

Kalaitzakis, M.E. & Pearce, R.K.B. (2009). The morbid anatomy of dementia in Parkinson's disease. *Acta Neuropathologica, 118,* 587-598.

Kalbe, E., Calabrese, P. Kohn, N., Hilker, R., Riedel, O., Wittchen, H.-U., Dodel, R., Otto, J., Eberbach,G. & Kessler, J. (2008). Screening for cognitive deficits in Parkinson's disease with the Parkinson neuropsychometric dementia assessment (PANDA) instrument. *Parkinsonism and Related Disorders, 14,* 93-101.

Kamrowska, A. (2009). Depresja w chorobie Parkinsona. (Depression in Parkinson's disease). *Polski Merkuriusz Lekarski, XXVII(158),* 170-172. Article in Polish.

Kanda, F., Oishi, K., Sekiguchi, K., Kuga, A., Kobessho, H., Shirafuji, T., Higuchi, M., Ishihara, H. (2008). Characteristics of depression in Parkinson's disease: evaluating with Zung's Self-Rating Depression Scale. *Parkinsonism and Related Disorders,14(1),* 19-23.

Kane, R.A. & Penrod, J.D. (1995). Toward a caregiving policy for the aging family. In R.A. Kane & J.D. Penrod (Eds.). *Family caregiving in an aging society: Policy perspectives* (pp.140-170). Thousand Oaks, CA: Sage.

Kang, G.A., Bronstein, J.M., Masterman, D.L., Redelings, M., Crum, J.A. & Ritz, B. (2005). Clinical characteristics in early Parkinson's disease in a central California population-based study. *Movement Disorders, 20(9),* 1133-1142.

Kapitza, I.G., Kalinina, T.S., Nerobkova, L.N., Voronina, T.A., Klodt, P.M., Narkevich,V.B. & Kudrin, V.S. (2008). Relationship between the severity of hypokinesia induced by neurotoxin 1-methyl-4-phenyl-1,2,3,6-tetrahydropyridine and neurochemical changes in brain structures of C57B1/6 mice. *Bulletin of Experimental Biology and Medicine, 146 (1),* 52-55.

Karantzas, G.C., Evans, L. and Foddy, M. (2010) The role of attachment in current and future parent caregiving. *Journal of Gerontology, 65B*(5), 573-580.

Karlsen, K.H., Larsen, J.P., Tandberg, E. & Jørgensen, K. (1999). Fatigue in patients with Parkinson's disease. *Movement Disorders, 14(2),* 237-241.

Karlsen, K.H., Tandberg, E., Aarsland, D. & Larsen, J.P. (2000). Health related quality of life in Parkinson's disease: A prospective longitudinal study. *Journal of Neurology, Neurosurgery and Psychiatry, 69,* 584-589.

Karnofsky, D.A. & Burchenal, J.H. (1949). The Clinical Evaluation of Chemotherapeutic Agents in Cancer. In C.M. MacLeod (Ed.), *Evaluation of Chemotherapeutic Agents* (p.196). Columbia University Press.

Kaszniak, A.W., Trosset, M.W., Bondi, N.W. & Bayles, K.A. (1992). Procedural learning of Parkinson's disease patients in a serial reaction time task. *Journal of Clinical and Experimental Neuropsychology, 14,* 51.

Katon, W. (1996). The impact of major depression on chronic medical illness. *General Hospital Psychiatry, 18(4),* 215-219.

Kehagia, A.A., Barker, R.A. & Robbins, T.W. (2010). Neuropsychological and clinical heterogeneity of cognitive impairment and dementia in patients with Parkinson's disease. *The Lancet Neurology, 9(12),* 1200-1213.

Kehagia, A.A., Barker, R.A. & Robbins, T.W. (2013). Cognitive Impairment in Parkinson's Disease: The Dual Syndrome Hypothesis. *Neurodegenerative Diseases, 11(2),* 79-92.

Kendall, E. & Buys, N. (1998). An integrated model of psychosocial adjustment following acquired disability. *Journal of Rehabilitation, 64*, 16-20.

Kennedy, I. (2003). Patients are experts in their own field. *British Medical Journal, 326*, 1276-1277.

Kenny, D.A. (2012). Mediation. http://www.davidakenny.net/cm/mediate.htm.

Kenny, D. A., Kashy, D. A., & Bolger, N. (1998). Data analysis in social psychology. In D. Gilbert, S. Fiske, & G. Lindzey (Eds.), *The Handbook of Social Psychology* (Vol. 1, 4th ed., pp. 233-265). Boston, MA: McGraw-Hill.

Kim, J., Knight, B.G. & Flynn Longmire, C.V. (2007) The role of familism values in stress and coping processes among African Americans and white dementia caregivers: effects on mental and physical health. *Health Psychology, 26*, 564-576.

Kim, K.S., Kim, B.J., Kim, K.H., Choe, M.A., Yi, M., Hah, Y.S., Chung, S.J., & Kwon, S.H. (2007). Subjective and objective caregiver burden in Parkinson's disease. *Taehan Kanho Hakhoe Chi, 37*(2), 242-248.

Kim, S.E., Choi, J.Y., Choe, Y.S., Choi, Y. & Lee, W.Y. (2003). Serotonin transporters in the midbrain of Parkinson's disease patients: a study with ^{123}I-beta-CIT SPECT. N. *Nuclear Medicine*, *44,* 870-876.

Kim, Y. & Carver, C.S. (2007). Frequency and difficulty in caregiving among spouses of individuals with cancer: effects of adult attachment and gender. *Psycho-Oncology, 16*, 714-723.

Kim, Y., Carver, C.S., Deci, E.L. & Kasser, T. (2008). Adult attachment and psychological well-being in cancer caregivers: the meditational role of spouses' motives for caregiving. *Health Psychology, 27*(2), S144-S154.

Kim, Y., Kashy, D.A. & Evans, T.V. (2007). Age and attachment style impact stress and depressive symptoms among caregivers: a prospective investigation. *Journal of Cancer Survival, 1,* 35-43.

Kirkpatrick, L.A. & Davies, K.E. (1994). Attachment style, gender and relationship stability: A longitudinal analysis. *Journal of Personality and Social Psychology, 66,* 502-512.

Kirkpatrick, L.A., & Hazan, C. (1994). Attachment styles and close relationships: A four-year prospective study. *Personal Relationships, 1,* 123-142.

Kirsch-Darrow, L., Fernandez, H.F., Marsiske, M., Okun, M.S. & Bowers, D. (2006). Dissociating apathy and depression in Parkinson's disease. *Neurology*, 67, 33-38.

Kitwood, T. (1997). *Dementia reconsidered: the person comes first.* Buckingham, Philadelphia: Open University Press.

Kleiner-Fisman, G., Herzog, J. Fisman, D.N., Tamma, F., Lyons, K.E., Pahwa, R., Lang, A.E. & Deuschl, G. (2006). Subthalamic nucleus deep brain stimulation: summary and meta-analysis of outcomes. *Movement Disorders*, 21(suppl. 14), S290-S304.

Klepac, N., Trkulja, V. & Relja, M. (2008). Nondemented Parkinson disease patients. Is cognitive performance associated with depressive difficulties? *Cognitive Behavioural Neurology, 21(2),* 87-91.

Klos, K.J., Bower, J.H., Josephs, K.A., Matsumoto, J.Y. & Ahlskog, J.E. (2005). Pathological hypersexuality predominantly linked to adjuvant dopamine agonist therapy in Parkinson's disease and multiple system atrophy. *Parkinsonism and Related Disorders, 11*(6), 381-386.

Koerts, J., Leenders, K.L., Koning, M., Bouma, A. & van Beilen, M. (2008). The assessment of depression in Parkinson's disease. *European Journal of Neurology, 15,* 487-492.

Koller, W.C. (1984). Disturbance of recent memory function in parkinsonian patients on anticholinergic therapy. *Cortex, 20,* 307-311.

Koller, W.C., Vetere-Overfield, B., Gray, C., Alexander, C., Chin, T., Dolezal, J., Hassanein, R. & Tanner, C. (1990). Environmental risk factors in Parkinson's disease. *Neurology*, 40, 1218-1221.

Konorski, J. (1969). *Integracyjna działalność mózgu.* (The integrated activity of the brain). Warszawa, Polskie Wydawnictwo Naukowe. In Polish.

Konstam, V., Holmes, W., Wilczeński, F., Baliga, S., Lester, J. & Priest, R. (2003). Meaning in the lives of caregivers of individuals with Parkinson's disease. *Journal of Clinical Psychology in Medical Settings, 10*(1), 17-25.

Kosberg, J.I. & Cairl, R.E. (1986). The Cost of Care Index: a case management tool for screening informal care providers. *The Gerontologist, 26*(3), 273-278.

Kostic, V.S., Agosta, F., Petrovic, I., Galantucci, S., Spica, V. Jecmenica-Lukic, M. & Filippi, M. (2010). Regional patterns of brain tissue loss associated with depression in Parkinson's disease. *Neurology, 75(10),* 857-863.

Kostíc, V.S., Filipović, S.R., Lecić, D., Momcilović, D., Sokić, D. & Sternić (1994). Effect of age at onset on frequency of depression in Parkinson's disease. *Journal of Neurology, Neurosurgery & Psychiatry,57,*1265-1267.

Kotzbauer, P.T., Trojanowski, J.Q. & Lee, V.M. (2001). Lewy body pathology in Alzheimer's disease. *Journal of Moelcular Neuroscience, 17(2),* 225-232.

Krach, P. & Brooks, L.A. (1995). Identifying the responsibilities and needs of working adults who are primary caregivers. *Gerontological Nursing, 2,* 41-50.

Kraepelin, E. (1915). *Psychiatrie* (8th edition). Leipzig: Verlag Von Johann Ambrosius Barth.

Kramer, B.J. (1993a). Expanding the conceptualization of caregiver coping: the importance of relationship-focused coping strategies. *Family Relations*, *42*(4), 383-391.

—. (1993b). Marital history and the prior relationship as predictors of positive and negative outcomes among wife caregivers. *Family Relations*, *42*(4), 367-375.

Kramer, B.J. & Kipnis, S. (1995). Eldercare and work-role conflict: toward an understanding of gender differences in caregiver burden. *The Gerontologist, 35*(3), 340-8.

Kramer, B.J. & Vitaliano, P.P. (1994). Coping: A review of the theoretical frameworks and the measures used among caregivers of individuals with dementia. *Journal of Gerontological Social Work, 23*(1/2), 151-174.

Kramer, J.H., Levin, B.E., Brandt, J. & Delis, D.C. (1989). Differentiation of Alzheimer's, Huntington's and Parkinson's disease patients on the basis of verbal learning characteristics. *Neuropsychology, 3,* 111-120.

Kubler-Ross, E. (1969). *On death and dying*. New York: Macmillan.

Kuhn, W., Müller, T., Gerlach, M., Sofic, E., Fuchs, G., Heye, N., Prautsch, R. & Przuntek, H. (1996). Depression in Parkinson's disease: biogenic amines in CSF of "de novo" patients. *Journal of Neural Transmission, 103(12),*1441-1445.

Kulisevsky, J. & Pagonabarraga, J. (2009). Cognitive impairment in Parkinson's disease: tools for diagnosis and assessment. *Movement Disorders, 24(8),* 1103-1110.

Kulkantrakorn, K. & Jirapramukpitak, T. (2007). A prospective study in one year cumulative incidence of depression after ischemic stroke and Parkinson's disease: a preliminary study. *Journal of Neurological*

Sciences, 263, 165-168.

Kunce, L.J. & Shaver, P.R. (1994). An attachment-theoretical approach to caregiving in romantic relationships. In K. Bartholomew & D. Perlman (Eds.), *Advances in personal relationships* (Vol. 5, pp. 205-237). London: Jessica Kingsley.

Kuopio, A.M., Marttila, R.J., Helenius, H., Toivonen, M. & Rinne, U.K. (2000). The quality of life in Parkinson's disease. *Movement Disorders, 15(2),* 216-223.

Kuran W. (2002). *Żyję z chorobą Parkinsona*. Wydawnictwo Lekarskie, PZWL, Warszawa. (In Polish).

Kuscu, M.K., Dural, U., Onen, P., Yasa, Y., Yayla, M., Basaran, G., Turhal, S. & Bekiroglu, N. (2009). The association between individual attachment patterns, the perceived social support, and the psychological well-being of Turkish informal caregivers. *Psycho-Oncology, 18*, 927-935.

Kuzis, G., Sabe, L., Tiberti, C., Leiguarda,R. & Starkstein, S.E. (1997). Cognitive functions in major depression and Parkinson's disease. *Archives of Neurology*, 54, 982-986.

Lai, D.W.L. & Thomson, C. (2011). The impact of perceived adequacy of social supporton caregiving burden of family caregivers. *Families in Society: The Journal of Contemporary Social Services*, 92(1), 99-106.

Lamura, G., Mnich, E., Nolan, M., Wojszel, B., Krevers, B., Mestheneos, L., & Döhner, H; EUROFAMCARE Group (2008). Family carers' experiences using support services in Europe: empirical evidence from the EUROFAMCARE study. *The Gerontologist, 48*(6), 752-771.

Lamura, G., Wojszel, B., Mnich, E., Krevers, B., McKee, K. & Mestheneos, E. (2006). Experiences and Preferences of Family Carers in the Use of Care and Support Services. In EUROFAMCARE Consortium (Eds). *Services for Supporting Family Carers of Elderly People in Europe: Characteristics, Coverage and Usage. Trans-European Survey Report.* Hamburg: Hamburg University Medical Centre of Hamburg-Eppendorf.

Landes, A.M., Sperry, S.D., Strauss, M.E., & Geldmacher, D.S. (2001). Apathy in Alzheimer's disease. *Journal of the American Geriatric Society, 49*(12), 1700-1707.

Lang, A.E. (2011). A critical appraisal of the premotor symptoms of Parkinson's disease: potential usefulness in early diagnosis and design of neuroprotective trials. *Movement Disorders,* 26(5), 775-783.

Lang, A.E. & Lozano, A.M. (1998). Parkinson's disease. *New England Journal of Medicine*, 339, 1130-1143.

Lang, F.R., & Carstensen, L.L. (1994). Close emotional relationships in late life: further support for proactive aging in the social domain. *Psychology of Aging, 9*(2), 315-24.

Lange, K.W., Robbins, T.W., Marsden, C.D., James, M., Owen, A.M. & Paul, G.M. (1992). L-dopa withdrawal in Parkinson's disease selectively impairs cognitive performance in tests sensitive to frontal lobe dysfunction. *Psychopharmacology, 107,* 394-404.

Lange, K.W., Sahakian, B.J., Quinn, N.P., Marsden, C.D. & Robbins, T.W. (1995). Comparison of executive and visuospatial memory function in Huntington's disease and dementia of Alzheimer-type matched for degree of dementia. *Journal of Neurology, Neurosurgery and Psychiatry, 58,* 598-606.

Lawrence, R.H., Tennstedt, S.L. & Assman, S.F. (1998). Quality of the caregiver – care recipient relationship: does it offset negative consequences of caregiving for family caregivers? *Psychology and Aging, 13*(1), 150-158.

Lawrence, V., Murray, J., Samsi, K. & Banerjee, S. (2008). Attitudes and support needs of black Caribbean, south Asian and white British carers of people with dementia in the UK. *The British Journal of Psychiatry, 193,* 240-246.

Lawton, M.P. & Brody, E.M. (1969). Assessment of older people: self-maintaining and instrumental activities of daily living. *The Gerontologist, 9,* 179-186.

Lawton, M. P., Kleban, M. H., & Di Carlo, E. (1984). Psychological well-being in the aged: Factorial and conceptual dimensions. *Research & Aging, 6*(1), 67-97.

Lawton, M.P., Kleban, M.H., Moss, M., Rovine, M., & Glicksman, A. (1989). Measuring caregiving appraisal. *Journal of Gerontology, 44B*(3), P61-P71.

Lawton, M.P., Moss, M., Kleban, M.H., Glicksman, A., & Rovine, M. (1991). A two-factor model of caregiving appraisal and psychological well-being. *Journal of Gerontology, 46B*(4), P181-P189.

Lazarus, R. (1993). Coping theory and research: Past, present and future. *Psychosomatic Medicine, 55,* 234-247.

Lazarus, R. & DeLongis, A. (1982). Psychological stress and coping in aging. *American Psychologist, 38,* 245-254.

Lazarus, R. & Folkman, S. (1984). *Stress, Appraisal and Coping*. New York: Springer.

Lazarus, L.W., Newton, N., Cohler, B., Lesser, J. & Schweon, C. (1987). Frequency and presentation of depressive symptoms in patients with primary degenerative dementia. *American Journal of Psychiatry. 144*(1), 41-45.

Leentjens, A.F.G. (2004). Depression in Parkinson's disease: conceptual issues and clinical challenges. *Journal of Geriatric Psychiatry and Neurology*, *17,*120-126.

Leentjens, A.F., Dujardin,K., Marsh, L., Martinez-Martin, P., Richard, I.H., Starkstein, S.E., Weintraub, D., Sampaio, C., Poewe, W., Rascol, O., Stebbins, G.T. & Goetz, C.G. (2008). Anxiety rating scales in Parkinson's disease: critique and recommendations. *Movement Disorders, 23(14)*, 2015-2025.

Leentjens, A.F.G., Lousberg, R. & Verhey, F.R.J. (2001). The psychometric properties of the Hospital Anxiety and Depression Scale in patients with Parkinson's disease. *Acta Neuropsychiatrica, 13,* 83-85.

Leentjens, A.F.G., Marinus, J., Van Hilten, J.J., Lousberg, R. & Verhey, F.R.J. (2003). The contribution of somatic symptoms to the diagnosis of depressive disorder in Parkinson's disease: a discriminant analytic approach. *The Journal of Neuropsychiatry and Clinical Neurosciences*, *15,* 74-77.

Leentjens, A.F.G., Verhey, F.R.J., Lousberg, R., Spitsbergen, H. & Wilmink, F.W. (2000). The validity of the Hamilton and Montgomery-Åsberg Depression Rating Scales as screening and diagnostic tools for depression in Parkinson's disease. *International Journal of Geriatric Psychiatry*, *15,* 644-649.

Leentjens, A.F.G., Verhey, F.R.J., Luijckx, G.J. & Troost, J. (2000). The validity of the Beck Depression Inventory as a screening and diagnostic instrument for depression in patients with Parkinson's disease. *Movement Disorders*, *15(6),* 1221-1224.

Leentjens, A.F., Vreeling, F.W., Luijckx, G.J. & Verhey, F.R. (2003). SSRIs in the treatment of depression in Parkinson's disease. *International Journal Geriatric Psychiatry,18(6),* 552-554.

Lee, T.M., Chan, C.C., Ho, S.L. & Li, L.S. (2005). Prose memory in patients with idiopathic Parkinson's disease. *Parkinsonism and Related Disorders. 11(7),* 453-8.

Lees, A.J. (1981). Early diagnosis of Parkinson's disease. *British Journal of Hospital Medicine, 26*(5), 511-2, 517-8.

—. (2005). Alternatives to levodopa in the intial treatment of early Parkinson's disease. *Drugs and Aging*, 22,731-740.

Lees, A.J. & Smith, E. (1983). Cognitive deficits in the early stages of Parkinson's disease. *Brain*, *106,* 257-270.

Leiber, L., Plumb, M.M., Gerstenzang, M.L. & Holland, J. (1976). The communication of affection between cancer patients and their spouses. *Psychosomatic Medicine, 38,* 379-389.

Leiknes, I., Tysnes, O.B., Aarsland, D. & Larsen, J.P. (2010). Caregiver distress associated with neuropsychiatric problems in patients with early Parkinson's disease: the Norwegian ParkWest study. *Acta Neurologica Scandinavica, 122*(6), 418-424.

Lemert, E. (1967). *Human deviance, social problems, and social control.* Englewood Cliffs, N.J.: Prentice-Hall.

Leroi, I., Harbishettar, V., Andrews, M., McDonald, K., Byrne, E.J. & Burns, A. (2012). Carer burden in apathy and impulse control disorders in Parkinson's disease. *International Journal Geriatric Psychiatry, 27(2),*160-166.

Leroi, I., McDonald, K., Pantula, H. & harbishettar, V. (2012). Cognitive impairment in Parkinson's disease: impact on quality of life, disability and caregiver burden. *Journal of Geriatric Psychiatry and Neurology, 25,* 208-214.

Lesch, K.P. & Mössner, R. (1998). Genetically driven variation in serotonin uptake: is there a link to affective spectrum, neurodevelopmental, and neurodegenerative disorders? *Biological Psychiatry*, *44(3),* 179-192.

Levenson, R.W., Cartensen, L.L. & Gottman, J.M. (1993) Long-term marriage: age, gender and satisfaction. *Psychology and Aging, 8*, 301-313.

Levin, B.E. & Katzen, H.L. (1995). Early cognitive changes and nondementing behavioural abnormalities in Parkinson's disease. In W.J. Weiner & A.E. Lang (Eds.), *Advances in Neurology: Vol. 65. Behavioural Neurology of Movement Disorders* (pp. 85-95). New York: Raven Press.

Levin, B.E. & Katzen, H.L. (2005). Early cognitive changes and nondementing behavioral abnormalities in Parkinson's disease. *Advances in Neurology, 96*, 84-94.

Levin, B.E., Llabre, M.M. &Weiner, W.J. (1988). Parkinson's disease and depression: psychometric properties of the Beck Depression Inventory. *Journal of Neurology, Neurosurgery and Psychiatry, 51(11),* 1401-1404.

Levin, B.E., Llabre, B.M. & Weiner, W.J. (1989). Cognitive impairments associated with early Parkinson's disease. *Neurology, 39,* 557-561.

Levin, B.E., Llabre, M.M., Reisman, S., Weiner, W.J., Sanchez-Ramos, J., Singer, C., Brown, M.C. (1991). Visuospatial impairment in Parkinson's disease. *Neurology, 41(3),* 365-369.

Levy, G. (2007). The relationship of Parkinson disease with aging. *Archives of Neurology, 64(9),* 1242-1246.

Levy, G., Jacobs, D.M., Tang, M.X., Côté, L.J., Louis, E.D., Alfaro,B.,

Mejia, H., Stern, Y. & Marder, K. (2002). Memory and executive function impairment predict dementia in Parkinson's disease. *Movement Disorders, 17(6),* 1221-1226.

Levy, G., Tang, M.X., Côté, L.J., Louis, E.D., Alfaro,B., Mejia, Stern, Y. & Marder, K. (2000). Motor impairment in PD: relationship to incident dementia and age. *Neurology, 55(4),* 539-544.

Levy, G., Tang, M.X., Louis, E.D., Côté, L.J., Alfaro,B., Mejia, H., Stern, Y. & Marder, K. (2002). The association of incident dementia with mortality in PD. *Neurology, 59,* 1708-1713.

Lewis, M.L., Hepburn, K., Narayan, S. & Kirk, L.N. (2005) Relationship matters in dementia caregiving. *American Journal of Alzheimer's Disease and Other Dementias, 20*(6): 341-347.

Lewis, S.J.G., Dove, A., Robbins, T.W., Barker, R.A. & Owen, A.M. (2003). Cognitive impairments in early Parkinson's disease are accompanied by reductions in activity in frontostriatal neural circuitry. *The Journal of Neuroscience, 23(15),* 6351-6356.

Lewis, S.J.G, Slabosz, A., Robbins, T.W., Barker, R.A. & Owen, A.M. (2005). Dopaminergic basis for deficits in working memory but not attentional set-shifting in Parkinson's disease. *Neuropsychologia, 43(6),* 823-832.

Lewy, F.H. (1923). *Die Lehre vom tonus und der Bewegung zugleich systematische Untersuchungen zur Klijik, Physiologie, Pathologie und Pathogenese der Paralysis agitans.* Berlin: Springer Verlag.

Lezak, M.D., Howieson, D.B. & Loring, D.W. (2004). *Neuropsychological Assessment* (4th ed.). New York: Oxford University Press.

Lieberman A. (2006). Depression in Parkinson's disease -- a review. *Acta Neurologica Scandinavica,113(1)*, 1-8.

Lieberman, A.N. (1974). Parkinson's disease: a clinical review. *American Journal of Medical Sciences, 267(2),* 66-80.

Lieberman, A., Dziatolowski, M., Kupersmith, M., Serby, M., Goodgold, A., Korein J. & Goldstein, M. (1979). Dementia in Parkinson disease. *Annals of Neurology*, *6,* 355-359.

Lifton, R.J. (1988). Understanding the traumatised self. In J.P. Wilson, Z. Harel & B. Kahana (Eds.). *Human adaptation to extreme stress* (pp.7-31). New York: Plenum.

Lim, S.Y. & Lang, A.E. (2010). The nonmotor symptoms of Parkinson's disease--an overview. *Movement Disorders*, *25, Suppl. 1,* S123-30.

Link, B.G., Cullen, F.T., Frank, J. & Wozniack, J.F. (1987). The social rejection of former mental patients: Understanding why labels matter. *American Journal of Sociology, 92*, 461-500.

Litvan, I., Bhatia, K.P., Burn, D.J., Goetz, C.G., Lang, A.E., McKeith, I., Quinn, N., Sethi, K.D., Shults C. & Wenning, G.K. (2003). SIC task force appraisal of clinical diagnostic criteria for Parkinsonian disorders. *Movement Disorders, 18*, 467-486.

Litvan, I., Mohr, E., Williams, J., Gomez, C. & Chase, T.N. (1991). Differential memory and executive functions in demented patients with Parkinson's and Alzheimer's disease. *Journal of Neurology, Neurosurgery and Psychiatry, 54(1),* 25-29.

Livneh, H. & Antonak, R.F. (1997). *Psychosocial adaptation to chronic illness and disability*. Gaithersburg, Maryland: Aspen Publishers Incorporated.

Livneh, H. & Martz, E. (2007). An introduction to coping theory and research. In E.Martz & H.Liveneh, *Coping with chronic illness and disability. Theoretical, empirical and clinical aspects* (pp. 3-28). New York: Springer.

Lloret, S.P., Rossi, M., Merello, M., Rascol, O. & Cardinali, D.P. (2011). Nonmotor symptoms groups in Parkinson's disease patients: results of a pilot, exploratory study. *Parkinson's disease*, article ID: 473579, doi:10.4061/2011/473579.

Local Government Association (2012). White Paper on Social Care and Funding Update LGA On-the-day briefing 11 July 2012. Retrieved from: http://www.local.gov.uk/web/guest/briefings-and-responses/-/journal_content /56/10171/3644927/ARTICLE-TEMPLATE

Locke, H.J. & Wallace, K.M. (1959). Short marital adjustment and prediction tests: their reliability and validity. *Marriage and Family Living, 21,* 251-255.

Logsdon, R.G. & Teri, L. (1995). Depression in Alzheimer's disease patients: caregivers as surrogate reporters. *Journal of the American Geriatrics Society, 43(2),* 150-155.

Lojek, E. (1999). Zaburzenia emocjonalne w wybranych chorobach struktur podkorowych mózgu. (Emotional disorders in subcortical diseases). In A. Herzyk & A. Borkowska (Eds). *Neuropsychologia emocji: poglady, badania, klinika (pp. 131-150).* Lublin: Wydawnictwo UMCS. In Polish.

Lökk, J. (2008). Caregiver strain in Parkinson's disease and the impact of disease duration. *European Journal Physical and Rehabilitation Medicine, 44(1),* 39-45.

Longmire, C.V.F & Knight, R.G. (2011). Confirmatory factor analysis of a brief version of the Zarit Burden Interview in black and white dementia caregivers. *The Gerontologist, 51(4),* 453-462.

Looi, J.C.L., Matias, M. & Ruzich, M.J. (2005). Conceptualization of depression in Parkinson's disease. *Neuropsychiatric Disease and Treatment, 1(2),* 135-143.

Loranger, A.W., Goodell, H., McDowell, F.H., Lee, J.E. & Sweet, R.D. (1972). Intellectual impairment in Parkinson's syndrome. *Brain, 95,* 405-412.

Losada, A., Marquez-Gonzalez, M., Knight, B.G., Yanguas, J., Sayegh, P., Romero-Moreno, R. (2010). Psychosocial factors and caregivers' distress: effects of familism and dysfunctional thoughts. *Aging and Mental Health, 14(2)*, 193-202.

Lowe, J.S., Mayer, R.J. & Landon, M. (1996). Pathological significance of Lewy bodies in dementia. In R. Perry, I. McKeith & E.Perry (Eds.). *Dementia with Lewy bodies.*(pp. 195-203). New York: Cambridge University Press.

Lubkin, I.M. & Larsen, P.D. (2006). *Chronic Illness. Impact and Interventions* (6th edition). Boston, Toronto, London, Singapore: Jones and Bartlett Publishers.

Luria A.R. (1976). *Problemy neuropsychologii i neurolingwistyki* (Basic Problems of Neurolinguistics). Warszawa: Państwowe Wydawnictwo Naukowe. (In Polish).

Lyonette, C. & Yardley, L. (2003). The influence on carer wellbeing of motivations to care for older people and the relationship with the care recipient. *Ageing and Society,23,*487-506.

Lyons, K.S., Sayer, A.G., Archbold, P.G., Hornbrook, M.C. & Stewart, B.J. (2007) The enduring and contextual effects of physical health and depression on care dyad mutuality. *Research in Nursing and Health, 30,* 84-98.

Lyons, K.S., Stewart, B.J., Archbold, P.G., & Carter, J.H. (2009). Optimism, pessimism, mutuality, and gender: predicting 10-year role strain in Parkinson's disease spouses. *The Gerontologist, 49*(3), 378-387.

Lyons, K.S., Stewart, B.J., Archbold, P.G., Carter, J.H. & Perrin, N.A. (2004) Pessimism and optimism as early warning signs for compromised health for caregivers of patients with Parkinson's disease. *Nursing Research, 53*(6): 354-362.

Lyons, K.S., Zarit, S.H., Sayer, A.G. & Whitlatch, C.J. (2002) Caregiving as a dyadic process: perspectives from caregivers and receivers. *Journal of Gerontology, 57B*(3), P195-P204.

Machin, E. (1984) A survey of the behaviour of the elderly and their supporters at home. Unpublished M.Sc. thesis, University of Birmingham, U.K. (1980). In C. Gilleard (Ed.) *Living with dementia.* London: Croom Helm.

Macht, M., Schwarz, R., & Ellgring, H. (2005). Patterns of psychological problems in Parkinson's disease. *Acta Neurologica Scandinavica, 111,* 95-101.

Mackinnon, D.P., Warsi, G. & Dwyer, J.H. (1995). A Simulation Study of Mediated Effect Measures. *Multivariate Behavioural Research, 30(1),* 41.

MacNeil, G., Kosberg, J.I., Durkin, D.W., Dooley, W.K., Decoster, J., & Williamson, G.M. (2010). Caregiver mental health and potentially harmful caregiving behavior: the central role of caregiver anger. *The Gerontologist, 50(1),* 76-86.

Magai, C. (2001). Emotions over the life span. In J.E. Birren & K.W. Schaie (Eds.), *Handbook of Psychology of Aging* (5th edition, p.419;). London, UK; Academic Press, Elsevier.

—. (2008). Attachment in middle and later life. In J. Cassidy & P. Shaver (Eds.), *Handbook of attachment: Theory, research and applications* (2nd edition, chapter 24). New York, Guilford Press.

Magai, C. & Cohen, C.I. (1998). Attachment style and emotion regulation in dementia patients and their relation to caregiver burden. *Journal of Gerontology, 53B(3),* P147-P154.

Magai, C., Cohen, C.I., Culver, C., Gomberg, D., & Malatesta, C. (1997). Relation between premorbid personality and patterns of emotion expression in mid- to late-stage dementia. *International Journal of Geriatric Psychiatry, 12*(11), 1092-9.

Magai, C., Cohen, C., Milburn, N., Thorpe, B., McPherson, R. & Peralta, D. (2001). Attachment styles in older European American and African American adults. *Journal of Gerontology, 56B*, S28-S35.

Magai, C., Cohen, C.I. Milburn, N., Thorpe, B., McPherson, R., Peralta, D. & Evans-Ross, A. (1999). Paper presented at the Gerontological Society of America, San Fransico.

Magai, C., Distal. N. & Liker, R. (1995). Emotion socialization, attachment and patterns of adult emotional traits. *Cognition and Emotion, 9,* 461-481.

Magai, C., Hunziker, Mesias, W. & Culver, L.C. (2000) Adult attachment styles and emotional biases. *International Journal of Behavioural Development, 24*, 301-309.

Magai, C. & McFadden, S.H. (1995) *The role of emotions in social and personality development: history, theory and research*. New York: Plenum Press.

Magai, C., & Passman, V. (1997). The interpersonal basis of emotional behavior and emotion regulation in adulthood. In M.P. Lawton & K.W. Schaie (Eds.), *Annual Review of Gerontology and Geriatrics, (Vol.17,* pp.104-137). New York: Springer.

Maher, J. & Green, H. (2002). *Carers 2000*. London: Office for National Statistics.

Mahoney, F.I. & Barthel, D.W. (1965). Functional evaluation: the BARTHEL index. *Maryland State Medical Journal, 14,* 61-65.

Mahoney, A.H., Dalby J.T. & King, M.C. (1998). Cognitive failures and stress. *Psychological Reports*, *82,* 1432-1434.

Mahoney, A.H., Regan, C., Katona, C. & Livingstone, G. (2005). Anxiety and depression in family caregivers of people with Alzheimer Disease. *American Journal of Geriatric Psychiatry, 13(9),* 795-801.

Maier, W., Buller, R., Philipp, M. & Heuser, I. (1988). The Hamilton Anxiety Scale: reliability, validity and sensitivity to change in anxiety and depressive disorders. *Journal of Affective Disorders*, *14*(1), 61-68.

Majerovitz, S.D. (1995). Role of family adaptability in the psychological adjustment of spouse caregivers to patients with dementia. *Psychology and Aging, 10,* 447-457.

Manni, R., Terzaghi, M., Pacchetti, C. & Nappi, G. (2007). Sleep disorders in Parkinson's disease: facts and new perspectives. *Neurological Sciences, 28,* S1-S5.

Marder, K., Leung, D., Tang, M., Bell, K., Dooneief, G., Côté, L., Stern, Y. & Mayeux, R. (1991). Are demented patients with Parkinson's disease accurately reflected in prevalence surveys? A survival analysis. *Neurology,41(8),* 1240-1243.

Marder, K., Tang, M.X., Côté, L., Stern, Y. & Mayeux, R. (1995). The frequency and associated risk factors for dementia in patients with Parkinson's disease. *Archives of Neurology, 52,* 695-701.

Marie, R.M., Barre, L., Dupuy, B., Viader, F., Defer, G. & Baron, J.C. (1999). Relationships between striatal dopamine denervation and frontal executive tests in Parkinson's disease. *Neuroscience Letters, 260,* 77-80.

Markham, C.H., Treciokas, L.J. & Diamond, S.G. (1974). Parkinson's disease and levodopa. A five-year follow-up and review. *Western Journal of Medicine, 121(3),* 188-206.

Markiewicz, D., Reis, M. & Gold, D.P. (1997) An exploration of attachment styles and personality traits in caregiving for dementia patients. *International Journal of Aging and Human Development, 45,* 111-132.

Markus, H. & Nurius, P. (1986). Possible selves. *American Psychologist, 41*(9), 954-969.

Marriott, A., Donaldson, C., Tarrier, N. & Burns, A. (2000). Effectiveness of cognitive behavioural family intervention in reducing the burden of care in carers of patients with Alzheimer's disease. *British Journal of Psychiatry, 176*, 557-562.

Marsh, G.G. & Markham, C.H. (1973). Does levodopa alter depression and psychopathology in Parkinsonism patients? *Journal of Neurology, Neurosurgery and Psychiatry*, *36,* 925-935.

Marsh, G.G., Markham, C.M. & Ansel, R. (1971). Levodopa's awakening effect on patients with Parkinsonosm. *Journal of Neurology, Neurosurgery and Psychiatry, 34,* 209-218.

Marsh, L., McDonald, W.M., Cummings, J., Ravina, B. and the NINDS/NIMH Work Group on Depression and Parkinson's Disease. (2006). Provisional Diagnostic Criteria for depression in Parkinson's disease: report of an NINDS/NIMH work group. *Movement Disorders, 21(2),* 148-158.

Marsh, L., Williams, J.R., Rocco, M., Grill, S., Munro, C., Dawson, T.M. (2004). Psychiatric comorbidities in patients with Parkinson disease and psychosis. *Neurology, 63*(2), 293-300.

Martilla, R.G. & Rinne, U.K. (1976). Dementia in Parkinson's disease. *Acta Neurologica Scandinavica, 54,* 431-441.

Martilla, R.G., Rinne, U.K. & Martilla, R.J. (1991). Progression and survival in Parkinson's disease. *Acta Neurologica Scandinavica, 84(S136),* 24-28.

Martin, G.N. (1998). Apraxias and other motor systems disorders. In *Human Neuropsychology*, (p.260). Harlow, England: Prentice Hall.

Martin, M. (1983). Cognitive failure: Everyday and laboratory performance. *Bulletin of the Psychonomic Society*, *21,* 97-100.

Martin, W.E., Loewenson, R.B., Resch, J.A. & Baker, A.B. (1973). Parkinson's disease. Clinical analysis of 100 patients. *Neurology. 23(8),* 783-790.

Martin-Carrasco, M., Otermin, P., Perez-Camo, V., Aguera, L., Martin, M.J., & Gobartt, A.L., Pons, S., & Balana, M. (2010), EDUCA study: Psychometric properties of the Spanish version of the Zarit Caregiver Burden Scale. *Aging and Mental Health, 14*(6), 705-711.

Martinez-Martin, P., Arroyo, S., Rojo-Abuin, J.M., Rodriguez-Blazquez, C., Frades, B., de Pedro Cuesta, J,; Longitudinal Parkinson's Disease Patient Study (Estudio longitudinal de pacientes con enfermedad de Parkinson-ELEP) Group. (2008). Burden, perceived health status, and mood among caregivers of Parkinson's disease patients. *Movement Disorders, 23*(12), 1673-1680.

Martinez-Martin, P., Benito-Leon, J., Alonso, F., Catalan, M.J., Pondal, M. & Zamarbide, I. (2004). Health-related quality of life evaluation by proxy in Parkinson's disease: approach using PDQ-8 and EuroQoL-

5D. *Movement Disorders, 19,* 312-318.

Martínez-Martín, P., Benito-León, J., Alonso, F., Catalán, M.J., Pondal, M., Zamarbide, I., Tobías, A. & de Pedro, J. (2005). Quality of life of caregivers in Parkinson's disease. *Quality of Life Research, 14*(2), 463-472.

Martínez-Martín, P., Forjaz, M.J., Frades-Payo, B., Rusiñol, A.B., Fernández-García, J.M., Benito-León, J., Arillo, V.C., Barberá, M.A., Sordo, M.P. & Catalán, M.J. (2007). Caregiver burden in Parkinson's disease. *Movement Disorders, 22*(7), 924-931.

Massano, J. & Garrett, C. (2012). Deep brain stimulation and cognitive decline in Parkinson's disease: a clinical review. *Frontiers in Neurology, 3, art.. 66*, 1-13.

Massman, P.J., Delis, D.C., Butters, N., Levin, B.E. & Salmon, D.P. (1990). Are all subcortical dementias alike?: Verbal learning and memory in Parkinson's and Huntington's disease patients. *Journal of Clinical and Experimental Neuropsychology, 12,* 729-744.

Mast, M.E. (1995). Adult uncertainty in illness: A critical review of research. *Scholarly Inquiry for Nursing Practice: An International Journal, 9*(1), 3-24.

Mathews, C.G. & Haaland, K.Y. (1979). The effect of symptom duration on cognitive and motor performance in parkinsonism. *Neurology*, *29,* 951-956.

Matison, R., Mayeux, R., Rosen, J. & Fahn, S. (1982). "Tip-of-the-tongue" phenomenon in Parkinson's disease. *Neurology, 32(5),* 567-570.

Maurin, J.T. & Boyd, C.B. (1990). Burden of mental illness on the family: A critical review. *Archives of Psychiatric Nursing, 4,* 99-107.

Mausbach, B.T., Aschbacher, K., Patterson, T. L., Ancoli-Israel, S., von Känel, R., Mills, P.J., Dimsdale, J. E., Grant, I. (2006) Avoidant coping partially mediates the relationship between patient problem behaviors and depressive symptoms in spousal Alzheimer caregivers. *American Journal of Geriatric Psychiatry, 14*(4), 299-306.

Mayberg, H.S. (2003). Modulating dysfunctional limbic-cortical circuits in depression: towards development of brain-based algorithms for diagnosis and optimized treatment. *British Medical Bulletin*, *65,* 193-207.

Mayberg, H.S., Starkstein, S.E., Sadzot, B., Preziosi, T., Andrezejewski, P.L., Dannals, R.F., Wagner, H.N. Jr. & Robinson, R.G. (1990). Selective hypometabolism in the inferior frontal lobe in depressed patients with Parkinson's disease. *Annals of Neurology*, *28(1),* 57-64.

Mayeux, R. (1984) Behavioural manifestations of movement disorders.

Neurologic Clinics, *2(3),* 527-540.

Mayeux, R., Stern Y., Cote, L. & Williams, J.B.W. (1984). Altered serotonin metabolism in depressed patients with Parkinson's disease. *Neurology*, *34,* 642-646.

Mayeux, R., Stern, Y., Rosen, J. & Leventhal, J. (1981). Depression, intellectual impairment and Parkinson's disease. *Neurology*, *31,* 645-650.

Mayeux, R., Stern, Y., Sano, M., Côté, L. & Williams, J.B. (1987). Clinical and biochemical correlates of bradyphrenia in Parkinson's disease. *Neurology, 37(7),* 1130-1134.

Mayeux, R., Stern, Y., Williams, J.B.W., Cote, L. Frantz, A. & Dyrenfurth, I. (1986). Clinical and biochemical features of depression in Parkinson's disease. *American Journal of Psychiatry*, *43,* 756-759.

McBride, M., Morioka-Douglas, N., & Yeo, G. (1996). Aging and health: Asian and Pacific Islander American elders (2nd ed). SGEC Working Paper Series # 3, Ethnogeriatric Reviews. Stanford, CA: Stanford Geriatric Education Center.

McDonald, W.M., Holtzheimer, P.E., Haber, M., Vitek, J.L., McWhorter, K. & DeLong, M. (2006). Validity of the 30-item Geriatric Depression Scale in patients with Parkinson's disease. *Movement Disorders*, *21(10),* 1618-1622.

McDonald, W.M., Richard, I.H. & DeLong, M.R. (2003). Prevalence, etiology and treatment of depression in Parkinson's disease. *Biological Psychiatry*, *54,* 363-375.

McKeith, I.G., Dickson, D.W., Lowe, J., Emre, M., O'Brien, J.T., Feldman, H., et al.; Consortium on DLB (2005). Diagnosis and management of dementia with Lewy bodies: third report of the DLB Consortium. *Neurology, 65*, 1863-1872.

McLeod, J.D. (1993). Spouse concordance for depressive disorders in a community sample. *Journal of Affective Disorders, 27*(1), 43-52.

McMillan, S.C. (2005). Interventions to facilitate family caregiving at the end of life. *Journal of Palliative Medicine, 8, Supplement 1,* S132-S139.

McNamara, P., Durso, R. & Brown, A. (2003). Relation of 'sense of self' to executive function performance in Parkinson's disease. *Cognitive Behavioural Neurology, 14,* 139-148.

McNamara, P., Durso, R. & Harris, E. (2008). Alterations of the sense of self and personality in Parkinson's disease. *International Journal of Geriatric Psychiatry, 23*, 79-84.

McRae, C., Diem, G., Vo, A., O'Brien, C. & Seeberger, L. (2002). Reliability of measurements of patient health status: a comparison of physician, patient, and caregiver ratings. *Parkinsonism and Related Disorders, 8,* 187-192.

McRae, C., Fazio, E., Hartsock, G., Kelley, L., Urbanski, S. & Russell, D. (2009). Predictors of loneliness in caregivers of persons with Parkinson's disease. *Parkinsonism and Related Disorders, 15*(8), 554-557.

McRae, C., Sherry, P. & Roper, K. (1999). Stress and family functioning among caregivers of persons with Parkinson's disease. *Parkinsonism and Related Disorders, 5*(1-2), 69-75.

Meara, J., Bhowmick, B.K. & Hobson, P. (1999). Accuracy of diagnosis in patients with presumed Parkinson's disease. *Age and Ageing, 28*(2), 99-102.

Meara, J., Mitchelmore, E. & Hobson, P. (1999). Use of the GDS-15 Geriatric Depression Scale as a screening instrument for depressive symptomatology in patients with Parkinson's disease and their carers in the community. *Age and Ageing, 28,* 35-38.

Meier, M. & Martin, W.E. (1970). Intellectual changes associated with levodopa therapy. *Journal of the American Medical Association, 213*(3), 465-466.

Melzer, T.R., Watts, R., MacAskill, M.R., Pitcher, T.L., Livingston, L., Keenan, R.J., Dalrymple-Alford, J.C. & Anderson, T.J. (2012). Grey matter atrophy in cognitively impaired Parkinson's disease. *Journal of Neurology, Neurosurgery and Psychiatry*, 83(2), 188-194.

Menza, M., Marin, H., Kaufman, K., Mark, M. & Lauritano, A.B. (2004). Citalopram treatment of depression in Parkinson's disease: the impact on anxiety, disability and cognition. *The Journal of Neuropsychiatry and Clinical Neurosciences, 16,* 315-319.

Menza, M.A. & Mark, M.H. (1994). Parkinson's disease and depression: the relationship to disability and personality. *Journal of Neuropsychiatry and Clinical Neuroscience, 6*(2), 165-169.

Menza, M.A., Robertson-Hoffman, D.E. & Bonapace, A.S. (1993). Parkinson's disease and anxiety: comorbidity with depression. *Biological Psychiatry, 34(7),* 465-470.

Menza, M.A., Sage, J., Marshall, E., Cody, R. & Duvoisin, R. (1990). Mood changes and "On-Off" phenomena in Parkinson's Disease. *Movement Disorders, 5,* 148-151.

Merschdorf, U., Berg, D., Csoti, I., Fornadi, F., Merz, B., Naumann, M., Becker, G. & Supprian, T. (2003). Psychopathological symptoms of depression in Parkinson's disease compared to major depression. *Psychopathology, 36,* 221-225.

Meyler, D., Stimpson, J.P., & Peek, M.K. (2007). Health concordance within couples: a systematic review. *Social Science and Medicine, 64*(11), 2297-2310.

Mickelson, K.D., Kessler, R.C. & Shaver, P.R. (1997) Adult attachment in a nationally representative sample. *Journal of Personality and Social Psychology, 74*, 1092-1106.

Middleton, F.A. & Strick, P.L. (2000). Basal ganglia and cerebellar loops: motor and cognitive circuits. *Brain Research Review, 31(2-3),* 236-250.

Miesen, B. (1992) Attachment theory and dementia. In G. Jones & B. Miesen (Eds.), *Caregiving in dementia: Research and applications* (Vol. 1, pp. 38-56). London: Routledge.

Miller, B., & Montgomery, A. (1990). Family caregivers and limitations in social activities. *Research in Aging. 12*(1), 72-93.

Miller, E. (1971). On the nature of the memory disorder in presenile dementia. N*europsychologia, 9,* 75-81.

—. (1984). *Recovery and management of neuropsychological impairments*. Chichester: John Wiley & Sons.

—. (1985). Possible frontal impairment in Parkinson's disease: a test using a measure of verbal fluency. *British Journal of Clinical Psychology, 24,* 211-212.

Miller, E., Berrios, G.E. & Politynska, B.E. (1987). The adverse effect of benzhexol on memory in Parkinson's disease. *Acta Psychiatrica Scandinavica, 76:* 278-282.

Miller, E., Berrios, G.E. & Politynska, B. (1996). Caring for someone with Parkinson's disease: Factors that contribute to distress. *International Journal of Geriatric Psychiatry, 11,* 263-268.

Miller, E. & Morley, S. (1986). *Investigating abnormal behavior*. London: Weidenfeld & Nicolson.

Miller, E. & Morris, R.G.(1993). *The psychology of dementia*. Chichester: John Wiley & Sons Ltd.

Miller, N.E. (1980). The measurement of mood in senile brain disease: examiner ratings and self-reports. *Proceedings of the Annual Meeting of the American Psychopathological Association. 69,* 97-122.

Miller, N., Noble, E., Jones, D., Allcock, L. & Burn, D.J. (2008). How do I sound to me? Perceived changes in communication in Parkinson's disease. *Clinical Rehabilitation, 22(1),*14-22.

Mindham R.H.S. (1970). Psychiatric symptoms in Parkinsonism. *Journal of Neurology, Neurosurgery and Psychiatry, 33,* 188-191.

Mindham, R.H.S., Marsden, C.D. & Parkes, J.D. (1976). Psychiatric symptoms during L-dopa therapy for Parkinson's disease and their relationship to physical disability. *Psychological Medicine, 6,* 23-33.

Minuchin, S. (1974). *Families and family therapy.* Cambridge, MA.: Harvard University Press.

Miodek, A., Szemraj, P., Kocur, J. & Ryś, A. (2007). Masked depression-history and present days. *Polski Merkuriusz Lekarski, 23(133),* 78-80. (In Polish).

Mitrani, V.B., Lewis, J.E., Feaster, D.J., Czaja, S.J., Eisdorfer, C., Schulz, R., Szapocznik, J. (2006). The role of family functioning in the stress process of dementia caregivers: a structural family framework. *The Gerontologist, 46*(1), 97-105.

Mittelman, M.S., Brodaty, H., Wallen, A.S., & Burns, A. (2008). A three-country randomized controlled trial of a psychosocial intervention for caregivers combined with pharmacological treatment for patients with Alzheimer disease: effects on caregiver depression. *American Journal of Geriatric Psychiatry, 16*(11), 893-904.

Mjones, H. (1949). Paralysis agitans, a clinical and genetic study. *Acta Neurologica Scandinavica, (Supplement), 54,*1-195.

Mohr, E., Juncos, J., Cox, C., Litvan, I., Fedio, P. & Chase, T.N. (1990). Selective deficits in cognition and memory in high-functioning parkinsonian patients. *Journal of Neurology, Neurosurgery and Psychiatry, 53,* 603-606.

Monahan, D.J. & Hooker, K. (1997). Caregiving and social support in two illness groups. *Social Work, 42(3),* 278-287.

Monat, A., & Lazarus, R.S. (Eds.) (1985). *Stress and Coping: An anthology*. New York: Columbia University Press.

Monini, P., Tognetti, A., Cinque, R., Di Franco, F., & Bartorelli, L. (2001) The importance of awareness: an experience of small support groups for the caregivers of Alzheimer's disease patients. *Archives of Gerontology, 33*(suppl. 7.), 267-271.

Monnot, M., Brosey, M. & Ross, E. (2005). Screening for dementia: family caregiver questionnaires reliably predict dementia. *Journal of the American Board of Family Practice*, *18,* 240-256.

Montagu, A. (1989). *Growing young*. (2nd edition). Granby, M.A.: Bergin & Garvey Publishers.

Montgomery, R.J.V. (1989). Investigating caregiver burden. In K.S. Markides & C.L. Cooper (Eds.). *Aging, Stress and Health* (pp. 201-218). Chichester, John Wiley & Sons.

Montgomery R.J.V. & Borgatta E. (1985). *Family support project.* Final report to the Administration on Aging.

Montgomery R.J.V. & Borgatta E.F. (1987). *Effects of alternative family support strategies*. Final report to the Health Care Financing Administration.

Montgomery, R.J.V., Gonyea, J.G. & Hooyman N.R. (1985) Caregiving and the experience of subjective and objective burden. *Family Relations, 34*(1), 19-26.

Montgomery R.J.V., Stull, D.E. & Borgatta E.F. (1985). Measurement and the analysis of burden. *Research on Aging, 7*(1), 137-152.

Montgomery, S.A. & Asberg, M. (1979). A new depression scale designed to be sensitive to change. *British Journal of Psychiatry,134,* 382-389.

Montse, A., Pere, V., Carme, J., Francesc, V. & Eduardo, T. (2001). Visuospatial deficits in Parkinson's disease assessed by judgement of line orientation test: error analyses and practice effects. *Journal of Clinical and Experimental Neuropsychology, 23(5),* 592-598.

Moons, P. (2004). Why call it health-related quality of life when you mean perceived health status? *European Journal of Cardiovascular Nursing, 3,* 275-277.

Moons, P., Budts, W. & De Geest, S. (2006). Critique on the conceptualization of quality of life: A review and evaluation of different conceptual approaches. *International Journal of Nursing Studies, 43,* 891-901.

Moore, S. & Knowles, S. (2006). Beliefs and knowledge about parkinson's disease. *E-Journal of Applied Psychology: Clinical and Social Issues, 2,*15-21.

Morris, H.R. (2005). Genetics of Parkinson's disease. *Annals of Medicine, 37(2),* 86-96.

Morris, R.G., Downes, J.J. & Robbins, T.W. (1990). The nature of the dysexecutive syndrome in Parkinson's disease. In K.J. Gilhooly, M.T.G. Keane, R.H. Logie & G. Erdos (Eds.) *Lines of Thinking: Reflections on the Psychology of Thought. Vol. 2.* (pp.247-258). Chichester: John Wiley & Sons.

Morris, R.G., Downes, J.J., Sahakian, B.J., Evenden, J.L., Heald, A. & Robbins, T.W. (1988). Planning and spatial working memory in Parkinson's disease. *Journal of Neurology, Neurosurgery and Psychiatry, 51,* 757-766.

Morris, L.W., Morris, R.G. & Britton, P.G. (1988) The relationship between marital intimacy, perceived strain and depression in spouse caregivers of dementia sufferers. *British Journal of Medical Psychology, 61*, 46-53.

Morris, R.G., Woods, R.T., Davies, K.S., & Morris, L.W. (1991). Gender differences in carers of dementia sufferers. *British Journal of Psychiatry, 10*(Suppl.), 69-74.

Mortimer, J.A. Pirozzolo, F.J., Hansch, E.C. & Webster, D.D. (1982). Relationship of motor symptoms to intellectual deficits in Parkinson disease. *Neurology, 32,* 133-137.

Moss, M., Albert, M.S., Butters, N. & Payne, M. (1986). Differential patterns of memory loss among patients with Alzheimer's disease, Huntington's disease and alcoholic Korsakoff syndrome. *Archives of Neurology, 43,* 239-246.

Moustafa, A.A., Herzallah, M.M. & Gluck, M.A. (2013). Dissociating the cognitive effects of levodopa versus dopamine agonists in a neurocomputational model of learning in Parkinson's disease. *Neurodegerative Diseases, 11(2),* 102-111.

Movement Disorder Society Task Force on Rating Scales for Parkinson's Disease. (2003). The Unified Parkinson's Disease Rating Scale (UPDRS): status and recommendations. *Movement Disorders, 18(7),* 738-750.

Müller-Thomsen, T., Arlt, S., Mann, U., Mass, R. & Ganzer, S. (2005). Detecting depression in Alzheimer's disease: evaluation of four different scales. *Archives of Clinical Neuropsychology, 20(2),* 271-276.

Murphy, B.H., Schofield, J., Nankervis, S., Bloch, H., Herrman, H. & Singh, (1997). Women in multiple roles: the emotional impact of caring for aging parents. *Ageing and Society, 17*(3), 277-291.

Murray, J.B. (1996). Depression in Parkinson's disease. *Journal of Psychology, 130,* 659-667.

Murphy, J.M., Olivier, D.C., Monson, R.R., Sobol, A.M. & Leighton, A.H. (1988). Incidence of depression and anxiety: The Stirling County study. *American Journal of Public Health, 78,* 534-540.

Murray, J. & Livingston, (1998). A qualitative study of adjustment to caring for an older spouse with a psychiatric illness. *Ageing and Society, 18(6),* 659-671.

Murrell, S.A. & Meeks, S. (1992). Depressive symptoms in older adults: Predispositions, resources and life expectancies. In K.W. Schaie & M.P. Lawton (Eds.), *Annual Review of Gerontology and Geriatrics* (pp. 216-286). New York, NY: Springer.

Muslimovic, D., Post, B., Speelman, J.D. & Schmand, B. (2005). Cognitive profile of patients with newly diagnosed Parkinson's disease. *Neurology, 65,* 1239-1245.

Mutch, W.J., Dingwall-Fordyce, I., Downie, A.W., Paterson, J.G. & Roy, S.K. (1986). Parkinson's disease in a Scottish city. *British Medical Journal, 292*, 534-536.

Muthane, U.B., Swamy, H.S., Satishchandra, P., Subhash, M.N., Rao, S. & Subbakrishna, D. (1994). Early onset Parkinson's disease: are juvenile- and young-onset different? *Movement Disorders, 9(5),* 539-544.

Mylne, A.O. Griffiths, C., Rooney, C. & Doyle, P. (2009). Trends in Parkinson's disease related to mortality in England and Wales, 1993-2006. *European Journal of Neurology, 16(9),* 1010-1016.

Myslobodsky, M., Lalonde, F. & Hicks, L. (2001). Are patients with Parkinson's disease suicidal? *Journal of Geriatric Psychiatry & Neurology, 14,* 120-124.

Naarding, P., Leentjens, A.F.G., van Kooten, F. & Verhey, F.R.J. (2002). Disease-specific properties of the Hamilton Rating Scale for depression in patients with stroke, Alzheimer's dementia and Parkinson's disease. *The Journal of Neuropsychiatry and Clinical Neurosciences, 14,* 329-334.

Naismith, S.L., Pereira, M., Shine, J.M. & Lewis, S.J.G. (2011). How well do caregivers detect mild cognitive change in Parkinson's disease? *Movement Disorders, 26*(1), 161-164.

National Alliance for Caregiving in collaboration with AARP (2009). *Caregiving in the United States.* Retrieved: http://www.caregiving.org/data/Caregiving_in_the_US_2009_full_report.pdf

National Institutes of Health Consensus Conference. (1991/1992) Diagnosis and treatment of depression in late life. *Consensus Statement. 9*(3), 1-27.

Neary, M. (2012). What price carer's assessments? Retrieved from: http://thesmallplaces.blogspot.com/2012/03/mark-neary-what-price-arers.html.

Nelson, H.E. & McKenna P. (1975). The use of current reading ability in the assessment of dementia. *British Journal of Social and Clinical Psychology, 14,* 259-267.

Nicoletti, A., Luca, A., Raciti, L., Contrafatto, D., Bruno, E., Dibilio, V., Sciacca, G., Mostile, G., Petralia, A., Zappia, M. (2013). Obsessive compulsive personality disorder and Parkinson's disease. *PLoS One, 8(1)*:e54822. doi: 10.1371/journal.pone.0054822.

Nijhof, G. (1995). Parkinson's disease as a problem of shame in public appearance. *Sociology of Health and Illness, 17*(2), 193-205.

—. (1996). Uncertainty and lack of trust with Parkinson's disease. *European Journal of Public Health, 6*(1), 58-63.

Nilsson, F.M., Kessing, L.V. & Bowling, T.G. (2001). Increased risk of developing Parkinson's disease for patients with major affective disorder: a register study. *Acta Psychiatrica Scandinavica, 104,* 380-386.

Nilsson, F.M., Kessing, L.V., Sørensen, T.M., Andersen, P.K. & Bolwig, T.G. (2002). Major depressive disorder in Parkinson's disease: a register-based study. *Acta Psychiatrica Scandinavica, 106,* 202-211.

Noelker, L.S., & Poulshock, S.W.(1984). Intimacy: factors affecting its development among members of a home for the aged. *International Journal of Aging and Human Development, 19*(3), 177-190.

Nolan, M. Grant, G. & Keady, J. (1996). Satisfactions of caring: the neglected dimension. In M. Nolan, G.Grant & J. Keady (Eds.). *Understanding Family Care: A multidimensional model of caring and coping.* (pp. 82-106). Buckingham, Philadelphia: Open University Press.

Nolan, G., Keady, J., Grant, G. & Lundh, U. (2003). Introduction: why another book on family care? In M. Nolan, U. Lundh, G. Grant & J. Keady (Eds.), *Partnerships in Family Care: understanding the caregiving career* (pp.1-12). Maidenhead, Philadelphia: Open University Press.

Nolan, M., Lundh, U., Grant, G. & Keady, J. (2003). *Partnerships in Family Care: understanding the caregiving career.* Maidenhead, Philadelphia: Open University Press.

Noonan, A.E. & Tennstedt, S.L. (1997). Meaning in caregiving and its contribution to caregiver wellbeing. *The Gerontologist, 37*(6), 785-794.

Norman, S., Tröster, A.I., Fields, J.A. & Brooks, R. (2002). Effects of depression and Parkinson's disease on cognitive functioning. *The Journal of Neuropsychiatry and Clinical Neurosciences*, *14,* 31-36.

Norton, M.C., Piercy, K.W., Rabins, P.V., Green, R.C., Breitner, J.C.S., Østbye, T., Corcoran, C., Welsh-Bohmer, K.A., Lyketsos, C.G. & Tschanz, J.T. (2009) Caregiver-recipient closeness and symptom progression in Alzheimer disease. The Cache County Dementia Progression Study. *Journal of Gerontology, Psychological Sciences, 64B*(5), P560-P568.

Nourhashémi, F., Andrieu, S., Sastres, N., Ducassé, J.L., Lauque, D., Sinclair, A.J., Albarède, J.L., &Vellas, B.J. (2001). Descriptive analysis of emergency hospital admissions of patients with Alzheimer disease. *Alzheimer's Disease and Associated Disorders, 15*(1), 21-25.

Nussbaum, M., Treves, T.A., Inzelberg, R., Rabey, J.M. & Korczyn, A.D. (1998). Survival in Parkinson's disease: the effect of dementia. *Parkinsonism and Related Disorders, 4,*179-181.

O'Brien, J.T., Firbank, M.J., Mosimann, U.P., Burn, D.J. & McKeith, I.G. (2005). Change in perfusion, hallucinations and fluctuations in consciousness in dementia with Lewy bodies. *Psychiatry Research, 139(2),* 79-88.

O'Connor, E.J., McCabe, M.P. & Firth, L. (2008) The impact of neurological illness on marital relationships. *Journal of Sex and Marital Therapy, 34,* 115-132.

Oehlberg, K., Barg, F.K., Brown, G.K., Taraborelli, D., Stern, M.B. & Weintraub, D. (2008). Attitudes regarding the etiology and treatment of depression in Parkinson's disease: A qualitative study. *Journal of Geriatric Psychiatry & Neurology, 21(2),* 123-132.

Ogden, J.A., Growdon, J.H. & Corkin, S. (1990). Deficits on visuospatial tests involving forward planning in high-functioning parkinsonians. *Neuropsychiatry, Neuropsychology and Behavioural Neurology, 3,* 125-139.

Oguru, M., Tachibana, H., Toda, K., Okuda, B. & Oka, N. (2010). Apathy and depression in Parkinson disease. *Journal of Geriatric Psychiatry and Neurology, 23(1),* 35-41.

O'Halloran, J., Miller, G.C. & Britt, H. (2004). Defining chronic conditions for primary care with ICPC-2. *Family Practice, 21(4)*, 381-386.

Okamoto, K., Hasebe, Y. & Harasawa, Y. (2007). Caregiver psychological characteristics predict discontinuation of care for disabled elderly at home. *International Journal of Geriatric Psychiatry, 22,*1110-1114.

Olanow, C.W., Stern, M.B. & Sethi, K. (2009). The scientific and clinical basis for the treatment of Parkinson disease. *Neurology*, *72,* S1-S136.

Olshansky S.J., Rudberg M.A., Carnes B.A., Cassel C.K., Brody J.A. (1991). Trading off longer life for worsening health. *Journal of Ageing and Health.* 3,194-216.

Olton, D.S., Becker, J.T. & Handelman, G.E. (1979) Hippocampus, space and memory. *Behavioural and Brain Sciences, 2,* 315-365.

O'Reilly, F., Finnan, F., Allwright, S., Davey Smith, G. & Ben-Shlomo, Y. (1996). The effects of caring for a spouse with Parkinson's disease on social, psychological and physical well-being. *British Journal of General Practice*, *46,* 507-512.

Osborn, D.P., Fletcher, A.E., Smeeth, L., Stirling, S., Nunes, M., Breeze, E., Siu-Woon, Nq. E., Bulpitt, C.J., Jones, D. & Tulloch, A. (2002). Geriatric Depression Scale scores in a representative sample of 14,545 people aged 75and over in the United Kingdom: results from the MRC Trial of Assessment and Management of Older People in the Community. *International Journal of Geriatric Psychiatry*, *17(4),* 375-382.

O'Shaughnessy, M., Lee, K & Lintern, T. (2010). Changes in the couple relationship in dementia care: Spouse carers' experiences. *Dementia, 9*(2), 237-258.

Osiejuk-Lojek, E. (1998). Deficyty neuropsychologiczne w chorobie Parkinsona. (Neuropsychological deficits in Parkinson's disease). In A.Herzyk & Kądzielawa, D. (Eds.) *Związek mózg-zachowanie w ujęciu neuropsychologii klinicznej (pp.191-215).* Lublin: Wydawnictwo UMCS. In Polish.

Ostwald, S.K., Hepburn, K.W., Caron, W., Burns, T. & Mantell, R. (1999). Reducing caregiver burden: a randomized psychoeducational intervention for caregivers of persons with dementia. *The Gerontologist,39(3),* 299-309.

Owen, A.M. (2004). Cognitive dysfunction in Parkinson's disease: the role of frontostriatal circuitry. *Neuroscientist, 10(6),* 525-537.

Owen, A.M., Beksinska, M., James, M., Leigh, P.N., Summers, B.A., Marsden, C.D., Quinn, N.P., Sahakian, B.J. & Robbins, T.W. (1993). Visuospatial memory deficits at different stages of Parkinson's disease. *Neuropsychologia, 31,* 627-644.

Owen, A.M., Downes, J.J., Sahakian, B.J., Polkey, C.E. & Robbins, T.W. (1990). Planning and spatial working memory following frontal lobe lesions in man. *Neuropsychologia, 28,* 1021-1034.

Owen, A.M., Doyon, J., Dagher, A., Sadikot, A. & Evans, A.C. (1998). Abnormal basal ganglia outflow in Parkinson's disease identified with PET. Implications for higher cortical functions. *Brain, 121 (Pt 5),* 949-965.

Owen, A.M., Doyon, J., Petrides, M. & Evans, A.C. (1996). Planning and spatial working memory: a positron emission tomography study in humans. *European Journal of Neuroscience, 8,* 353-364.

Owen, A.M., Iddon, J.L., Hodges, J.R., Summers, B.A. & Robbins, T.W. (1997). Spatial and non-spatial working memory at different stages of Parkinson's disease. *Neuropsychologia*, *35,* 519-532.

Owen, A.M., James, M., Leigh, P.N., Summers, B.A., Marsden, C.D., Quinn, N.P., Lange, K.W. & Robbins, T.W. (1992). Fronto-striatal cognitive deficits at different stages of Parkinson's disease. *Brain, 115,* 1727-1751.

Owen, A.M., Roberts, A.C., Hodges, J.R., Summers, B.A., Polkey, C.E. & Robbins, T.W. (1993). Contrasting mechanisms of impaired attentional set-shifting in patients with frontal lobe damage or Parkinson's disease. *Brain, 116 (Pt 5),* 1159-1175.

Owen, A.M., Roberts, A.C. Polkey, C.E., Sahakian, B.J. & Robbins, T.W. (1991). Extra-dimensional versus Intra-dimensional set shifting performance following frontal lobe excisions, temporal lobe excisions or amygdalo-hippocampectomy in man. *Neuropsychologia, 29(10),* 993-1006.

Owen, A.M., Sahakian, B.J., Semple, J., Polkey, C.E. & Robbins, T.W. (1995). Visuo-spatial short-term recognition memory and learning after temporal lobe excisions, frontal lobe excisions or amygdalo-hippocampectomy in man. *Neuropsychologia, 33(1),* 1-24.

Oxtoby, M. (1982). *Parkinson's disease patients and their social needs: A survey of patients in contact with the Parkinson's Disease Society.* London: Parkinson's Disease Society.

Pąchalska, M. (2007). *Neuropsychologia Kliniczna: Urazy mózgu,* vol.2. (Clinical Neuropsychology: Brain Injuries), Warszawa: Wydawnictwo Naukowe PWN. In Polish.

Pahwa, R., Factor, S.A., Lyons, K.E., Ondo, W.G., Gronseth, G., Bronte-Stewart, H., Hallett, M., Miyasaki, J., Stevens, J. & Weiner, W.J. (2006). Practice parameter: treatment of Parkinson's disease with motor fluctuations and dyskinesia (an evidence based review): report of the Quality Standards Subcommittee of the American Academy of Neurology. *Neurology, 66,* 983-995.

Pahwa, R., Lyons, K.E., McGuire, D., Silverstein, P., Zwiebel, F., Robischon, M. & Koller, W.C. (1997). Comparison of standard carbidopa-levodopa and sustained-release carbidopa-levodopa in Parkinson's disease: pharmacokinetic and quality-of-life measures. *Movement Disorders, 12(5)*, 677-681.

Pagonabarraga, J., Kulisevsky, J., Llebaria, G., Garcia-Sanchez, C., Pascual-Sedano, B. & Gironell, A. (2008). Parkinson's disease-cognitive eating scale: a new cognitive scale specific for Parkinson's disease. *Movement Disorders, 23(7),* 998-1005.

Pal, P.K., Thennarasu, K., Fleming, J., Schulzer, M., Brown, T. & Calne, S.M. (2004) Nocturnal sleep disturbances and daytime dysfunction in patients with Parkinson's disease and in their caregivers. *Parkinsonism and Related Disorders, 10*(3), 157-168.

Pålhagen, S.E., Carlsson, M., Curman, E., Wålinder, J. & Granérus, A.K. (2008). Depressive illness in Parkinson's disease-indication of a more advanced and widespread neurodegenerative process? *Acta Neurologica Scandinavica, 117(5),* 295-304.

Papadopoulos, F.C., Petridou, E., Argyropoulou, S., Kontaxakis, V., Dessypris, N., Anastasiou, A., Katsiardani, K.P., Trichopoulos, D. & Lyketsos, C. (2005). Prevalence and correlates of depression in late life: a population based study from a rural Greek town. *International Journal of Geriatric Psychiatry, 20(4),* 350-357.

Papapetropoulos, S., Gonzalez, J., Lieberman, A. Villar, J.M. & Mash, D.C. (2005). Dementia in Parkinson's disease: a post-mortem study in a population of brain donors. *International Journal of Geriatric Psychiatry, 20*, 418-422.

Parker, G. (1992). Counting care: numbers and types of informal carers. In J. Twigg (Ed.). *Carers, Research and Practice*. London: HMSO.

Parker, G. (1993). *With this body: Caring and disability in marriage*. Buckingham: Open University Press.

Parker, G. & Lawton, D. (1994). *Different Types of Care, Different Types of Carer. Evidence From The General Household Survey*. London: HMSO.

Parker, R.M., Schaller, J. & Hansmann, S. (2003). Catastrophe, chaos and complexity models and psychosocial adjustment to disability. *Rehabilitation Counselling Bulletin, 46,* 234-241.

Parkinson, J. (1817). *An essay on the shaking palsy*. London, Sherwood, Neely & Jones.

Parkinson's U.K. (2012a). Website at: http://www.parkinsons.org.uk/.

—. (2012b). Website at: http://www.parkinsons.org.uk/about_us/policy_and_campaigns1/policy/policy_statements/carers_policy_statement.asx

Passafiume, D., Boller, F. & Keefe, M.C. (1986). Neuropsychological impairment in patients with Parkinson's disease. In I. Grant & K.M. Adams (Eds.) *Neuropsychological assessment of neuropsychiatric disorders* (pp. 374-383). New York: Oxford University Press.

Patrick, H.T. & Levy, D.M. (1922). Parkinson's Disease. A clinical study of 146 cases. *Archives of Neurology and Psychiatry, 7,* 711-720.

Patterson, T.L., Semple, S.J., Shaw, W.S., Yu, E., He, Y., Zhang, M.Y., Wu, W., & Grant I. (1998). The cultural context of caregiving: a comparison of Alzheimer's caregivers in Shanghai, China and San Diego, California. *Psychological Medicine, 28*(5), 1071-1084.

Paulus, W. & Jellinger, K. (1991). The neuropathologic basis of different clinical subgroups of Parkinson's disease. *Journal of Neuropathology and Experimental Neurology*, *50(6),* 743-755.

Paulus, W. & Trenkwalder, C. (1998). Imaging of nonmotor symptoms in Parkinson syndromes. *Clinical Neuroscience, 5(2),*115-120.

Pearlin, L.I., Mullan, J.T., Semple, S.J. & Skaff, M.M. (1990). Caregiving and the stress process. An overview of concepts and their measures. *The Gerontologist*, *30B(5),* P583-P591.

Pereira do Prado, R.C. & Barbosa, E.R. (2005). Depression and Parkinson's disease: study of 60 cases. *Arquivos Neuropsiquiatria*, *63(3-B),* 766-771.

Perneger, T.V. (1998). What's wrong with Bonferroni adjustments. *British Medical Journal, 316 (7139),* 1236.

Perren, A., Schmid, R., Herrmann, S. & Wettstein, A. (2007). The impact of attachment on dementia-related problem behaviour and spousal caregivers' well-being. *Attachment and Human Development, 9*(2), 163-178.

Perry, R.J. & Hodges, J.R. (2000) Differentiating frontal and temporal variant frontotemporal dementia from Alzheimer's disease. *Neurology, 54,* 2277-2284.

Pfeiffer, E. (1979). A short psychiatric evaluation schedule: a new 15-item monotonic scale indicative of functional disorder. In *Brain Function in Old Age: Proceedings of Bayer Symposium VII* (pp. 228-236).New York: Springer-Verlag.

Phillips, L. (2006). Dropping the bomb: The experience of being diagnosed with Parkinson's disease. *Geriatric Nursing, 27*(6), 362-369.

Piccinni, A., Marazziti, D., Veltri, A., Ceravolo, R., Ramacciotti, C., Carlini, M., Del Debbio, A., Schiavi, E., Bonuccelli, U. &, Dell'osso, L. (2012). Depressive symptoms in Parkinson's disease. *Comprehensive Psychiatry, 53(6),*727-731.

Piccirilli, M., D'Alessandro, P., Finali, G. & Piccinin, G.L. (1994). Neuropsychological follow-up of Parkinsonian patients with and without cognitive impairment. *Dementia, 5*(1), 17-22.

Pickard, L., (2001). Carer break or carer blind? Policies for informal carers in the U.K. *Social Policy and Administration, 35*(4), 441-458.

—. (2002). The decline of intensive intergenerational care of older people in Great Britain, 1985-1995. *Population trends*, 110, 31-41.

Pickard, L.,Wittenberg, R.,Comas-Herrera, A., Davies & Darton, R. (2000) Relying on informal care in the new century? Informal care for elderly people in England to 2031. *Ageing & Society, 20*(6), 745-772.

Pierret, J. (2003) The illness experience: State of knowledge and perspectives for research. *Sociology of Health and Illness, 25,* 4-22.

Pilling, S., Anderson, I., Goldberg, D., Meader, N., Taylor, C. & Two Guideline Development Groups. (2009). Depression in adults, including those with a chronic physical health problem: summary of NICE guidance. *British Medical Journal*, *339*:b4108.

Pillon, B., Deweer, B., Agid, Y. & Dubois, B. (1993). Explicit memory in Alzheimer's, Huntington's and Parkinson's diseases. *Archives of Neurology, 50,* 374-379.

Pillon, B., Dubois, B., Lhermitte, F. & Agid, Y. (1986). Heterogeneity of cognitive impairment in progressive supranuclear palsy, Parkinson's disease and Alzheimer's disease. *Neurology, 36,* 1179-1185.

Pillon, B., Dubois, B., Ploska, A. & Agid, Y. (1991). Severity and specificity of cognitive impairment in Alzheimer's. Huntington's and Parkinson's diseases and progressive supranuclear palsy. *Neurology, 41(5),* 634-643.

Pinder, R. (1988). Striking Balances: Living with Parkinson's disease.In R. Anderson & M.Bury (Eds.). *Living with Chronic illness. The experience of patients and their families* (pp.67-88). London: Unwin Hyman.

—. (1990). What to expect: information and the management of uncertainty in Parkinson's disease. *Disability and Society, 5*(1), 77-92.

—. (1992). Coherence and incoherence: doctors' and patients' perspectives on the diagnosis of Parkinson's disease. *Sociology of Health and Illness, 14,* 1-22.

Pinquart, M. & Sörensen, S. (2003a). Associations of stressors and uplifts of caregiving with caregiver burden and depressive mood: a meta-analysis. *Journal of Gerontology, 58B*(2), P112-P128.

Pinquart, M., & Sörensen, S. (2003b). Differences between caregivers and noncaregivers in psychological health and physical health: A meta-analysis. *Psychology and Aging, 18(2),* 250-267.

Pinquart, M. & Sörensen, S. (2005). Caregiving distress and psychological health of caregivers. In K. V. Oxington (Ed.), *Psychology of stress* (pp. 165–206). New York: Nova Science Publishers Inc.

Pinquart, M. & Sörensen, S. (2006). Gender differences in caregiver stressors, social resources, and health: an updated meta-analysis. *Journal of Gerontology, , 61B*(1), P33-P45.

Pinquart, M. & Sorensen, S. (2007) Correlates of physical health of informal caregivers: a meta-analysis. *Journal of Gerontology, 62B,* P126-P137.

Piovezan, M.R., Teive, H.A.G., Piovesan, E.J., Mader, M.J. & Werneck, L.C. (2007). Cognitive function assessment in idiopathic Parkinson's disease. *Arquivos de Neuro-Psiquiatria, 65(4-A),* 942-946.

Pirozzolo, F.J., Hansch, E.C., Mortimer, J.A., Webster, D.D. & Kuskowski, M.A. (1982). Dementia in Parkinson's disease: A neuropsychological analysis. *Brain and Cognition, 1,* 71-83.

Pirozzolo, F.J., Swihart, A.A., Rey, G., Mahurin, R., & Jankovic, J. (1993). Cognitive impairments associated with Parkinson's disease and other movement disorders. In J. Jankovic & E. Tolosa (Eds.).

Parkinson's disease and movement disorders, (2nd ed., pp. 493-510). Baltimore: Williams and Wilkins.

Platt, S. (1985). Measuring the burden of psychiatric illness on the family: an evaluation of some rating scales. *Psychological Medicine, 15*(2), 383-393.

Platt, S. & Hirsch, S. (1981).The effects of brief hospitalization upon the psychiatric patient's household. *Acta Psychiatrica Scandinavica, 64,* 199-216.

Pluck, G.C. & Brown, R.G. (2002). Apathy in Parkinson's disease. *Journal of Neurology, Neurosurgery & Psychiatry, 73,* 636-642.

Plumb, M.M. & Holland, J. (1977). Comparative studies of psychological function in patients with advanced cancer-1. Self reported depressive symptoms. *Psychosomatic Medicine, 39,* 264-276.

Poliakoff, E. & Smith-Spark, J.H. (2008). Everyday cognitive failures and memory problems in Parkinson's patients without dementia. *Brain and Cognition*, *67,* 340-350.

Politynska, B., Berrios G. & Lewko J. (1995). Neuropsychiatric aspects of subarachnoid haemorrhage: A review. *Neurology, Psychiatry and Brain Research*, *3,* 111-120.

Politynska B., Mariak Z., Lewko J. (1999). The influence of post-traumatic syndrome in determining capacity to return to work after closed head injury. *Roczniki Akademii Medycznej w Białymstoku, 44,* 141-150.

Poletti, M. & Bonuccelli, U. (2012). Personality traits in patients with Parkinson's disease: assessment and clinical implications. *Journal of Neurology, 259(6),* 1029-1038.

Pollina, L.K., Greene, A. L., Tunick, R.H. & Puckett, J.M. (1993). Dimensions of everyday memory in late adulthood. *Current Psychology: Research and Reviews*, *12,* 46-56.

Pollock, M. & Hornabrook, R.W. (1966). The prevalence, natural history and dementia of Parkinson's disease. *Brain*, 89(3), 429-488.

Ponce, F.A. & Lozano, A.M. (2010). The most cited works in Parkinson's disease. *Movement Disorders, 26(3),* 380-390.

Pontone, G.M., Williams, J.R., Anderson, K.E., Chase, G., Goldstein S.A., Grill, S., Hirsch, E.S., Lehmann, S., Little, J.T., Margolis, R.L., Rabins, P.V., Weiss, H.D. & Marsh, L. (2009). Prevalence of anxiety disorders and anxiety subtypes in patients with Parkinson's disease. *Movement Disorders*, *24(9),* 1333-1338.

Post, B., Speelman, J.D. & de Haan, R.J. on behalf of the CARPA study group. (2008). Clinical heterogeneity in newly diagnosed Parkinson's disease. *Journal of Neurology*, *255(5),* 716-722.

Pot, A.M., Deeg, D.J.H. & Knipscheer, C.P.M. (2001) Institutionalisation of demented elderly: the role of caregiver characteristics. *International Journal of Geriatric Psychiatry, 16,* 273-280.

Poulshock, S.W. & Deimling, G.T. (1984). Families caring for elders in residence: issues in the measurement of burden. *Journal of Gerontology*, *39*(2), 230-239.

Powell, R. (2003). Psychometric properties of the Beck Depression Inventory and the Zung Self Rating Depression Scale in adults with mental retardation. *Mental Retardation, 41(2),* 88-95.

Prado, R.C. & Barbosa, E.R. (2005). Depression in Parkinson's disease: study of 60 cases. *Arquivos Neuropsiquiatria*, *63,* 766-771.

Pratt, C.C., Schmall, V.L., Wright, S. & Cleland, M. (1985). Burden and coping strategies of caregivers to Alzheimer's patients. *Family Relations, 34,* 27-33.

Price, H. J., & Levy, K. A. (1990). Variables influencing burden in spousal and adult child primary caregivers of persons with Alzheimer's disease in the home setting. *American Journal of Alzheimer's Disease and Other Dementias* : *5* (1), 34-42.

Probst, A., Bloch, A. & Tolnay, M. (2008). New insights into the pathology of Parkinson's disease: does the peripheral autonomic system become central? *European Journal of Neurology,15(suppl. 1),* 1-4.

Pruchno, R.A., Burant, C.J. & Peters, N.D. (1997). Understanding the well-being of care receivers. *The Gerontologist, 37,* 102-109.

Pruchno, R.A., & Potashnik, S.L. (1989). Caregiving spouses. Physical and mental health in perspective. *Journal of the American Geriatric Society, 37*(8), 697-705.

Pruchno, R.A. & Resch, N.L. (1989a). Aberrant behaviours and Alzheimer's disease. Mental health effects on spouse caregivers. *Journal of Gerontology, Social Sciences, 44,* S177-S182.

Pruchno, R.A. & Resch, N.L. (1989b). Mental health of caregiving spouses: coping as mediator, moderator or main effect? *Psychology and Aging, 4(4),* 454-463.

Purves, D., Augustine, G.J., Fitzpatrick, D., Katz, L.C., LaMantia, A.S., McNamara, J.O. & Williams, S.M. (2001). *Neuroscience*, 2nd edition., Massachusetts, Sinauer Associates, Inc.

Quayhagen, M.P. & Quayhagen, M. (1988) Alzheimer's stress: coping with the caregiving role. *The Gerontologist, 28*, 391-396.

Quinn, C., Clare, L. & Woods, R.T. (2012). What predicts whether caregivers of people with dementia find meaning in their role? *International Journal of Geriatric Psychiatry, 27(11,)* 1195-1202.

Quintana, S.M. & Maxwell, S.E. (1999). Implications of recent developments in structural equations modelling for counselling psychology. *The Counseling Psychologist, 27*, 485-527.

Rabbit, P., & Abson, V. (1990). "Lost and Found": Some logical and methodological limitations of self-report questionnaires as tools to study cognitive ageing. *British Journal of Psychology, 81,* 1-16.

Rabins, P.R., Mace, N. & Lucas, M.J. (1982). The impact of dementia on the family. *Journal of the American Medical Association, 248,* 333-335.

Rabinstein, A.A. & Shulman, L.M. (2001). Management of behavioural and psychiatric problems in Parkinson's disease. *Parkinsonism and Related Disorders*, *7,* 41-50.

Rafal, R.D., Posner, M.I., Walker, J.A. & Friedrich, F.J. (1984). Cognition and the basal ganglia. Separating mental and motor components of performance in Parkinson's disease. *Brain, 107*, 1083-1094.

Rahman, S., Griffin, H.J., Quinn, N.P. & Jahanshahi, M. (2008). Quality of life in Parkinson's disease: The relative importance of the symptoms. *Movement Disorders, 23*(10), 1428-1434.

Ramaker, C., Marinus, J., Stiggelbout, A.M. & van Hilten, B.J. (2002). Systematic evaluation of rating scales for impairment and disability in Parkinson's disease. *Movement Disorder*, *17,* 867-876.

Randolph, C., Mohr, E. & Chase, T.N. (1993). Assessment of intellectual functioning in dementing disorders: Validity of WAIS-R short forms for patients with Alzheimer's, Huntington's and Parkinson's disease. *Journal of Clinical and Experimental Neuropsychology, 15,* 743-753.

Rankin, E. D., Haut, M.W. & Keefover, R.W. (2001) Current marital functioning as a mediating factor in depression among spouse caregivers in dementia. *Clinical Gerontologist, 23*(3/4), 27-44.

Rappley, I., Gitler, A.D., Selvy, P.E., LaVoie, M.J., Levy, B.D., Brown, H.A., Lindquist, S. & Selkoe, D.J. (2009). Evidence that α-synuclein does not inhibit phospholipase D. *Biochemistry*, *48,* 1077-1083.

Raskin, S.A., Sliwinski, M. & Borod, J.C. (1992). Clustering strategies on tasks of verbal fluency in Parkinson's disease. *Neuropsychologia, 30,* 95-99.

Raudonis, B.M. (2006). Palliative Care. In I.M. Lubkin & P.D. Larsen (Eds.). *Chronic Illness. Impact and Interventions* (6th edition). (pp. 537-554). Boston, Toronto, London: Jones and Bartlett Publishers.

Ravina, B., Camicioli, R., Como, P.G., Marsh, L., Jankovic, J., Weintraub, D. & Elm, J. (2007). The impact of depressive symptoms in early Parkinson's disease. *Neurology*, *69(4),* 342-347.

Ravina, B., Elm, J., Camicioli, R., Como, P.G., Marsh, L., Jankovic, J. & Weintraub, D. (2009). The course of depressive symptoms in early Parkinson's disease. *Movement Disorders*, *24(9),* 1306-1311.

Razali, R., Ahmad, F., Rahman, F.N., Midin, M., & Sidi, H. (2011). Burden of care among caregivers of patients with Parkinson disease: a cross-sectional study. *Clinical Neurology and Neurosurgery, 113*(8), 639-643.

Ready, R., Ott, B. & Grace, J. (2004). Validity of informant reports about AD and MCI patients' memory. *Alzheimer's Disease and Associated Disorders, 18,* 11-16.

Reid, W.G., Broe, G.A., Hely, M.A., Morris, J.G., Williamson, P.M., O'Sullivan, D.J., Rail, D., Genge, S. & Moss, N.G. (1989). The neuropsychology of de novo patients with idiopathic Parkinson's disease: the effects of age of onset. *International Journal of Neurosciences, 48(3-4),* 205-217.

Reijnders, J.S., Ehrt, U., Weber, W.E., Aarsland, D. & Leentjens, A.F. (2008). A systematic review of prevalence studies of depression in Parkinson's disease. *Movement Disorders*, *23,* 183-189.

Reijnders, J.S., Lousberg, R. & Leentjens, A.F. (2010). Assessment of depression in Parkinson's disease: the contribution of somatic symptoms to the clinimetric performance of the Hamilton and Montgomery-Asberg rating scales. *Journal of Psychosomatic Research,68(6),* 561-565.

Reinhard, S.C., & Horowitz, A.V. (1995). Caregiving burden: differentiating the content and consequences of family caregiving. *Journal of Marriage and the Family, 57,* 741-750.

Reitan, R.M. & Boll, T.J. (1971). Intellectual and cognitive functions in Parkinson's disease. *Journal of Consulting and Clinical Psychology, 37(3),* 364-369.

Rektorová, I., Rector, I., Bares, M., Dostál,V., Ehler, E., Fanfrdlová, Z., Fiedler, J., Klajblová, H., Kulist'ák, P., Ressner, P., Svátová, J., Urbánek, K., Velísková, J. (2003). Pramipexole and pergolide in the treatment of depression in Parkinson's disease: a national multicentre prospective randomized study. *European Journal of Neurology*, *10(4),* 399-406.

Remy, P., Doder, M., Lees, A., Turjanski, N. & Brooks, D. (2005). Depression in Parkinson's disease: loss of dopamine and noradrenaline innervation in the limbic system. *Brain*, *128(6),* 1314-1322.

Reynolds, N.C., & Montgomery, G.K. (1987). Factor analysis of Parkinson's impairment. An evaluation of the final common pathway. *Archives of Neurology, 44*(10), 1013-1016.

Rezak, M. (2007). Current pharmacotherapeutic treatment options in Parkinson's disease. *Disease-A-Month*, *53,* 214-222.

Richard, I.H., Justus, A.W. & Kurlan, R. (2001). Relationship between mood and motor fluctuations in Parkinson's disease. *Journal of Neuropsychiatry and Clinical Neurosciences*, *13(1),* 35-41.

Richard, I.H., Schiffer, R.B. & Kurlan, R. (1996). Anxiety and Parkinson's disease. *Journal of Neuropsychiatry and Clinical Neurosciences, 8(4)*, 383-392.

Richter, P., Werner, J., Bastine, R., Heerlein, A., Kick, H. & Sauer H. (1997). Measuring treatment outcome by the Beck Depression Inventory. *Psychopathology, 30(4),* 234-240.

Rickards, H. (2005). Depression in neurological disorders: Parkinson's disease, multiple sclerosis and stroke. *Journal of Neurology, Neurosurgery and Psychiatry*, *76,* 48-52.

Riedel, O., Dodel, R., Deuschl, G., Klotsche, J., Förstl, H., Heuser, I., Oertel, W., Reichmann, H., Riederer, P., Trenkwalder, C. & Wittchen, H.U. (2011). Depression and care dependency in Parkinson's disease: Results from a nationwide study of 1449 outpatients. *Parkinsonism and Related Disorders,18(5),* 598-601.

Riedel, O., Klotsche, J., Spottke, A., Deuschl, G., Förstl, H., Henn, F., Heuser, I., Oertel, W., Reichmann, H., Riederer, P., Trenkwalder, C., Dodel, R. & Wittchen, H.U. (2008). Cognitive impairment in 873 patients with idiopathic Parkinson's disease. Results from the German Study on Epidemiology of Parkinson's Disease with Dementia (GEPAD). *Journal of Neurology*, 255(2), 255-264.

Riley, D.E. (2002). Reversible transvestic fetishism in a man with Parkinson's disease treated with selegiline. *Clinical Neuropharmacology, 25*(4), 234-237.

Rinaldi, P., Spazzafumo, L., Mastriforti, R., Mattioli, P., Marvardi, M., Polidori, M.C., Cherubini, A., Abate, G., Bartorelli, L., Bonaiuto, S., Capurso, A., Cucinotta, D., Gallucci, M., Giordano, M., Martorelli, M., Masaraki, G., Nieddu, A., Pettenati, C., Putzu, P., Tammaro, V.A., Tomassini, P.F., Vergani, C., Senin, U. & Mecocci, P.; Study Group on Brain Aging of the Italian Society of Gerontology and Geriatrics (2005). Predictors of high level of burden and distress in caregivers of demented patients: results of an Italian multicenter study. *International Journal of Geriatric Psychiatry, 20*(2), 168-174.

Ring, H.A., Bench, C.J., Trimble, M.R., Brooks, D.J., Frackowiak, R.S. & Dolan, R.J. (1994). Depression in Parkinson's disease. A positron emission study. *British Journal of Psychiatry, 165(3),* 333-339.

Robbins, T.W. (2010). From behaviour to cognition: Functions of mesostriatal, mesolimbic and mesocortical dopamine systems. In L.L. Iversen, S.D. Iversen, S.B. Dunnett, A. Bjorklund (Eds.). *Dopamine Handbook* (pp.203-214). New York: Oxford University Press.

Robbins, T.W., James, M., Lange, K.W., Owen, A.M., Quinn, N.P. & Marsden, C.D. (1992). Cognitive performance in multiple system atrophy. *Brain, 115(1),* 271-291.

Robbins, T.W., James, M., Owen, A.M., Sahakian, B.J., McInnes, L. & Rabbitt, P. (1994). Cambridge Neuropsychological Test Automated Battery (CANTAB): a factor analytic study of a large sample of normal elderly volunteers. *Dementia, 5(5),* 266-281.

Robbins, T.W., Owen, A.M. & Sahakian, B.J. (1999). The neuropsychology of basal ganglia disorders: an integrative cognitive and comparative approach. In M.A. Ron and A.S. David (Eds.), *Disorders of Brain and Mind,* (pp.57-79). Cambridge: Cambridge University Press.

Roberts, A.C., Robbins, T.W. & Everitt, B.J. (1988). The effects of intra-dimensional and extra-dimensional shifts on visual discrimination learning in humans and non-human primates. *Quarterly Journal of Experimental Psychology, 40B,* 321-341.

Robinson, B.C. (1983). Validation of a caregiver strain index. *Journal of Gerontology, 38*(3), 344-348.

Rodda, J., Walker, Z. & Carter, J. (2011). Depression in older adults. *British Medical Journal*, *343,* 683-687.

Rodin, G. & Voshart K. (1986). Depression in the medically ill: an overview. *American Journal of Psychiatry*, *143,* 696-705.

Rodríguez-Violante, M., Cervantes-Arriaga, A., Berlanga-Flores, C. & Ruiz-Chow, A. (2012). Prevalence and determinants of depression in Mexican patients with Parkinson's disease. *Clinical Neurology and Neurosurgery, 114(10),* 1293-1296.

Rogers, R.D., Sahakian, B.J., Hodges, J.R., Polkey, C.E., Kennard, C. & Robbins, T.W. (1998). Dissociating executive mechanisms of task control following frontal lobe damage and Parkinson's disease. *Brain, 121(5),* 815-842.

Rojo, A., Aguilar, M., Garolera, M.T., Cubo, E., Navas, I. & Quintana, S. (2003). Depression in Parkinson's disease: clinical correlates and outcome. *Parkinsonism and Related Disorders*, *10,* 23-28.

Roland, K.P., Jenkins, M.E., & Johnson, A.M. (2010). An exploration of the burden experienced by spousal caregivers of individuals with Parkinson's disease. *Movement Disorders, 25*(2), 189-193.

Roland, K., Johnson, A.M. & Jenkins, M.E. (2011). Identifying and managing caregiver burden among spouses of individuals with Parkinson's disease. *Journal of Current Clinical Care,* 33-39.Available at: http://works.bepress.com/andrewjohnson/1

Rosenbaum, R.B. (2006). *Understanding Parkinson's disease. A personal and professional view*. Westport, Connecticut: Praeger Publishers.

Rosser, R. (1988). A health index and output measure. In S.R. Walker & R.M. Rosser (Eds.). *Quality of life: Assessment and application.* Lancaster, PA: MIT Press.

Rossor, M.N. (1981). Parkinson's disease and Alzheimer's disease as disorders of the isodendritic core. *British Medical Journal (Clinical Research & Education), 283(6306),* 1588-1590.

Rothbard, J.C. & Shaver, P.R. (1994). Continuity of attachment across the lifespan. In M.B. Sperling & W.H. Berman (Eds.), *Attachment in adults: Clinical and developmental perspectives* (pp.31-71). New York: Guilford Press.

Rowe, J., Stephan, K.E., Friston, K., Frackowiak, R., Lees, A. & Passingham, R. (2002). Attention to action in Parkinson's disease: impaired effective connectivity among frontal cortical regions. *Brain, 125,* 276-289.

Ruberg, M., Ploska, A., Javoy-Agid, F. & Agid, Y. (1982). Muscarinic binding and choline acetyltransferase activity in Parkinsonian subjects with reference to dementia. *Brain Research, 232(1),*129-139.

Sacks, O. (1999). *Awakenings*. London: Picador.

Sacks, O.W., Kohl, M.S., Messeloff, C.R. & Schwartz, W.F. (1972). Effects of levodopa in Parkinsonian patients with dementia. *Neurology, 22(5),* 516-519.

Sadeh, M., Braham, J. & Modan, M. (1982). Effects of anticholinergic drugs on memory in Parkinson's disease. *Archives of Neurology, 39,* 666-667.

Sagar, H.J., Cohen, N.J., Sullivan, E.V., Corkin, S. & Growdon, J.H. (1988). Remote memory function in Alzheimer's disease and Parkinson's disease. *Brain, 111,* 185-206.

Sagar, H.J., Sullivan, E.V., Gabrieli, J.D.E., Corkin, S. & Growdon, J.H. (1988). Temporal ordering deficits and short term memory deficits in Parkinson's disease. *Brain, 111,* 525-539.

Sahakian, B.J., Downes, J.J., Eagger, S., Evenden, J.L., Levy, R., Philpot, M., Roberts, A.C. & Robbins, T.W. (1990). Sparing of attentional relative to mnemonic function in a subgroup of patients with dementia of the Alzheimer type. *Neuropsychologia, 28(11),* 1197-1213.

Sahakian, B.J., Morris, R.G., Evenden, J.L., Heald, A., Levy, R., Philpot, M. & Robbins, T.W. (1988). A comparative study of visuospatial memory and learning in Alzheimer-type dementia and Parkinson's disease, *Brain, 111*, 695-718.

Sahakian, B.J. & Owen, A.M. (1992). Computerised assessment in neuropsychiatry using CANTAB: discussion paper. *Journal of the Royal Society of Medicine, 85,* 399-402.

Saint-Cyr, J.A., Taylor, A.E. & Lang, A.E. (1988). Procedural learning and neostriatal dysfunction in man. *Brain, 111,* 941-959.

Salmon, D.P. & Butters, N. (1995). Neurobiology of skill and habit learning. *Current Opinion in Neurobiology, 5,* 184-190.

Salmon, P. (2002). *Psychology of medicine and surgery. A guide for psychologists, counsellors, nurses and doctors*. Chichester: John Wiley & Sons, Ltd.

Samii, A., Nutt, J.G. & Ransom, B.R. (2004). Parkinson's disease. *Lancet, 363(9423),* 1783-1793.

Samuel, M., Maidment, I., Boustani, M. & Fox, C. (2006). Clinical management of Parkinson's disease dementia: Pitfalls and progress. *Advances in Psychiatric Treatment*, *12*, 121-129.

Sanders, C., Donovan, J. & Dieppe, P. (2002). The significance and consequences of having painful and disabled joints in older age: co-existing accounts of normal and disrupted biographies. *Sociology of Health and Illness, 24*(2), 227-253.

Sanford, J.R.A. (1975). Tolerance of debility in elderly dependants by supporters at home: its significance for hospital practice. *British Medical Journal, 3*, 471-475.

Santamaria, J., Tolosa, E. & Valles, A. (1986). Parkinson's disease with depression: a possible subgroup of idiopathic parkinsonism. *Neurology*, *36,* 1130-1133.

Savundranayagam, M.Y., Hummert M.L. & Montgomery, R.J. (2005). Investigating the effects of communication problems on caregiver burden. *Journal of Gerontology, 60B*(1), S48-S55.

Savundranayagam, M.Y., Montgomery, R.J. & Kosloski, K. (2011). A dimensional analysis of caregiver burden among spouses and adult children. *The Gerontologist, 51*(3), 321-31.

Sayegh, P. & Knight, B.G. (2011) The effects of familism and cultural justification on the mental and physical health of family caregivers. *Journal of Gerontology, 66B*(1): P3-P14.

Schacter, D.L., (1987). Implicit memory: History and current status. *Journal of Experimental Psychology: Learning, Memory and Cognition, 13,* 501-518.

Schag C.C., Heinrich R.L. & Ganz P.A.(1984). Karnofsky performance status revisited: Reliability, validity, and guidelines. *Journal of Clinical Oncology. 2,* 187-193.

Scheife, R.T., Schumock, G.T., Burstein, A., Gottwald, M.D. & Luer, M.S. (2000). Impact of Parkinson's disease and its pharmacological treatment on quality of life and economic outcomes. *American Journal of Health Systems Pharmacology, 57*, 953-962.

Schelosky, L. & Poewe, W. (1994). Life expectancy and disability in Parkinson disease. *Versicherungsmedizin, 46*(4), 119-122.

Schiffer, R.B., Kurlan, R., Rubin, A. & Boer, S. (1988). Evidence for atypical depression in Parkinson's disease. *American Journal of Psychiatry*, *145,* 1020-1022.

Schneider, J.W. & Conrad, P. (1981). Medical and sociological typologies: the case of epilepsy. *Social Science and Medicine, Part A., 15*(3 Pt 1), 211-219.

Schneider, J., Murray, J., Banerjee, S. & Mann, A. Eurocare: a cross-national study of co-resident spouse carers for people with Alzheimer's disease: I – Factors associated with carer burden. (1999). *International Journal of Geriatric Psychiatry*. *14*(8), 651-661.

Schrag, A. (2006). Quality of life and depression in Parkinson's disease. *Journal of the Neurological Sciences*, *248,* 151-157.

Schrag, A., Barone, P., Brown, R.G., Leentjens, A.F.G., McDonald, W.M., Starkstein, S., Weintraub, D., Poewe, W., Rascol, O., Sampaio, C., Stebbins, G.T. & Goetz, C.G. (2007). Depression rating scales in Parkinson's disease: critique and recommendations. *Movement Disorders*, *22*(8), 1077-1092.

Schrag, A., Ben-Shlomo, Y. & Quinn, N. (2002). How valid is the clinical diagnosis of Parkinson's disease in the community? *Journal of Neurology, Neurosurgery and Psychiatry*, *73*(5), 529-534.

Schrag, A., Hovris, A., Morley, D., Quinn, N. & Jahanshahi, M. (2006). Caregiver-burden in Parkinson's disease is closely associated with psychiatric symptoms, falls, and disability. *Parkinsonism and Related Disorders*, *12*(1), 35-41.

Schrag, A., Jahanshahi, M. & Quinn, N. (2000). What contributes to quality of life in patients with Parkinson's disease? *Journal of Neurology, Neurosurgery and Psychiatry, 69*(3), 308-312.

Schrag, A., Jahanshahi, M. & Quinn, N. (2001). What contributes to depression in Parkinson's disease? *Psychological Medicine*, *31,* 65-73.

Schrag, A., Morley, D. Quinn, N. & Jahanshahi, M. (2004) Impact of Parkinson's disease on patients' adolescent and adult children. *Parkinsonism and Related Disorders, 10*, 391-397.

Schrag, A. & Quinn, N. (2000). Dyskinesias and motor fluctuations in Parkinson's disease. A community based study. *Brain, 123,* 2297-2305.

Schrag, A. & Schott, J.M. (2006). Epidemiological, clinical and genetic characteristics of early-onset parkinsonism. *Lancet Neurology, 5*(4), 355-363.

Schulz, R. & Beach, S.R. (1999). Caregiving as a risk factor for mortality. The caregiver health effects study. *Journal of the American Medical Association, 282,* 2215-2219.

Schulz, R., Boerner, K., Shear, K., Zhang, S. & Gitlin, L. (2006). Predictors of complicated grief among dementia caregivers: A prospective study of bereavement. *American Journal of Geriatric Psychiatry, 14,* 650-658.

Schulz, R., Martire, L.M. & Klinger, J.N. (2005). Evidence-based caregiver interventions in geriatric psychiatry. *Psychiatric Clinics of North America, 28,* 1007-1038.

Schulz, R., O'Brien, A.T., Bookwala, J. & Fleissner, K. (1995). Psychiatric and physical morbidity effects of dementia caregiving: prevalence, correlates, and causes. *The Gerontologist. 35*(6),771-791.

Schulz, R., & Sherwood, P.R. (2008). Physical and mental health effects of family caregiving. *American Journal of Nursing, 108*(9 Suppl), 23-27.

Schulz, R., Visintainer, P. & Williamson G.M. (1990). Psychiatric and physical morbidity effects of caregiving. *Journal of Gerontology, 45*(5), 181- 191.

Schulz, R. & Williamson, G.M. (1997). The measurement of caregiver outcomes in Alzheimer disease research. *Alzheimer Disease and Associated Disorders,11* Supplement 6, 117-124.

Schumacher, K.L., Stewart, B.J. & Archbold, P.G. (2007) Mutuality and preparedness moderate the effects of caregiving demand on cancer family caregiver outcomes. *Nursing Research*, 56, 425-433.

Schumacher, K.L., Stewart, B.J., Archbold, P.G., Caparro, M., Mutuale, F. & Agrawal, S. (2008) Effects of caregiving demand, mutuality and preparedness on family caregiver outcomes during cancer treatment. *Oncology Nursing Forum, 35*, 49-56.

Schuurman, A.G., Van den Akker, M., Ensinck, K.T.J.L., Metsemakers, J.F.M., Knottnerus, J.A., Leentjens, A.F.G. & Buntinx, F. (2002). Increased risk of Parkinson's disease after depression. *Neurology, 58*, 1501-1504.

Schwab, R.S. & England, A.C. (1958). Parkinson's disease. *Journal of Chronic Diseases*, *8*(4), 488-509.

Schwab, R.S. & England, A.C. (1969). Projection techniques for evaluating surgery in Parkinson's disease. Paper presented at the Third Symposium on Parkinson's Disease, May 20-22, 1968 Royal College of Surgeons in Edinburgh.

Scott, W.K., Edwards, K.B., Davis, D.R., Cornman, C.B., & Macera, C.A. (1997). Risk of institutionalisation among community long-term care clients with dementia. *The Gerontologist*, *37,* 46-51.

Scott, J., Roberto, K.A., & Hutton, J. (1986). Families of Alzheimer's victims: Family support to caregivers. *Geriatrics Digest, 8*, 22-23.

Secker, D.L. & Brown, R.G. (2005). Cognitive behavioural therapy (CBT) for carers of patients with Parkinson's disease: a preliminary randomised controlled trial. *Journal of Neurology, Neurosurgurgery and Psychiatry, 76*(4), 491-497.

Secretaries of State (1989). *Caring for people: Community care in the next decade and beyond.* Cm849. London: HMSO.

Segal, D.L., Needham, T.N. & Coolidge, F.L. (2009). Age differences in attachment orientations among younger and older adults: evidence from two self-report measures of attachment. *International Journal of Aging and Human Development, 69*(2), 119-132.

Seiler, S., Perleth, B., Gasser, T., Ulm, G., Oertel, W. & Ellgring, H. (1992). Partnership and depression in Parkinson's disease. *Behavioural Neurology, 5*, 75-81.

Semple, S.J. (1992) Conflict in Alzheimer's caregiving families: its dimensions and consequences. *The Gerontologist, 32,* 648-655.

Seng, B.K., Luo, N., Ng, W.Y., Lim, J., Chionh, H.L., Goh, J., & Yap, P. (2010). Validity and reliability of the zarit Burden Interview in assessing caregiving burden. *Annals Academy of Medicine of Singapore, 39*(10), 758-763.

Seppi, K., Weintraub, D., Coelho, M., Perez-Lloret, S., Fox, S.H., Katzenschlager, R., Hametner, E.M., Poewe, W., Rascol, O., Goetz, C.G. & Sampaio, C. (2011). The Movement Disorder Society Evidence-Based Medicine Review Update: Treatments for the non-motor symptoms of Parkinson's disease. *Movement Disorders, 26,* Supplement 3, S42-80.

Shallice, T. (1982). Specific impairments of planning. *Philosophical Transactions of the Royal Society, Series B, 298,* 199-209.

Shapiro, M.A., Chang, Y.L., Munson, S.K., Okun, M.S. & Fernandez, H.H. (2006). Hypersexuality and paraphilia induced by selegiline in Parkinson's disease: report of 2 cases. *Parkinsonism and Related Disorders, 12*(6), 392-395.

Shapiro, M.B. (1961). A method for measuring psychological changes specific to the individual psychiatric patient. *British Journal of Medical Psychology, 34*, 151-155.

Shaw, K.M., Lees, A.J. & Stern, G.M. (1980). The impact of treatment with levodopa on Parkinson's disease. *Quarterly Journal of Medicine. 49*(195), 283-293.

Sheikh, J.I. & Yesavage, J.A. (1986). Geriatric Depression Scale (GDS): recent evidence and development of a shorter version. *Clinical Gerontology*, *5,* 165-173.

Sheridan, M.R., Flowers, K.A. & Hurrell, J. (1987). Programming and execution of movement in Parkinson's disease. *Brain, 110,* 1247-1271.

Shim, B., Landerman, L.R. & Davis, L. (2011). Correlates of care relationship mutuality among carers of people with Alzheimer's and Parkinson's disease. *Journal of Advanced Nursing, 67(8),* 1729-1738.

Shimamura, A.P., Salmon, D.P., Squire, L.R. & Butters, N. (1987). Memory dysfunction and word priming in dementia and amnesia. *Behavioural Neuroscience, 101,* 347-351.

Shin, H., Lee, J., Youn, J., Kim, J.S. & Cho, J.W. (2012). Factors contributing to spousal and offspring caregiver burden in Parkinson's disease. *European Neurology, 67(5),* 292-296.

Shin, H., Youn, J., Kim, J.S., Lee, J., & Cho, J.W. (2012). Caregiver burden in Parkinson disease with dementia compared to Alzheimer disease in Korea. *Journal of Geriatric Psychiatry and Neurology, 25(4),* 222-226.

Shontz, F.C. (1975). *The psychological aspects of physical illness and disability.* New York: Macmillan.

—. (2003). Rehabilitation psychology, then and now. *Rehabilitation Counselling Bulletin, 46,*176-181.

Shrout, P.E. & Bolger, N. (2002). Mediation in experimental and nonexperimental studies: new procedures and recommendations. *Psychological Methods, 7(4),* 422-445.

Shulman, L.M., Taback, R.L., Bean, J. & Weiner, W.J. (2001). Comorbidity of the nonmotor symptoms of Parkinson's disease. *Movement Disorders, 16(3)*, 507-510.

Shulman, L.M., Taback, R.L., Rabinstein, A.A. & Weiner, W.J. (2002). Non-recognition of depression and other non-motor symptoms in Parkinson's disease. *Parkinsonism and Related Disorders*, *8,* 193-197.

Shumway, M., Sentell, T., Unick, G. & Bamberg, W. (2004). Cognitive complexity of self-administered depression measures. *Journal of Affective Disorders*, *83,* 191-198.

Siderof, A. & Stern, M. (2006). Clinical trials with rasagiline: evidence for short-term and long-term effects. *Neurology*, *66,* S80-S88.

Siegert, R.J., Jackson, D.M., Tennant, A. & Turner-Stokes, L. (2010). Factor analysis and Rasch analysis of the Zarit Burden Interview for acquired brain injury carer research. *Journal of Rehabilitation Medicine, 42(4),* 302-309.

Silberman, C.D., Laks, J., Capitao, C.F., Rodrigues, C.S., Moreira, I. & Engelhardt, E. (2006). Recognizing depression in patients with Parkinson's disease; accuracy and specificity of two depression rating scales. *Arquivos Neuropsiquiatria*, *64(2-B),* 407-411.

Silbert, L.C. & Kaye, J. (2010). Neuroimaging and cognition in Parkinson's disease dementia. *Brain Pathology, 20(3),* 646-653.

Simpson, J.A., Rholes, W.S. & Nelligan, J.S. (1992). Support seeking and support giving within couples in an anxiety-provoking situation: The role of attachment styles. *Journal of Personality and Social Psychology, 62*, 434-446.

Sinding, C. & Wiernikowski, J. (2008). Disruption foreclosed: older women's cancer narratives. *Health (London), 12*(3), 389-411.

Singh, N., Pillay, V. & Choonara, Y.E. (2007). Advances in the treatment of Parkinson's disease. *Progress in Neurobiology, 81,* 29-44.

Singleton, S.S. (2001). Depression and quality of life: a patient's perspective. *Journal of Clinical Psychiatry, 62,* Supplement 26, 22.

Sink, K.M., Holden, K.F., & Yaffe, K. (2005) Pharmacological treatment of neuropsychiatric symptoms of dementia: A review of the evidence. *Journal of the American Medical Association, 293,* 596-608.

Skapinakis, P., Bakola, E., Salanti, G., Lewis, G., Kyritsis, A.P. & Mavreas, V. (2010). Efficacy and acceptability of selective serotonin reuptake inhibitors for the treatment of depression in Parkinson's disease: a systematic review and meta-analysis of randomized controlled trials. *BMC Neurology, 10:*49, 1-11.

Skeie, G.O., Muller, B., Haugarvoll, K., Larsen, J.P. & Tysnes, O.B. (2013). Parkinson disease: Associated disorders in the Norwegian population based incident ParkWest study. *Parkinsonism and Related Disorders, 19*, 53-55.

Skolnick, A. (1986). Early attachment and personal relationships across the life course. *Life Span Development and Behaviour, 7,* 173-206.

Slabosz, A., Lewis, S.J., Smigasiewicz, K., Szymura, B., Barker, R.A. & Owen, A.M. (2006). The role of learned irrelevance in attentional set-shifting impairments in Parkinson's disease. *Neuropsychology, 20*(5), 578-588.

Slaughter, J.R., Slaughter, K.A., Nichols, D. Holmes, S.E. & Martens, M.P. (2001). Prevalence, clinical manifestations, etiology and treatment of depression in Parkinson's disease. *Journal of Neuropsychiatry and Clinical Neurosciences*, *13*(2), 187-196.

Sławek, J. (2008). Późne powikłania ruchowe w chorobie Parkinsona. *Polski Przegląd Neurologiczny*, *4*(3), 119-124. (In Polish)

Smith, E.E. & Jonides, J. (1999). Storage and executive processes in the frontal lobes. *Science, 283,* 1657-1661.

Smith, G.R., Williamson, G.M., Miller, L.S. & Schulz, R. (2011). Depression and quality of informal care: a longitudinal investigation of caregiving stressors. *Psychological Aging, 26*(3), 584-591.

Smith, M.C. (1996). Illness, sickness and disease. In M.C. Smith & A.I. Wertheimer (Eds.). *Social and behavioral aspects of pharmaceutical care* (pp. 21-40). Binghamton, New York: Pharmaceutical Products Press (The Haworth Press Incorporated).

Smith, M.C., Goldman, W.P., Janer, K.W., Baty, J.D. & Morris, J.C. (1998). Cognitive speed in nondemented Parkinson's disease. *Journal of the International Neuropsychology Society, 4*(6), 584-92.

Snaith, R.P., Bridge, G.W.K. & Hamilton, M. (1976). The Leeds scales for the self-assessment of anxiety and depression. *British Journal of Psychiatry*, *128,* 156-165.

Snaith, R.P. & Zigmond, A.S. (1986). The hospital anxiety and depression scale. *British Medical Journal, 292*(6516), 344.

Sobel, M.E.(1990). Effect analysis and causation in linear structural equation models. *Psychometrika, 55(3),* 495-515.

—. (1982). Asymptotic confidence intervals for indirect effects in structural equations models. In S.Leinhart (Ed.) *Sociological methodology* (pp. 290-312). San Francisco: Jossey-Bass.

Söderlin, M.K., Hakala, M. & Nieminen, P. (2000). Anxiety and depression in a community-based rheumatoid arthritis population. *Scandinavian Journal of Rheumatology*, *29*(3), 177-183.

Sohlberg, M.M. & Mateer, C.A. (1989). *Introduction to Cognitive Rehabilitation. Theory and Practice.* New York: Guilford Press.

Sohlberg, M.M. & Mateer, C.A. (2001). *Cognitive Rehabilitation: An integrative neuropsychological approach.* New York: Guilford Press.

Somerfield, M.R. & McCrae, R.R. (2000). Stress and coping research. Methodological challenges, theoretical advances and clinical applications. *American Psychologist, 55*(6), 620-625.

Son, J., Erno, A., Shea, D.G., Femia, E.E., Zarit, S.H., & Stephens. M.A. (2007). The caregiver stress process and health outcomes. *Journal of Aging and Health, 19*(6), 871-887.

Sorensen, S., Pinquart, M. & Duberstein, P. (2002). How effective are interventions with caregivers? An updated meta-analysis. *The Gerontologist, 42*(3), 356-372.

Sörensen, S., Webster, J.D. & Roggman, L.A. (2002). Adult attachment and preparing to provide care for older relatives. *Attachment and Human Development, 4(1),*84-106.

Spica, V., Pekmezovic, T., Svetel, M. & Kostic, V.S. (2013). Prevalence of non-motor symptoms in young-onset versus late-onset Parkinson's disease. *Journal of Neurology, 260(1),* 131-137.

Spitznagel, M.B., Tremont, G., Davis, J.D. & Foster, S.M. (2006). Psychosocial predictors of dementia caregiver desire to institutionalize: Caregiver, care recipient and family relationship factors. *Journal of Geriatric Psychiatry and Neurology, 19*(1), 16-20.

Sprecher, S. (1992). How men and women expect to feel and behave in response to inequity in close relationships. *Social Psychology Quarterly, 55*, 57-69.

Squire, L.R. (1987). *Memory and brain.* New York: Oxford University Press.

Stacy, M. (2002) Sleep disorders in Parkinson's disease: epidemiology and management. *Drugs and Aging. 19(10),* 733-739.

Standaert, D.G. & Stern, M.B. (1993). Update on the management of Parkinson's disease. *Medical Clinics of North America, 77(1),* 169-183.

Stanley-Hermanns, M. & Engebretson, J. (2010). Sailing the stormy seas: The illness experience of persons with Parkinson's disease. *The Qualitative Report, 15(2),* 340-369.

Starkstein, S.E., Berthier, M.L., Bolduc, P.L., Preziosi, T.J. & Robinson, R.G. (1989). Depression in patients with early versus late onset of Parkinson's disease. *Neurology*, *39,* 1441-1445.

Starkstein S.E., Bolduc, P.L., Mayberg, H.S., Preziosi, T.J. & Robinson, R.G. (1990). Cognitive impairments and depression in Parkinson's disease: a follow-up study. *Journal of Neurology, Neurosurgery and Psychiatry*, *53(7),* 597-602.

Starkstein, S., Dragovic, M., Jorge, R., Brockman, S., Merello, M., Robinson, R.G., Bruce, D. & Wilson, M. (2011). Diagnostic criteria for depression in Parkinson's disease: A study of symptom patterns using latent class analysis. *Movement Disorders*, *26(12),* 2239-2245.

Starkstein, S.E., Mayburg, H.S., Leiguarda, R., Preziosi, T.J. & Robinson, R.G. (1992). A prospective longitudinal study of depression, cognitive decline and physical impairments in patients with Parkinson's disease. *Journal of Neurology, Neurosurgery and Psychiatry*, *55,* 377-382.

Starkstein, S.E., Mayburg, H.S., Preziosi, T.J., Andrzejewski, P., Leiguarda, R. & Robinson, R.G. (1992). Reliability, validity and clinical correlates of apathy in Parkinson's disease. *Journal of Neuropsychiatry and Clinical Neuroscience, 4,* 134-139.

Starkstein, S.E., Petracca, G., Chemerinski, E., Tesón, A., Sabe, L., Merello, M. & Leiguarda, R. (1998). Depression in classic versus akinetic-rigid Parkinson's disease. *Movement Disorders*, *13(1),* 29-33.

Starkstein, S.E., Preziosi, T.J., Bolduc, P.L. & Robinson, R.G. (1990). Depression in Parkinson's disease. *Journal of Nervous and Mental Diseases, 178(1)*, 27-31.

Starkstein, S.E., Preziosi, T.J., Forrester, A.W. & Robinson, R.G. (1990). Specificity of affective and autonomic symptoms of depression in Parkinson's disease. *Journal of Neurology, Neurosurgery and Psychiatry, 53(10),* 869-873.

Starkstein, S.E. & Robinson, R.G. (1991). Dementia of depression in Parkinson's disease and stroke. *Journal of Nervous and Mental Disease*, *179*(10), 593-601.

Steadman, P.L., Tremont, G. & Duncan Davis J. (2007) Premorbid relationship satisfaction and caregiver burden in dementia caregivers. *Journal of Geriatric Psychiatry and Neurology, 20*(2): 115-119.

Steele, H., Phibbs, E. & Woods, R.T. (2004). Coherence of mind in daughter caregivers of mothers with dementia: links with their mothers' joy and relatedness on reunion in a strange situation. *Attachment and Human Development, 6*(4), 439-450.

Stella, F., Banzato, C.E., Quagliato, E.M., Viana, M.A. & Christofoletti, G. (2009). Psychopathological features in patients with Parkinson's disease and related caregivers' burden. *International Journal Geriatric Psychiatry, 24*(10), 1158-1165.

Stephens, M.A., Norris, V.K., Kinney, J.M., Ritchie, S.W., & Grotz, R.C. (1988). Stressful situations in caregiving: relations between caregiver coping and well-being. *Psychology of Aging, 3*(2), 208-209.

Stern, M., Dulaney, E. and Gruber, S.B., Golbe, L., Bergen, M., Hurtig, H., Gollomp, S. & Stolley, P. (1991). The epidemiology of Parkinson's disease. A case-control study of young-onset and old-onset patients. *Archives of Neurology*, *48(9),* 903–907.

Stern, G. & Lees, A. (1982). *Parkinson's disease: the facts*. Oxford University Press, Oxford.

Stern,Y., Marder, K., Tang, M.X. & Mayeux, R. (1993). Antecedent clinical features associated with dementia in Parkinson's disease. *Neurology, 43*(9), 1690-1692.

Stern, Y., Richards, M., Sano, M. & Mayeux, R. (1993). Comparison of cognitive changes in patients with Alzheimer's and Parkinson's disease. *Archives of Neurology, 50,* 1040-1045.

Stewart, D.C. & Sullivan,T.J. (1982). Illness behavior and the sick role in chronic disease. The case of multiple sclerosis. *Social Science and Medicine, 16(15)*, 1397-1404.

Stirling, C., Andrews, S., Croft, T., Vickers, J., Turner, P, & Robinson, A. (2010). Measuring dementia carers' unmet need for services--an exploratory mixed method study. *BMC Health Service Research,* 10, 122.

St Pierre, J., Craven, R.F. & Bruno, P. (1986). Late life depression: a guide for assessment. *Journal of Gerontological Nursing,12(7)*, 5-10.

Stuckey, J.C., Neundorfer, M.M. & Smyth, K.A. (1996). Burden and well-being: the same coin or related currency. *The Gerontologist, 36*(5), 686-693.

Stull, D.E. (1988) A dyadic approach to predicting well-being in later life. *Research on Aging, 10* (1), 81-101.

Stull, D.E., Kosloski, K. & Kercher, K. (1994) Caregiver burden and generic well-being: opposite sides of the same coin? *The Gerontologist, 34*(1), 88-94.

Stuss, D.T. & Alexander, M.P. (2008). Is there a dysexecutive syndrome? In J. Driver, P. Haggard & T. Shallice, (Eds.), *Mental Processes in the Human Brain*, (pp.225-248), New York: Oxford University Press.

Suchman, E. (1965). Stages of illness and medical care. *Journal of Health and Human Behaviour, 6,* 114-128.

Sullivan, E.V. & Sagar, H.J. (1991). Double dissociation of short-term and long-term memory for nonverbal material in Parkinson's disease and global amnesia. A further analysis. *Brain,114 (Pt 2),* 893-906.

Sutcliffe, C., Cordingley, L., Burns, A., Mozley, C.G., Bagley, H., Huxley, P. & Challis, D. (2000). A new version of the geriatric depression scale for nursing and residential home populations: the geriatric depression scale (residential) (GDS-12R). *International Psychogeriatrics, 12(2),* 173-181.

Syndulko, K., Gilden, E.R., Hansch, E.C., Potvin, A.R., Tourtellotte, W.W. & Potvin, J.H. (1981). Decreased verbal memory associated with anti-cholinergic treatment in Parkinson's disease patients. *International Journal of Neuroscience, 14,* 61-66.

Szepietowska, M.E. & Misztal, H. (1999). Neuropsychologiczny opis zaburzeń emocjonalnych w polskim piśmiennictwie klinicznym. (Neuropsychological analysis of emotional dysfunctions in the Polish clinical literature). In A. Herzyk & A. Borkowska (Eds).

Neuropsychologia emocji: poglady, badania, klinika (pp. 83-105). Lublin, Wydawnictwo Uniwersytetu Marii Curie-Skłodowskiej. Chapter in Polish.

Takeshita, S., Kurisu, K., Trop, L., Arita, K., Akimitsu, T. & Verhoeff, N.P. (2005). Effect of subthalamic stimulation on mood state in Parkinson's disease: evaluation of previous facts and problems. *Neurosurgical Reviews, 28(3)*, 179-186.

Talland, G.A. (1962). Cognitive function in Parkinson's disease. *The Journal of Nervous and Mental Disease*, 135, 196-205.

Tam, C.W., Burton, E.J., McKeith, I.G., Burn, D.J. & O'Brien, J.T. (2005). Temporal lobe atrophy on MRI in Parkinson disease with dementia: a comparison with Alzheimer disease and dementia with Lewy bodies. *Neurology, 64(5),* 861-865.

Tan, L.C.S. (2012). Mood disorders in Parkinson's disease. *Parkinsonism and Related Disorders*, *18S1,* S74-S76.

Tan, S.K., Hartung, H., Sharp, T. & Temel, Y. (2011). Serotonin-dependent depression in Parkinson's disease: a role for the subthalamic nucleus? *Neuropharmacology,61(3),* 387-399.

Tandberg, E., Larsen, J.P., Aarsland, D. & Cummings, J.L. (1996). The occurrence of depression in Parkinson's disease. A community-based study. *Archives of Neurology, 53,* 175-179.

Tandberg, E., Larsen, J.P., Aarsland, D., Laake, K. & Cummings, J.L. (1997). Risk factors for depression in Parkinson disease. *Archives of Neurology, 54(5),* 625-630.

Tandberg, E., Larsen, J.P. & Karlsen, K.A. (1998). A community-based study of sleep disorders in patients with Parkinson's disease. *Movement Disorders, 13,* 895-899.

Tanji, H., Anderson, K.E., Gruber-Baldini, A.L., Fishman, P.S., Reich, S.G., Weiner, W.J. & Shulman, L.M. (2008). Mutuality of the marital relationship in Parkinson's disease. *Movement Disorders, 23*(13), 1843-1849.

Tapiola, T., Alafuzoff, I., Herukka, S.K., Parkkinen, L., Hartikainen, P., Soininen, H. & Pirttilä, T. (2009). Cerebrospinal fluid {beta}-amyloid 42 and tau proteins as biomarkers of Alzheimer-type pathologic changes in the brain. *Archives of Neurology, 66(3)*, 382-389.

Tarnopolsky, A., Hand, D.J., McLean, E.K., Roberts, H. & Wiggins, R.D. (1979). Validity and uses of a screening questionnaire (GHQ) in the community. *British Journal of Psychiatry, 134,* 508-515.

Taylor, A.E., Saint-Cyr, J.A. & Lang, A.E. (1986). Frontal lobe dysfunction in Parkinson's disease. The cortical focus of neostriatal outflow. *Brain, 109,* 845-883.

Taylor, A.E., Saint-Cyr, J.A., Lang, A.E. & Kenny, F.T. (1986). Parkinson's disease and depression: a critical re-evaluation. *Brain*, 109, 279-292.

Taylor, A.E., Saint-Cyr, J.A. & Lang, A.E. (1990). Memory and learning in early Parkinson's disease: evidence for a "frontal lobe syndrome". *Brain and Cognition, 13,* 211-232.

Tekin, S. & Cummings, J.L. (2002). Frontal-subcortical neuronal circuits and clinical neuropsychiatry: an update. *Journal of Psychosomatic Research, 53(2),* 647-654.

Tessa, C., Giannelli, M., Della Nave, R., Lucetti, C., Berti, C., Ginestroni, A., Bonuccelli U. & Masacalchi, M. (2008). A whole-brain analysis in de novo Parkinson disease. *American Journal of Neuroradiology*, *29,* 674-680.

Thane, P., (2009). Memorandum submitted to the House of Commons' Health Committee Inquiry: Social Care. Retrieved from: www.historyandpolicy.org/ docs/thane_social_care.pdf

Thanvi, B.R., Munshi, S.K., Vijaykumar, N. & Lo, T.C.N. (2003). Neuropsychiatric non-motor aspects of Parkinson's disease. *Postgraduate Medicine Journal*, *79,* 561-565.

The Columbia Encyclopedia, 6th ed.. 2011. L-dopa. Retrieved July 07, 2012 from Encyclopedia.com: http://www.encyclopedia.com/doc/1E1-ldopa.html

The Global Parkinson's Disease Survey Steering Committee. (2002). Factors impacting on quality of life in Parkinson's disease: results from an international survey. *Movement Disorders, 17,* 60-67.

The Guardian (2010). http://www.guardian.co.uk/society/2010/mar/31/free-care-elderly-lords-bill

The Law Commission (2010). *Adult Social Care*. Law Com No. 326. London: The Stationery Office.

—. (2012). *Adult Social Care*. Commentary on the publication of the draft bill, retrieved from: http://lawcommission.justice.gov.uk/areas/adult-social-care.htm

The National Archives (2012). Carer's Allowance. http://webarchive.nationalarchives.gov.uk/+/www.direct.gov.uk/en/caringforsomeone/moneymatters/dg_10012522.

The Resource Implications Study Group of the Medical Research Council study of cognitive function and ageing [RIS MRC CFAS], (2000). Psychological morbidity among informal caregivers of older people: a 2-year follow-up study. *Psychological Medicine, 30(4),* 943-955.

Thomas, P., Ingrand, P., Lalloue, F., Hazif-Thomas, C., Billon, R., Viéban, F., & Clément, J.P. (2004). Reasons of informal caregivers for institutionalizing dementia patients previously living at home: the Pixel study. *International Journal of Geriatric Psychiatry, 19*(2), 127-35.

Thommessen B., Aarsland D., Braekhus A., Oksengaard A.R., Engedal K. & Laake K. (2002). The psychosocial burden on spouses of the elderly with stroke, dementia and Parkinson's disease. *International Journal of Geriatric Psychiatry*, *17,* 78-84.

Thompson, A.W., Liu, H., Hays, R.D., Katon, W.J., Rausch, R., Diaz, N., Jacob, E.L., Vassar, S.D. & Vickrey, B.G. (2011). Diagnostic accuracy and agreement across three depression assessment measures for Parkinson's disease. Parkinsonism and Related Disorders. 17(1), 40-45.

Thompson, R.L., Lewis, S.L., Murphy, M.R., Hale, J.M., Blackwell, P.H., Acton, G.J., Clough, D.H., Patrick, G.J. & Bonner, P.N. (2004). Are there sex differences in emotional and biological responses in spousal caregivers of patients with Alzheimer's disease? *Biological Research for Nursing, 5*(4), 319-330.

Thrall, J.H. (2005) Prevalence and costs of chronic disease in a health care system structured for treatment of acute illness. *Radiology, 235*(1), 9-12.

Timonen, M. & Liukkonen, T. (2008). Management of depression in adults. *British Medical Journal*, *336(7641),* 435-439.

Tindall, L.R. and Huebner, R.A. (2009). The impact of an application of telerehabilitation technology on caregiver burden. *International Journal of Telerehabilitation, 1(1),* 3-7.

Tinker, A.,Wright, F., McCreadie, C., Askham, J., Hancock, R. & Holmans, A. (1999). *Alternative models of care for older people.* Royal Commission on long term care. With respect to old age: Long term care – rights and responsibilities. Research vol.2. Cm4192-II/2. London: TSO.

Tison, F., Barberger-Gateau, P., Dubroca, B., Henry, P & Dartiques, J.F. (1997). Dependency in Parkinson's disease: a population-based survey in nondemented elderly subjects. *Movement Disorders, 12(6)*, 910-915.

Tobin, S. & Kulys, R. (1981). The family in the institutionalisation of the elderly. *Journal of Social Issues, 37,* 145-157.

Todes, C.J., & Lees, A.J. (1985). The pre-morbid personality of patients with Parkinson's disease. *Journal of Neurology, Neurosurgery & Psychiatry, 48*(2), 97-100.

Torti, F.M., Gwyther, L.P., Reed, S.D., Friedman, J.Y. & Schulman, K.A. (2004). A multinational review of recent trends and reports in dementia caregiver burden. *Alzheimer's Disease and Associated Disorders, 18*(2), 99-109.

Townsend, A.L. & Franks, M.M. (1995). Binding ties: Closeness and conflict in adult children's caregiving relationships. *Psychology and Aging, 10*, 343-351.

Travis, L., Binder, J., Bliwise, N., & Horne-Moyer, L. (2001). Changes in clients' attachment styles over the course of time-limited psychotherapy. *Psychotherapy, 38(2),* 149-159.

Tremont, G., Duncan Davis, J. & Bishop, D.S. (2006) Unique contribution of family functioning in caregivers of patients with mild to moderate dementia. *Dementia and Geriatric Cognitive Disorders, 21(3),* 170-174.

Tröster, A.I., Fields, J.A. Paolo, A.M. & Koller, W.C. (1996). Performance of individuals with Parkinson's disease on the Vocabulary and Information subtests of the WAIS-R as a neuropsychological instruments. *Journal of Clinical Geropsychology, 2,* 215-223.

Tröster, A.I., Heindel, W.C., Salmon, D.P. & Butters, N. (1989). Category fluency performance in Parkinson's disease with and without dementia. *The Clinical Neuropsychologist, 3,* 284.

Tröster, A.I., Paolo, A.M., Lyons, K.E., Glatt, S.L., Hubble, J.P. & Koller, W.C. (1995). The influence of depression on cognition in Parkinson's disease: a pattern of impairment distinguishable from Alzheimer's disease. *Neurology*, *45,* 672-676.

Tröster, A.I., Salmon, D.P., McCullough, D. & Butters, N. (1989). A comparison of the category fluency deficits associated with Alzheimer's and Huntington's disease. *Brain and Language, 37,* 500-513.

Tsai, C.H., Lu, C.S., Hua, M.S., Lo, W.L. & Lo, S.K. (1994). Cognitive dysfunction in early onset parkinsonism. *Acta Neurologica Scandinavica, 89,* 9-14.

Tulving, E. (1983). *Elements of episodic memory*. London: Oxford University Press.

Tumas, V., Rodrigues, G.G.R., Farias, T.L.A. & Crippa, J.A.S. (2008). The accuracy of diagnosis of major depression in patients with Parkinson's disease. *Arquivos Neuropsiquiatria*, *66(2-A),* 152-156.

Turner, M.A., Moran, N.F. & Kopelman, M.D. (2002). Subcortical dementia. *The British Journal of Psychiatry, 180,* 148-151.

Twaddle, A. (1973). Illness and Deviance. *Social Science and Medicine, 7,* 751-762.

Tweedy, J.R., Langer, K.G., & McDowell, F.H. (1982). The effect of semantic relations on the memory deficit associated with Parkinson's disease. *Journal of Clinical Neuropsychology, 4*(3), 235-247.

Twenge, J.M. (2001). Changes in women's assertiveness in response to status and roles: a cross-temporal meta-analysis, 1931-1993. *Journal of Personality and Social Psychology, 81(1),* 133-145.

Twigg, J. (1992). Carers in the service system. In J. Twigg (Ed.) *Carers: research and practice*. London: HMSO.

—. (1998). Informal care and older people. In M. Bernard & J. Phillips (Eds.). *The social policy of old age.* London: Centre for Policy on Ageing.

Twigg, J. & Atkin, K. (1994). *Carers Perceived: policy and practice in informal care*. Buckingham: Open University Press.

Tylee A, Walters P. (2007). Underrecognition of anxiety and mood disorders in primary care: why does the problem exist and what can be done? *Journal of Clinical Psychiatry*, *68 Suppl. 2,* 27-30.

Uekermann, J., Daum., Peters, S., Wiebel, B., Przuntek, H. & Muller, T. (2003). Depressed mood and executive dysfunction in early Parkinson's disease. *Acta Neurologica Scandinavica, 107(5),* 341-348.

Uitti, R.J., Tanner, C.M., Rajput, A.H., Goetz, C.G., Klawans, H.L. & Thiessen, B. (1989). Hypersexuality with antiparkinsonian therapy. *Clinical Neuropharmacology, 12*(5), 375-383.

Ulstein, I., Wyller, T.B., & Engedal, K. (2007). High score on the Relatives Stress Scale, a marker of possible psychiatric disorder in family carers of patients with dementia. *International Journal of Geriatric Psychiatry, 22*, 195-202.

Välimäki, T.H., Vehviläinen-Julkunen, K.M., Pietilä, A.M., & Pirttilä, T.A. (2009). Caregiver depression is associated with a low sense of coherence and health-related quality of life. *Aging and Mental Health, 13*(6), 799-807.

Van Den Eeden, S.K., Tanner, C.M., Bernstein, A.L., Fross, R. D., Leimpeter, A. Bloch, D.A. & Nelson, L.M. (2003). Incidence of Parkinson's disease: variation by age, gender and race/ethnicity. *American Journal of Epidemiology*, *157(11),* 1015-1022.

Van der Hoek, T.C., Bus, B.A., Matui, P., van der Marck, M.A., Esselink, R.A. & Tendolkar, I. (2011). Prevalence of depression in Parkinson's disease: effects of disease stage, motor subtype and gender. *Journal Neurological Sciences, 310(1-2)*, 220-224.

Van Durme, T., Macq, J., Jeanmart, C. & Gobert, M. (2012). Tools for measuring the impact of informal caregiving of the elderly: A literature review. *International Journal of Nursing Studies, 49(4),* 490-504.

Van Ijzendoorn, M.H., Kroonenberg, P.M. (1988). Cross-cultural patterns of attachment: A meta-analysis of the strange-situation. *Child Development, 59,* 147–156.

Van Rooden, S.M., Colas, F., Martínez-Martín, P., Visser, M., Verbaan, D., Marinus, J., Chaudhuri ,R.K., Kok, J.N. & van Hilten, J.J. (2011). Clinical subtypes of Parkinson's disease. *Movement Disorders, 26(1),* 51-58.

Van Rooden, S.M., Heiser, W.J., Kok, J.N., Verbaan, D., van Hilten, J.J. & Marinus J. (2010) The identification of Parkinson's disease subtypes using cluster analysis: a systematic review. *Movement Disorders, 25(8),* 969-978.

Van Rooden, S.M., Visser, M., Verbaan, D., Marinus, J. & van Hilten, J.J. (2009a). Motor patterns in Parkinson's disease: a data-driven approach. *Movement Disorders, 24(7)*, 1042-1047.

Van Rooden, S.M., Visser, M., Verbaan, D., Marinus, J., & van Hilten, J.J. (2009b). Patterns of motor and non-motor features in Parkinson's disease. *Journal of Neurology, Neurosurgery and Psychiatry, 80(8),* 846-850.

Van Spaendonck, K.P., Berger, H.J., Horstink, M.W., Buytenhuijs, E.L. & Cools, A.R. (1996). Executive functions and disease characteristics in Parkinson's disease. *Neuropsychologia, 34,* 617-626.

Varanese, S., Perfetti, B., Ghilardi, M.F. & Di Roco, A. (2011). Apathy, but not depression, reflects inefficient cognitive strategies in Parkinson's disease. *PLoS ONE, 6(3),*1-6.

Vaughan, I. (1986). *Ivan: Living with Parkinson's disease*. London: Macmillan.

Veiga, B.A., Borges, V., Silva, S.M., Goulart Fde, O., Cendoroglo, M.S. & Ferraz, H.B. (2009). Depression in Parkinson's disease: clinical-epidemiological correlates and comparison with a controlled group of non-parkinsonian geriatric patients. *Revista Brasileira de Psiquiatria. 31(1),* 39-42.

Veazey, C., Aki, S.O.E., Cook, K.F., Lai, E.C. & Kunik, M.E. (2005). Prevalence and treatment of depression in Parkinson's disease. *Journal of Neuropsychiatry and Clinical Neurosciences*, *17(3),* 310-323.

Vilariño-Güell, C., Wider, C., Ross, O.A., Dachsel, J.C., Kachergus, J.M., Lincoln, S.J., Soto-Ortolaza, A.I., Cobb, S.A., Wilhoite, G.J., Bacon, J.A., Behrouz, B., Melrose, H.L., Hentati, E., Puschmann, A., Evans, D.M., Conibear, E., Wasserman, W.W., Aasly, J.O., Burkhard, P.R., Djaldetti, R., Ghika, J., Hentati, F., Krygowska-Wajs, A., Lynch, T., Melamed, E., Rajput, A., Rajput, A.H., Solida, A., Wu, R.M., Uitti, R.J., Wszolek, Z.K., Vingerhoets, F. & Farrer, M.J. (2011). VPS35 Mutations in Parkinson Disease. *The American Journal of Human Genetics*, 89(1), 162-167.

Vilas, D., Pont-Sunyer, C. & Tolosa, E. (2012). Impulse control disorders in Parkinson's disease. *Parkinsonism and Related Disorders, 18S1,* S80-S84.

Visser, M., Leentjens. A.F., Marinus, J., Stiggelbout, A.M. & van Hilten, J.J. (2006). Reliability and validity of the Beck depression inventory in patients with Parkinson's disease. *Movement Disorders, 21(5),* 668-672.

Vitaliano, P.P., DeWolfe, D.J., Maiuro, R.D., Russo, J., & Katon, W. (1990). Appraised changeability of a stressor as a modifier of the relationship between coping and depression: a test of the hypothesis of fit. *Journal of Personality and Social Psychology, 59*(3), 582-592.

Vitaliano, P.P, Russo, J., Young, H.M., Becker, J., & Maiuro, R.D. (1991). The screen for caregiver burden. *The Gerontologist, 31*(1), 76-83.

Vitaliano, P.P., Zhang, J. & Scanlan, J.M. (2003). Is caregiving hazardous to one's physical health? A meta-analysis. *Psychological Bulletin, 129*(6), 946-972.

Voon, V., Hassan, K., Zurowski, M., Duff-Canning, S., de Souza, M., Fox, S., Lang, A.E. & Miyasaki, J. (2006). Prospective prevalence of pathologic gambling and medication association in Parkinson's disease. *Neurology*, *66,* 1750-1752.

Wade, D.T., & Collin, C. (1988). The Barthel ADL Index: a standard measure of physical disability? *International Disability Studies, 10*(2), 64-67.

Wagle, A.C., Berrios, G.E. & Ho, L. (1999). The Cognitive Failures Questionnaire in Psychiatry. *Comprehensive Psychiatry*, *40*(6), 478-484.

Walshe, F.M.R. (1955). A clinical analysis of the paralysis agitans syndrome. In: James Parkinson. M. Critchley (Ed.) London, MacMillan.

Walters, A.H., Oyebode, J.R. & Riley, G.A. (2010) The dynamics of continuity and discontinuity for women caring for a spouse with dementia. *Dementia, 9*(2), 169-189.

Warburton, J.W. (1967a). Depressive symptoms in Parkinson patients referred for thalamotomy. *Journal of Neurology, Neurosurgery and Psychiatry*, *30,* 368-370.

—. (1967b). Memory disturbance and the Parkinson syndrome. *British Journal of Medical Psychology, 40,*169-171.

Waters, E., Weinfield, N.S., & Hamilton, C.E. (2000). The stability of attachment security from infancy to adolescenceand early adulthood: General discussion. *Child Development, 71*(3), 703-706.

Watkins, E.S. & Oppenheimer, D.R. (1962). Mental disturbances after thalamolysis. *Journal of Neurology, Neurosurgery and Psychiatry*, *25,* 243-250.

Watson, L., Lewis, C. & Fillenbaum, G. (2005). Asking family about memory loss. Is it helpful? *Journal of General Internal Medicine, 20,* 28-32.

Watson, L.C., Lewis, C.L., Moore, C.G., & Jeste, D.V. (2011). Perceptions of depression among dementia caregivers: findings from the CATIE-AD trial. *International Journal of Geriatric Psychiatry, 26*(4), 397-402.

Watts, F.N. (Ed.) (1993). *Neuropsychological perspectives on emotion.* Hove, U.K., Lawrence Erlbaum Associates, Publishers.

Wear, H.J., Wedderburn, C.J., Mioshi, E., Williams-Gray, C.H., Mason, S.L., Barker, R.A. & Hodges, J.R. (2008). The Cambridge Behavioural Inventory Revised. *Dementia & Neuropsychologia*, *2(2),* 102–107.

Webster, D., (1968). Critical analysis of the disability in Parkinson's disease. *Modern Treatment*, *5,* 257-258.

Webster, J.D. (1997). Attachment style and well-being in elderly adults: a preliminary investigation. *Canadian Journal on Aging, 16*, 101-111.

Wechsler, D. (2008). Wechsler Adult Intelligence Scale—*4th Edition* (WAIS-4®) San Antonio, TX: Harcourt Assessment.

Weinfield, N., Sroufe, L.A., & Egeland, B. (2000). Attachment from infancy to young adulthood in a high risk sample: Continuity, discontinuity and their correlates. *Child Development, 71*, 695-702.

Weingartner, H., Burns, S., Diebel, R. & Lewitt, P.A. (1984). Cognitive impairments in Parkinson's disease: Distinguishing between effort-demanding and automatic cognitive processes. *Psychiatry Research, 11,* 223-235.

Weintraub, D. (2009). Impulse control disorders in Parkinson's disease: prevalence and possible risk factors. *Parkinsonism and Related Disorders*, *15S3,* S110-S113.

Weintraub, D. & Burn, D.J. (2011). Parkinson's disease: the quintessential neuropsychiatric disorder. *Movement Disorders*, *26*(6), 1022-1031.

Weintraub, D., Comella, C.L. & Horn, S. (2008). Parkinson's disease. Part 2: Treatment of motor systems. *The American Journal of Managed Care*, *14,* S49-S58.

Weintraub, D., Dietz, N., Duda, J.E., Wolk, D.A., Doshi, J., Xie, S.X., Davatzikos, C., Clark, C.M. & Siderowf, A. (2012). Alzheimer's disease pattern of brain atrophy predicts cognitive decline in Parkinson's disease. *Brain, 135(Pt 1),* 170-180.

Weintraub, D., Koester, J., Potenza, M.N., Siderowf, A.D., Stacy, M., Voon, V., Whetteckey, J., Wunderlich, G.R. & Lang, A.E. (2010). Impulse control disorders in Parkinson’s disease. *Archives of Neurology*, *67(5),* 589-595.

Weintraub, D., Moberg, P.J., Culbertson, W.C., Duda, J.E. & Stern, M.B. (2004). Evidence for impaired encoding and retrieval memory profiles in Parkinson’s disease. *Cognitive and Behavioural Neurology, 17(4):* 195-200.

Weintraub, D., Moberg, P.J., Duda, J.E., Katz, I.R. & Stern, M.B. (2003). Recognition and treatment of depression in Parkinson’s disease. *Journal of Geriatric Psychiatry and Neurology*, *16,* 178-183.

Weintraub, D., Moberg, P.J., Duda, J.E., Katz, I.R. & Stern, M.B. (2004). Effect of psychiatric and other non-motor symptoms on disability in Parkinson’s disease. *Journal of the American Geriatrics Society*, *52(5),* 784-788.

Weintraub, D., Morales, K.H., Moberg, P.J., Bilker, W.B., Balderston, C., Duda, J.E., Katz, I.R. & Stern, M.B. (2005). Antidepressant studies in Parkinson’s disease: a review and meta-analysis. *Movement Disorders, 20(9),* 1161-1169.

Weintraub, D., & Nirenberg, M.J. (2013). Impulse control related disorders in Parkinson’s disease. *Neurodegenerative Diseases, 11(2),* 63-71.

Weintraub, D., Oehlberg, K.A., Katz, I.R. & Stern, M.B. (2006). Test characteristics of the 15-item Geriatric Depression Scale and Hamilton Depression rating Scale in Parkinson’s disease. *American Journal of Geriatric Psychiatry*, *14,* 169-175.

Weintraub, D. & Stern, M.B. (2009). Recognizing psychiatric and cognitive complications in Parkinson’s Disease. Retrieved from: www.medscape.org/viewarticle/590850.

Weissman, M.M., Bland, R.C., Canino, G.J., Faravelli, C., Greenwald, S., Hwu, H.G., Joyce, P.R., Karam, E.G., Lee, C.K., Lellouch, J., Lépine, J.P., Newman, S.C., Rubio-Stipec, M., Wells, J.E., Wickramaratne, P.J., Wittchen, H. & Yeh, E.K. (1996). Cross-national epidemiology of major depression and bipolar disorder. *Journal of the American Medical Association, 276(4),* 293-299.

Wermuth, L. & Stenager, E. (1995). Sexual problems in young patients with Parkinson's disease. *Acta Neurologica Scandinavica, 91*(6):453-455.

Werner, P., Mittelman, M.S., Goldstein, D. & Heinik, J. (2012). Family stigma and caregiver burden in Alzheimer's disease. *The Gerontologist, 52*(1), 89-97.

Whiting, J.B. & Crane, D.R. (2003). Distress and divorce: establishing cutoff scores for the marital status inventory. *Contemporary Family Therapy*, *25*(2), 195-205.

Whitlatch, C.J., Zarit, S.H. & von Eye, A. (1991). *The Gerontologist, 31(1),* 9-14.

Whittemore, R. & Dixon, J. (2008). Chronic illness: the process of integration. *Journal of Clinical Nursing, 17*(7B),177-187.

Whittington, C.J., Podd, J. & Kan, M.M. (2000). Recognition memory impairment in Parkinson's disease: power and meta-analyses. *Neuropsychology,14(2)*, 233-46.

Wichowicz, H. (2009). Zaburzenia psychiczne towarzyszące chorobie Parkinsona. *Psychiatria w Praktyce Klinicznej, 2(1),* 1-14. (Article in Polish).

Wiglesworth, A., Mosqueda, L., Mulnard, R., Liao, S., Gibbs, L, & Fitzgerald, W. (2010). Screening for abuse and neglect of people with dementia. *Journal of the American Geriatric Society, 58*(3), 493-500.

Wild, B., Herzog, W., Schellberg, D., Lechner, S., Niehoff, D., Brenner, H., Rothenbacher, D., Stegmaier, C. & Raum, E. (2012). Association between the prevalence of depression and age in a large representative German sample of people aged 53 to 80 years. *International Journal of Geriatric Psychiatry*, *27(4),* 375-381.

Williams, A.M. (1979). The quantity and quality of marital interaction related to marital satisfaction: a behavioural analysis. *Journal of Applied Behaviour Analysis*, *12,* 665-678.

Williams, J.R., Hirsch, E.S., Anderson, K., Bush, A.L., Goldstein, S.R., Grill, S., Lehmann, S., Little, J.T., Margolis, R.L., Palanci, J., Pontone, G., Weiss, H., Rabins, P. & Marsh, L. (2012). A comparison of nine scales to detect depression in Parkinson disease: which scale to use? *Neurology, 78(13)*, 998-1006.

Williams, S.J. (2000). Chronic illness as biographical disruption or biographical disruption as chronic illness? Reflections on a core concept. *Sociology of Health and Illness, 22*(1), 40-67.

Williams-Gray, C.H., Evans, J.R., Goris A., Foltynie, T., Ban, M., Robbins, T.W., Brayne, C.E.G., Kolachana B.S., Weinberger, D.R., Sawcer, S.J. & Barker, R.A. (2009). The distinct cognitive syndromes of Parkinson's disease: 5 year follow-up of the CamPaIGN cohort. *Brain, 132,* 2958-2969.

Williams-Gray, C.H., Foltynie, T., Brayne, C.E.G., Robbins, T.W. & Barker, R.A. (2007). Evolution of cognitive dysfunction in an incident Parkinson's disease cohort. *Brain, 130,* 1787-1798.

Williams-Gray, C.H., Mason, S.L., Evans, J.R., Foltynie, T., Barker, R.A. (2012). The CamPaIGN study of incident Parkinson's disease: Natural history over the first 10 years [abstract]. *Movement Disorders, 27* (Suppl. 1), 1596.

Williamson, G.M., Shaffer, D.R. & The Family Relationships in Late Life Project. (2001). Relationship quality and potentially harmful behaviours by spousal caregivers: how we were then, how we are now. *Psychology and Aging, 16(2),* 217-226.

Williamson, G.M., & Schulz, R. (1990). Relationship orientation, quality of prior relationship and distress among caregivers of Alzheimer's patients. *Psychology and Aging, 5,* 502-509.

Williamson, G.M., Schulz, R., Bridges, M.W. & Behan, A.M. (1994). Social and psychological factors in adjustment to limb amputation. *Journal of Social Behavior and Personality, 9,* 249-268.

Wilson, B., Gracey, F., Evans, J.J & Bateman, A. (2009). *Neuropsychological rehabilitation: Theory, models, therapy and outcome.* Cambridge, UK: Cambridge University Press.

Wilson, R.S., Kaszniak, A.W., Klawans, H.L., Garron, D.C. (1980). High speed memory scanning in parkinsonism. *Cortex, 16*(1), 67-72.

Wilson, S.A.K. (1912). Progressive lenticular degeneration: a familial nervous disease associated with cirrhosis of the liver. *Brain, 34,* 295-509.

Wistow, G., Knapp, M., Hardy, B., Forder,J., Kendall, J. & Manning,R. (1996). Social care markets: Progress and Prospects. Buckingham, Open University Press.

Wolf, S.M. & Davis, R.L. (1973). Permanent dementia in idiopathic Parkinsonism treated with levodopa. *Archives of Neurology, 29(4),* 276-278.

Wolinsky, F.D., Callahan, C.M., Fitzgerald, J.F., & Johnson, R,J. (1992). The risk of nursing home placement and subsequent death among older adults. *Journal of Gerontology, 47*(4), S173-S182.

Wolters, E.Ch. (2008). Variability in the clinical expression of Parkinson's disease. *Journal of the Neurological Sciences, 266,* 197-203.

Wooten, G.F., Curries, L.J., Bovbjerg, V.E., Lee, J.K. & Patrie, J. (2004). Are men at greater risk for Parkinson's disease than women? *Journal of Neurology, Neurosurgery and Psychiatry, 75*, 637-639.

World Health Organization (1980). *International classification of impairments, disabilities and handicaps.* Geneva: World Health Organization.

Wright, J.M. & Keller-Byne, J. (2005). Environmental determinants of Parkinson's disease. *Archives of Environmental and Occupational Health, 60*(1), 32-38.

Wright, L.K. (1991) The impact of Alzheimer's disease on the marital relationship. *The Gerontologist, 31*(2), 224-237.

Wright, M.J., Burns, R.J., Geffen, G.M. & Geffen, L.B. (1990). Covert orientation of visual attention in Parkinson's disease: an impairment in the maintenance of attention. *Neuropsychologia, 28(2),* 151-159.

Wright, S.J. & Kirby, A. (1999). Deconstructing conceptualizations of adjustment to chronic illness: A proposed integrative framework. *Journal of Health Psychology, 4*(2), 259-272.

Yaffe, K., Fox, P., Newcomer, R., Sands, L., Lindquist, K., Dane, K. & Covinsky, K.E. (2002). Patient and caregiver characteristics and nursing home placement in patients with dementia. *Journal of the American Medical Association, 287*, 2090-2097.

Yamamoto, M. (2001). Depression in Parkinson's disease: its prevalence, diagnosis and neurochemical background. *Journal of Neurology, 248*(Suppl. 3), III/5-III/11.

Yan, E., & Kwok, T. (2011). Abuse of older Chinese with dementia by family caregivers: an inquiry into the role of caregiver burden. *International Journal of Geriatric Psychiatry, 26*(5), 527-535.

Yates, M.E., Tennstedt, S., & Chang, B.H. (1999). Contributors to and mediators of psychological well-being for informal caregivers. *Journal of Gerontology, 54B*(1), P12-P22.

Yee, J.L. & Schulz, R. (2000). Gender differences in psychiatric morbidity among family caregivers: A review and analysis. *The Gerontologist, 40*(2), 147-164.

Yesavage, J.A., Brink, T.L., Rose,T.L., Lum, D., Huang, V., Adey, M. & Von Leirer, O. (1982-83). Development and validation of a geriatric depression screening scale: a preliminary report. *Journal of Psychiatric Research, 17(1),* 37-49.

Yip, A.G., Brayne, C., Matthews, F.E.; MRC Cognitive Function and Ageing Study (2006). Risk factors for incident dementia in England and Wales: The Medical Research Council Cognitive Function and Ageing Study. A population-based nested case-control study. *Age and Ageing. 35(2),* 154-160.

Yoshida, K.K. (1993). Reshaping of self: A pendular reconstruction of self and identity among adults with traumatic spinal cord injury. *Sociology of Health and Illness, 15,* 217-245.

Youdim, M.B.H. & Riederer, P. (1997). Understanding Parkinson's disease. *Scientific American, 276*(1), 52-59.

Young, J.T. (2004). Illness behaviour: a selective review and synthesis. *Sociology of Health and Illness, 26*(1), 1-31.

Yu, M., Roane, D.M., Miner, C.R., Fleming, M. and Rogers, J.D. (2004) Dimensions of sexual dysfunction in Parkinson's disease. *American Journal of Geriatric Psychiatry, 12,* 221-226.

Zarit, S.H. (1989). Editorial. Do we need another "Stress and caregiving" study? *The Gerontologist, 29*(2), 147-148.

Zarit, S.H., Johansson, L., & Jarrott, S.E. (1998). Family caregiving: Stresses, social programs and clinical interventions. In I.H. Nordhus, G. VandenBos, S. Berg & P. Fromholt (Eds.), *Clinical geropsychology* (pp. 345-360). Washington, D.C.: American Psychological Association Books.

Zarit, S.H., Orr, N. & Zarit J.M. (1985). *The hidden victims of Alzheimer's disease: families under stress.* New York: University Press.

Zarit, S.H., Pearlin, L.I. & Schaie, K.W. (1993). *Caregiving systems. Formal and informal helpers.* Hillsdale, New Jersey: Lawrence Erlbaum Associates, Publishers.

Zarit, S.H., Reever, K.E. & Bach-Peterson, J. (1980). Relatives of the impaired elderly: Correlates of feelings of burden. *The Gerontologist, 20*(6), 649-655.

Zarit, S.H., Todd, P.A. & Zarit, J.M. (1986). Subjective burden of husbands and wives as caregivers: a longitudinal study. *The Gerontologist, 26,* 260-266.

Zemore, R. & Eames, N. (1979). Psychic and somatic symptoms of depression among young adults, institutionalized aged and noninstitutionalized aged. *Journal of Gerontology, 34*(5), 716-722.

Zetusky, W.J., Jankovic, J. & Pirrozzolo, F.J. (1985). The heterogeneity of Parkinson's disease: clinical and prognostic implications. *Neurology, 35*, 522-526.

Zgaljardic, D.J., Borod, J.C., Foldi, N.S. & Mattis P. (2003). A review of the cognitive and behavioral sequelae of Parkinson's disease: relationship to frontostriatal circuitry. *Cognitive Behavioural Neurology, 16*(4), 193-210.

Zgaljardic, D.J., Borod, J.C., Foldi, N.S., Mattis, P.J., Gordon, M.F., Feigin, A. & Eidelberg, D. (2006). An examination of executive dysfunction associated with frontostriatal circuitry in Parkinson's disease. *Journal of Clinical and Experimental Neuropsychology, 28,* 1127-1144.

Zhang, F., & Labouvie-Vief, G. (2004). Stability and fluctuation in adult attachment style over a 6-year period. *Attachment and Human Development, 6*, 419-437.

Zhao, Y.J., Wee, H.L., Chan, Y.H., Seah, S.H., Au, W.L., Lau, P.N., Pica, E.C., Li, S.C., Luo, N. & Tan, L.C. Progression of Parkinson's disease as evaluated by Hoehn and Yahr stage transition times. *Movement Disorders, 25*(6), 710-716.

Ziabreva, I., Ballard, C.G., Aarsland, D., Larsen, J.P., McKeith, I.G., Perry, R.H. & Perry, E.K. (2006). Lewy body disease: Thalamic cholinergic activity related dementia and parkinsonism. *Neurobiology of Aging, 27,* 433-438.

Zigmond, A.S. & Snaith, R.P. (1983). The hospital anxiety and depression scale. *Acta Psychiatrica Scandinavica, 67(6),* 361-370.

Zigmond, M.J. & Burke, R.E. (2002). Pathophysiology of Parkinson's disease. In K.L. Davis, D. Charney, J.T. Coyle & C. Nemeroff, (Eds), *Neuropsychopharmacology: The Fifth Generation of Progress*, American College of Neuropsychopharmacology.

Zimmerman, M., Posternak, M.A. & Chelminski, I. (2005). Is it time to replace the Hamilton Depression Rating Scale as the primary outcome measure in treatment studies of depression? *Journal of Clinical Psychopharmacology, 25,* 105-110.

Zung, W.W. (1965). A self-rating depression scale. *Archives of General Psychiatry*, *12,* 63-70.

INDEX